Video Atlas of Upper and Lower Airway Management

SECOND EDITION

Wanda M. Popescu, MD, FASA

Professor of Anesthesiology
Department of Anesthesiology
Yale School of Medicine
New Haven, Connecticut

Lena N. Glowka, MD

Assistant Professor of Anesthesiology
Department of Anesthesiology
Frank H. Netter MD School of Medicine
at Quinnipiac University
North Haven, Connecticut

Nicole E. Ginsberg, MD

Assistant Professor of Anesthesiology
Department of Anesthesiology
Yale School of Medicine
New Haven, Connecticut

William H. Rosenblatt, MD

Professor of Anesthesiology
Department of Anesthesiology
Yale School of Medicine
New Haven, Connecticut

Wolters Kluwer

Philadelphia • Baltimore • New York • London
Buenos Aires • Hong Kong • Sydney • Tokyo

Acquisitions Editor: Keith Donnellan
Development Editor: Ashley Fischer
Editorial Coordinator: Priyanka Alagar, Bhavani Ganesan
Production Project Manager: Matthew West
Design Coordinator: Stephen Druding
Manufacturing Coordinator: Lisa Bowling
Prepress Vendor: Aptara, Inc.

Second edition

9 8 7 6 5 4 3 2 1

Printed in the United States of America

Cataloging-in-Publication Data available on request from the Publisher

ISBN: 978-1-9751-9776-6

shop.LWW.com

MPP1225

To my children, Alexandra and Daniel, my husband, Radu, my father, Dan, and my beloved mother, Dori, who lives on in my heart:

Your love has carried me, your support has lifted me, and your steadfast belief in me has been my foundation. This journey has never been mine alone—I share this achievement with all of you, with all my love.

—Wanda M. Popescu

I dedicate my work on this book to Dr. Arthur Wayne Glowka, my father and lifelong English professor who taught me the art of concise writing. A huge thank you to my husband Dr. Terrence Feldheim for his unwavering, enthusiastic support of my career and for keeping me company through many hours of editing.

—Lena N. Glowka

I dedicate this book to Ellie and Jake—the two halves of my heart. Your joy and smiles bring light to every single day of my life. And to my love, David—thank you for your unwavering belief in me, for walking beside me on every journey, and for keeping us all well fed along the way.

—Nicole E. Ginsberg

I dedicate my work in this book to my colleagues at Yale School of Medicine and Yale New Haven Hospital in Anesthesiology, Surgery and Nursing, as well as the members of our ancillary and support staff without whom our clinical duties would be impossible to perform.

—William H. Rosenblatt

Foreword

A difficult airway in the setting of a patient needing anesthesia and surgery epitomizes a critical, stressful situation. The patient's life is on the line, the time to manage the problem is limited, and the relative rarity and variable constellation of factors prevents a "one size fits all" solution.

How do you manage an acute challenging emergency? It is best to be well prepared, have a lot of experience, and be able to adapt to the situation at hand. The book *Video Atlas of Upper and Lower Airway Management* provides a useful tool to accomplish this. It is based on real-life experiences and practical guidance from expert clinicians who have been around the block many times before.

The book is organized to facilitate preparation. It is easy to locate the specific challenge that the case involves. Nuances and variations of the situation and approaches are provided so one can think through what might happen, and plan to have relevant resources at hand.

How do you gain experience on the fly when faced with a rare but critical event? This book provides a solution. Because it is based on real-life experiences and management by expert clinicians, one has the ability to not only read, but also watch and experience the event. It is written by esteemed teachers with a focus on imparting skills to others. Reviewing the potential challenges and solutions gets one incredibly close to having been in the situation before.

Any critical rare event requires an ability to think on your feet and adapt the approach to the specific realities that are encountered. By comprehensively discussing multiple approaches and tools to manage a situation, it provides the user with the ability to assess how to change the original plan when specifics of the case make it suboptimal.

In summary, this book provides a unique tool. It is not something one needs every day, but that doesn't affect the value. When encountering a difficult airway, the resource this book provides is priceless.

Frank Detterbeck, MD
Professor of Thoracic Surgery
Yale School of Medicine
New Haven, Connecticut

Preface

It is with great enthusiasm that we present the second edition of the *Video Atlas of Upper and Lower Airway Management Techniques*. The title of the book has been purposefully updated to emphasize the extensive collection of videos and images designed to provide readers with a richer, more practical understanding of the scenarios and techniques described. This edition introduces new chapters that highlight updated approaches to the difficult airway, as well as novel devices and management techniques—including the groundbreaking use of extracorporeal membrane oxygenation (ECMO) to support particularly challenging airway clinical situations.

In this edition, Dr. William H. Rosenblatt has assumed the sole role of video editor. Nearly every chapter now includes video material drawn from a database of more than 2,000 patients, primarily from Yale New Haven Hospital, with select contributions from authors at other institutions. These videos are intended not to mirror the accompanying text, but to serve as complementary resources—offering alternative approaches, unique clinical findings, or parallel procedures that broaden the reader's perspective. Many chapters now include two videos, along with an expanded selection of images. In the few situations where appropriate patient videos were not available, mannequins or models were used. Editing has been applied to clarify or shorten procedures for educational purposes. With rare exceptions, all editing was completed by the editors, and any inquiries or concerns should be directed to us.

This second edition also marks the expansion of the editorial team, with the addition of Dr. Lena N. Glowka and Dr. Nicole E. Ginsberg. Their dedication to refining chapters and harmonizing the writing style across the book has been invaluable. We extend our deepest gratitude to all contributing authors—especially our resident and fellow collaborators—for their commitment to presenting state-of-the-art airway management.

We are equally grateful to our partners at Wolters Kluwer. Keith Donnellan once again championed the vision for this book and secured its support, while Ashley Fischer guided us through the intricacies of the editorial process. The broader team dedicated countless hours to bring this project to fruition.

The *Video Atlas of Upper and Lower Airway Management Techniques* embodies the proverb, "It takes a village." We hope this edition not only enhances your understanding of airway management but also provides meaningful clinical benefit in your practice.

Wanda M. Popescu, MD, FASA
Lena N. Glowka, MD
Nicole E. Ginsberg, MD
William H. Rosenblatt, MD

Acknowledgments

The editors thank the following companies and persons for aiding with the completion of this project through the loan of expertise or equipment:

Nicole Aaronson, MD
Frank Detterbeck, MD
Michael Lerner, MD
David Karus, MD
Christopher Schutt, MD
Daniel Kinney, MD

The operating room staff, surgeons, and anesthesia providers of Yale New Haven Hospital

Verathon Corporation
Ambu Corporation
Teleflex Corporation
Karl Storz Endoscopy
Intersurgical
Cook Critical Care
Mercury Medical
Fisher & Parkel HealthCare
Uescope
Medtronic
Fujifilm/Sonosite
Through The Cords
VBM

Contents

PART A: UPPER AIRWAY

SECTION I: Basic Airway Evaluation and Management Procedures

SECTION II: Difficult Airway Management

SECTION III: Advanced Airway Procedures

SECTION IV: Special Clinical Situations

SECTION V: Head and Neck Patient and Procedures

PART B: LOWER AIRWAY

SECTION I: Interventional Pulmonology

Glossary

Throughout this volume, chapter authors were encouraged, but not required to use the following abbreviations. When authors chose to use a different abbreviation, it is defined within the chapter.

Bronchial blocker = BB
Continuous positive airway pressure = CPAP
Double-lumen tube = DLT
Diffusing capacity of the lung for carbon monoxide = DLCO
Endotracheal tube = ETT
Flexible bronchoscope = FB
Flexible intubating scope = FIS
Forced expiratory volume in 1 second = FEV1
Gum Elastic Bougie = GEB
Laryngeal mask airway = LMA
One-lung ventilation = OLV
Operating room = OR
Peak airway pressure = PAP
Positive end-expiratory pressure = PEEP
Rapid sequence induction = RSI
Supraglottic airway = SGA
Tracheal Tube = TT
Video-assisted thoracoscopic surgery = VATS

Basem B. Abdelmalak, MD, FASA, SAMBA-F
Professor of Anesthesiology
Director of Anesthesia for Bronchoscopy
Department of General Anesthesiology
Anesthesiology Institute
Cleveland Clinic
Cleveland, Ohio

Anoushka Afonso, MD
Vice Chair, Faculty Affairs
Department of Anesthesiology and Critical Care
Memorial Sloan Kettering Cancer Center
New York, New York

Felice Eugenio Agrò, MD
Full Professor
Department of Anesthesia and Intensive Care
University Hospital Campus Bio-Medico
Rome, Italy

Shamsuddin Akhtar, MD
Professor
Department of Anesthesiology and Pharmacology
Yale School of Medicine
New Haven, Connecticut

Khalid G. Al Abdul Raheem, MD
Anesthesiologist
Department of Anesthesiology
Advocate Aurora Healthcare
Milwaukee, Wisconsin

F. Luke Aldo, DO
Cardiac Anesthesiologist
Department of Anesthesiology
Integrated Anesthesia Associates
Hartford, Connecticut

Laura J. Alexander, MD
Anesthesiologist
Department of Anesthesiology
Lahey Health & Medical Center
Burlington, Massachusetts

Michael Alperovich, MD, MSc
Associate Professor
Department of Surgery
Yale School of Medicine
New Haven, Connecticut

Diana Anca, MD
Associate Professor
Attending Anesthesiologist
Department of Anesthesiology
Weill Cornell Medicine
New York, New York

Michael Ancuta, MD
Assistant Professor
Associate Vice Chair of Clinical Operations
Department of Anesthesiology
Yale School of Medicine
New Haven, Connecticut

Andres De Lima Arboleda, MD
Assistant Professor
Department of Anesthesiology
Yale School of Medicine
New Haven, Connecticut

Valerie E. Armstead, MD, MAUB
Professor of Anesthesiology
Department of Anesthesiology
Lewis Katz School of Medicine at Temple University
Philadelphia, Pennsylvania

Sherif Assaad, MD
Associate Professor of Anesthesiology
Department of Cardiothoracic Anesthesiology
Cleveland Clinic Lerner College of Medicine of Case Western Reserve University School of Medicine
Staff Anesthesiologist
Department of Cardiothoracic Anesthesiology
Cleveland Clinic
Cleveland, Ohio

Rita Asuquo, BS, MD
Department of Anesthesiology
Yale New Haven Hospital
New Haven, Connecticut

Paul Baker, MBChB, MD, FANZCA
Associate Professor
Department of Anesthesiology
University of Auckland
Auckland, New Zealand

Neil S. Ballard, MD
Professor
Department of Anesthesiology and Perioperative Medicine
The University of Texas, MD Anderson Cancer Center
Houston, Texas

Trevor M. Banack, MD
Associate Professor
Vice Chair, Clinical Operations
Department of Anesthesia
Yale School of Medicine
New Haven, Connecticut

Bartlomiej Bartkowiak, MD
Clinical Fellow, Pediatric Anesthesiology
Department of Anesthesiology
Yale New Haven Hospital
New Haven, Connecticut

Andres R. Brenes Bastos, MD
Assistant Professor
Department of Anesthesiology
Yale School of Medicine
New Haven, Connecticut

Elizabeth C. Behringer, MD
Cardiac Surgical Intensivist—Anesthesiologist Division of Cardiovascular Surgery and Critical Care
Kaiser Permanente Los Angeles
Los Angeles, California

Lauren C. Berkow, MD, FASA
Professor of Neuroanesthesiology
Department of Anesthesiology
University of Florida College of Medicine
Gainesville, Florida

Randal S. Blank, MD, PhD
Professor of Anesthesiology
Department of Anesthesiology
University of Virginia School of Medicine
Charlottesville, Virginia

Morten Bøttger, MD, MBA
Senior Consultant
Department of Anesthesiology, Centre of Head and Orthopedics
Copenhagen University Hospital Rigshospitalet
Copenhagen, Denmark

Ruma Bose, MD
Fellowship Director
Department of Anesthesiology, Critical Care and Pain Medicine
Beth Israel Deaconess Medical Center
Boston, Massachusetts

Kyle Bramley, MD
Associate Professor of Medicine (Pulmonary)
Department of Pulmonary, Critical Care and Sleep Medicine
Yale School of Medicine
New Haven, Connecticut

Jay B. Brodsky, MD
Professor
Department of Anesthesiology, Pain and Perioperative Medicine
Stanford University School of Medicine
Stanford, California

Arne Budde, MD
Professor of Anesthesiology
Department of Anesthesiology and Perioperative Medicine
Penn State Health
Hershey, Pennsylvania

Valentin Calu, MD, PhD, Consultant Surgeon
Associate Professor of Surgery
Department of General Surgery
Carol Davila University of Medicine and Pharmacy Elias Emergency University Hospita
Bucharest, Romania

Javier H. Campos, MD
Executive Medical Director, Perioperative Services
Department of Anesthesia
University of Iowa Health Care
Iowa City, Iowa

Zyad J. Carr, MD
Associate Professor
Department of Anesthesiology
Yale School of Medicine
New Haven, Connecticut

Yen Chow, MD
Physician
Department of Emergency
Thunder Bay Regional Health Sciences Center
Thunder Bay, Ontario, Canada

Joseph Cicenia, MD
Physician
Department of Pulmonary Medicine
Cleveland Clinic
Cleveland, Ohio

Richard M. Cooper, BSc, MSc, MD, FRCPC
Professor Emeritus
Department of Anesthesiology and Pain Medicine
University of Toronto
Toronto, Ontario, Canada

Abdulrahman Dardeer, FCAI
Physician
Department of Anaesthetics and Critical Care
Watford General Hospital
Watford, London

Yi Deng, MD
Assistant Professor
Department of Anesthesiology
Baylor College of Medicine
Houston, Texas

Justine Denomme, BMSc, MD, FRCPC
Anesthesiologist
Department of Anesthesia
McMaster University
Hamilton, Ontario, Canada

Prianka Desai, MD

Anesthesiologist
Department of Anesthesiology
Ascension Seton Medical Center Austin
Austin, Texas

Michiel de Wolf

Anesthetist
Department of Anesthesia
Maastricht University Medical Center
Maastricht, The Netherlands

Andrew Dhanasopon, MD

Associate Professor
Department of Thoracic Surgery
Yale School of Medicine
New Haven, Connecticut

Grace F. Donzelli, MD

Assistant Professor
Department of Anesthesia and Perioperative Care
UCSF School of Medicine
San Francisco, California

D. John Doyle, MD, PhD, DPhil

Professor of Anesthesiology
Department of Anesthesiology Institute
Cleveland Clinic
Cleveland, Ohio

James C. DuCanto, MD

Staff Anesthesiologist
Department of Aurora Medical Group
Advocate Aurora Healthcare
Milwaukee, Wisconsin

Madalina Dutu, MD, PhD

Associate Professor of Anesthesia
Consultant Anesthetist at ICU Department at University Emergency Center
Department of Anesthesia and Intensive Care
Carol Davila University of Medicine and Pharmacy
Bucharest, Romania

Jan Ehrenwerth, MD

Professor Emeritus
Department of Anesthesiology
Yale School of Medicine
New Haven, Connecticut

Amr Elmoheen, MD

Fellowship of the Royal College of Emergency Medicine
Consultant Emergency Medicine
Department of Emergency Medicine
Hamad Medical Corporation
Doha, Qatar

Jessica L. Feinleib, MD, PhD

Assistant Professor of Anesthesiology
Department of Anesthesiology
Yale School of Medicine
National Course Director, Veterans Health Administration Out of Operating Room Airway Management
Veterans Health Administration National Simulation Center
Veterans Health Administration
New Haven, Connecticut

Terrence Feldheim, MD, MA

Assistant Professor
Cardiac Anesthesiogist
Department of Anesthesiology
Yale New Haven Hospital
New Haven, Connecticut

Andrew Fisher, MD

Assistant Professor
Department of Anesthesia and Perioperative Medicine
Medical University of South Carolina
Charleston, South Carolina

Lorraine J. Foley, MD, MBA

Clinical Assistant Professor of Anesthesia
Anesthesia Medical Director
Department of Anesthesia
Tufts University School of Medicine
Shields Ambulatory Surgical Center
Boston, Massachusetts

Arthur R. Formanek III, MD

Instructor
Department of Anesthesiology
Harvard Medical School
Mass General Brigham
Boston, Massachusetts

S. Zach Frabitore, MD

Cardiothoracic Anaesthesiologist
Department of Anesthesia Associates of Gainesville
Northeast Georgia Medical Center
Gainesville, Georgia

Gyorgy Frendl, MD, PhD

Associate Professor
Department of Anesthesiology
Harvard Medical School
Mass General Brigham
Boston, Massachusetts

Larissa I. Galante, MSN, BSN, CRNA

Nurse Anesthetist
Department of Anesthesia
New York Presbyterian Weill—Cornell Medical Center
New York, New York

Richard E. Galgon, MD, MS

Staff Anesthesiologist
Department of Anesthesia
Dean Medical Group
SSM Health St. Mary's Hospital—Janesville
Janesville, Wisconsin

Theresa A. Gelzinis, MD
Professor
Department of Anesthesiology and Perioperative Medicine
University of Pittsburgh School of Medicine
Pittsburgh, Pennsylvania

Manuel Granell Gil, PhD, MD
Professor of Anesthesiology
Head, Section of Anesthesiology
Anesthesiology Unit
Departments of Surgery, Anesthesiology, Critical Care and Pain Relief
University of Valencia
Consorcio Hospital General Universitario de Valencia
Valencia, Spain

Lena N. Glowka, MD
Assistant Professor
Department of Anesthesiology
Frank H. Netter MD School of Medicine at Quinnipiac University
North Haven, Connecticut

Sapna Govindan, MD
Instructor in Anesthesia, Critical Care, and Pain Medicine
Department of Anesthesia
Beth Israel Deaconess Medical Center
Boston, Massachusetts

Loreta Grecu, MD
Associate Professor of Anesthesiology
Department of Anesthesiology
Duke University School of Medicine
Duke University Medical Center
Durham, North Carolina

Carin A. Hagberg, MD
Chief Academic Officer
Department of Anesthesiology and Perioperative Medicine
The University of Texas MD Anderson Cancer Center
Houston, Texas

Keith Haller, DO
Pediatric Anesthesiologist
Department of Anesthesiology
Northwell Lenox Hill Hospital
New York, New York

Ankie Hamaekers, MD, PhD
Anesthesiologist
Department of Anesthesiology and Pain Therapy
Maastricht University Medical Center
Maastricht, The Netherlands

Satoshi Hanada, MD, MBA, FASE
Professor of Clinical Anesthesia
Department of Anesthesia
Indiana University School of Medicine
Indianapolis, Indiana

Philip M. Hartigan, MD
Director of Thoracic Anesthesia
Department of Anesthesiology
Brigham and Women's Hospital
Boston, Massachusetts

David W. Healy, MD, FRCA, FASA
Professor of Anesthesiology
Department of Anesthesiology
University of Michigan Medical School
Ann Arbor, Michigan

Jagtar Singh Heir, DO
Professor of Perioperative Medicine, Cardiovascular Anesthesiology
Department of Anesthesiology and Perioperative Medicine
The University of Texas MD Anderson Cancer Center
Houston, Texas

Andrew Herlich, DMD, MD, FAAP, FASA
Professor Emeritus
Department of Anesthesiology and Perioperative Medicine
University of Pittsburgh School of Medicine
Pittsburgh, Pennsylvania

Adriana Herrera, MD
Assistant Professor
Department of Anesthesiology
Yale School of Medicine
New Haven, Connecticut

Katherine Herrera, MD
Fellow
Department of Anesthesiology
Albert Einstein College of Medicine
Montefiore Medical Center
Bronx, New York

Kenneth N. Hiller, MD
Private Practice
Department of Anaesthesiology
Memorial Hermann
Houston, Texas

Matthew B. Hirsch, MD
Attending Surgeon
Department of Otolaryngology
San Diego Ear, Nose and Throat Specialists
Carlsbad, California

Bryan Husta, MD
Program Director
Department of Pulmonary Medicine
Mayo Clinic
Jacksonville, Florida

Jaime B. Hyman, MD
Associate Professor of Anesthesiology
Department of Anesthesiology
Yale School of Medicine
New Haven, Connecticut

Haitham Ibrahim, MD

Assistant Professor
Department of Anesthesiology
Yale School of Medicine
New Haven, Connecticut

Ann Marie Melookaran Iliff, MD

Adjunct Assistant Professor
Department of Anesthesiology and Perioperative Medicine
University of Missouri School of Medicine
Columbia, Missouri

Narasimhan Jagannathan, MD, MBA

Professor and Chief Anesthesiology
Department of Pediatric Anesthesiology
Phoenix Children's Hospital
Phoenix, Arizona

Tim Ting Han Jen, MD, FRCPC

Clinical Assistant Professor
Department of Anesthesiology, Pharmacology and Therapeutics
University of British Columbia
Vancouver, British Columbia, Canada

Douglas Milano-Johnson, MS, PA-C

Physician Assistant
Department of Critical Care
New York Presbyterian
New York, New York

Emily Kahn, MD

Anesthesiologist
Department of Anesthesiology
Northwell Health
Huntington, New York

Or Kalchiem-Dekel, MD

Assistant Professor of Medicine
Department of Section of Interventional Pulmonology
Memorial Sloan Kettering Cancer Center
New York, New York

Sergey Karamnov, MD

Division Chief, Thoracic Anesthesia
Department of Anesthesia and Perioperative Medicine
University of Massachusetts
Worcester, Massachusetts

Darpan Kayastha, MD

Department of Otorhinolaryngology, Head and Neck Surgery
Yale New Haven Health
New Haven, Connecticut

Akhil Khosla, MD

Physician
Department of Pulmonary, Critical Care and Sleep Medicine
Yale School of Medicine
New Haven, Connecticut

P. Allan Klock Jr, MD

Professor and Chairman
Department of Anesthesia and Critical Care
The University of Chicago Pritzker School of Medicine
Chicago, Illinois

Helga Komen, MD, MBA

Assistant Professor
Department of Anesthesiology
Washington University School of Medicine
St. Louis, Missouri

Michael S. Kristensen, MD

Consultant
Department of Anesthesia
Rigshospitalet, Copenhagen University Hospital
Copenhagen, Denmark

Viji Kurup, MD

Professor
Department of Anesthesiology
Yale School of Medicine
New Haven, Connecticut

Roberto Larios, MD

Physician
Department of Emergency Medicine and Critical Care
Lowell General and UMASS Health Alliance Hospitals
Lowell and Leominster, Massachusetts

Kyuho Lee, MD, PhD

Assistant Professor
Department of Anesthesiology and Pain Medicine
Yonsei University College of Medicine
Seoul, Republic of Korea

Rainer Lenhardt, MD

Professor
Department of Anesthesiology
University of Louisville School of Medicine
Louisville, Kentucky

Richard M. Levitan, MD

Attending Physician
Department of Emergency Medicine
Littleton Regional Hospital
Littleton, New Hampshire

Ramneek Maan, MD

Fellow
Department of Anesthesiology
Yale School of Medicine
New Haven, Connecticut

Seth Manoach, BS, MD

Associate Professor of Clinical Medicine
Division of Pulmonary and Critical Care Medicine
Department of Medicine
Weill Cornell Medicine
Director, Medical ICU
NewYork-Presbyterian Lower Manhattan Hospital
New York, New York

Lynette J. Mark, MD
Professor
Anesthesiology and Critical Care Medicine
Johns Hopkins Medical Institutions
Baltimore, Maryland

Archer Kilbourne Martin, MD
Professor
Chair
Division of Cardiovascular and Thoracic Anesthesiology
Mayo Clinic
Jacksonville, Florida

Vincent J. Mase Jr, MD
Assistant Professor of Surgery
Department of Thoracic Surgery
Yale School of Medicine
New Haven, Connecticut

Sarah McDonald, MSc, MD, FRCPC
Anesthesiologist
Department of Anesthesiology and Pain Medicine
University of Toronto
Toronto, Ontario, Canada

Gaetane C. Michaud, MD, MS
Professor of Medicine
Department of Medicine and Cardiothoracic Surgery
USF Health Morsani College of Medicine
Tampa, Florida

Katherine A. Michelini, MD
Anesthesiologist
Integrated Anesthesia Associates
St. Vincent's Hospital
Bridgeport, Connecticut

Sabrina Migliorelli, MD
Anesthesiologist
Department of Anesthesiology and Intensive care unit
Fondazione Policlinico Universitario Campus Bio-Medico
Rome, Italy

Thomas C. Mort, MD
Senior Anesthesiologist
Department of Anesthesiology
Hartford Hospital
Hartford, Connecticut

Gabrielle Musci
Assistant Professor
Department of Anesthesia and Perioperative Medicine
Medical University of South Carolina
Charleston, South Carolina

Abbas Mustafa, MD, PhD
Professor, Senior Consultant
Department of Clinical Imaging, Diagnostic Radiology
Hamad Medical Corporation
Doha, Qatar

Karl Nazareth, MD
Anesthesiologist
Department of Anesthesiology
US Anesthesia Partners
Sugar Land, Texas

Vojislava Neskovic, MD, PhD, DEAA
Professor
Anesthesiologist
Department of Anesthesia and Intensive Care Clinic
Military Medical Academy
Belgrade, Serbia

Ha V. Nguyen, MD
Attending Anesthesiologist
Department of Anesthesiology
El Camino Hospital
Mountain View, California

Andrew Notarianni, MD
Assistant Professor of Anesthesiology
Department of Anesthesiology
Yale School of Medicine
New Haven, Connecticut

Adriana D. Oprea, MD
Associate Professor of Anesthesiology
Department of Anesthesiology
Yale School of Medicine
New Haven, Connecticut

Irene Osborn, MD
Professor
Department of Anesthesiology
Albert Einstein College of Medicine
Bronx, New York

Anup Pamnani, MD
Assistant Professor of Anesthesiology
Department of Anesthesiology
Weill Cornell Medicine
New York, New York

Giuseppe Pascarella, MD
Consultant Anesthetist
Department of Anesthesia and Intensive care
Fondazione Policlinico Universitario Campus Bio-Medico
Rome, Italy

Boris Paskhover, MD
Chief of Facial Plastics
Department of Otolaryngology
Rutgers Biomedical Health Science
Newark, New Jersey

Anil Patel, MBBS, PhD, FRCA
Consultant Anaesthetist
Department of Anaesthesia
University College London Hospitals
London, England

Bhoumesh Patel, MD
Anesthesiologist and Cardiac Intensivist
Hackensack Meridian Health
Neptune, New Jersey

John B. Pawlowski, MD, PhD
Anesthesiologist
Department of Anesthesiology, Critical Care and Pain Medicine
Beth Israel Deaconess Medical Center
Boston, Massachusetts

Alessia Pedoto, MD, FASA
Professor of Clinical Anesthesiology
Department of Anesthesiology and Critical Care Medicine
Memorial Sloan Kettering Cancer Center
New York, New York

Albert C. Perrino Jr, MD
Professor of Anesthesiology
Chief, Anesthesiology
Department of Anesthesiology
Yale School of Medicine
Department of VA Connecticut Healthcare
New Haven, Connecticut

Mariel Poole, MD, MPH
Assistant Professor of Anesthesiology
Department of Anesthesiology
Yale School of Medicine
New Haven, Connecticut

Elizabeth S. Reinhart, MD
Anesthesiologist
Department of Anesthesiology
ProMedica Toledo Hospital
Toledo, Ohio

Claudia Fernandez Robles, MD
Assistant Professor of Anesthesiology
Department of Anesthesiology
Yale School of Medicine
New Haven, Connecticut

William H. Rosenblatt, MD
Professor of Anesthesiology
Department of Anesthesiology
Yale School of Medicine
New Haven, Connecticut

Jennifer E. Sainsbury, MBBS
Consultant Anesthetist
Department of Anesthesia and Perioperative Medicine
Freeman Hospital
Newcastle upon Tyne, England

Jeffrey J. Schwartz, BS, MD
Associate Professor of Anesthesiology
Department of Anesthesiology
Yale School of Medicine
New Haven, Connecticut

Paul J. Schwartz, DMD
Oral and Maxillofacial Surgeon
Anesthesiologist
Department of Oral and Maxillofacial Surgery
Private Practice
Wendell, North Carolina

Mert Senturk, MD
Professor
Department of Anesthesiology
Acibadem University School of Medicine
Istanbul, Turkey

Nabil A. Shallik, MD
Associate Professor
Department of Clinical Anesthesia
Qatar University
Weill Cornell Medical College in Qatar
Tanta University
Doha, Qatar

Melissa S. Shears, MD, FRCPC
Fellow
Department of Anesthesiology
Yale School of Medicine
New Haven, Connecticut

Cliff Shelton, MBChB, PhD, FRCA
Consultant
Department of Anesthesia
Wythenshawe Hospital
Manchester, England

Jodi Sherman, MD
Associate Professor of Anesthesiology
Department of Anesthesiology
Yale School of Public Health
Yale School of Medicine
New Haven, Connecticut

Ralph L. Slepian, MD
Professor of Clinical Anesthesiology
Vice Chair, Department of Anesthesiology
Department of Anesthesiology
Weill Cornell Medicine
New York, New York

Peter Slinger, MD, FRCPC
Professor
Department of Anesthesia
University of Toronto
Toronto, Ontario, Canada

Radu Stoica, MD, PhD
Associate Professor
Head, Department of Anesthesia and ICU
Department of Anesthesia and ICU
Monza Oncology Hospital
Bucharest, Romania

Anika Sud, BMBCh, FRCA
Consultant Anaesthetist
Nuffield Department of Anaesthetics
Oxford University Hospitals NHS Foundation Trust
Oxford, England

Christopher Szabo, MD
Associate Professor of Clinical Anesthesiology
Department of Anesthesiology
Yale School of Medicine
New Haven, Connecticut

Guy Talmor, MD
Physician
Department of Otolaryngology
Sutter Health
Santa Rosa, California

Wendy H. L. Teoh, MBBS, FANZCA
Senior Consultant
Department of Private Anaesthesia Practice
Private Anaesthesia Practice
Singapore, Singapore

Eryn Thiele, MD
Assistant Professor
Department of Anesthesiology
University of Virginia School of Medicine
Charlottesville, Virginia

Christian R. Tilley, MD
Department of Anesthesiology
Weill Cornell Medicine
New York, New York

Lisa K. Torres, MD, MS
Assistant Professor of Medicine
Division of Pulmonary and Critical Care Medicine
Department of Medicine
NewYork-Presbyterian/Weill Cornell Medical Center
New York, New York

Paula Trigo, MD
Consultant Anesthesiologist
Department of Anesthesiologist
Southern New Hampshire Medical Center
Nashua, New Hampshire

Hisashi Tsukada, MD, PhD
Assistant Professor
Department of Surgery
Brigham and Women's Hospital
Boston, Massachusetts

James Turnbull, MBChB
Consultant Anaesthesiologist
Department of Anaesthesia
University College London Hospitals
London, London

Brooks V. Udelsman, MD, MHS
Assistant Professor of Surgery
University of Southern California
Los Angeles, California

Felipe Urdaneta, MD, FASA
Clinical Professor Anesthesiology
Department of Anesthesiology
University of Florida College of Medicine
North Florida/South Georgia Veterans Health System
Gainesville, Florida

Sonia Vaida, MD
Professor of Anesthesiology and Perioperative Medicine
Department of Anesthesiology
Pennsylvania State University College of Medicine
Hershey, Pennsylvania

Eric L. Vu, MD, MSCI
Medical Director, Pediatric Cardiovascular Anesthesiology
Department of Pediatric Anesthesiology
Northwestern University Feinberg School of Medicine
Ann and Robert H. Lurie Children's Hospital
Chicago, Illinois

Ashutosh Wali, MBBS, MD, FFARCSI
Professor of Anesthesiology
Department of Anesthesiology
Baylor College of Medicine
Houston, Texas

Anna M. Weyand, MD
Physician
Department of Anesthesiology
U.S. Anesthesia Partners of Colorado
HealthOne
Denver, Colorado

Robert White, MD, MS
Assistant Professor of Anesthesiology
Department of Anesthesiology
Weill Cornell Medicine
New York, New York

Lauren C. Williams, MD
Resident
Division of Otolaryngology Head and Neck Surgery
Department of Surgery
Yale School of Medicine
New Haven, Connecticut

David T. Wong, MD
Anesthesiologist
Department of Anesthesia
University of Toronto
Toronto Western Hospital
Toronto, Ontario, Canada

Nwanmegha Young, MD
Associate Professor
Department of Surgery
Yale School of Medicine
New Haven, Connecticut

Hany A. Zaki, MD, MRCEM
Assistant Professor
Department of Emergency Medicine
Qatar University
Doha, Qatar

PART A UPPER AIRWAY

SECTION I BASIC AIRWAY EVALUATION AND MANAGEMENT PROCEDURES

Decision Making in the 2022 Difficult Airway Guidelines

1

William H. Rosenblatt

1 Describe in detail the device or technique.

It goes without saying, though it is often said, that the most important job of the anesthesia provider is management of the airway. The modern airway armamentarium provides this clinician with an array of tools and techniques to manage both normal and highly distorted patient airways. In large data studies, the low failure rates of core airway procedures (tracheal intubation, facemask ventilation, and supraglottic ventilation) and the application of advanced techniques (eg, awake intubation) prove that the occurrence of failed airway and rescue invasive airway in the elective operating room suite should be extraordinarily low. Unfortunately, the rate of emergency invasive airway rescue is higher than would be expected and is in great part attributed to poor evaluation and decision making. This cause of airway management failure has been highlighted in both analyses of the American Society of Anesthesiologists' (ASA) Closed Claims Project and the Fourth National Project of the Royal College of Anaesthetists.

Clinician training and experience, the context in which care is delivered, and the availability of equipment and skill will vary, often on a case-by-case basis. Developing a plan for airway management must consider these factors alongside physical, physiologic, and historical patient information.

2 Where or when is the device used in airway management?

In 2022, the fourth iteration of the ASA Guidelines on Management of the Difficult Airway was released. A major change in the Guidelines' algorithm was the inclusion of a decision tree tool to help the clinician choose between two airway management pathways: awake intubation and airway management after the induction of anesthesia (see Chapter 28: The 2022 Difficult ASA Difficult Airway Infographic—Adult). This tool appears as part of the ASA Difficult Airway Algorithm, as well as Part 1 of the ASA's new Airway Infographic.

This decision tree tool, as it appears in the ASA Airway Infographic, is shown in Figure 1.1. Though this tool starts with an assessment of the difficulty of tracheal intubation, it does not assume that the clinician's anesthetic plan includes general anesthesia. Analysis of airway-related claims in the ASA's closed claims project, has noted that airway management may become necessary during the course of a regional anesthetic (due to block failure or other patient's issues). A full evaluation of the patient's airway should take place, and a backup airway management plan should be determined in all cases.

Because the archetypical airway management is most often considered tracheal intubation, ease of laryngoscopy and intubation is first considered. The experience and preferences of the individual tasked with managing the airway are important to risk assessment, and therefore, direct or indirect laryngoscopy may be considered. Patient evaluation, available instrumentation, the operator's experience with that instrument, and other contextual factors are included in the assessment. If the clinician assesses that there is no risk of difficulty, they are directed to the management after the induction of anesthesia pathway. The clinician is confident that, if needed, the archetypical airway management technique can be applied. This does not imply that tracheal intubation is the primary plan. It may be the plan, or a rescue plan. Likewise, if the clinician's judgment was faulty and tracheal intubation is delayed, requires other instrumentation, or proves impossible, the Infographic as well as the Difficult Airway Algorithm provide rescue pathways. Because unforeseen pathology or other issues could render what was assessed as a straightforward procedure difficult, evaluation of all airway management core techniques should take place.

If, on assessment, it is determined that there is any risk that laryngoscopy and tracheal intubation could be at all difficult (eg, require more time or maneuvers than normally expected), other means of airway support are

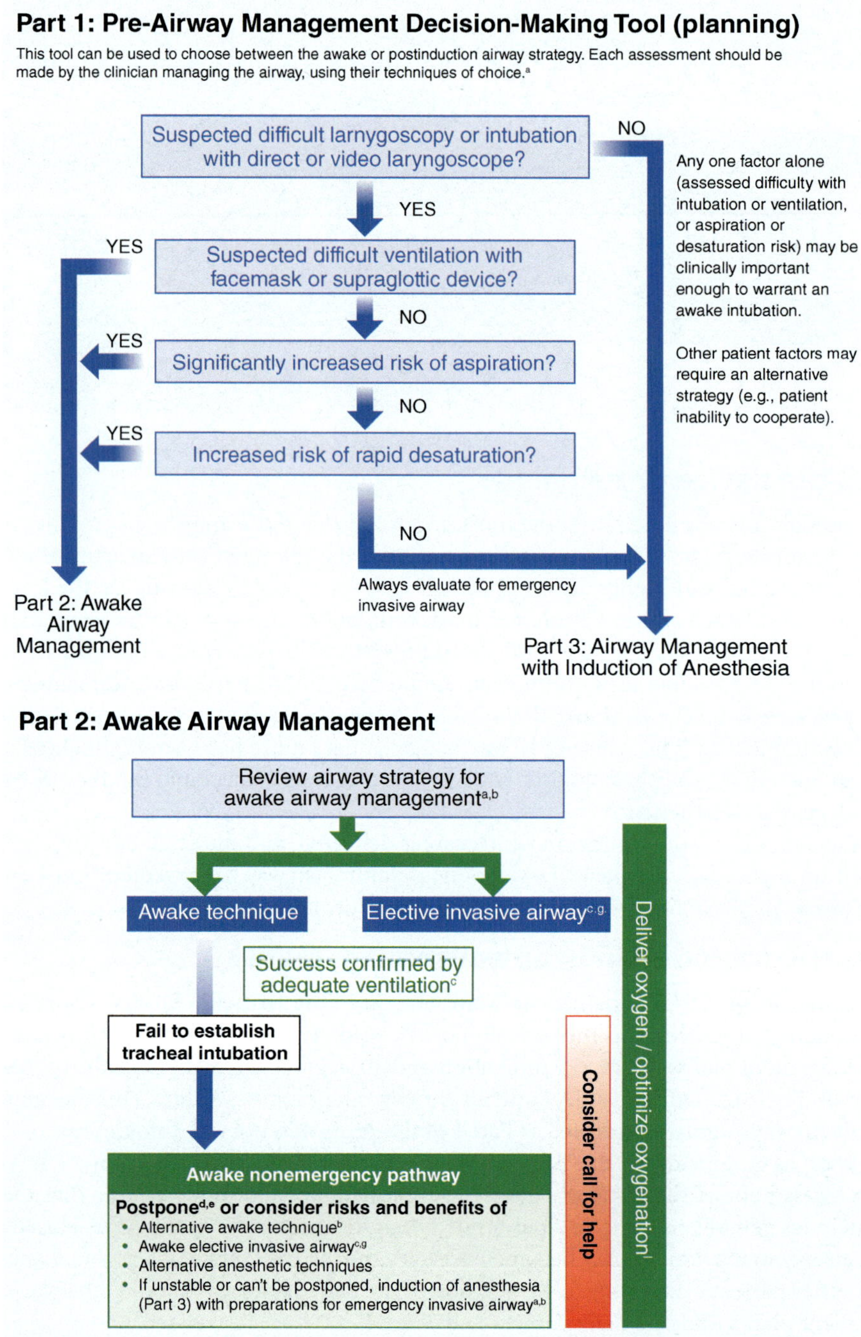

Figure 1.1. The decision tree tool of the ASA difficult airway infographic aids the individual clinician in choosing between the two pathways of airway management, awake intubation or airway management after the induction of anesthesia. (Reprinted with permission from Apfelbaum JL, Hagberg CA, Connis RT, et al. 2022 American Society of Anesthesiologists practice guidelines for management of the difficult airway. *Anesthesiology*. 2022;136(1):31–81. Copyright © 2021 The American Society of Anesthesiologists.)

considered. The ability to care for the patient's airway with a facemask or supraglottic ventilation is assessed. As with laryngoscopy and intubation, this must be considered within the limitations of the operator's experience and other contextual factors enumerated above. If the answer to this question is "yes," then a juncture of potential for difficult intubation and potential for difficult ventilation has been reached. Because this defines an emergency pathway, anesthetic induction is ill advised, and the awake intubation pathway is recommended. Highlighted here is the importance of the serial evaluation and risk assessment embedded in the decision tree tool. Though any one core technique of airway management may not appear impossible to apply, the assessment that both intubation and ventilation have any risk of failing directs the clinician toward awake intubation.

If there is no concern by the operator regarding the successful application of a facemask or supraglottic ventilation, the second question is answered "no," and the aspiration risk is now considered. If there is an increased risk of aspiration of gastric contents in a patient whose airway may not be secured rapidly and efficiently, the induction of general anesthesia could be hazardous and the awake intubation arm is chosen. Otherwise, if the stomach is considered functionally empty (there is no apparent aspiration risk), and the risk of an unprotected airway is acceptable, the final question is considered.

If ventilation (facemask or supraglottic) is believed to be achievable in the patient in whom laryngoscopy and intubation might fail, and this ventilation can be applied with minimal or no aspiration risk, the operator still must consider the potential harm that could follow if an error in judgment has been made. The patient who is systemically healthy and can be thoroughly preoxygenated will tolerate a moderate period of apnea, during which alternative techniques of tracheal intubation or noninvasive ventilation can be attempted. In the rare circumstance where intubation and both mask and supraglottic device ventilation all fail after multiple attempts, the patient may remain well oxygenated and permit controlled invasive airway rescue. The airway management after the induction of anesthesia pathway is entered with the knowledge that, should airway management fail, corrective measures can be applied in a controlled manner. Patients who might not have as robust a reserve (eg, intrapulmonary shunt, increased metabolic rate, obesity, pregnancy) are less tolerant of apnea, and, when appropriate, the awake intubation pathway is chosen.

Though both the Guidelines' Infographic and the Difficult Airway Algorithm include all of the above assessment points, the two differ in including assessment of the ease of performing emergency invasive access. Whereas the Infographic asks the clinician to always evaluate for an emergency invasive airway, the Difficult Airway Algorithm formally includes this in the decision process. In the latter, a patient who may experience delay in achieving tracheal intubation and who appears difficult to perform an invasive airway on, is directed toward awake intubation.

Safe anesthetic care demands a thorough and thoughtful consideration of those factors which tax the skill of the anesthesia provider in light of patient conditions, resource availability, and their own experience, both recent and remote. The decision tree tool guides the choice of airway management by isolating the primary airway management factors—laryngoscopy and intubation, facemask and supraglottic ventilation, aspiration risk, and apnea tolerance risk. Pre- and postmanagement, isolating these elements during assessment, and using them to construct a rational plan, allows the clinician to precisely explain and document a strategy for patient care.

- The ASA Difficult Airway Guidelines include a premanagement decision tree tool to help clinicians choose an airway management pathway—this tool should be used before any anesthetic.
- Intubation, ventilation, aspiration risk, and oxyhemoglobin desaturation risk should all be evaluated as separate elements prior to anesthetic induction.
- Patients at risk of difficult intubation and ventilation failure or aspiration, or rapid oxyhemoglobin desaturation should be managed with awake intubation.
- Following the decision tree tool allows the clinician to explain their choice of airway management pathway (Figure 1.2 and **Video 1.1**).

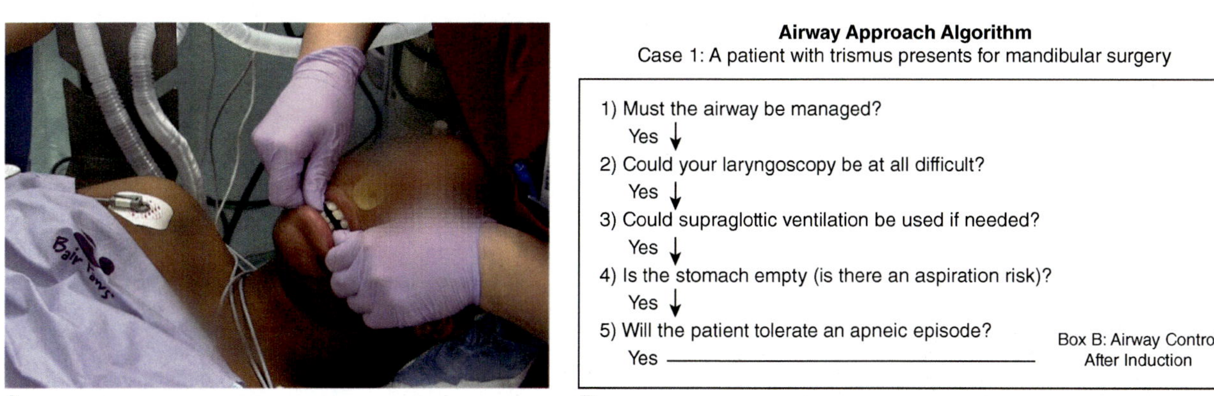

Figure 1.2. A: Patient with near-complete trismus. Following the ASA decision tree tool, two anesthesiologists may develop two very different plans (**B**) for airway management based on whether or not they assess that the patient can be safely mask ventilated.

Suggested Readings

Joffe AM, Ramaiah R, Donahue E, et al. Ventilation by mask before and after the administration of neuromuscular blockade: a pragmatic non-inferiority trial. *BMC Anesthesiol.* 2015;15:134.

Kheterpal S, Healy D, Aziz MF. Incidence, predictors, and outcome of difficult mask ventilation combined with difficult laryngoscopy. *Anesthesiology.* 2013;119(6):1360–1369.

Peterson GN, Domino KB, Caplan RA, Posner KL, Lee LA, Cheney FW. Management of the difficult airway: closed claims database. *Anesthesiology.* 2005;102:33–39.

Rosenblatt WH. The airway approach algorithm: A decision tree for organizing preoperative airway information. *J Clin Anesth.* 2004;16:312–316.

The 2022 Difficult ASA Difficult Airway Guidelines Recommendations Update

2

Andrew Fisher

1 Describe in detail the device or technique.

Originally published in 1992, the Practice Guidelines for Management of the Difficult Airway have shifted alongside the evolution of the practice of anesthesia. This evolution between the Practice Guidelines in 2013 and the most recently published in 2022 is no exception. With the ever-changing world of airway management and current practices, the modification and additions to our guidelines here reflect the current practice of airway management. The decision making guided by the Difficult Airway Algorithm will be discussed in detail elsewhere in this text (see Chapter 1: Decision Making in the 2022 Difficult Airway Guidelines).

2 Where or when is the device used in airway management?

The utilization of the Difficult Airway Algorithm can be applied to every patient encounter, as a thorough practitioner can run through the algorithm on a theoretical basis to ensure adequate preparedness for their anesthetic airway management. The application of these new guidelines reaches from the preoperative examination of the patient, the intraoperative management of airway securement and extubation, to the postoperative management of nonoperating room extubation and follow-up care. The approach to an expected or confirmed difficult airway necessitates an intimate understanding of the guidelines described in the 2022 American Society of Anesthesiologists (ASA) Difficult Airway Guidelines. Similarly, all practitioners should be familiar with these guidelines in the case of an unanticipated difficult airway.

3 What distinguishes this device or technique from similar airway management methods?

In a discussion of how the 2022 guidelines differ from it is predecessor, it seems natural to note the composition of the ASA-appointed task force who spearheaded the update to the guidelines. The ASA-appointed task force members have expanded from 10 to 15 and have, for the first time, included international participants with members representing Italy, Switzerland, India, and Ireland. In addition to this new international viewpoint among the ASA-appointed task force, the buildout of pediatric guidelines alongside adult guidelines deserves note. The pediatric difficult airway will be discussed in a separate section of this text. In addition to the increased number and diversification of the task force members, the number of expert consultants included in the guideline surveys has increased. In 2013, 66 expert consultants were polled, and that number ballooned to over 159 in 2022.

The core of these guidelines lies in the ASA Difficult Airway Algorithm. This infographic and cognitive aid deserves attention, as slight modifications reflect a diversion of emphasis from the ASA task force. Beyond the initial differences in the algorithm layout regarding preoperative airway evaluation and decision aids on patient selection for an intubation attempt while the patient is awake, three differences in the new guideline should be noted: the emphasis of optimizing oxygenation throughout attempted awake intubation, the recommendation to limit intubation attempts, and the awareness of the passage of time in a cannot intubate, cannot ventilate (CICV) scenario. All three concepts and recommendations are new additions to the 2022 algorithm. Though all three are previously addressed throughout the 2013 guidelines, they are not included in the 2013 algorithm. This new inclusion of three vital recommendations speaks to the importance of these recommendations from the task force.

New subsection organization within the 2022 guidelines include the discussion of Unanticipated and Emergency Difficult Airway Management, separate from the Anticipated Difficult Airway Management. The vastly different clinical scenarios between an anticipated, well-planned difficult airway and an emergent, unanticipated difficult airway cannot be understated. For the ASA task force to separately discuss this dichotomy underlines the importance of preparedness for emergency unanticipated difficult airway, also referred to as cannot intubate, cannot ventilate (CICV). Important additions to this CICV subsection include recommendations on the management of an unanticipated difficult airway with invasive procedures. The task force recommends a skilled practitioner be the provider to perform the procedure. This recommendation should enfranchise practitioners to utilize learning resources like simulation-based learning to gain these skills in a controlled environment. The task force also recommends a secondary plan for airway securement be discussed and deliberated when an invasive approach is utilized. This is an important addition to these guidelines because it highlights the importance of both comfort in performing multiple invasive airway securement techniques and the introduction of extracorporeal membrane oxygenation when available. Both of these recommendations are new and guide practitioners on individual skill-based preparedness training and institutional support systems to optimize unexpected difficult airways.

The ASA task force's inclusion of Human Factors Relevant to Difficult Airway Management deserves discussion. The information conveyed in this table is new to the guidelines and addresses the burgeoning school of thought that practitioners' performance in emergency situations can be optimized if individual and institutional metrics are themselves optimized. This table's information touches on practitioner-specific and external factors' relation to airway management. The broad topics discussed in this section encourage practitioners to advocate for the creation of care models or changes to their current model to help optimize difficult airway management. In addition, these recommendations can help individual practitioners in their negotiation for practice specifics (ie, burnout prevention and work–life balance).

The Portable Storage Unit, colloquially known as the difficult airway cart, is integral to an airway expert's ability to provide safe airway management in diverse care environments. The 2022 guidelines recommended items for the difficult airway cart largely mirror the 2013 guidelines, but new additions merit mention. Most noteworthy in these additions: the addition of jet ventilation equipment. Though the use of oral and transtracheal jet ventilation is discussed in the 2013 guidelines, the task force's new inclusion of this equipment in the difficult airway cart emphasizes the role jet ventilation can play in the management of a difficult airway. Duggan et al. published a systematic review of the use of transtracheal jet ventilation in the CICV clinical scenario. They note multiple studies describing its use and utility, while recognizing the statistically significant rate of complications (ie, barotrauma and device failure). Despite the incidence of complications, transtracheal and oral jet ventilation provides an entirely unique airway management tool and can prove a vital component in the management of both anticipated and unanticipated difficult airways. Beyond this inclusion, additions like nasal and oral airways, nasal cannula, topical anesthetics, and a laminated cognitive aid in the case of a difficult airway provide a more complete arsenal for the anesthesiologist to expedite and optimize management of a difficult airway.

Author Caveats

The integration of simulation-based learning can increase practitioner comfort and patient outcomes in the setting of both anticipated and unanticipated difficult airways.

- The 2022 guidelines were shaped from the start with the first-time inclusion of international task force members, additional task force members, and a higher number of expert consultants.
- The 2022 guidelines and the included algorithm for difficult airway emphasize optimizing oxygenation while performing an awake intubation and reducing the number of intubation attempts when performing an unanticipated difficult airway.
- New additions to the management of invasive airways include recommendations that an invasive airway procedure should be performed by a trained practitioner and a secondary plan (ie, ECMO) for this invasive airway procedure should be contemplated and discussed.

Suggested Readings

American Society of Anesthesiologists Task Force on Management of the Difficult Airway. Practice guidelines for management of the difficult airway: an updated report by the American Society of Anesthesiologists Task Force on management of the difficult airway. *Anesthesiology*. 2003;98(5):1269–1277.

Apfelbaum JL, Hagberg CA, Connis RT, et al. 2022 American Society of Anesthesiologists practice guidelines for management of the difficult airway. *Anesthesiology*. 2022;136(1):31–81.

Duggan LV, Ballantyne Scott B, Law JA, Morris IR, Murphy MF, Griesdale DE. Transtracheal jet ventilation in the 'can't intubate can't oxygenate' emergency: a systematic review. *Br J Anaesth*. 2016;117 Suppl 1:i28–i38.

Preoperative Endoscopic Airway Evaluation

3

Anup Pamnani • Ralph L. Slepian

1 Describe in detail the device or technique.

The American Society of Anesthesiologists' Difficult Airway Practice Guidelines recommend a three-component approach to airway evaluation, including history, physical examination, and additional evaluation as needed. When patients present with upper airway lesions or for airway surgery, preoperative endoscopic airway evaluation (PEAE) can provide information not available on routine history and external physical examination.

Airway lesions can severely disrupt the airway anatomy and function, and render tracheal intubation, and mask or supraglottic airway (SGA) ventilation difficult. Their location (frequently the base of tongue, the posterior pharynx, and the laryngeal structures) makes them difficult to appreciate by conventional airway assessment techniques. Symptoms related to respiration and swallowing can be misleading as lesions may become more obstructive once neuromuscular blockade is employed. PEAE allows for the close examination of these airway lesions and can aid the clinician in airway management decisions, such as the necessity of an awake intubation (AI) versus a standard induction technique.

Prior to PEAE, a routine preoperative airway assessment is performed. This consists of an airway history that includes review of previous intubation records, symptoms of airway compromise, recent food intake, and risk factors for aspiration. The external physical examination assesses predictors of difficult intubation and difficult mask or SGA ventilation. Medical conditions that may impact airway management, such as obstructive sleep apnea, lung diseases, congenital diseases, and their associated anatomic abnormalities, are also assessed.

When planning for nasopharyngoscopic endoscopic examination, the patient should be screened for nasal pathology such as chronic epistaxis, nasal polyps, and obstructed passages. In addition, any available previous imaging studies should be reviewed, such as a head CT or MRI. If the patient has undergone prior endoscopic examination in the surgeon's office, it may be helpful to review their previous experience, including their level of discomfort with the procedure.

PEAE is performed with the patient in the semirecumbent or sitting position. A vasoconstrictor (eg, oxymetazoline spray or 4% cocaine-soaked pledgets) is applied to both nostrils, which is followed by application of topical analgesia. Three to five milliliters of lidocaine 4% solution, dispensed via a mucosal atomizer device, should provide effective analgesia for the airway.

A small (2.5- to 3.5-mm) flexible fiberoptic intubating scope (FIS) is inserted into a nare that has been suitably prepared and then advanced below the inferior turbinate until the epiglottis is visualized. The FIS is then used to examine the vallecula and the base of the tongue. The laryngeal apparatus is inspected, including the true and false vocal cords and the arytenoids. Direct contact with the epiglottis is avoided. The patient may be asked to phonate in order to assess movement of the vocal cords and the size of the laryngeal inlet. Lateral movement of the FIS allows for examination of pyriform sinuses.

Occasionally, PEAE may also be performed using the oral approach. An oropharyngeal airway device that allows for introduction of a FIS, such as the William or Ovassapian airway, coated with 4% lidocaine jelly to anesthetize the tongue, may be used to assist the procedure. Care must be used to ensure that any devices introduced into the mouth do not disrupt the airway lesion. Oral airway devices are contraindicated when vascular and friable lesions are present at the base of the tongue.

When performing PEAE, the site of the lesion, degree of vascularity, and any anatomic disruption of the airway should be noted. The clinician performing the examination assesses whether a single-plane optical path leads to the laryngeal inlet. Multiplane paths to the laryngeal inlet may portend difficulty with FIS-aided intubation, and consideration should be given to an AI technique. Moorthy et al. suggest a grading system to aid the decision process. Patients with lower grade lesions (grades 0 to 1), characterized by clearly visible vocal folds and normal vocal function, are intubated using a standard induction technique. Intermediate lesions (grade 2a, b), characterized by partially visible vocal folds and hoarse voice on examination, may require AI depending on the clinician's assessment of difficulty visualizing the laryngeal inlet. High-grade lesions (grades 3 to 4), characterized by a significantly obscured laryngeal inlet and difficulty breathing on examination, are typically subject to AI.

The location of pathologic lesions can also be assessed with regard to suitability for the placement of supraglottic devices. This assessment can be particularly valuable in predicting the difficulty of rescue ventilation which is not apparent by external physical examination.

2 Where or when is this technique used in airway management?

PEAE can be particularly helpful in evaluating patients with known or suspected airway pathology. Rosenblatt et al. have shown that the use of PEAE changed the airway management plan in 26% of patients presenting for obstructive airway surgery. This included a reduction in unnecessary AI and discovery of unexpectedly severe airway pathology that required AI. In lieu of AI, PEAE may guide the decision process for the induction of anesthesia while maintaining spontaneous ventilation during the intubation attempt.

3 What distinguishes this technique from similar airway management methods?

PEAE can be a vital part of the airway expert's armamentarium; however, it may differ significantly from a similar evaluation carried out by surgical consultants in the presurgical visit. Although surgical evaluation of the airway pathology includes an assessment of airway patency, it is typically focused on staging of disease, assessment of regional spread, preservation of function, the type and timing of surgical intervention and obtaining biopsies, among other things.

PEAE performed by the airway consultant specifically assesses for obstacles to airway management. It provides information that can identify necessary airway equipment, predict difficulty with placement of ventilation devices, and can aid the decision-making process for securing the airway. This information may not necessarily be elicited from external physical examination, the surgical consultant's evaluation, or static imaging studies. Keep in mind that a "good airway" has different meanings to the anesthesia team and the surgeon.

It is important that the findings of PEAE not be assessed in isolation. Results from such examination must always be considered in the context of a comprehensive airway assessment. The assessment must account for comorbidities that can impact airway management, ease of ventilation, risk of aspiration, and the patient's ability to tolerate apnea. The information provided by PEAE should supplement, not substitute for, a rational and comprehensive approach to airway management. In this regard, an algorithm that organizes preoperative airway information into a decision tree can be particularly useful (see Chapter 1: Decision Making in the 2022 Difficult Airway Guidelines, Figure 3.1, and **Video 3.1** for additional details).

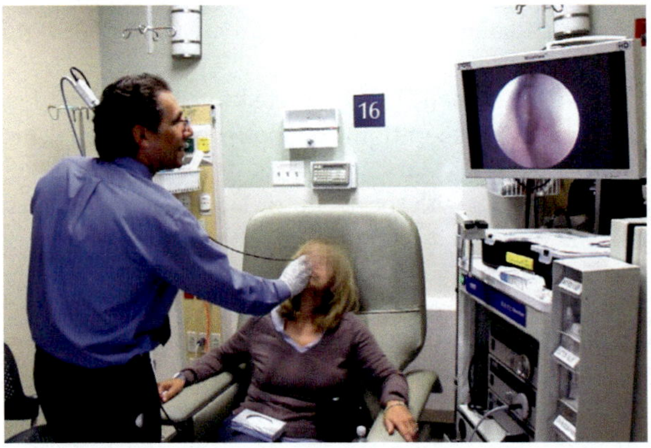

Figure 3.1. Preoperative endoscopic airway examination takes place during a preadmission clinic visit. Note that as a routine exam, there is no monitoring or intravenous access, and both the patient and the examiner are in street clothes.

- PEAE can be used to determine whether a standard or AI approach should be taken for the patient with a potentially difficult airway.
- A brief nasal application of a vasoconstrictor and a small amount of topical anesthetic is typically applied before nasoendoscopy. Occasionally an oral technique for PEAE may be viable if nasal endoscopy is contraindicated.
- A clear path to the airway, the absence of bleeding or friable lesions, and a finding of no difficulty with potential mask/SGA ventilation will generally lead to choosing a standard induction technique.
- A similar examination may have been performed by the surgeon, but may be missing information important to the airway specialist.
- *See Figure 3.2 and* ***Video 3.2*** *for additional details.*

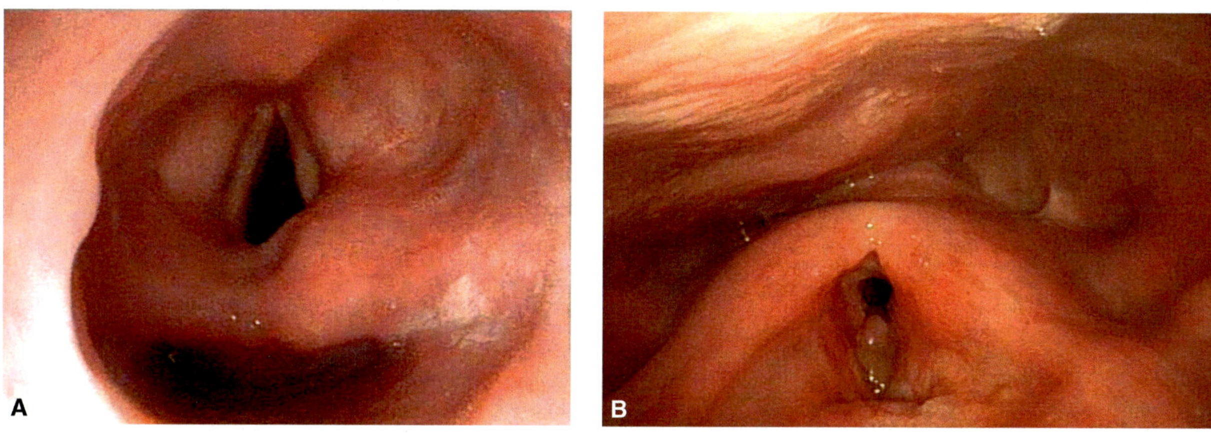

Figure 3.2. **A:** Preoperative endoscopy in a patient who has received chemoradiation for upper airway cancer reveals pharyngeal stenosis. **B:** Vocal cord cancer and the degree of laryngeal obstruction are revealed during preoperative endoscopy.

Suggested Readings

Apfelbaum JL, Hagberg CA, Connis RT, et al. 2022 American Society of Anesthesiologists practice guidelines for management of the difficult airway. *Anesthesiology*. 2022;136(1):31–81.

Chu EA, Kim YJ. Laryngeal cancer: Diagnosis and preoperative work-up. *Otolaryngol Clin North Am*. 2008;41(4):673–695.

Moorthy SS, Gupta S,Laurent B, Weisberger EC. Management of airway in patients with laryngeal tumors. *J Clin Anesth*. 2005; 17(8):604–609.

Rosenblatt W, Ianus AI, Sukhupragarn W, Fickenscher A, Sasaki C. Preoperative endoscopic airway examination (PEAE) provides superior airway information and may reduce the use of unnecessary awake intubation. *Anesth Analg*. 2011;112(3):602–607.

Rosenblatt WH, Yanez ND. A decision tree approach to Airway Management Pathways in the 2022 difficult airway algorithm of the American Society of Anesthesiologists. *Anesth Analg*. 2022;134(5):910–915.

Thekdi AA, Ferris RL. Diagnostic assessment of laryngeal cancer. *Otolaryngol Clin North Am*. 2002;35(5):953–969.

4 Virtual Endoscopy of the Human Airway

Nabil A. Shallik • Abdulrahman Dardeer • Amr Elmoheen •
Abbas Mustafa • Hany A. Zaki

1 Describe in detail the device or technique.

The complex anatomy of the upper airway has made proper assessment and evaluation a challenge. This is further complicated by pathologic lesions, and prior therapies such as surgical intervention or radiation treatment. A special concern is the utility of radiologic assessment. Before the era of computer tomography (CT), plain radiography, conventional tomography, and barium studies, as well as laryngography, were commonly employed. The superimposition effect of different anatomical structures in plain radiography hinders the proper visualization of airway-related structures. This issue was partially solved by the introduction of CT, at the expense of increased radiation exposure to the patient. Virtual endoscopy (VE) is a method of generating two-dimensional (2D) and three-dimensional (3D) images, similar to those obtained with conventional endoscopic (CE) examination, by reformatting thin volumetric axial CT raw data to produce a video-like construction of the upper airway. The resulting data file gives the clinician an endoscopic-like view of the normal and pathologic anatomy of the airway. The introduction of multirow detector computed tomography (MDCT) scanners has made it possible to acquire high-resolution images of the upper, central, and segmental airways within a short time, which can subsequently be reconstructed into elegant and distinguished 2D reformation and 3D images, including internal virtual endoscopic renderings that closely simulate images from CE or real endoscopy (RE).

There are many techniques for generating the flight path during VE, including manual camera movement, semiautomatic path planning, and automatic path planning. In manual camera movement, the position, field of view, and focal point of the camera are interactively changed by the operator, with software providing collision detection to keep the camera within the potential cavity of the lumen. In semiautomatic path generation (also known as key-framing), the operator specifies key path points that have unique special and directional coordinates and field of view, which are connected by cubic splines.

In automatic flight path, at a rate of 25 to 30 frames per second, the computer generates an uninterrupted, approximated flight route connecting the key views. The flight path is automatically computed after the operator designates an initial, and one or more end points by computing the centerline of the imaged structure.

The typical flight path is planned through the air containing nostrils, nasal cavities, natural drainage pathways, and ostia of paranasal sinuses to the oropharynx, down to the trachea, and then passing through different segments of the airway. While showing the partially transparent nasopharyngeal borders, the soft tissue can be made transparent in order to visualize the underlying bone morphology and preoperatively evaluate key structures.

During VE navigation, pyriform sinuses, aryepiglottic folds, and vocal cords can be appreciated, down to the trachea and carina (Figures 4.1 and 4.2).

2 Where or when is the device used in airway management?

VE can be used whenever a detailed 2D or 3D exam of the middle and distal columns of the airway is needed to assess the risk of difficult airway management. Though a VE file can be obtained in any patient (when the processing software is available), its reconstruction from existing CT data makes this technique especially attractive to reduce the cost, discomfort, and risk associated with CE or unforeseen airway failures.

3 What distinguishes this device or technique from similar airway management methods?

For the clinician tasked with evaluating and managing a difficult airway, VE offers advantages over CE. Because the VE "video" is constructed from diagnostic CT scans, it does not add an invasive procedure to the evaluation of the patient, therefore presenting no additional risk or discomfort. In addition, VE may allow perspectives of the airway not physically duplicated by any other means, for instance, visualization of the posterior choana, posterior nares, and Eustachian tubes orifices. It can also assess for subglottic extensions of laryngeal neoplasm, and can navigate and fly-through in the caudocephalic direction as well as through narrow segment areas where CE cannot pass due to the relatively large caliber of the physical endoscope.

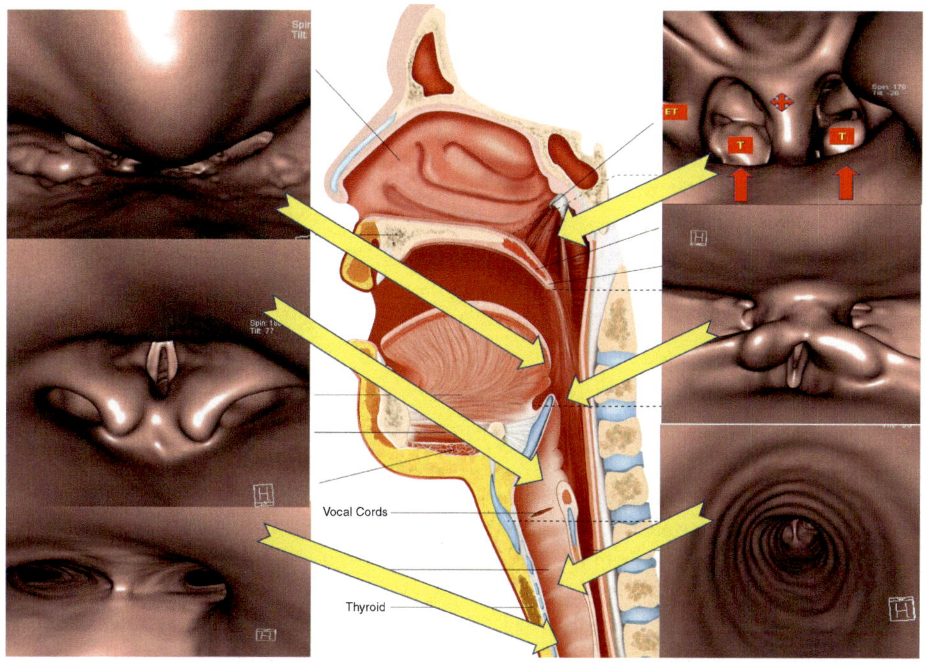

Figure 4.1. Still images of the normal human airway using virtual endoscopy. (Images courtesy of Dr. Nabil Shallik.)

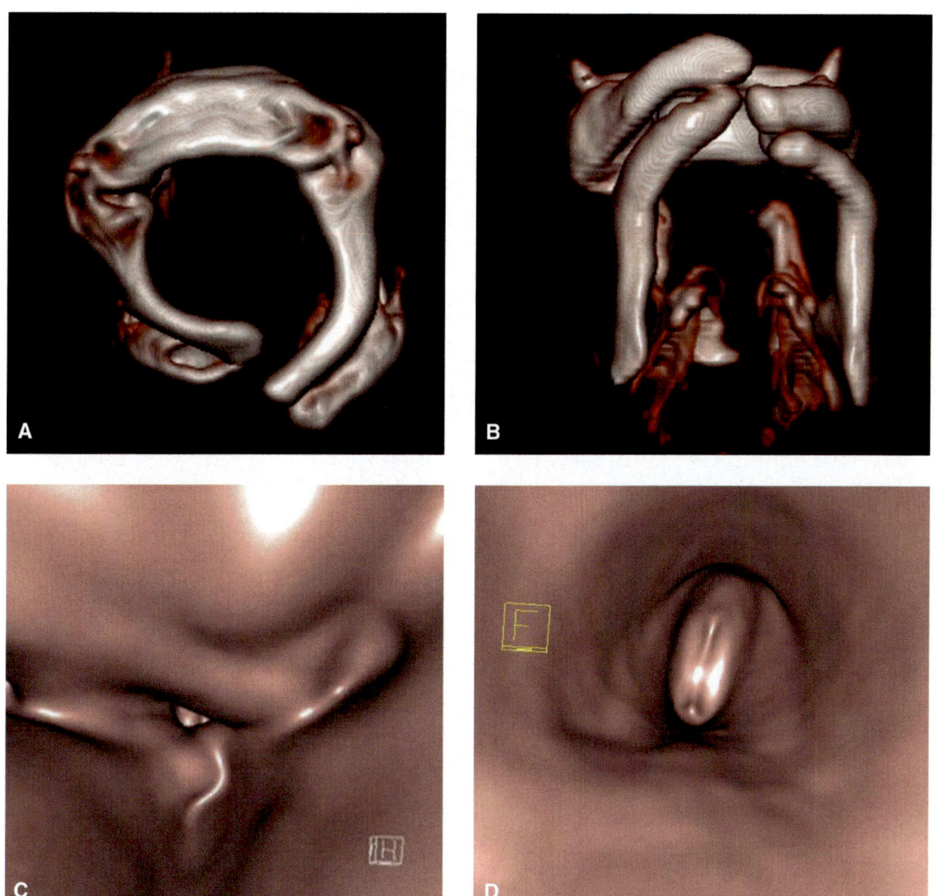

Figure 4.2. **A** and **B** show the superior thyroid cornu share the same process, which was seen by the 3D images. **C:** Virtual endoscopy (VE) shows a significant airway narrowing at the level of hyoid bone from a caudal to cranial view. **D:** VE shows a significant airway narrowing at the level of hyoid bone from a cranial to caudal view. (Images courtesy of Dr. Nabil Shallik.)

Author Caveats

Despite the advantages, VE has its own flaws. As compared to CE, VE is still less sensitive in the visualization of superficial lesions of the mucosal lining. VE cannot be used to assess mucosa, perform biopsies, or therapeutic maneuvers. Presence of retained mucus or blood can be falsely reported as tracheobronchial stenosis or a foreign body. Furthermore, the diameter of the airway on the CT depends on the respiratory cycle, therefore, stenosis of tracheobronchial tree may be underestimated. In some cases, such as tracheomalacia, assessment should be during both inspiration and expiration, which can be challenging to achieve in infants and children. VE does not show the segmental and subsegmental parts of the tracheobronchial tree. It could be difficult, or even impossible, to detect some dynamic airway lesions such as immobile vocal cords. Finally, it may require 5 to 10 minutes to reconstruct the VE file from the available CT data.

- The airway manager planning to use VE in their practice should establish its availability prior to the presentation of potential patients.
- VE, when available, poses decreased risk and discomfort to the patient, as compared to CE.
- It is helpful to orient the image to correspond with a CE view.
- VE is a powerful tool in the diagnosis of airway-related pathologies and planning of treatment strategies.
- The development of higher resolution CT data files will eventually improve VE ability to help the clinician assess mucosal lesions.
- *See Figure 4.3 and* ***Video 4.1*** *for additional details.*

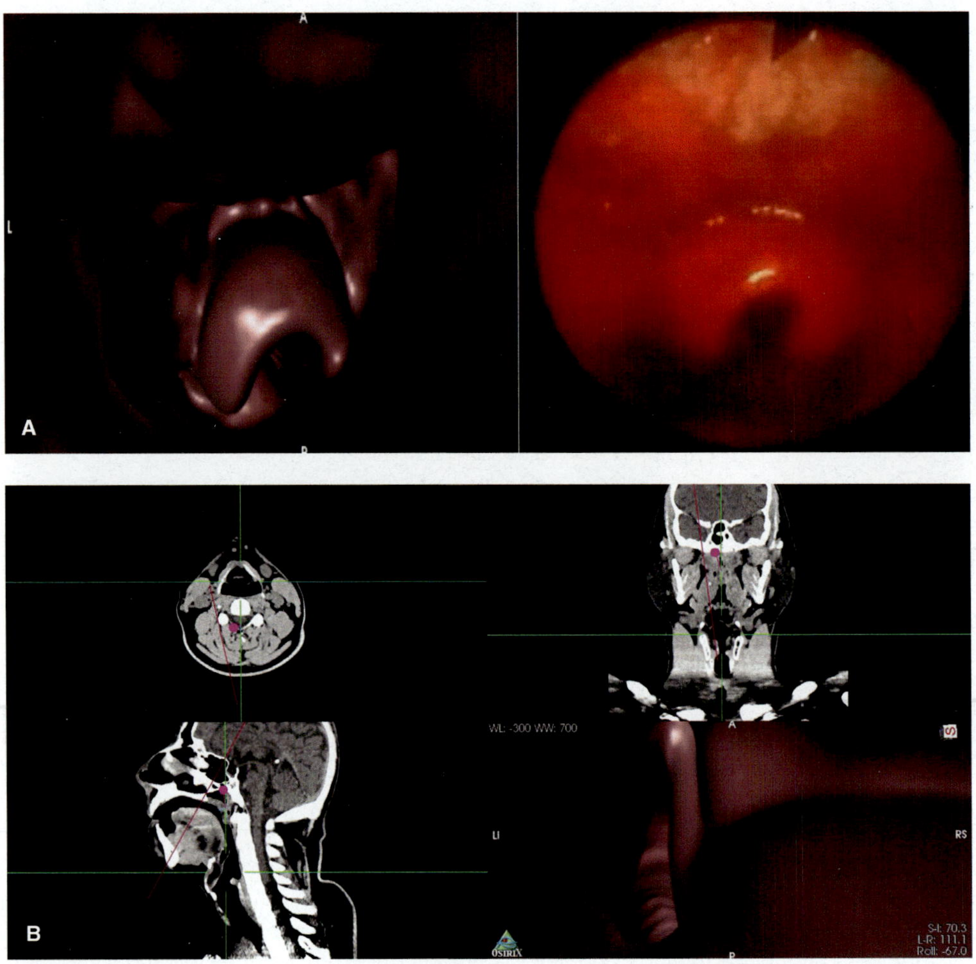

Figure 4.3. A, B: Virtual endoscopy and traditional endoscopy image of epiglottitis.

Suggested Readings

Ganaw AEA. Role of virtual endoscopy and 3-D reconstruction in airway assessment of critically ill patients. In: Shallik NA, Moustafa AH, Marcus MAE, eds. *Virtual Endoscopy and 3D Reconstruction in the Airways*. Springer; 2019.

Moustafa AH, Shallik NA. Radiological evaluation of the airway: one-stop shop. In: Shallik NA, Moustafa AH, Marcus MAE, eds. *Virtual Endoscopy and 3D Reconstruction in the Airways*. Springer; 2019.

Ragheb AS, EL-Gerby KM, Ahmed AF, El-Anwar MW, El-monaem SA. Conventional endoscopy versus virtual laryngoscopy in assessment of laryngeal lesions. *Egypt J Radiol Nuc Med.* 2013;44(3):497–503.

Shallik N, Haidar H, Dogan Z, et al. Circular hyoid bone: the first reported case in literature. *Trends Anaesth Crit Care.* 2017;16:27–28.

Shallik N, Zaghw A, Dogan Z, Rahman W. The use 3D reconstructive and virtual endoscopy for upper airway images in post-traumatic airway stenosis. *Trends Anaesth Crit Care.* 2017;16:16–17.

Song SG, Seo JJ, Chung TW, et al. Virtual endoscopy using spiral CT in patients with carcinomas of the hypopharynx and larynx. *J Korean Radiol Soc.* 2000;42(5):715–720.

Yunus M. Helical CT scan with 2D and 3D reconstructions and virtual endoscopy versus conventional endoscopy in the assessment of airway disease in neonates, infants and children. *J Pak Med Assoc.* 2012;62(11):1154–1160.

5 Difficult Airway Letter

Lynette J. Mark • Lorraine J. Foley

Clinical Scenario: A 49-year-old woman presents for elective laparoscopic-assisted vaginal hysterectomy under general anesthesia. The patient is 5′8″ tall and weighs 250 pounds. On airway examination, she has a Mallampati class II oropharyngeal view and prominent front teeth. The patient is induced for general anesthesia with propofol. Mask ventilation is found to be slightly difficult and an oral airway is placed. Intubation is attempted with direct laryngoscopy with a Macintosh blade and a grade III Cormack and Lehane view is obtained. A second intubation attempt is made with a Miller blade—a grade IIb view was obtained. Intubation with a bougie is unsuccessful. A third attempt with a video laryngoscopy is made. The patient's vocal cords are visualized and a 7.0 endotracheal tube is placed without difficulty. Tracheal intubation is verified with continuous capnography and bilateral breath sounds. At the end of the procedure, the patient is extubated without difficulty. In the postanesthesia care unit, the patient is informed that she has a difficult airway and that she should inform future health care providers of this.

1 I have already documented in the patient's anesthesia records details about the difficult airway. Why should I provide a Difficult Airway Letter to the patient?

Guidelines from the American Society of Anesthesiologists (ASA) regarding patients with difficult airways recommend examining previous anesthetic records, if available, during preoperative assessments, documenting the presence and nature of the difficult airway in patient medical records, informing the patient about the difficulty encountered, and evaluating and following the patient for potential adverse events related to difficult airway management. Difficult airway information provided verbally to patients or family members before or at discharge may not be retained. Additionally, details pertaining to difficult airway management would probably be beyond a layman's understanding, therefore, a letter will help patients retain and share information.

Comprehensive Difficult Airway Letters are invaluable for individual hospital registries and interhospital communications. Communicating difficult airway information to the patient with a letter enables that patient to help future providers be better prepared for airway management, as this will provide the pertinent information.

2 What should be included in a Difficult Airway Letter?

Some practitioners tend to limit the Difficult Airway Letter to a generic one, advising their patient to inform future care providers that they have a "difficult airway" (Figure 5.1). Although providers appreciate this alert, more detailed information would be beneficial. We recommend that the following comprehensive information be included in the Difficult Airway Letter to the patient:

- Date and institution where difficult airway was identified
- Provider contact information
- Patient characteristics, such as anatomic features, body mass index, and significant comorbidities
- Type of difficulty encountered (mask ventilation, ventilation with supraglottic apparatus, intubation, extubation
- Unsuccessful and successful techniques with best laryngeal visualization
- Implications for future care
- Recommendations for registration with an emergency notification service

Dear Patient,

As we discussed during our postoperative visit, you underwent general anesthesia (completely asleep for surgery). This required a breathing tube to be placed in your windpipe to deliver oxygen to your lungs, heart, brain and other vital organs. When the breathing tube was inserted, it was difficult to place the breathing tube in your windpipe. This is referred to as a "Difficult Airway."

Now that we know that you have a "Difficult Airway," it is important that you do the following to help protect yourself.

1. Tell your primary care physician or family doctor that you have a "Difficult Airway."
2. Tell your family and others of your choosing that you have a "Difficult Airway" in case they need to provide this information on your behalf.
3. If you are to have surgery, tell your anesthesiologist that you have a "Difficult Airway." Show your anesthesiologists the attached form that contains all the medical details needed to manage your difficult airway.
4. You are strongly advised to enroll in the The MedicAlert Foundation's Registry for Difficult Airway/Intubation.
   a. Fill out the attached MedicAlert Foundation application for enrollment and send a copy of the "Difficult Airway" information form and membership fee along with it.
   b. After you enroll, you will receive an ID number, wallet card with the MedicAlert Foundation toll-free phone number, and a custom engraved "Difficult Airway/I" metal emblem on a necklace or bracelet.
   c. Your "DIFFICULT AIRWAY "information will be in the Registry at the MedicAlert Foundation, which has safeguards for patient confidentiality.
   d. In an emergency or if you have surgery, your "DIFFICULT AIRWAY" information can be accessed by your health care provider or any provider 24 hours a day, 7 days a week, at no charge.

I have informed you of your DIFFICULT AIRWAY because it is extremely important that you are aware of the difficulties in placing a breathing tube. Please keep this letter in a safe place for future reference.

I cannot emphasize enough how important it is for you to wear a MedicAlert emblem bracelet or necklace. It could be lifesaving! If you are unable to afford the enrollment fee, please let me know and I can write a letter for a waiver of the fee. Please contact me if you have any questions or desire further information.

Sincerely,
Staff Physician Anesthesiologist
Hospital
Address
Phone:

DIFFICULT AIRWAY MEDICAL INFORMATION FORM [apply patient sticker]

____ was found to have a "DIFFICULT AIRWAY"
on ____/____/____ at ____
MR#______________________________ Telephone# ______________________________

Mask Ventilation: _______ Easy _______ Difficult _______ Impossible
_______ Difficult Intubation _______ Difficult Laryngoscopy _______ Failed Intubation

Physical Exam: Reason for Difficulty

Height:_______ Weight:_______
Mouth Opening: _______ cm
Teeth: _______ prominent _______edentulous
Thyromental Distance: _______ <6 cm
Other____

Mallampati Class (I–IV): _______
Neck Extension: _______ full _______ limited
Large Tongue:_______
Anterior Larynx:_______

DETAILS OF AIRWAY MANAGEMENT
Mask Ventilation: _______ oral a/w _______ nasal a/w _______ 2 person technique
Success achieved with patient:
_______ awake _______ asleep _______ muscle relaxant used _______ muscle relaxant not used
_______ Intubation was unsuccessful
Rating Cormack/Lehane Laryngoscopy View: _______
(I—full view of glottis opening, II—epiglottis and arytenoids, III—tip of soft palate, IV-only soft palate)
SEQUENCE OF EVENTS
ATTEMPT 1: Device Used:_______________ Grade Laryngoscopy: __________
_______ Successful _______ Unsuccessful
ATTEMPT 2: Device Used:_______________ Grade Laryngoscopy: __________
_______ Successful _______ Unsuccessful
ATTEMPT 3: Device Used:_______________ Grade Laryngoscopy: __________
_______ Successful _______ Unsuccessful
ADDITIONAL COMMENTS:

Figure 5.1. Sample patient letter and form.

3 Our institution does not have a Difficult Airway Letter. What resources are available to us?

Various airway societies, including the Society for Airway Management (SAM) of the United States of America, the Difficult Airway Society of the United Kingdom, the Danish Airway Society, and the Austrian Airway Society, provide templates for Difficult Airway Letters.

4 Why would I recommend the MedicAlert Difficult Airway/Intubation Registry to my patient?

The MedicAlert Foundation, founded in 1956 as a nonprofit organization to provide a comprehensive emergency medical identification service for over 6 million people worldwide, was endorsed by the ASA in 1979. In collaboration with the Anesthesia Advisory Council, the National Difficult Airway/Intubation Registry was established in 1992. The registry offers a uniform recording system for the difficult airway, standardized "Dear Patient" and "Dear Practitioner" letters, a 24-hour response service, and a patient identification emblem. In 1996, SAM endorsed this registry and over 12,000 patients have been enrolled in it. Approximately 12% of these patients have attached "Dear Patient" letters from more than 150 institutions. The institutions represent private, academic, and military settings from almost every state in the United States.

5 What is the current state of clinical practice in terms of providing a Difficult Airway Letter to the patient and future directions?

A Difficult Airway Letter template is available through SAM at https://samhq.com/airway-lead-material/. SAM is in the process of developing a national consensus statement to facilitate improved communication of difficult airways to patients and, ultimately, to future health care providers in an effort to decrease adverse events and promote patient safety. (*See Figure 5.2 and* ***Video 5.1*** *for additional details.*)

- The Difficult Airway Letter is an effective mechanism for patient follow-up.
- Difficult Airway Letter templates are readily available through MedicAlert and SAM. The letter to the patient should be comprehensive and answer the question "what information would I like to receive from a patient that would facilitate my ability to manage his/her airway?"
- The MedicAlert Difficult Airway Registry provides a long-term, 24/7 emergency response identification service for difficult airway patients and health care providers.
- A copy of the Difficult Airway Letter should be sent to the patient's surgeon and primary care physician.

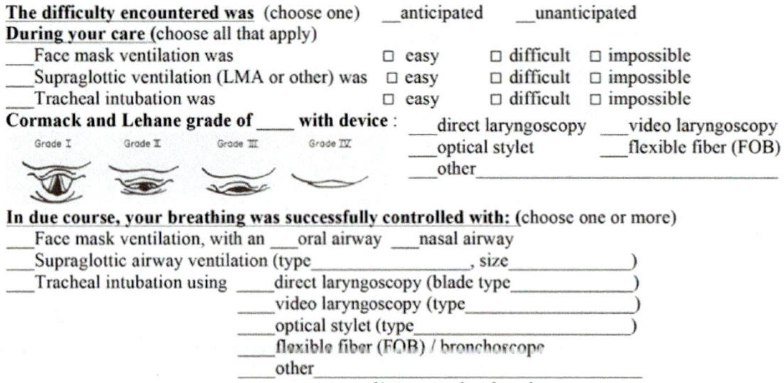

The difficulty encountered was (choose one) __anticipated __unanticipated
During your care (choose all that apply)
___Face mask ventilation was ☐ easy ☐ difficult ☐ impossible
___Supraglottic ventilation (LMA or other) was ☐ easy ☐ difficult ☐ impossible
___Tracheal intubation was ☐ easy ☐ difficult ☐ impossible
Cormack and Lehane grade of ____ with device : ___direct laryngoscopy ___video laryngoscopy ___optical stylet ___flexible fiber (FOB) ___other________
Grade I Grade II Grade III Grade IV

In due course, your breathing was successfully controlled with: (choose one or more)
___Face mask ventilation, with an ___oral airway ___nasal airway
___Supraglottic airway ventilation (type__________, size__________)
___Tracheal intubation using ____direct laryngoscopy (blade type__________)
____video laryngoscopy (type__________)
____optical stylet (type__________)
____flexible fiber (FOB) / bronchoscope
____other__________
____never secured/attempts abandoned__________

Figure 5.2. The institutional airway letter given to the patient should, at minimum, include elements of the airway physical exam, method of induction, the devices used, the anatomy seen, and the final management method and result.

Suggested Readings

American Society of Anesthesiologists Task Force on Management of the Difficult Airway. Practice guidelines for management of the difficult airway: a report by the American Society of Anesthesiologists Task Force on Management of the Difficult Airway. *Anesthesiology*. 1993;78(3):597–602.

Apfelbaum JL, Hagberg CA, Caplan RA, et al. Practice guidelines for management of the difficult airway: an updated report by the American Society of Anesthesiologists Task Force on management of the difficult airway. *Anesthesiology*. 2013;118(2):251–270.

Mark LJ, Akst S, Michelson J. General considerations of anesthesia and management of the difficult airway. In: Cummings CW, ed. *Cumming's Otolaryngology Head and Neck Surgery*. 4th ed. Mosby; 2004.

Mark LJ, Foley LA, Michelson JD. Effective dissemination of critical information: The MedicAlert National Difficult Airway/Intubation Registry. In: Hagberg CA, ed. *Benumof's Airway Management*. 3rd ed. Mosby; 2012:1094–1105.e2.

Mark LJ, Schauble J, Gibby G, et al. The national difficult airway/intubation registry, Medic Alert Foundation. In: Benumof JL, ed. *Airway Management: Principles and Practice*. Mosby; 1996.

MedicAlert Foundation. 2014. http://www.medicalert.org.

Trentman TL, Frasco PE, Milde LN. Utility of letters sent to patients after difficult airway management. *J Clin Anesth*. 2004; 16(4):257–261.

6 Routine Mask Ventilation

Richard E. Galgon

1 Describe in detail the device or technique.

The standard face mask (FM) most commonly in use today is a disposable, symmetrical device consisting of a transparent dome with a centered 22-mm universal connector and a soft cushion as the interface between the device and the patient's face. The generic one-handed face mask ventilation (FMV) technique is implemented with the "E-C" grip. The face-seal is applied by the thumb and index finger on the dome of the mask ("C"), while the remaining three fingers spread over the mandible ("E") with the fourth finger applied at the angle of the jaw, instituting the airway maneuver. The generic one-handed FMV technique is a suboptimal and asymmetric technique. The FMV technique is optimized by using either a one-handed, symmetrical "power-grip" technique or a two-handed technique, while also placing the patient in the sniffing position and using oropharyngeal and/or nasopharyngeal airways.

2 Where or when is this device or technique used in airway management?

The FM is a ubiquitous tool readily available in any circumstance where oxygenation/ventilation may be needed. In the operating room, it is used for preoxygenation, ventilation after induction, and before insertion of an advanced airway device, for general anesthesia in short procedures, after emergence from general anesthesia, and in any emergent situation where oxygenation is needed.

3 What distinguishes this device or technique from similar airway management methods?

The FM's effectiveness relies on the provider's skill and knowledge to provide a seal with the face and to relieve airway obstruction, both during inspiration and expiration.

Airway patency is affected by the manipulation of two movable bony structures: the cervical spine (chin lift/head extension) and the temporomandibular joints (mandibular advancement/jaw thrust). Both maneuvers stretch the anterior neck structures and, by increasing the distance between the chin and sternum and the chin and cervical spine, respectively, pull the tongue, larynx, epiglottis, hyoid bone, and associated soft tissues off the posterior pharynx, increasing the cross-sectional area of the upper airway ("active" increase of pharyngeal airway). The most effective airway maneuver is the two-handed triple-airway maneuver (chin lift/head extension, jaw thrust, and opening the mouth).

FMV is a dynamic process with the potential for airway obstruction to occur during inspiration and/or expiration. During inspiration (without an oral or nasopharyngeal airway), the nasal route may be obstructed at the nasal passages, soft palate, tongue, epiglottis, and/or glottis. Insertion of an oropharyngeal airway will support some of the obstructing soft tissues (tongue) and will commit to an oral route of ventilation, bypassing superior obstruction sites. During expiration (without an oral or nasopharyngeal airway), the primary site of obstruction is the soft palate. As the egress of air is blocked, the chest rises but does not fall (breath stacking), there is no expiratory end-tidal CO_2, and when the mask is removed, a forceful egress of gas occurs through the mouth. The use of an oropharyngeal airway will bypass the soft-palate obstruction during expiration. An optimal FMV technique includes strategies to improve ventilation and to limit stomach inflation by keeping PAP low (~20 to 25 cm H_2O). An inadequate technique increases the risks for gastric insufflation and regurgitation and aspiration, generates hypoventilation, risking hypoxia and hypercapnia, and causes facial, eye, and nerve injuries.

Author Caveats

The clinician should practice FMV based on ergonomics and physiology.

1. Know the Limitations of the "E-C" Technique: The face-seal ("C") is suboptimal as the dome of the mask is controlled only by two fingers of the left hand often resulting in a consistent leak on the right side of the mask. The leak may force the operator to increase downward pressure, pushing the chin toward the chest and inducing an iatrogenic airway obstruction. The airway maneuver (the "E" on the mandible) was never validated. Both validated airway maneuvers (chin lift and jaw thrust) are two-handed techniques applied during expired air resuscitation (eg, mouth to mouth). Support of the mandible by one hand ("E") is

suboptimal. In adult patients, the jaw thrust generated by the fourth finger at the mandibular angle is ineffective as it is asymmetric and cannot implement bilateral translation of the temporomandibular joints.

2. Implement an Optimal Seal Using a Power Grip: The ergonomic principles of the hand-tool interaction require full contact between the hand (the grip) and the device (FM). This is realized by placing the web of the left hand between digits 1 and 2 around the ventilator connector. These two digits will reach and control the right side of the dome while the rest of the fingers (3, 4, and 5) perform a chin lift. The hypothenar eminence will control the left, and the thenar eminence the posterior part of the dome.
3. Maximize the Patency of the Upper Airway with a Measurable Chin-Lift/Head-Tilt Maneuver: An effective chin lift/head extension can be estimated subjectively by (maximizing) the stretch of the chin–sternum space and objectively by the measurable angle between the longitudinal axis of the head surface and the longitudinal axis of the FM (~42 degrees) (Figure 6.1). An FM designed for a power grip and chin lift/head extension is the Ergonomic Face Mask.

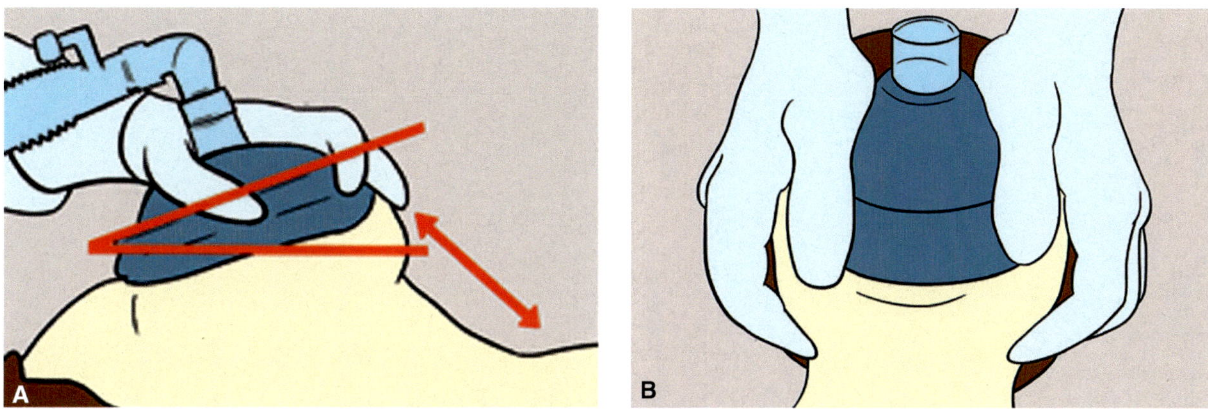

Figure 6.1. A, B: Objective assessment of the one-handed face mask ventilation technique.

4. Make an Objective Assessment of the FMV Effectiveness: As a rule of thumb in adult patients, an optimal FMV technique should generate low tidal volumes (~300 to 500 cc) with low airway pressure (~20 cm H_2O) and a capnogram tracing with plateau. Numerical values should be routinely used to define FMV "difficulty" (eg, an attempt with an airway pressure of 30 cm H_2O, a tidal volume of 50 cc, and a capnogram without plateau).
5. Maximize the Use of Airway Accessories: Oral and nasopharyngeal airways should be used immediately once an optimal FMV attempt is objectively confirmed as difficult or inadequate. Additional attempts at FMV without the use of one or more of these accessories in this situation wastes valuable time and oxygen reserve.

- An effective FMV technique relies on the provider's skill and knowledge to generate a perfect seal between the FM and the patient and to relieve airway obstruction both during inspiration and expiration.
- *See Figure 6.2 and* **Video 6.1** *for additional details.*

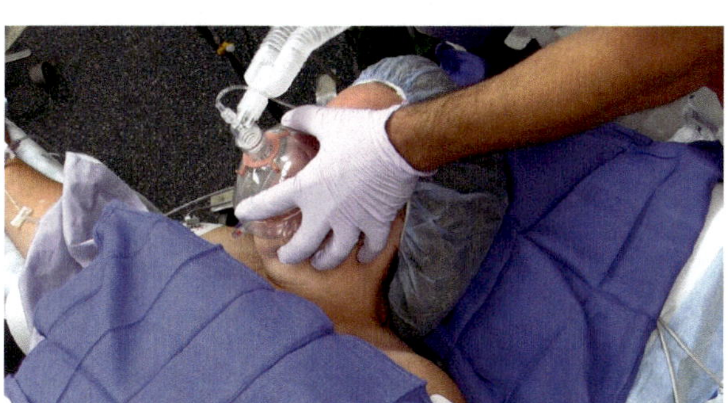

Figure 6.2. Routine mask ventilation. *See* ***Video 6.1*** *for further detail.*

Suggested Readings

Buffungton CW, Wells CMQ, Soose RJ. Expiratory upper airway obstruction caused by the soft palate during bag mask ventilation. *Open J Anesthesiol.* 2012;2:38–44.

Matioc AA. An anesthesiologist's perspective on the history of basic airway management: the "modern" era, 1960 to present. *Anesthesiology.* 2019;130:686–711.

Paal P, Goedecke A, Brugger H, et al. Head position for opening the upper airway. *Anaesthesia.* 2007;62:227–230.

Wenzel V, Idris AH, Dorges V, et al. The respiratory system during resuscitation: a review of the history, risk of infection during assisted ventilation, respiratory mechanics, and ventilation strategies for patients with an unprotected airway. *Resuscitation.* 2001;49:123–134.

Difficult Mask Ventilation

7

Richard E. Galgon

Clinical Scenario: A 48-year-old obese woman presents for elective cholecystectomy. Her body mass index (BMI) is 45. Though she snores loudly, she has not been diagnosed with obstructive sleep apnea. She is being successfully treated for gastroesophageal reflux disease. Her airway examination appears otherwise normal. After preoxygenation for 3 minutes with a tight-fitting face mask, she is induced with propofol. Mask ventilation proves impossible.

1 What are the anesthetic and airway management considerations for this case?

The incidence of the difficult face mask ventilation (DMV) ranges between 0.03% and 18%, depending on the population and airway management location. Langeron et al. describe five predictors for DMV—increased BMI, history of snoring/obstructive sleep apnea, lack of teeth, presence of beard, and age >55. The presence of at least two of these risk factors indicates a high likelihood of DMV. Other authors have described additional predictors: limited mandibular protrusion test, male gender, airway masses/tumors, history of radiation therapy, short thyromental distance, Mallampati score 3 to 4, and a history of failed direct laryngoscopy. The possibility of a DMV should trigger the preoperative evaluation of the triple-airway maneuver: mandibular advancement (mandibular teeth in front of the maxillary teeth), neck extension (chin up with mouth closed), and mouth opening. Other factors may affect mask ventilation in the morbidly obese patient (eg, a restrictive pulmonary function pattern on spirometry, increased oxygen consumption, and reduced pulmonary compliance).

2 How would you manage the airway in this case?

Though this case involves a patient whose DMV was encountered after anesthetic induction, all patients at risk should be properly readied. Thorough preoxygenation, head elevated positioning, and possibly continuous positive airway pressure should be employed prior to induction (see Chapter 54: Positioning of the Morbidly Obese Patient).

Postinduction DMV creates a critical situation that requires immediate response. Early recognition and prompt action is paramount. The decision to proceed is dictated by the speed of desaturation and the level of experience and skill of the practitioner:

1. Ensure neuromuscular blockade (NMB).
2. Position the patient in a backup position and pursue ventilation by switching to a two-handed face mask ventilation (FMV) technique with oropharyngeal and/or nasopharyngeal airway, instituting the triple-airway maneuver (see above). The one-handed FMV attempt without an oropharyngeal airway in a morbidly obese patient with history of snoring is very likely to fail. A two-handed FMV will provide a greater upper airway patency (bilateral jaw thrust) and can be implemented by a single provider assisted by an anesthesia ventilator, using pressure-controlled ventilation mode set to limit peak inspiratory airway pressure to avoid stomach inflation. The two-handed technique can also be provided by two practitioners, with one handling the face mask (seal and airway maneuver) and the other ventilating and monitoring the PAP The use of an oropharyngeal airway is critical as the oral ventilation route will bypass the retropalatal obstruction. A nasopharyngeal airway inserted postinduction can be maintained in situ and used in the postextubation period. The assistant can prepare for the next step.
3. Pursue ventilation with a supraglottic airway (SGA) device of choice. Pending available variations, a second-generation SGA with design features to optimize the oropharyngeal seal and enable gastric decompression is preferred.
4. Abandon ventilation and follow with an intubation attempt.

Regarding NMB timing, clinicians may remain divided on whether it is necessary to confirm adequate mask ventilation before the administration of neuromuscular blocking drugs (NMBDs). Recent research, performed on patients with "normal airways," does suggest rocuronium facilitates, or at least does not deteriorate FMV, while succinylcholine is associated with airway dilatation during pharyngeal fasciculation. It is unknown if NMB would help an "impossible" FMV situation. The ability to mask ventilate is a dynamic process determined by the patient's anatomy and position during induction, devices available, technique (one- or two-handed), experience, and drugs (depth of anesthesia, short- or long-acting muscle relaxants, rocuronium with sugammadex). A muscle relaxant will ensure glottic patency, optimize direct (and possibly indirect) intubation, facilitate positive-pressure ventilation (by decreasing pulmonary compliance), and may help the insertion of an SGA. Nevertheless, it can induce an iatrogenic airway obstruction by the relaxation and collapse of the upper airway, especially in obese patients. In this context, the decision to use an NMB before or after FMV remains an individual decision built into the general airway management strategy of a specific patient.

The author's choice would be to induce the patient with propofol and succinylcholine, then manage the airway with a two-handed FMV technique (ramped position, maximal triple-airway maneuver, oropharyngeal airway) followed by an indirect laryngoscopy intubation attempt in the presence of difficult or impossible FMV.

3 What are the potential hazards and complications in regard to the airway?

Unrecognized stomach inflation generated by aggressive FMV technique, resulting in high PAPs, will further burden ventilation attempts, and expose the patient to the risk of aspiration. FMV is a dynamic process and DMV/impossible mask ventilation may occur immediately postinduction, after a failed airway instrumentation attempt, or postextubation.

4 What distinct airway device might be used in this case, and what are the special considerations?

The need to have the difficult airway cart available cannot be overstated. A large array of SGAs have been evaluated in the ventilation of the morbidly obese and DMV patients. It may be advantageous to choose an SGA with a gastric drain (as mentioned in the previous section) to be able to access the stomach.

- Patients who are at risk of DMV should be properly positioned and preoxygenated.
- Many clinicians use early NMBs to facilitate mask ventilation.
- Two- and three-handed mask ventilation should be employed, as well as oral and/or nasal airway as indicated (Figure 7.1).
- When FMV is very difficult or impossible, proceeding immediately to an SGA or tracheal intubation is recommended.
- *See* ⊙ ***Video 7.1*** *for additional details.*

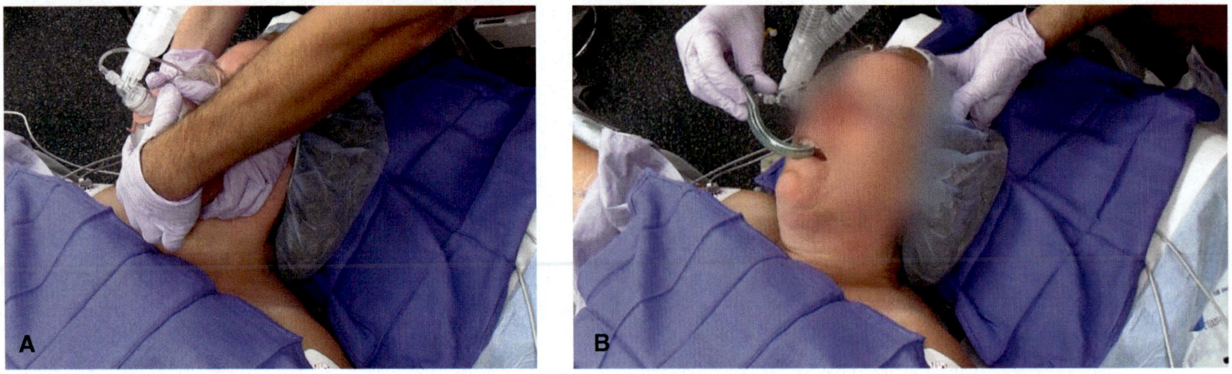

Figure 7.1. **A:** A three-handed mask grip is used in a difficult to mask-ventilate patient. **B:** An oral airway is placed to facilitate anesthesia face mask ventilation. Other options, including nasal trumpets, may be employed at the discretion of the airway manager.

Suggested Readings

El-Orbany M, Woehlck HJ. Difficult mask ventilation. *Anesth Analg.* 2009;109(6):1870–1880.

Ikeda A, Isono S, Sato Y, et al. Effects of muscle relaxants on mask ventilation in anesthetized persons with normal upper airway anatomy. *Anesthesiology.* 2012;117:487–493.

Joffe AM, Hetzel S, Liew EC. A two-handed jaw-thrust technique is superior to the one-handed "E-C clamp" technique for mask ventilation in apneic unconscious person. *Anesthesiology.* 2010;113:873–879.

Langeron O, Masso E, Huraux C, et al. Prediction of difficult mask ventilation. *Anesthesiology.* 2000;92:1229–1236.

Law JA, Duggan LV, Asselin M, et al. Canadian Airway Focus Group updated consensus-based recommendations for management of the difficult airway: part 1. Difficult airway management encountered in an unconscious patient. *Can J Anaesth.* 2021;68(9):1373–1404.

Sato Y, Ikeda A, Ishikawa T, et al. How can we improve mask ventilation in patients with obstructive sleep apnea during anesthesia induction? *J Anesth.* 2013;27:152–156.

Warters RD, Szabo TA, Spinale FG, et al. The effect of neuromuscular blockade on mask ventilation. *Anaesthesia.* 2011;66:163–167.

8 Direct Laryngoscopy and the Pogo Score

Richard M. Levitan

1 Describe in detail the device or technique.

Direct laryngoscopy (DL) is the creation of a direct line-of-sight to the larynx using a rigid blade. The two primary structures that must be manipulated in order to directly expose the larynx are the tongue and the epiglottis. Anatomic variables that can affect laryngoscopic exposure include mouth opening, dentition, and cervical spine positioning.

DL is fundamentally dependent on the quality of illumination and the operator's visual acuity. Proper positioning, a stepwise approach to tongue and epiglottis control, and an overall understanding of mechanics are required for procedural success.

Straight laryngoscopy blades displace a smaller amount of tissue than do curved blades. They are best used with a paraglossal approach, keeping the proximal portion of the blade in the right corner of the mouth, and not impacting the central dental arch or teeth. The small flange size of most straight blades does not allow sweeping of the tongue. The epiglottis is elevated directly with the tip of the blade. Tube delivery should be from the extreme right side of the mouth, avoiding the barrel of the blade, which would block the line of sight. The Miller design, created in 1941, is the most common of the straight blades. It has a small flange height and a flattened D-shaped barrel. Straight blades are commonly used in infants and children who tend to have a relatively small displacement space. Because of the very small tube size relative to the blade lumen size, tube delivery with straight blades is easier in children compared to adults.

In 1943, Macintosh observed that direct visualization of the larynx could sometimes be obtained with a Boyle-Davis mouth gag, an instrument commonly used by otolaryngologists. Its curved laryngoscope blade design has a natural fit against the curvature of the tongue. It lifts the epiglottis by indirect pressure on the hyoepiglottic ligament at the base of the vallecula.

Intubation via DL can be broken down into three components: (1) epiglottoscopy; (2) laryngeal exposure; and (3) tube delivery.

The epiglottis is roughly halfway between the tongue and the glottic opening. Unlike any other laryngeal landmark, it has a horizontally oriented edge. Head positioning, specifically elevation of the head until the ear and sternal notch are aligned, and keeping the face plane parallel to the ceiling, are critical to avoid pivoting the tongue base and epiglottis against the hypopharyngeal posterior wall. Atlanto-occipital extension impedes epiglottis elevation, narrows the space for laryngeal exposure, and prevents maximal mouth opening. In a supine orientation, head-elevated positioning is fundamental for the mechanics of laryngoscopy and vital for proper preoxygenation and passive apneic oxygenation, since it reduces alveolar collapse and improves functional residual capacity (FRC). The most useful mechanism of improving laryngeal view, after the epiglottis has been identified, is for the operator to apply direct pressure on the larynx. This bimanual laryngoscopy technique pushes the larynx down into the operator's line of sight. When using a curved blade, bimanual manipulation also optimizes the tip position in the vallecula and more effectively transmits force to the hyoepiglottic ligament. A second technique to improve the view after epiglottis identification is to increase head elevation. This improves mouth opening, shortens the distance to the glottis, and aligns the laryngoscopic view and cervical trachea with the natural forward inclination of the thoracic trachea.

Several systems of describing laryngeal exposure have been developed. The POGO (percentage of glottic opening) score was developed for grading laryngoscopic images. A full exposure (100%) spans from the anterior commissure to the interarytenoid notch; partial visualization is given a number estimated between 1% and 99%. POGO scoring allows categorization of laryngeal view in a detailed manner, and it has been used in numerous studies of video laryngoscopes.

The general principle of tube delivery is to avoid placing the tube directly in the line of sight, and instead, to approach the larynx from below. Stylets, shaped in a straight-to-cuff manner and stopping at the distal cuff, minimize the long-axis dimensions of the tube and maximize control and visibility of the tube tip. Angulation of the stylet at the proximal cuff should not exceed 35 degrees, otherwise the distal tip of the tube will impact the tracheal rings. With a left-facing beveled tube, tube rotation rightward helps if tracheal ring impaction occurs. Experienced operators can successfully intubate despite a low POGO score, by careful tube delivery and an advanced understanding of the posterior structures.

2 What distinguishes this device or technique from similar airway management methods?

There are many reasons why DL remains a fundamentally critical medical procedure despite newer indirect video and endoscopic methods of intubation. DL is fast, tube delivery is straightforward, and intubation succeeds more than 99.5% of the time. It is also especially effective in situations of bleeding and vomitus.

Author Caveats

The most common errors in DL are overrunning the epiglottis, and overgripping the laryngoscope (resulting in applying too much force early in the procedure). *See Figure 8.1 and* ***Video 8.1*** *for additional details.*

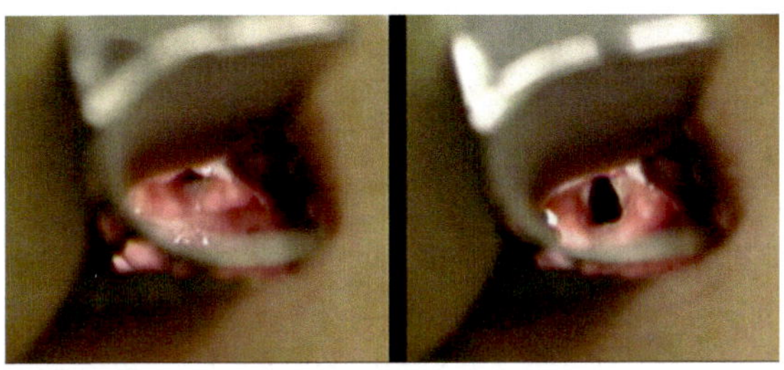

Figure 8.1. The view of the larynx using the AirwayCam demonstrating "overrunning" the epiglottis in the "left-handed image" that has been corrected on the right.

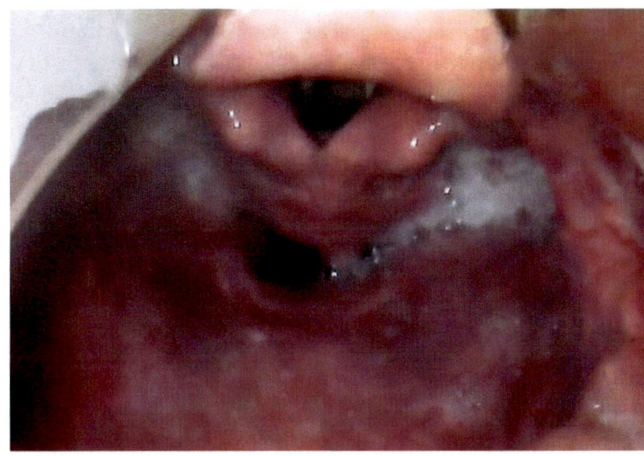

Figure 8.2. A POGO score of 50%.

- Expert laryngoscopists practice epiglottoscopy before seeking direct visualization of the larynx.
- Progressive visualization of landmarks is the key to success: uvula, epiglottis, posterior cartilages, glottic opening, and cords.
- Bimanual laryngoscopy and head elevation improve the mechanics of exposure and the visual line-of-sight to the target.
- The POGO score can be a statistically useful method of capturing differences in laryngeal exposure when studying direct and video laryngoscopy (*see Figure 8.2 and* ***Video 8.2*** *for additional details*).

Suggested Readings

Collins JS, Lemmens HJ, Brodsky JB, et al. Laryngoscopy and morbid obesity: a comparison of the "sniff" and "ramped" positions. *Obes Surg.* 2004;14:1171–1175.

Levitan RM, Everett WW, Kinkle WC, et al. Laryngeal view during laryngoscopy: a randomized trial comparing cricoid pressure, BURP, and bimanual laryngoscopy. *Ann Emerg Med.* 2006;47:548–555.

Levitan RM, Mechem CC, Ochroch EA, et al. Head Elevated Laryngoscopy Positioning (HELP): improving laryngeal exposure during laryngoscopy by increasing head elevation. *Ann Emerg Med.* 2003;41:322–330.

Levitan RM. *The Airway Cam Guide to Intubation and Practical Emergency Airway Management.* Airway Cam Technologies, Inc.; 2004.

Levitan RM. The mystique of direct laryngoscopy. *Respir Care.* 2007;52:21–23.

Ochroch AE, Kush S, Stuart S, et al. Assessment of laryngeal view in direct laryngoscopy: the percentage of glottic opening (POGO) score compared to Cormack and Lehane grading. *Can J Anesth.* 1999;46:987–990.

9 High-Flow Nasal Oxygen

Anika Sud • Anil Patel

1 Describe in detail the device or technique.

High-flow nasal oxygen (HFNO) is increasingly used in anesthetic practice and is recommended in several international airway guidelines as a means of optimizing oxygenation throughout airway management.

HFNO devices consist of an oxygen plus or minus air source and blender, water reservoir, flow meter, humidifier and heating system, heated noncondensing circuit, and patient interface. They deliver warmed, humidified, oxygen-air mix (FiO_2 0.21 to 1.0), at flow rates up to 70 L/min^{-1} to a patient via a specialized nasal cannula. Flow rates greater than 30 L/min^{-1} are considered ""high" flow, as this exceeds a patient's peak inspiratory flow rate (PIFR) at rest during "normal" tidal breathing (approximately 30 L/min^{-1}). When the HFNO flow rate exceeds a patient's PIFR, the HFNO system is converted from an open oxygen delivery system into a functionally closed system, thereby minimizing ambient gas entrainment. Importantly, a patient's PIFR increases in respiratory distress, and therefore the delivered HFNO flow rate should be correspondingly increased, to minimize the reduction in inspired FiO_2 (from entrainment of air), and hence FAO_2.

If HFNO device is delivering 100% O_2:

Mouth closed + (Nasal high-flow rate > PIFR) = FiO_2 of 1.0 delivered

2 Where or when is the device used in airway management?

HFNO has a broad range of applications in anesthesia in both the *spontaneously breathing patient*, when it is termed HFNO, and in the intentionally *apneic patient* when it is termed THRIVE (Transnasal Humidified Rapid-Insufflation Ventilatory Exchange). See Table 9.1 for additional details.

TABLE 9.1 Uses of HFNO and THRIVE in Anesthesia

HFNO (patient *spontaneously breathing*)	THRIVE (patient *apneic*)
1. **Preoxygenation**	1. **Peri-intubation** to extend the safe apneic window during the intubation process
2. **Procedural sedation** eg, awake tracheal intubation, endoscopy, ECT.	
3. **General anesthesia** for shared airway surgery where spontaneous ventilation is maintained	2. **Extended apnea application** to facilitate ear, nose, and throat (ENT) surgery
4. **Postextubation** and in recovery	

In this chapter, we focus on the role of THRIVE in airway management for enhancing oxygenation peri-intubation, and its extended apnea application to facilitate ENT surgery.

The physiologic mechanisms underlying THRIVE are incompletely understood but are thought to consist of: (1) apneic oxygenation and possibly (2) apneic ventilation. Apneic oxygenation extends the safe apnea time prior to desaturation and occurs with both low flow (eg, NODESAT technique, facemask, nasopharyngeal catheter) and high-flow oxygen systems. During apnea, provided a patent airway exists between the pharynx and the alveoli, the difference between the alveolar rate of oxygen uptake (250 mL/min^{-1}) and carbon dioxide excretion (10 mL/min^{-1}), produces a volume deficit in the alveoli (approximately 240 mL/min^{-1}). This generates a subatmospheric pressure gradient within the lower airway, drawing gas into the lungs, termed aventilatory mass flow or apneic oxygenation.

Apneic ventilation extends the safe apnea time while also, in some patient groups, having an effect on carbon dioxide clearance. Apneic ventilation only occurs with high-flow oxygen systems, but the mechanism underlying it is not fully understood. Apneic ventilation is thought to arise from an interaction between highly turbulent supraglottic flow vortices (generated by the HFNO stream in the upper airway) from the top end, and cardiogenic oscillations (pulsatile changes in airway gas flow which are synchronous with the cardiac cycle), from below. This interaction provides a means by which carbon dioxide could be removed from carina to pharynx, in the absence of respiratory movements. It is currently unclear whether apneic ventilation occurs in all adult patient groups, and it has not been demonstrated in pediatric patients.

THRIVE Peri-Intubation Use

THRIVE can be used to maintain arterial oxygenation and prolong the safe apnea time peri-intubation, thereby improving the margin of safety for securing the airway. HFNO can be used to preoxygenate the patient, and then, following induction of anesthesia, continued as THRIVE, providing apneic oxygenation and ventilation not only during apnea but also during laryngoscopy, so long as a patent airway is maintained. This is termed *per*oxygenation. Prolonging the safe apnea time reduces the time pressure on the anesthetist to achieve tracheal intubation. This potentially allows optimization of the human factor aspects of difficult airway management, improved performance, decision-making ability, and probability of success, and enhances opportunities and safety for airway management training (Figure 9.1).

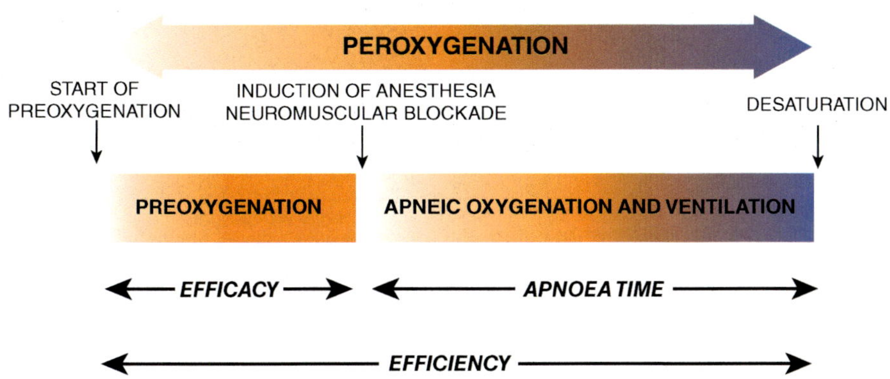

Figure 9.1. The underlying principles of peroxygenation, which includes preoxygenation and apneic oxygenation and ventilation. Efficacy describes the time during which preoxygenation achieves a predetermined end-tidal oxygen concentration before apnea commences. The apnea time is the time between the commencement of apnea and arterial oxygen desaturation. Efficiency is the combination of preoxygenation with apneic oxygenation and ventilation. (From Patel A, El-Boghdadly K. Apnoeic oxygenation and ventilation: go with the flow. *Anaesthesia*. 2020;75(8):1002–1005. Copyright © 2020 Association of Anaesthetists. Reprinted by permission of John Wiley & Sons, Inc.)

The safe apnea time achieved with THRIVE will vary between patient groups and clinical situations. Factors affecting the safe apnea time in patients undergoing THRIVE are: (i) alveolar oxygen content at the end of preoxygenation (FRC × FAO_2), (ii) magnitude of effect of mechanisms that will add oxygen to the reservoir during apnea (ie, apneic oxygenation and apneic ventilation), (iii) factors affecting the oxygen cascade, transport, and cellular uptake, and (iv) metabolic rate of oxygen consumption (Figure 9.2).

THRIVE Extended Apnea Application for ENT Surgery

A specialized use of THRIVE is its extended apnea application allowing "tubeless" anesthesia to facilitate airway surgery in patients with laryngeal or tracheal pathologies, for example, subglottic stenosis or tracheal and laryngeal papillomatosis. THRIVE in this extended apnea context has the advantages of providing an unobstructed view of the larynx, avoiding airway trauma related to tracheal intubation, and acting as an alternative to jet ventilation techniques.

A review of 15 THRIVE studies, including patients with difficult airways, in a shared airway setting found median apnea time ranged between 13 and 27 minutes, with THRIVE mostly terminated due to completion of the procedure. THRIVE was terminated earlier than planned due to desaturation (10% cases), hypercapnia (1.5% cases), and laryngospasm (0.3% cases). Eleven percent of patients required rescue ventilation with supraglottic jet ventilation, facemask ventilation, or intubation. Therefore, THRIVE is not a panacea for airway management. It is essential that there is a robust airway strategy and plan for managing a patient's airway and oxygenation if THRIVE fails. Measuring CO_2 during apnea is challenging, with transcutaneous CO_2 monitoring, arterial partial pressure CO_2, and $ETCO_2$ with a facemask on termination of THRIVE being used.

A. OXYGEN RESERVOIR AT END OF PREOXYGENATION

O_2 content in alveolar compartment = $PAO_2 \times FRC$
where:

1. ***$PAO_2 = (FiO_2 \times [P_{atm} - P_{H_2O}]) - PACO_2/R$***
   - FiO_2 delivered
   - Degree of air entrainment (nasal high-flow rate: nasal PIFR ratio, and nasal cannulae: nares ratio)
   - Degree of denitrogenation achieved
   - $PACO_2$ (inversely proportional to minute ventilation)
   - R (0.7–1.0 varies dependent on diet)

2. ***FRC***
   - ***Reduced***: obesity, pregnancy, pediatrics, restrictive lung disease, supine position
   - ***Increased***: head-up position, positive airway pressure (mouth open/closed), recruitment, obstructive lung disease
   - Proximity of closing volume to FRC

Alveolar reservoir is by far the largest oxygen compartment. Also consider arterial, venous, and tissue O_2.
eg, $CaO_2 = (1.34 \times [Hb] \times SaO_2) + (0.0225 \times PAO_2)$ kPa

B. MECHANISMS ADDING OXYGEN TO RESERVOIR DURING APNEA

1. ***Apneic oxygenation:***
   Magnitude of effect dependent upon:
   - Airway patency
   - Entrained FiO_2
   - Degree of denitrogenation achieved
2. ***Apneic ventilation:*** (oxygenation & partial removal of CO_2)
   Magnitude of effect dependent upon:
   - ***Turbulence from supraglottic flow vortices***
     - *Proportional to flow rate*
     - *Variable upper airway anatomy*
   - ***Magnitude of cardiogenic oscillations***
     - 'Cardiogenic stroke volume'
       - HR, cardiac contractility, pulmonary vascular compliance
       - $\uparrow PACO_2 \rightarrow +$ SNS $\rightarrow \uparrow$cardiac contractility $\rightarrow \uparrow$cardiogenic stroke volume

C. OXYGEN UPTAKE FROM ALVEOLI → ARTERIAL BLOOD

- V/Q matching (deadspace, shunt Q_S/Q_T)
- 1/diffusion barrier (Fick's)

D. OXYGEN DELIVERY (DO_2) AND CELLULAR UPTAKE

$DO_2 = CaO_2 \times CO$
- $CaO_2 = (1.34 \times [Hb] \times SaO_2) + (0.0225 \times PAO_2$ kPa)
- P_{50} (position) of oxy-Hb dissociation curve
  - pH, $PACO_2$, temperature, 2,3-DPG etc
- Bohr shift: increasing $PACO_2$ during apnoea

Apnea time (with patent airway) $\propto$ $\dfrac{\text{A} \times \text{B} \times \text{C} \times \text{D}}{\text{E}}$

E. OXYGEN CONSUMPTION (VO_2)

Increased: critical illness, pediatrics, obesity, pregnancy, hypermetabolic states, eg, thyrotoxicosis, fasciculations from suxamethonium

Figure 9.2. Conceptual framework of factors influencing apnea time with THRIVE. CaO_2, arterial O_2 content; CO, cardiac output; DO_2, O_2 delivery; FiO_2, fraction of inspired O_2; FRC, functional residual capacity; [Hb], hemoglobin concentration; $PACO_2$, alveolar CO_2 partial pressure; PAO_2, alveolar partial pressure of O_2; P_{atm}, atmospheric pressure; P_{H_2O}, standard vapor pressure of water; R, respiratory quotient; SaO_2, arterial O_2 saturation of hemoglobin; SNS, sympathetic nervous system; V/Q, ventilation/perfusion; PIFR, peak inspiratory flow rate. (Reprinted from Sud A, Patel A. THRIVE: five years on and into the COVID-19 era. *Br J Anaesth*. 2021;126(4):768–773. Copyright © 2021 British Journal of Anaesthesia. With permission.)

THRIVE is contraindicated in patients with aspiration risk, nasal trauma/epistaxis, airway/maxillofacial trauma, communication from nasal to intracranial space (pneumocephalus risk), conditions in which hypercarbia or hyperoxia are detrimental, and surgery using LASER or diathermy (Figure 9.3).

3 What distinguishes this device or technique from similar airway management methods?

See previous sections.

- A patent airway is a prerequisite for apneic oxygenation and ventilation to occur.
- Safe apnea time will differ in different patient groups.
- THRIVE can fail and should always be part of a wider airway strategy consisting of multiple plans.
- *See Figure 9.4 and* ***Videos 9.1*** *and* ***9.2*** *for additional details.*

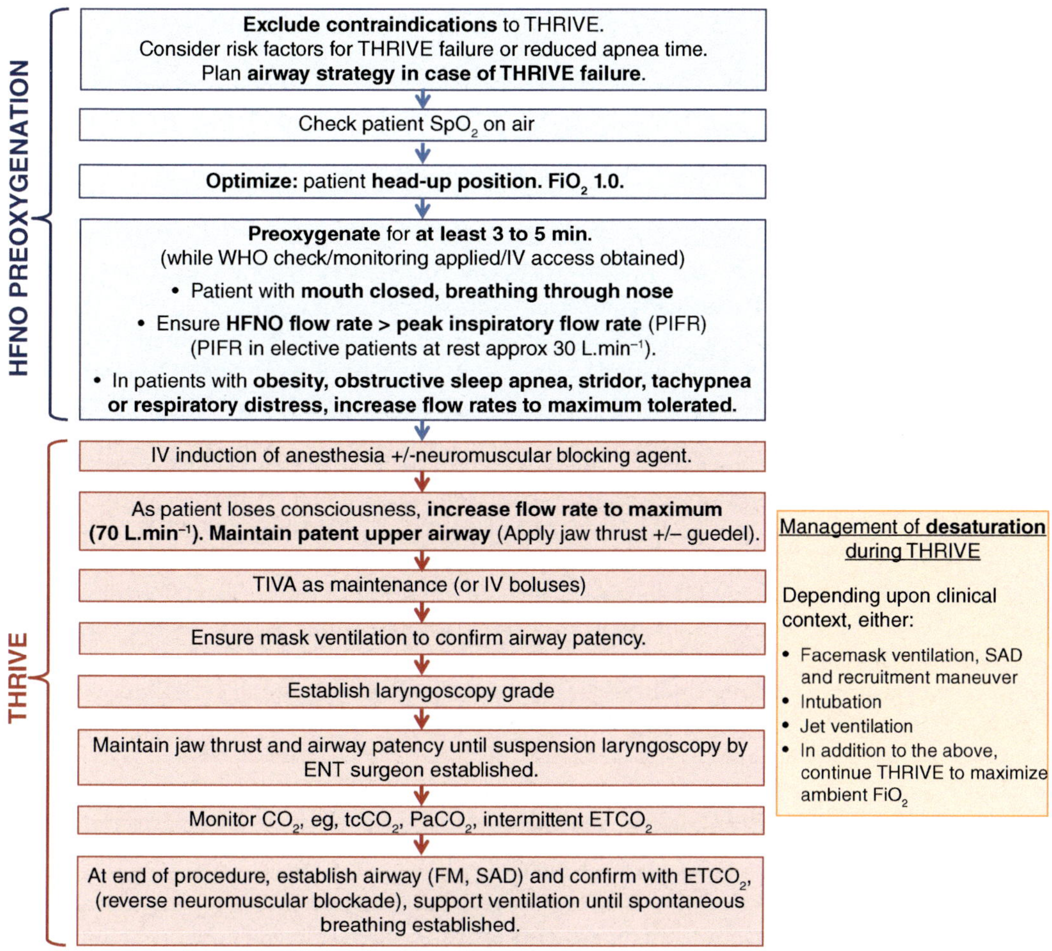

Figure 9.3. A practical outline of how to THRIVE for ENT surgery.

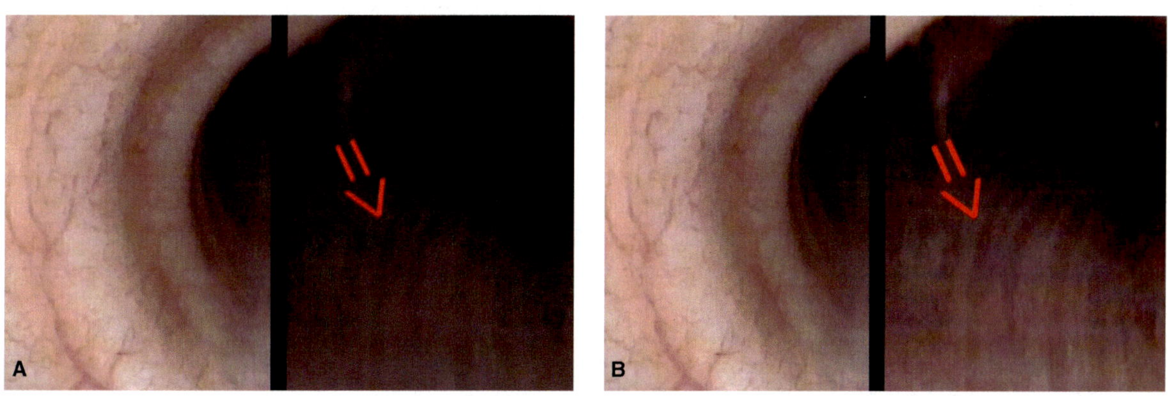

Figure 9.4. **A:** A patient for upper airway lesion biopsy under general anesthesia is kept apneic with total intravenous anesthesia and the airway is maintained with high-flow nasal oxygen. **B:** Cardiac oscillations (see **Video 9.1**) aid in driving CO_2 from the airway during apnea and high-flow nasal management.

Suggested Readings

Gustafsson I-M, Lodenius A, Tunelli J, et al. Apnoeic oxygenation in adults under general anaesthesia using Transnasal Humidified Rapid-Insufflation Ventilatory Exchange (THRIVE)—a physiological study. *Br J Anaesth*. 2017;118(4):610–617.

Huang L, Dharmawardana N, Badenoch A et al. A review of the use of transnasal humidified rapid insufflation ventilatory exchange for patients undergoing surgery in the shared airway setting. *J Anesth*. 2020;34(1):134–143.

Patel A, El-Boghdadly K. Apnoeic oxygenation and ventilation: go with the flow. *Anaesthesia*. 2020;75(8):1002–1005.

Patel A, Nouraei SAR. Transnasal Humidified Rapid-Insufflation Ventilatory Exchange (THRIVE): a physiological method of increasing apnoea time in patients with difficult airways. *Anaesthesia*. 2015;70(3):323–329.

Sud A, Patel A. THRIVE: five years on and into the COVID-19 era. *British Journal of Anaesthesia*. 2021;126(4):768–773.

10 Conversion from THRIVE to Tracheal Intubation

Bartlomiej Bartkowiak • William H. Rosenblatt

Clinical Scenario: A 64-year-old woman with recurrent adenoid cystic carcinoma of the salivary glands presents for direct laryngoscopy with biopsy and fine needle aspiration.

The patient's past airway management history includes multiple uneventful anesthetics with grade 1 face mask ventilation and successful intubations using video laryngoscopy. The patient denies any stridor, shortness of breath, or symptoms consistent with obstructive sleep apnea. On routine airway physical exam, the patient has a Mallampati class I oropharyngeal grade, the ability to bite the upper lip with the lower jaw, a thyromental distance greater than 3 fingerbreadths, and full range of motion of the neck with a normal pulmonary and cardiovascular exam. She weighs 58.5 kg and is 160 cm tall, with a calculated BMI of 22.85. General intravenous anesthesia with Transnasal Humidified Rapid-Insufflation Ventilatory Exchange (THRIVE) apneic oxygenation is planned.

In the operating room, induction of anesthesia and the initiation of the surgical procedure proceed uneventfully. However, after biopsy of the patient's lesion, brisk bleeding occurs. As the surgical team works to control the bleeding, oxygen saturation as measured by pulse oximetry begins to drop from 96% to 77%. The decision is made to tracheally intubate the patient; this is accomplished with a single attempt using a Glidescope, size 4 hyperangulated blade.

1 What are the anesthetic/airway management considerations for this case?

Head and neck surgery presents a particularly challenging set of circumstances for the anesthesiologist. The overlap of the surgical site and the airway requires close collaboration and excellent communication between the anesthesia and surgical teams. Because the patient's airway is often oriented away from the anesthesiologist, limits on immediate access necessitate enhanced vigilance—particularly when some procedures require the surgeon's manipulation of the position of the head and neck. Furthermore, the patient population undergoing head and neck surgery is likely to be older, have pulmonary and cardiac conditions, and present with difficult airways due to the nature of their disease and/or prior treatment (eg, surgical procedures and/or radiation therapy). Therefore, it is essential that a careful examination of the airway is performed and a well-considered anesthetic and airway management strategy is developed that takes into account both the needs of the anesthesiologist and surgeon.

With regards to the anesthetic management, the anesthesiologist needs to ensure excellent intraoperative analgesia, immobility, and a smooth emergence. Given the highly stimulating nature of laryngoscopic procedures, coupled with the robust innervation, reflexogenicity, and the vascularity of the involved tissues, opioid-based anesthetic techniques are often employed. For a short procedure with relatively minimal postoperative pain, like the one described in this clinical scenario, a total intravenous anesthesia (TIVA) approach using propofol and remifentanil is often employed. This allows for potent, airway-independent, short-acting analgesia/anesthesia with an excellent emergence profile that limits coughing and bucking. Given the use of rigid instruments and bronchoscopes in such procedures, immobilization with neuromuscular blocking agents (either succinylcholine or rocuronium with subsequent reversal) is often employed to ensure patient safety.

Since its introduction in 2015, Transnasal Humidified Rapid-Insufflation Ventilatory Exchange (THRIVE) has become an important airway management tool in the practice of head and neck anesthesia. As discussed in Chapter 9: High-Flow Nasal Oxygen, THRIVE refers to the administration of high-flow nasal oxygen therapy in apneic patients. The benefits of THRIVE in upper airway surgery are substantial as it is noninvasive and grants unimpeded airway access to the surgical team. Unfortunately, these benefits are tempered by the challenges of inefficient ventilation, an increased fire risk, and a lack of airway isolation that can result in aspiration of upper airway contaminants, and more significantly, intraoperative loss of airway patency resulting in hypoxia.

2 How would you manage the airway in this case?

The challenges introduced with THRIVE can be mitigated through a thorough understanding of the technique, proper patient selection, planning, and caution. An ideal candidate should have a patent airway, have a low risk for loss of airway patency, be free of significant respiratory pathology, and be at low risk for rapid desaturation (eg, nonmorbidly obese, critically ill, nor pregnant). A clear backup plan for securing the airway is critical; backup equipment needs to be prepared and readily available, and most importantly, the backup plans must be discussed with the surgical team prior to the induction of anesthesia. Vigilance and rapid recognition of desaturation events is important as pulse oximetry measurements can lag actual oxygen saturation levels by as much as 60 seconds. Once the decision is made to proceed to endotracheal intubation, any reasonable method of airway management is appropriate. This includes direct laryngoscopy, video-assisted laryngoscopy, flexible bronchoscopy, and the leverage of the surgical team's tools and access to the airway.

In this clinical scenario, prior to the initiation of the case, routine intubation equipment as well as a monsoon jet ventilator were prepared and placed within immediate reach of the anesthesia team. Although the scenario describes a situation where the patient is intubated using a Glidescope, multiple other approaches are possible. As an additional example, an alternative situation may play out as follows.

Noticing a drop in oxygen saturation in the setting of a high-risk situation, the anesthesiologist alerts the surgical team to the desaturation event. A suspension laryngoscope is placed into the oropharynx, while the anesthesiologist passes a previously prepared tracheal tube to the surgical team. The tracheal tube is then placed through the surgical suspension laryngoscope into the larynx under direct visualization. The tracheal tube cuff is inflated, the anesthesia circuit connected, and manual ventilation with an FiO_2 of 1.0 results in immediate return to a pulse oximetry saturation of 99%. The standard 15-mm connector of the tracheal tube is then removed, and a grasper is used to maintain the position of the endotracheal tube (ETT) while the suspension laryngoscope is removed. The circuit is then reattached to the ETT with subsequent initiation of manual, followed by mechanical ventilation (see **Video 10.1**; which documents the conversion from THRIVE to endotracheal intubation in a case similar to the clinical scenario). The surgery then proceeds without further issues.

3 What are other potential hazards in regard to the airway?

Due to the high flow of oxygen and the possibility of electrocautery and laser use in upper airway surgery, operating room personnel must be particularly alert to the possibility of fire during these procedures. For a fire to occur, the three elements of the fire triad must be present: (1) an oxidizer (such as oxygen gas), (2) an ignition source, and (3) fuel. For airway fires, the most common fuel source is the ETT itself; thus, the probability of fire inside the airway is significantly lessened by the use of THRIVE apneic oxygenation. However, there still exists a high risk of fire outside of the airway, and there is a case report of the ignition of a monopolar diathermy grip during palate surgery using THRIVE when an arc arose from the diathermy tip to a titanium implant. Therefore, it is important to discuss any plans for laser/electrocautery use with the surgical team, and to limit oxygen concentration to 30% or discontinue THRIVE and suction airway gases prior to use.

4 What other airway devices might be used in this case, and what are the special considerations?

In addition to the application of THRIVE, there are several other airway management options during upper airway procedures. These include mechanical ventilation through a small ETT, jet ventilation, apnea with intermittent ventilation, and (if no muscle relaxant agents are employed) spontaneous ventilation. Of these options, only the placement of an ETT secures and isolates the airway and allows for the use of inhalational anesthetics without significant environmental contamination. However, the use of an ETT presents the above-mentioned risk of airway fire and can limit surgical exposure. Fire risk can be mitigated with the use of specialized, laser-resistant tubes, and the inflation of the tube cuff with saline; however, even these tubes may ignite with prolonged laser exposure.

Jet ventilation refers to the use of a high-pressure (15 to 20 psi in adults) gas jet delivered through a specialized narrow and stiff cannula that is either positioned at the entrance of the larynx via an operating laryngoscope, or below the larynx via the cricothyroid membrane. This technique allows for effective oxygenation and ventilation for longer airway procedures. However, compared to THRIVE, this is a more invasive technique requiring provider expertise and care to avoid barotrauma and complications such as pneumomediastinum and pneumothorax.

- Even relatively short and uncomplicated head and neck procedures, such as laryngoscopy with biopsy, require a well-thought-out airway management plan and close collaboration between the anesthesia and surgical teams.
- THRIVE presents itself as a useful airway management tool in the practice of head and neck anesthesia; however, the lack of a "secure" airway can result in intraoperative loss of airway patency, resulting in hypoxia.
- The risks of THRIVE can be mitigated through proper technique, patient selection, and preparation with a clear backup plan for securing the airway that is formulated and discussed with the surgical team prior to induction of anesthesia.
- With proper planning and preparation, the transition from THRIVE to endotracheal can be performed rapidly and safely, allowing for a suitable margin of safety in the use of THRIVE apneic oxygenation in upper airway procedures.
- *See Figures 10.1 and 10.2 for additional details.*

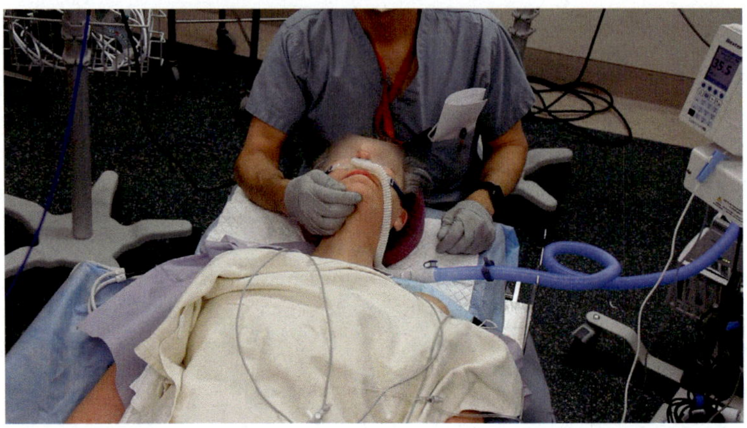

Figure 10.1. The patient is preoxygenated and undergoes intravenous induction of anesthesia with the THRIVE high-flow nasal cannula in place.

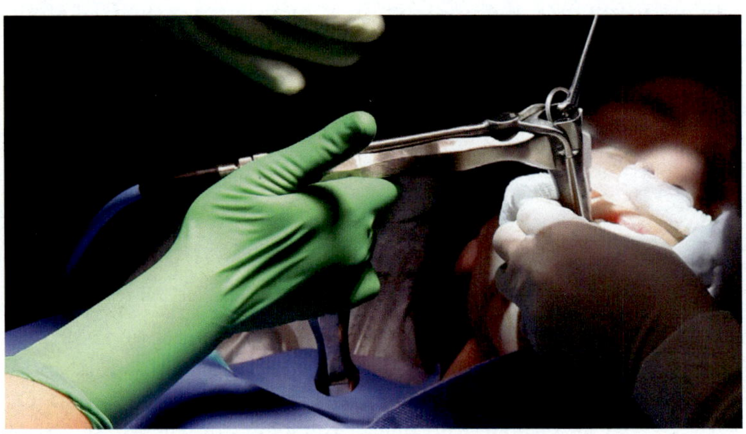

Figure 10.2. A tracheal tube has been inserted into the larynx via the surgical suspension laryngoscope, and an instrument is used to grab the proximal end. The suspension laryngoscope has been retreated off the tracheal tube. The grasper instrument stabilized the tracheal tube during the retreat.

Suggested Readings

Benninger MS, Zhang ES, Chen B, et al. Utility of transnasal humidified rapid insufflation ventilatory exchange for microlaryngeal surgery. *Laryngoscope*. 2021;131(3):587–591.

Huang L, Dharmawardana N, Badenoch A, et al. A review of the use of transnasal humidified rapid insufflation ventilatory exchange for patients undergoing surgery in the shared airway setting. *J Anesth*. 2020;34(1):134–143.

Jaffe RA, Schmiesing CA, Golianu B. *Anesthesiologist's Manual of Surgical Procedures*. 6th ed. Wolters Kluwer; 2020.

Nekhendzy V, Saxena A, Mittal B, et al. The safety and efficacy of transnasal humidified rapid-insufflation ventilatory exchange for laryngologic surgery. *Laryngoscope*. 2020;130(12):E874–E881.

Sud A, Patel A. THRIVE: five years on and into the COVID-19 era. *Br J Anaesth*. 2021;126(4):768–773.

Preparation for Awake Intubation

11

Ralph L. Slepian

1 Describe in detail the device or technique.

The technique of "awake intubation" may be misnamed. Dr Andranick Ovassapian, the founder of the Society for Airway Management, commented that the patient undergoing awake intubation should appear to sleep, but be aroused by verbal or other nonnoxious stimulation. Some authors have preferred to call the state "aware." The patient should be comfortable and should be able to obey commands and maintain oxygenation and ventilation and protect their own airway. In addition, sufficient analgesia of the upper airway must be achieved to allow examination and instrumentation by an oral or nasal route (when not contraindicated).

Awake intubation is not synonymous with flexible scope intubation. Virtually any device used to manage the airway of a patient under general anesthesia can be used in the awake patient.

Planning is an essential part of the technique and the anesthesia provider should have a predetermined plan for patient preparation and contingency plans for each step of preparation, as well as airway management.

Psychological Preparation

Most patients expect to be asleep or unconscious when the surgical procedure calls for general anesthesia. A frank discussion, including the reason awake intubation has been chosen, and assurances go a long way toward engendering a cooperative patient. Patient positioning can help reduce apprehension. Patients with airway pathology typically prefer a semiupright position (using wedges, pillows, or the maneuverability of the OR table). Not only will this often improve their breathing comfort, but it may also reduce the effects of gravity on the anesthesia provider's ability to access the airway.

Desiccation

When not contraindicated by glaucoma or a compromising atrial arrhythmia, early IM or IV application of a drying agent will increase the effectiveness of topical anesthetics and reduce obscuring secretions in the airway. Glycopyrrolate, 0.2 to 0.4 mg, is often chosen. Topical anesthesia of the upper airway (excluding the nose) should not be started until the patient subjectively feels drying. The dose may be repeated.

Sedation/Analgesia

Intravenous analgesia may be used judiciously: small, repeated doses of midazolam (1 to 2 mg in an average adult) and fentanyl (eg, 50 to 100 μg) or remifentanil or dexmedetomidine infusions. Following the principles enumerated above, it is better to undersedate and "add," than to lose the patient's cooperation and airway maintenance. Avoid compensating for poor analgesic block technique with oversedation.

Supplemental Oxygen Delivery

Oxygen administration should include oxygen delivery by nasal cannulae or other acceptable devices while allowing for the "awake intubation."

Topical/Local Analgesia

Many techniques have been described to anesthetize the nares, oral pharynx, and upper airway, including topical anesthetics and nerve blocks. If a nasal approach is planned, the nasal passages will additionally need to be prepared with a vasoconstrictor (eg, oxymetazoline).

My method of choice for anesthetizing the airway is quite simple and can usually be accomplished in about 10 minutes. Once the patient notes that the antisialogogue is effectively drying the oral secretions, steps 1 to 3 are followed:

1. 120 to 160 mg of 4% lidocaine solution is placed in a syringe loaded with an oral mucosa atomizer, such as the MADgic (Laryngo-Tracheal Mucosal Atomizer by Teleflex) (Figure 11.1A). The lidocaine is slowly sprayed onto the oropharynx, and the patient is asked to "swish and swallow." This process is repeated one to two times. It may be of help to hold the patient's tongue with a cotton gauze during the application.

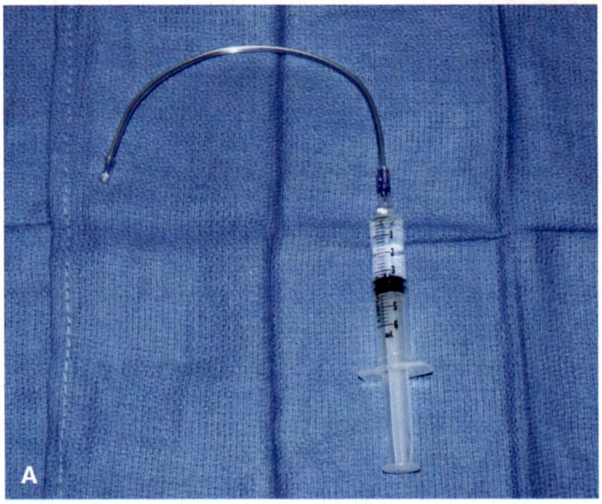

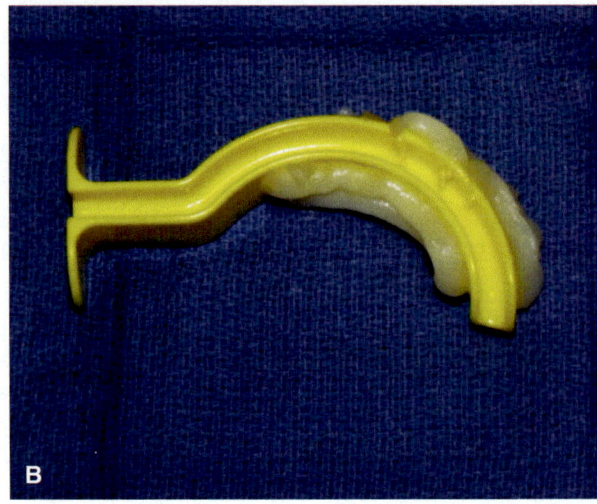

Figure 11.1. **A:** MADgic Atomizer. **B**: Lidocaine lollipop.

2. Apply 1 to 2 inches of lidocaine 5% ointment (100 mg/inch) to both sides of a standard oral airway. I like to think of this as a "lidocaine 5% lollipop" (Figure 11.1B). The goal is to have the patient suck on the airway and slowly, but steadily, continue to place the airway further and further into the patient's oropharynx. Continue until the oral airway is completely inserted without a gag reflex. The "lollipop" is removed.
3. While using a tongue depressor, the mucosal atomizer (with 4% lidocaine) is used to ensure that the more distal areas of the oropharynx are anesthetized. This atomization usually passes the vocal cords and will typically anesthetize the trachea. In addition, you may place the malleable atomizer into the oropharynx via the nasal passages. This will allow for atomized lidocaine 4% to be entrained into the trachea when the atomization is timed with inspiration. This typically negates the need for a transtracheal nerve block.

Careful attention should be paid to the total lidocaine dose. Less than 600 mg of topical lidocaine is safe in the adult patient.

Last, if care has been taken to choose awake intubation, the choice was made on the basis of safety. Awake intubation will undoubtedly require more time and effort than routine induction of anesthesia. The surgical team must be counseled to accept this, even if it requires some scheduling disruption. Early preparation of the patient (eg, explanation, desiccation, and initial airway analgesia applied in the preoperative area) will reduce delays.

2 Where or when is this device or technique used in airway management?

Awake intubation is one of the only two entry points into the American Society of Anesthesiologists Difficult Airway Algorithm. See Chapter 1: Decision Making in the 2022 Difficult Airway Guidelines for a decision-tree approach to choosing awake intubation.

- Awake intubation is a mandatory skill of the anesthesia provider.
- During awake intubation, the patient must be responsive to commands and able to maintain and protect their own airway.
- Supplemental oxygen delivery should be provided as needed.
- A methodical stepwise approach as outlined above should be developed and followed with contingency plans available.
- The entire OR team must be counseled on the rationale for awake intubation and any associated delays. Advanced planning will reduce delays.
- *See Figures 11.2, 11.3, and* ***Video 11.1*** *for additional details.*

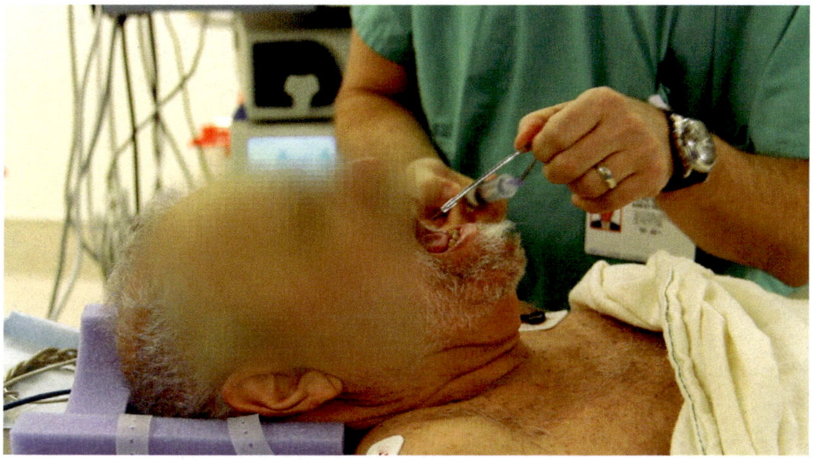

Figure 11.2. An oral airway generously covered with topical anesthetic ointment. Once placed in the oral cavity, the warming ointment will spread within the mouth, pharynx, and hypopharynx.

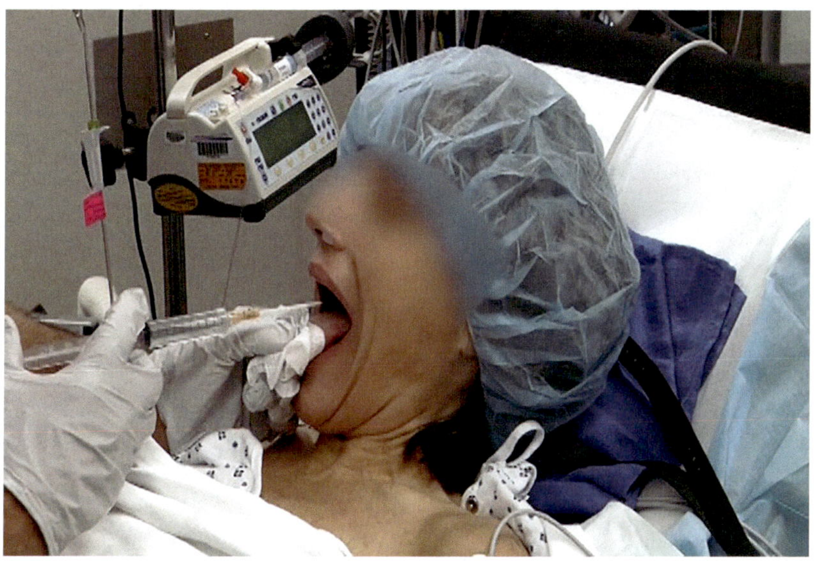

Figure 11.3. Tongue control with a folded gauze can not only expose anatomic targets, but also disable the patient's ability to swallow, thereby encouraging aspiration of topical anesthetics.

Suggested Readings

Apfelbaum JL, Hagberg CA, Connis RT, et al. 2022 American Society of Anesthesiologists Practice Guidelines for Management of the Difficult Airway. *Anesthesiology*. 2022;136:31–81.

Lebowitz PW, Shay H, Straker T, et al. Shoulder and head elevation improves laryngoscopic view for tracheal intubation in nonobese as well as obese individuals. *J Clin Anesth*. 2012;24(2):104–108.

12 Video Stylets in Awake Intubation

Andres R. Brenes Bastos

Clinical Scenario: The patient is a female with a known diagnosis of ankylosing spondylitis who presented to the ED with transvaginal bleeding in a remote location in a Latin American country. Due to the waitlists at the time of presentation, the patient had to wait 2 years for a surgical appointment. There was no bronchoscope available, so the anesthesiologist proceeded with an awake intubation utilizing the Levitan Stylet so as to not delay further surgical intervention.

1 Technique: Use of the Levitan Stylet for Awake Intubation

Patients who present for elective surgical procedures with an anticipated difficult airway are a challenge to the anesthesiologist and a test of their skill. Likewise, when the clinician does not have experience with these patients, nor the appropriate equipment, these cases may be highly stressful . Commonly, these clinical situations are managed with awake intubation, and most often with the use of a flexible intubation scope. However, these devices are expensive, may be fragile, and are not readily available in some resource-constrained settings. Optical stylets, on the other hand, tend to be more affordable, sturdy, portable, and have fewer maintenance needs. We will explore the option of awake intubation with the Levitan stylet (Figure 12.1).

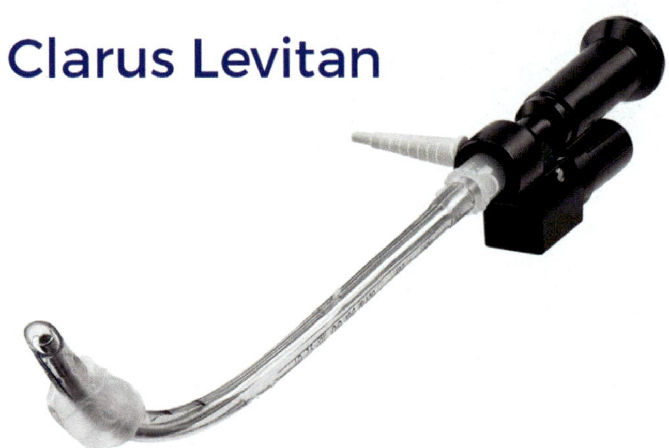

Figure 12.1. The Levitan optical stylet is a rigid, nonmalleable, intubating stylet originally designed to be used in conjunction with a direct laryngoscope. (Courtesy of Clarus-Medical, Minneapolis, MN.)

2 Describe in detail the device or technique.

The Levitan stylet shares many of the major features of other optical stylets, and is one of the simpler and less expensive devices available. The Shikani and Clarus Video System (Clarus-Medical, Minneapolis, MN), and the Bonfills (Karl Storz, Germany) are other examples of these devices. The Levitan is a malleable, rigid optical stylet that was initially designed by Dr. Richard Levitan as an aid to direct laryngoscopy in the emergency department. It replaces the ETT stylet and allows a view from the distal end of the ETT. It is built as a sealed single piece that connects to a light source (either a Green line laryngoscope handle or a Clarus proprietary Turbo LED light source), making it highly portable. It has a high-resolution eyepiece that can be used directly with the naked eye or can be fitted with a standard fiberoptic scope camera. There is a side port for oxygen insufflation, which can also be used with suction to remove debris and secretions at the tip of the stylet. A tracheal tube adapter holds the tracheal tube in place on the proximal stylet during intubation attempts. The stylet is 30 cm in total length and 5.01 mm in diameter, allowing it to work with a variety of ETT between 5.5

and 9.0 mm. Because of its short length, adult tracheal tubes require trimming of the proximal end (which can create a false impression of a deep intubation and subsequent inadvertent extubation).

3 Where or when is this device used in airway management?

Optical stylets can be used for both awake and asleep intubations. Most frequently, they are used via a midline or retromolar approach without laryngoscopy or as a stylet with optical capabilities during laryngoscopy for postinduction intubations. Optical stylets are useful for awake intubations (Figure 12.2 and **Video 12.1**). The midline or retromolar approach are the preferred techniques. This is especially beneficial when working with a patient with a smaller oral aperture. The stylet can be manipulated to change the curvature, allowing for the anatomical differences among patients. Its use minimizes pharyngeal stimulation and trauma. Once sedation and topicalization are achieved, the patient is requested to open the mouth and protrude the tongue. Phonation can be requested to increase the diameter of the airway when advancing the stylet. Under direct visualization of the airway, the stylet should aim to stay in the center and avoid contact with the mucosa. Stylet curvature can be modified between attempts to correct for patient anatomy. Once cord visualization is achieved, instillation of local anesthetic can be performed by advancing an epidural catheter through the oxygen port or simply squirting the drug into the port as it will flow through the ETT. Once the stylet tip is at the vocal cords or slightly past, the ETT can be advanced into the trachea, and positioning will be confirmed. There is some literature on the use of the Shikani stylet for awake nasal intubations.

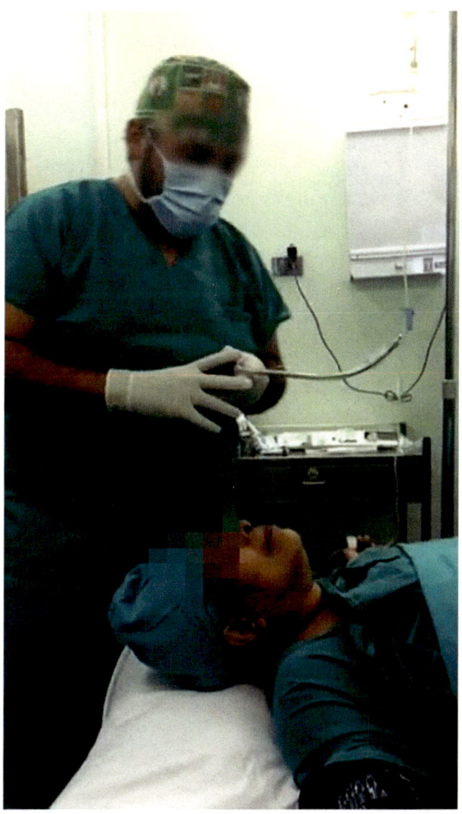

Figure 12.2. The author prepares to intubate an awake patient using the Levitan stylet.

Author Caveats

Due to the rigidity of the stylet, contact with the mucosa is more stimulating to the patient than that of a bronchoscope. Maneuvering the stylet requires significant dexterity and comfort in the absence of a laryngoscope. Defogging measures, such as placing the stylet in warm saline or antifogging solution, are essential but can be short lived.

- The Levitan Stylet and other optical stylets often cost a fraction of the price of a bronchoscope and are portable and lower maintenance.
- They are a good alternative for awake intubation in resource-limited settings.
- Optical stylets require less mouth opening than other intubating devices, which leads to less postoperative oropharyngeal discomfort than found with direct laryngoscopy.
- Optical stylets do not require a video tower, and the light source is portable and handheld.
- *See Figure 12.3 for additional details.*

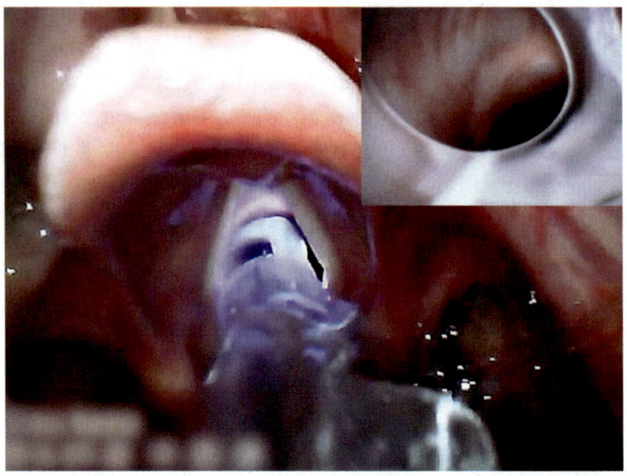

Figure 12.3. During a combined technique intubation, an imaging stylet is seen entering the larynx (image generated by a simultaneously used video laryngoscope). *Inset* shows the image from the stylet.

Suggested Readings

Kovacs G, Law AJ, Petrie D. Awake fiberoptic intubation using an optical stylet in an anticipated difficult airway. *Ann Emerg Med.* 2007;49(1):81–83.

Mahrous RSS, Ahmed AMM. The Shikani optical stylet as an alternative to awake fiberoptic intubation in patients at risk of secondary cervical spine injury: a randomized controlled trial. *J Neurosurg Anesthesiol.* 2018;30(4):354–358.

Ultrasound in Airway Evaluation

13

Wendy H. L. Teoh • Michael S. Kristensen

Ultrasound (US) in the evaluation of the airway for the purposes of identifying the cricothyroid membrane *before* further airway management and determining the ease of tracheal intubation, face mask ventilation, supraglottic airway (SGA) ventilation, and front-of-neck-airway access.

1 Describe in detail the device or technique.

Increasingly, US is being used in medicine to provide bedside imaging of internal structures. Though it has applications in airway evaluation, the inability of US to penetrate air limits its imaging field to structures from the skin to the most superficial parts of the underlying airway, for example, the posterior surface of the root of the tongue or the mucosal lining of the anterior trachea. Anything posterior to this "air–tissue border" cannot be imaged, and appears as artifact.

The floor of the mouth can be depicted by placing a linear US probe submentally in a transverse orientation. The probe is slid in a caudal direction from the tip of the chin to the hyoid bone. By increasing the depth of scanning, the entire body of the tongue can be imaged in the same manner. When a convex US probe is used, and slid from side to side, one can obtain a three-dimensional picture of the entire length of the tongue (Figure 13.1). If the subject's mouth is filled with water, the entire oral cavity is imaged, and even the soft and hard palate can be appreciated.

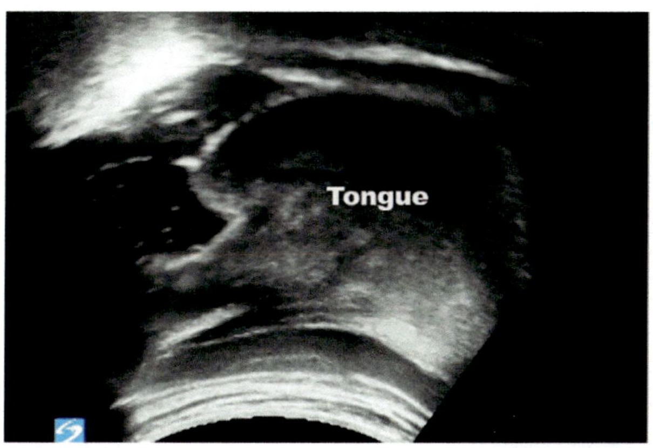

Figure 13.1. Submental ultrasound of tongue.

In the transverse midline plane, just cranial to the hyoid bone, the tongue base and the floor of the mouth, lingual tonsils, and the vallecula can be visualized. Just below the hyoid bone, the vallecula is seen. In this position, when the probe is angled caudally, the pre- and paraglottic spaces as well as the infrahyoid part of epiglottis are seen. The hyoid bone is visible on the transverse view as a superficial hyperechoic inverted U-shaped structure. On the sagittal and parasagittal views, the hyoid bone is visible in cross-section as a narrow, hyperechoic curved structure.

The thyrohyoid membrane provides a sonographic window through which a midline sagittal scan reveals the thyrohyoid ligament, the pre-epiglottic space containing echogenic fat, and posterior to this, a white line representing the laryngeal surface of the epiglottis. On the transverse view, the epiglottis is shaped as an inverted "C" and is related anteriorly to the hyperechoic pre-epiglottic space and lined posteriorly by a hyperechoic air–mucosa interface. Because of the superficial location of the larynx, US using a linear high-frequency transducer offers images of higher resolution than CT scanning.

In younger individuals with a noncalcified thyroid cartilage, the false and the true vocal cords can be visualized through the thyroid cartilage. In individuals with a calcified thyroid cartilage, the vocal cords and arytenoid cartilages can be seen by scanning from a point just cranial to the superior thyroid notch with a caudal probe angle, and by scanning from the midline and from each side of the cricothyroid membrane with the transducer angled cranially 30 degrees. The true vocal cords appear as two triangular hypoechoic structures lined by one distinct hyperechoic line, the air–tissue border. The false vocal cords lie parallel and cephalad to the true cords, and are more hyperechoic in appearance.

The cricothyroid membrane runs between the caudal border of the thyroid cartilage and the cephalad border of the cricoid cartilage, and its luminal surface is clearly seen on sagittal and parasagittal views as a hyperechoic band linking the hypoechoic thyroid and cricoid cartilages. If the cricothyroid membrane needs to be identified before anesthesia, and if palpation is not revealing, US can be performed in the following stepwise systematic manner.

With the patient lying supine, stand on the patient's right-hand side, facing the patient's head. Place a linear transducer transversely just above the suprasternal notch and note the trachea in the midline. A tracheal ring in the transverse plane is recognized as a horseshoe-shaped dark structure with a posterior strong hyperechoic white line, which is produced by the "air–tissue border." Move the transducer to the patient's right side so that the right border of the transducer corresponds to the midline of the trachea, and the US image of the trachea is truncated in half on the screen. While keeping the right end of the transducer in the midline of the trachea, the left end of the transducer is rotated into the sagittal plane, resulting in a longitudinal scan (Figure 13.2). Hypoechoic (ie, dark) tracheal rings will be seen. These lie atop the white hyperechoic air–tissue border, appearing as a "string-of-pearls." Move the transducer in a cranial direction, and the cricoid cartilage comes into view as a slightly elongated hypoechoic structure that is significantly larger and more anterior than the tracheal rings. While still holding the US transducer with your right hand, use your left hand to slide a needle under the transducer from under the patient's chin until the needle's shadow is in the middle between the caudal border of the thyroid cartilage and the cranial border of the cricoid cartilage. Remove the transducer. The position of the needle indicates the location of the distal border of the cricothyroid membrane. This exact point can be indicated with a skin marker, so that the cricothyroid membrane can be found later for emergency airway access, oxygen insufflation, jet ventilation, injection of local analgesics, or retrograde intubation, should the need arise.

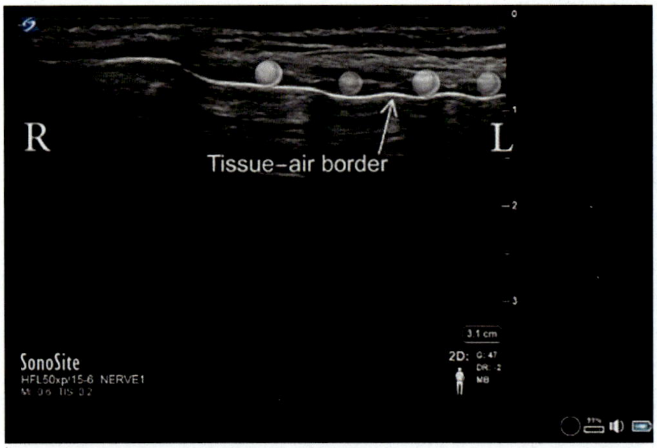

Figure 13.2. Longitudinal ultrasound of trachea with illustration of the "string of pearls" (ie, tracheal rings).

2 Where or when is this device or technique used in airway management?

When the clinician is suspicious that an airway issue may affect management, preanesthetic US examination can advantageously be applied in patients:

- Who have pathology, or symptoms of pathology, that may affect intubation or SGA function. Examples include subglottic hemangiomas, laryngeal stenosis, laryngeal cysts, respiratory papillomatosis, sialolithiasis, a pharyngeal pouch (Zenker diverticulum), and malignancies where their relationship with the airway can then be seen and quantified.
- In whom palpation of the trachea and cricothyroid membrane is challenging.
- In whom administration of local anesthetic through the cricothyroid membrane or blocking the superior laryngeal nerve is planned.
- In whom the knowledge of the tracheal diameter is crucial for tube-size selection.
- In whom one will subsequently use ultrasonography for direct confirmation of tracheal tube entrance into trachea.

- In whom you will perform tracheostomy and thus want to identify the ideal interspace between tracheal rings and anticipate the depth from the skin to trachea and avoid overlying blood vessels.

3 What distinguishes this device or technique from similar airway management methods?

US has many obvious advantages—it is safe, rapid, repeatable, portable, widely available, and provides real-time dynamic images. Several studies have evaluated its role in both the management of the airways and the diagnosis of upper and lower airway pathology.

- US can be performed by the anesthesiologist immediately prior to management.
- The airway and related structures can be depicted from the chin to midtrachea.
- The cricothyroid membrane can be localized before difficult airway management.
- The air–tissue interphase limits US to imaging structures superficial to the airway column.
- *See **Video 13.1** for additional details.*

Suggested Readings

Gomes SH, Simões AM, Nunes AM, et al. Useful ultrasonographic parameters to predict difficult laryngoscopy and difficult tracheal intubation-a systematic review and meta-analysis. *Front Med (Lausanne)*. 2021;8:671658.

Kristensen MS. Ultrasonography in the management of the airway. *Acta Anaesthesiol Scand*. 2011;55:1155–1173.

Kristensen MS, Teoh WH. The ultrasound probe in the hands of the anesthesiologist: a powerful new tool for airway management. *Anesthesiol News*. 2013;38(8):23–30.

Kristensen MS, Teoh WH. Ultrasound identification of the cricothyroid membrane: the new standard in preparing for front-of-neck airway access. *Br J Anaesth*. 2021;126(1):22–27

Kristensen MS, Teoh WH, Graumann O, Laursen CB. Ultrasonography for clinical decision-making and intervention in airway management: from the mouth to the lungs and pleurae. *Insights Imaging*. 2014;5(2):253–279.

Suhitharan T, Seevanayagam S, Parker FC, Teoh WH. Acute unilateral submandibular gland swelling associated with the laryngeal mask airway. *Singapore Med J*. 2013;54:e236–e239.

14 Ultrasound in Confirming Endotracheal Intubation

Michael S. Kristensen • Wendy H. L. Teoh

1 Describe in detail the device or technique.

During tracheal intubation, visualization of the tracheal tube passing the vocal cords and the detection of end-tidal CO_2 are considered the gold standards of verification. These standards may not always be possible to meet—for example, in the difficult laryngoscopy patient or the low-flow state, respectively. Ultrasonography (US) provides a new monitor to determine the success of tracheal intubation and has the added capability to detect bronchial intubation. During attempts at tracheal intubation, confirmation of the tracheal tube position within the trachea can be verified by US in two ways: US scans of the anterior neck during or immediately after intubation (direct detection) or by detecting ventilation at the pleural or diaphragmatic level.

Direct US scans of the anterior neck can be performed in three distinct areas: transversely, high on the neck at the level of the vocal cords/cricothyroid membrane where the dynamic, real-time tissue movement due to the tracheal tube can be detected; transversely, lower on the neck at the level of the suprasternal notch where both dynamic and static scanning are effective; and longitudinal scanning covering the visible length of trachea.

The authors recommend placing a linear transducer transversely on the neck immediately cranial to the suprasternal notch in the midline. The trachea is identified as a horseshoe-shaped, dark structure with a strong white line "tissue–air-border" artifact and a "comet-tail" artifact immediately posterior. The esophagus is seen posterolateral to the trachea on the patient's left side and has a "bullseye" appearance due to its concentric layers. Asking the patient to swallow will make the esophagus compress and expand, and thus aids in its identification. Intubation should then be performed. If the tracheal tube enters trachea, a brief "snowstorm" artifact may be seen as the tracheal tube touches the anterior tracheal wall. No artifact may be seen if a layer of air separates the tracheal tube from the mucosa, precluding conduction of the US beam to the tracheal tube. If the tracheal tube enters the esophagus, it will create a "tissue–air border" in the otherwise collapsed esophagus. This will appear as a strong white horizontal line that may repeat itself several times (like a flutter) due to "comet-tail"-like artifact. The esophagus will assume a shape similar to the trachea, and creates what is called the "double-trachea" sign. This test has a sensitivity of 86% to 100% for detecting esophageal intubation in emergency and cardiac arrest patients. If the tracheal tube is seen passing into the esophagus, it should be removed without initiating positive-pressure ventilation. Tracheal intubation may be reattempted as indicated. Successful intubation may or may not create an echo from trachea, so ventilation should be started as long as the tracheal tube is not appreciated in the esophagus.

Subsequently, the transducer is moved to the midaxillary line on either side of the patient's chest. The pleural line is identified, posterior to the rib shadows. During positive-pressure ventilation, a "lung-slide" sign should be visualized bilaterally. Lung sliding appears as a to-and-fro movement synchronous with ventilation. The movement is striking because the surrounding tissue is motionless. The detection of lung sliding can be enhanced by applying M-mode scanning, which highlights a clear distinction between a wave-like pattern located above the pleural line and a sand-like pattern below. This is referred to as the "seashore" or the "sandy beach" sign. Detecting unilateral lung sliding confirms the intra-airway location of the tracheal tube, but does not rule out mainstem bronchus intubation. In this situation, a contralateral lung-pulse sign can be sought. The lung pulse arises from the beating heart pushing the lung and the pleura with each heartbeat. If there is one-sided lung sliding and a contralateral lung pulse, then a mainstem intubation is likely, and the tracheal tube should be withdrawn gradually until bilateral lung sliding is present. If lung sliding cannot be detected on either side, but a lung pulse is present, the presence of esophageal intubation should be reconsidered, and appropriate remedies should be taken. If there is neither lung pulse nor lung sliding, then a pneumothorax should be suspected.

The sensitivity for US distinction between tracheal and mainstem bronchus intubation is less (69% to 78%) than that for esophageal and tracheal intubation. In accidental mainstem bronchus intubation, US scanning of the diaphragm will show no, or possibly paradoxical, motion on the side contralateral to the side of mainstem intubation.

Correct positioning of a double-lumen endotracheal tube can be evaluated by thoracic US. The US approach reaches same sensitivity and specificity as flexible scope bronchoscopy, but is more rapid.

2 Where or when is this device or technique used in airway management?

Accidental esophageal intubation can be recognized immediately when direct US scans are performed, and corrective actions can be taken before ventilation is initiated. This rapid diagnosis, independent of CO_2 monitoring, allows the clinician to avoid stomach insufflation. This makes the technique especially attractive in emergency presentations when the patient is known or assumed to have a full stomach.

Both the direct and the indirect confirmation by the US can be used in very–low-cardiac-output states or severe bronchospasm where capnography may fail in the face of successful tracheal intubation. In one study of 89 patients, capnography misdiagnosed 5 patients as having esophageal intubations, due to the absence of a capnography tracing.

US evaluation may also be helpful in noisy environments where auscultation may be difficult (eg, during critical care transport).

The clinician performing tracheal intubation should have multiple confirmation methods that allow the practitioner to adapt to a variety of clinical situations. In this regard, the US adds to the armamentarium of the airway manager.

Author Caveats

Subcutaneous emphysema can render airway US unreliable. Neck tumors and neck trauma may exclude direct US examination of the neck. Pneumothorax, pneumonia, or malignancy may make it impossible to use lung sliding on the affected side as an indicator of successful tracheal intubation.

- Esophageal intubation can be detected immediately by ultrasound scanning directly on the neck.
- We recommend direct scanning on the neck, followed by bilateral lung scanning for determining the tube location and function.
- Bilateral scanning of the lungs to some degree allows differentiation between tracheal and endobronchial intubation.
- A distinct advantage of US detection of esophageal intubation is the nonreliance on capnography.
- *See Figure 14.1 and* **Video 14.1** *for additional details.*

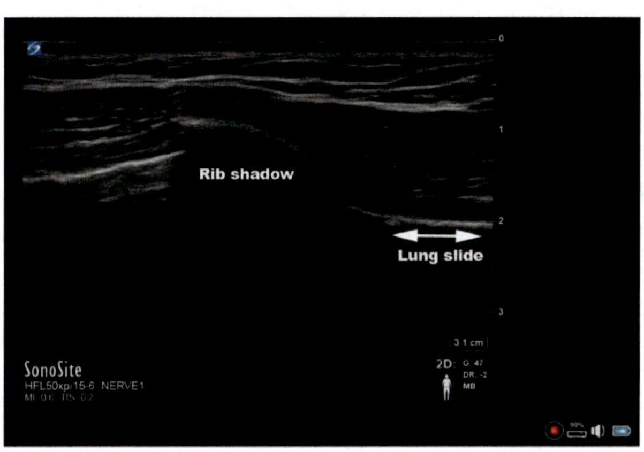

Figure 14.1. Lung slide is used to verify tracheal intubation but does not rule out bronchial intubation.

Suggested Readings

Abbasi S, Farsi D, Zare MA, Hajimohammadi M, Rezai M, Hafezimoghadam P. Direct ultrasound methods: a confirmatory technique for proper endotracheal intubation in the emergency department. *Eur J Emerg Med.* 2015;22(1):10–16.

Gottlieb M, Holladay D, Peksa GD. Ultrasonography for the confirmation of endotracheal tube intubation: a systematic review and meta-analysis. *Ann Emerg Med.* 2018;72(6):627–636.

Kristensen MS. Ultrasonography in the management of the airway. *Acta Anaesthesiol Scand.* 2011;55:1155–1173.

Kristensen MS, Teoh WHL, Grauman O, Laursen CB. Ultrasonography for clinical decision-making: from the mouth to the lungs and pleurae. *Insights Imaging.* 2014;5(2):253–279.

Men XQ, Yan XX. Tracheal ultrasound for the accurate confirmation of the endotracheal tube position in obese patients. *J Ultrasound Med.* 2020;39(3):509–513.

15 Reusable Versus Single-Use Devices: Environmental, Economic, and Public Health Considerations

Jodi Sherman • Cliff Shelton

1 Describe in detail the device or technique.

US hospitals generate more than 6 million tons of medical waste annually. Reliance on single-use disposable (SUD) medical equipment is proliferating in the United States and worldwide, often justified by reduction in the risk of health care–associated infections, this benefit is largely theoretical. The production, delivery, and waste management of SUDs require significant quantities of materials and energy, which are themselves linked to emissions that affect public health and worsen global warming. Waste reduction can save money directly via spending less on waste treatment and disposal, and indirectly through the prevention of supply production and transportation.

Traditional criteria for the selection and purchase of medical devices include safety for patients and staff, efficacy and ease of use, and capital and maintenance costs. Devices should also be compared along environmental and public health dimensions, using methods such as life cycle costing (LCC) and life cycle assessment (LCA) that consider the full costs and benefits of a product from "cradle to grave." Exposures and impacts that occur during raw material extraction, device production and packaging, transportation, use, reprocessing/sterilization, and waste disposal management of discarded materials are all included. Reusable and disposable models of several devices used in airway management have been compared across the entire life cycle, including supraglottic airways (SGAs), laryngoscopes, and breathing circuits.

2 Where or when is this device or technique used in airway management?

SGA: Eckelman et al. performed an LCA comparing 40 uses of a reusable Laryngeal Mask Airway (LMA) to 40 disposable LMAs. They found the reusable model to have fewer negative environmental effects in nearly all categories, typically contributing <50% of the impacts of single-use disposal models. The largest source of greenhouse gas (GHG) emissions for the single-use LMAs (23%) is the production and polymerization of polyvinyl chloride (PVC). SUD LMAs are primarily made of PVC, with diethylhexyl phthalate (DEHP) softener additives. The American Medical Association recently reaffirmed its commitment to encourage hospitals and health systems to reduce their use of PVC products, especially those containing DEHP, due to their toxic effects on developing fetuses and children. The majority (77%) of life cycle GHG emissions for the reusable LMA are due to steam autoclaving. Changes in the design and processing of both models can yield efficiencies—for reusables by optimizing loading of sterilization and for disposables by using alternative polymers.

There is no reported case of iatrogenic infection linked to a reusable SGA. Despite this, there appears to be a general perception that reusable SGAs have a safety profile inferior to that of SUD models. Patients who are highly infective may warrant the use of disposable devices; however, data do not support the broad adoption of disposables for all patients to mitigate the risk of infection.

Laryngoscopes: Some reusable laryngoscope handles require high-level disinfection (HLD) in their instructions for use. This can be achieved via in-house central sterilization and supply (CSS) processing; however, many institutions opt instead for SUD laryngoscopes. The life cycle GHG and financial impacts of various iterations of reusable and disposable laryngoscope assemblies were examined by Sherman et al. (Figure 15.1).

GHG impacts are readily influenced by laryngoscope handle material and processing practice. Significant benefits are seen from disinfecting reusable components between uses when compared to the GHG impacts created from disposing of single-use components after each use. Reusing steel components through CSS processing, as compared to SUD equivalents, were calculated to save between $675,000 and $869,000 per year at the U.S. study site, assuming 60,000 procedures per year. A similar study by Rouviere et al. (based on European data) identified savings in financial costs, GHGs, and raw mineral extraction requirements with reusable versus SUD laryngoscopes, affirming general findings.

Breathing circuits: In the United States, anesthesia breathing circuits are discarded after every use (and in some institutions, after any OR case, even if unused). In Europe and elsewhere, breathing circuits are routinely changed less frequently, ranging from once a day to once a week, except in select cases of known or presumed infectious patients. Microbial filters (usually combined with a heat and moisture exchanger) are placed in-between the circuit and the airway device, and discarded between patients. McGain et al. found that prolonging

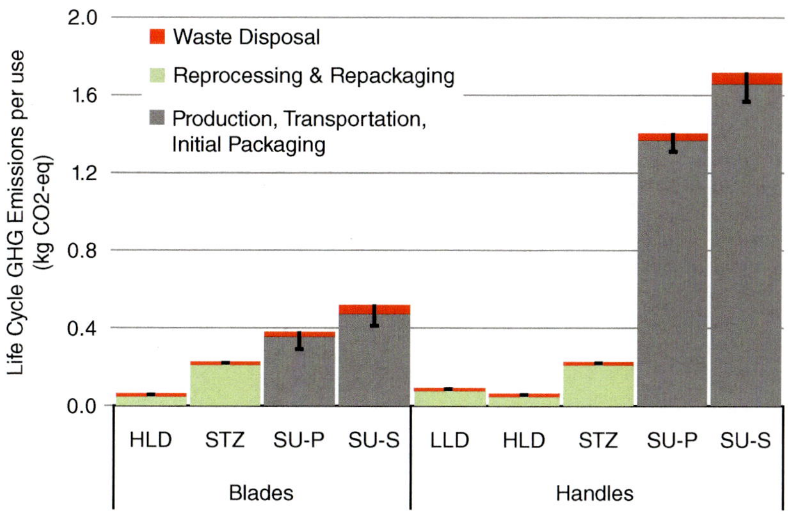

Figure 15.1. GWP impacts of single- and multiuse laryngoscopes. GHG, greenhouse gas; HLD, high-level disinfection; LLD, low-level disinfection; MU, multiuse (reusable); SUD, single-use disposable; STZ, sterilization. (Reprinted with permission from Sherman JD, Raibley LA IV, Eckelman MJ. Life cycle assessment and costing methods for device procurement: comparing reusable and single-use disposable laryngoscopes. *Anesth Analg.* 2018;127(2):434–443. Figure 2. Copyright © 2018 International Anesthesia Research Society.)

the interval between anesthesia breathing-circuit changes in this fashion results in financial, energy, and water savings, without any increase in significant microbial contamination rates. However, this simple change is hampered in the United States by institutional infection control policies that are out of keeping with other high-income systems.

Life cycle methodology can be incorporated into routine procurement committee value analytics. Facilities may discover in several instances that monies saved through choosing reusable alternatives justify hiring more cleaning staff, all while simultaneously reducing pollution and improving supply chain resilience.

- There is a paucity of evidence linking the transmission of infection to reusable airway devices.
- A device selection process should weigh environmental and public health impacts, in addition to traditional criteria.
- LCA and life cycle costing are modeling tools that quantify environmental impacts and costs of a product across the cradle to grave of manufacturing, use and reuse, through waste disposal management, to facilitate fair comparisons.
- *See Figure 15.2 and* ***Video 15.1*** *for additional detail.*

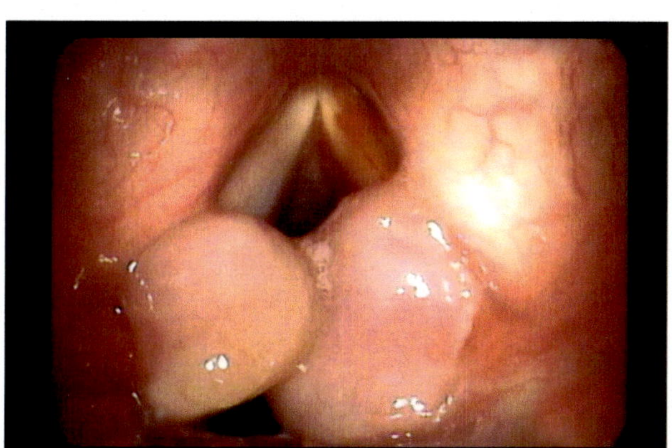

Figure 15.2. The components of a "single"-use laryngoscope.

Suggested Readings

Eckelman M, Mosher M, Gonzalez A, Sherman J. Comparative life cycle assessment of disposable and reusable laryngeal mask airways. *Anesth Analg.* 2012;114(5):1067–1072.

MacNeill A, Hopf H, Khanuja A, et al. A call for medical device industry transformation: toward a circular economy. *Health Affairs.* 2020;39(12):2071–2079.

McGain F, Algie CM, O'Toole J, et al. The microbiological and sustainability effects of washing anaesthesia breathing circuits less frequently. *Anaesthesia.* 2014;69(4):337–342.

Rouvière N, Chkair S, Auger F, Cuvillon P, Leguelinel-Blache G, Chasseigne V. Reusable laryngoscope blades: a more eco-responsible and cost-effective alternative. *Anaesth Crit Care Pain Med.* 2023;42(5):101276.

Sherman J, Gaal D. Materials management and pollution prevention. In: Frost E, ed. *Role of Anesthesiology in Global Health.* Springer; 2014:93–104.

Sherman J, Raibley L, Eckelman M. Life cycle assessment and costing methods for device procurement: comparing reusable and single-use disposable laryngoscopes. *Anesth Analg.* 2018;127(2):434–443.

Sherman J, Ryan S. Ecological responsibility in anesthesia practice. *Int Anesthesiol Clin.* 2010;48(3):139–151.

Nasal Intubation

16

Sonia Vaida

1 Describe in detail the device or technique.

Nasotracheal intubation may be required in several settings, including oral and maxillofacial surgery. A discussion with the surgical team should clarify the need for nasotracheal intubation, which can be performed in the awake or postinduction patient (see Chapter 1: Decision Making in the 2022 Difficult Airway Guidelines). Because nasotracheal intubation is associated with a unique set of concerns and complications, the rationale and consequences of choosing this route to secure the airway should be discussed with the patient preoperatively.

In addition to performing a routine airway assessment, physical and historical factors that may indicate difficult nasal access should be sought. A history of nasal pathology (eg, hereditary hemorrhagic telangiectasia, septum deviation, hypertrophy of turbinates, obstruction, chronic epistaxis, etc.), previous nasal surgery (eg, cleft nasal repair, pharyngoplasty, nasal septum repair, cosmetic reconstruction, etc.), and coagulopathies should be elicited. Facial trauma and concerns over incompetence of the bony nasal structures have long been considered an absolute contraindication to nasotracheal intubation. Examination of the nasal cavity using a flexible scope can help identify asymptomatic nasal obstruction and other anatomical defects.

With the goal of minimizing trauma to the mucosa, the nostrils are prepared for intubation with topical vasoconstrictors and lubricating gels. Both nostrils and nasal cavities should be prepared (if not contraindicated) to allow for a change in sides, should problems be encountered. Use of left-beveled tracheal tubes inserted via the right nostril can decrease the incidence and severity of epistaxis.

Topical vasoconstrictors help reduce epistaxis through vessel constriction and shrinking of the mucous membranes. Common agents include phenylephrine (0.25% to 1%) and oxymetazoline (0.05%) nasal drops. Phenylephrine, predominantly an $\alpha 1$-adrenergic agonist, can be systemically absorbed and cause hypertension, reflex bradycardia, and ventricular arrhythmias. Topical local anesthetics are used to reduce pain during awake nasotracheal intubation, and blunt intubation-induced hypertensive responses. Cocaine (4% to 10%) is often employed by otolaryngologists because of its analgesic and vasoconstricting actions. On the other hand, it has the disadvantage of stimulating the adrenergic receptors (by inhibiting the reuptake of norepinephrine) and causing increased cardiac contractility and hypertension. Dilation of the nostrils and nasal cavity can be achieved by inserting gradually increasing sizes of well-lubricated nasopharyngeal airways (eg, 30F to 36F). However, because both the medial and lateral walls of the nasal cavity are mechanically restricted by the nasal turbinates and septum, respectively, dilatation is limited and controversial, as it can increase the time for intubation and can cause trauma.

To diminish trauma, a smaller than otherwise recommended tracheal tube is chosen. The tracheal tube should be well coated with a water-soluble lubricant and thermosoftening of the tracheal tube (eg, by placing in warm water) should be considered. Overwarming can cause loss of the shape and integrity of the tracheal tube, and collapse of the tube lumen should be suspected if air-flow resistance or frank obstruction is encountered after intubation. An assortment of available tracheal tube designs has been suggested for use in nasotracheal intubation. The Ring–Adair–Elwin (RAE) tracheal tube has a preformed curve that positions the proximal circuit connector over the forehead and away from the surgical field. The RAE tube is also longer than the length of a standard oral ETT with the same diameter (Figure 16.1A). The Parker Flex-Tip tube (Figure 16.1B) has a soft, rounded, and flexible tapered tip designed to reduce trauma. The Endotrol (Figure 16.1C) has a wire lead connected to the distal tube tip through which the curve of the ETT can be exaggerated and the tip moved anteriorly.

The tracheal tube is inserted along the floor of the nose with the cuff completely deflated and lubricated. The vector of insertion should be perpendicular to the plane of the face, with the bevel facing laterally. The tube is advanced through the nose and nasopharynx into the oropharynx. Resistance to advancement is often encountered as the distal tracheal tube reaches the nasopharynx, and may not negotiate the turn into the oral pharynx. The following maneuvers can facilitate tracheal tube advancement: (1) gentle counterclockwise rotation of the tracheal tube; (2) tracheal tube withdrawal, head extension, and readvancement; and (3) changing to

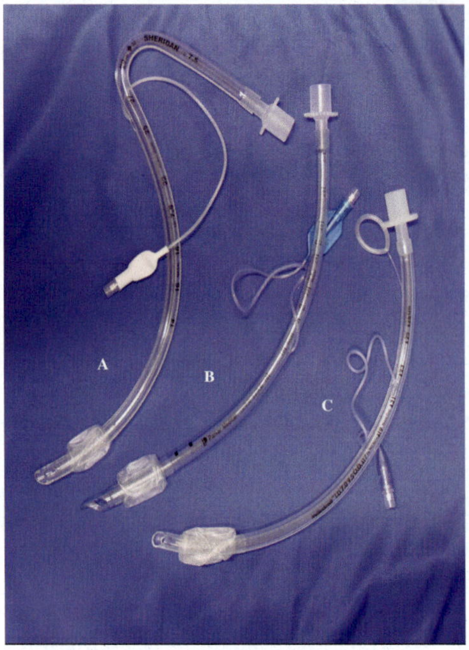

Figure 16.1. **A:** Nasal RAE. **B:** Parker Flex-Tip. **C:** Endotrol Tracheal Tubes.

a smaller-sized tracheal tube. Excessive insertion force can cause trauma and bleeding, and should be avoided during the procedure.

Once the tracheal tube reaches the oropharynx, its advancement into the larynx can be completed blindly or visually using direct or indirect laryngoscopy. Blind advancement is preferably performed with the patient breathing spontaneously in either an awake or anesthetic state. Tracheal tube placement may be guided by the breath sounds appreciated at the proximal tracheal tube and/or by external laryngeal palpation. Breath sounds intensify as the tracheal tube is passed into the glottis. Maneuvers that can help to align the tracheal tube with the glottis include jaw elevation to lift the epiglottis, neck flexion or rotation, and/or gentle tracheal tube rotation.

The tracheal tube can also be manipulated into the larynx under direct laryngoscopy, indirect laryngoscopy, video laryngoscopy, or by using fiberoptic guidance. Frequently, guidance with a Magill forceps is necessary, especially if the tracheal tube tip is located posterior to the glottic opening. Attention must be paid not to damage the tracheal tube cuff with the Magill forceps. Other maneuvers that can facilitate passage of the tracheal tube include inflating the cuff to elevate the tracheal tube bevel off the pharyngeal wall, advancing an intubating stylet through the tracheal tube, changes in head and neck position, or optimal external laryngeal manipulation.

2 Where or when is this device or technique used in airway management?

Nasotracheal intubation is indicated for the airway management of surgical procedures requiring unrestricted access to the oral cavity, oropharynx, the face, for intraoral pathology or cervical spine instability, and when there is limited mouth opening (trismus), or mandibular fracture. Surgical procedures which will end with surgical closure of the mouth (eg, malocclusion correction) will often also require nasotracheal intubation.

3 What distinguishes this device or technique from similar airway management methods?

The primary advantage of nasotracheal intubation is allowing an unobstructed oropharyngeal surgical field. An in situ nasotracheal tube is better tolerated by the awake patient than an orally inserted tube, and less cervical spine movement is needed during the intubation. Tracheal tube fixation is also easier. In addition, nasal placement avoids the potential for tracheal tube biting.

There are also several disadvantages to nasotracheal intubation. A smaller-sized ETT is used to avoid trauma, resulting in increased resistance to breathing and difficulty in suctioning. Epistaxis is a common complication.

Nasotracheal intubation is contraindicated in cases of suspected or confirmed skull base or facial bone fractures, or a defect in the bony skull (eg, previous transnasal transsphenoidal surgery), because of the risk of cranial vault penetration through the cribriform plate. Coagulopathy and anticoagulation therapy significantly increase the risk and severity of epistaxis. Pregnancy, hereditary hemorrhagic telangiectasia, and nasal obstruction are other common contraindications.

- Both nostrils should be prepared for intubation (if not contraindicated).
- Nasal intubation is contraindicated in cases of suspected or confirmed skull base or facial fractures.
- The most common complication of nasal intubation is epistaxis.
- *See Figure 16.2 and* ◉ ***Video 16.2*** *for additional detail.*

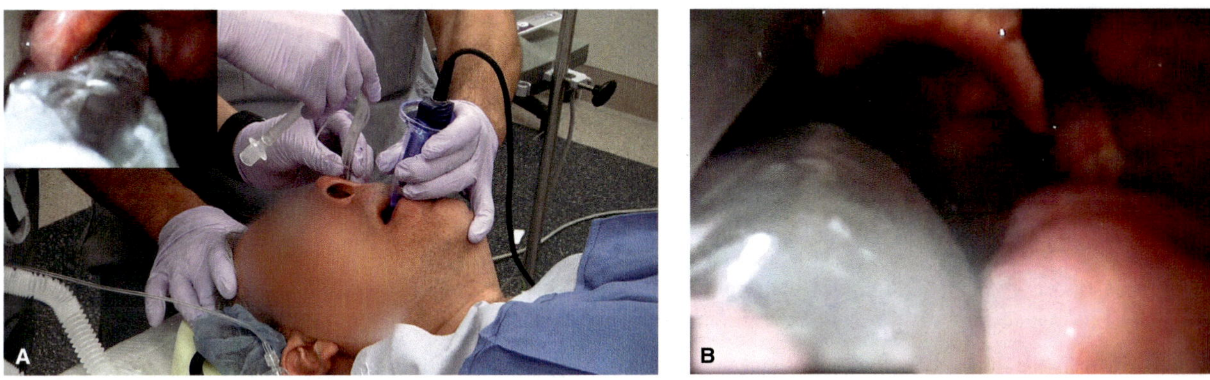

Figure 16.2. A, B: Nasotracheal intubation with use of a video laryngoscope. Rotation of the tracheal tube may be needed to move the bevel off of the cricoid cartilage.

Suggested Readings

Coe TR, Human M. The peri-operative complications of nasal intubation: a comparison of nostril side. *Anaesthesia*. 2001;56:447–450.

Hall CEJ, Shutt LE. Nasotracheal intubation for head and neck surgery. *Anaesthesia*. 2003;58:249–256.

Puchner W, Drabauer L, Kern K, et al. Indirect versus direct laryngoscopy for routine nasotracheal intubation. *J Clin Anesth*. 2011;23:280–285.

Tan YL, Wu ZH, Zhao BJ, Ni YH, Dong YC. For nasotracheal intubation, which nostril results in less epistaxis: right or left?: A systematic review and meta-analysis. *Eur J Anaesthesiol*. 2021;38:1180–1186.

Tong JL, Tung A. A randomized trial comparing the effect of fiberoptic selection and guidance versus random selection, blind insertion, and direct laryngoscopy, on the incidence and severity of epistaxis after nasotracheal intubation. *Anesth Analg*. 2018;127:485–489.

17 Optical Stylets

James C. DuCanto • Yen Chow

1 Describe in detail the device or technique.

Optical stylets are metal-reinforced, self-contained endoscopes that are placed within the lumen of the tracheal tube and serve as a guide for intubation. These devices are used as imaging guides at the distal end of the tracheal tube, in contrast to flexible endoscopes, which serve as a conduit for tracheal tube delivery after its placement into the airway. Most optical stylets have a standard 32-mm diameter eyepiece, which will accept an endoscopy camera head, and typically incorporate a self-contained light source or a fiberoptic light cord for use with an external light source (eg, Shikani and Levitan scopes, Clarus Medical, Minneapolis, MN; Bonfils Stylet, Karl Storz, El Segundo, CA). A commonly manufactured endoscope diameter is 5.0 mm, allowing the use of tracheal tubes as small as 5.5-mm internal diameter (ID). Pediatric-sized devices are also available.

Optical stylets may be used for tracheal tubes in a variety of ways:

1. Midline approach or retromolar approach
2. Alongside a conventional laryngoscope or a video laryngoscope, when an adequate view cannot be obtained with the primary device
3. Through an SGA of the laryngeal mask (LM) variety
4. Cricothyrotomy delivery device for a Melker 5.0-mm ID cricothyrotomy catheter
5. For inspection of the vocal cords and supra- and subglottic areas prior to extubation

Optical stylets are typically utilized in recognized difficult airway cases as a supplemental device for tracheal intubation alongside direct laryngoscopy or video laryngoscopy, or alternatively through an SGA. They may also be used in patients with normal airways, as their use can limit pharyngeal trauma and reduce the severity of sore throat as compared to direct laryngoscopy. The ability to have a view from the tip of the optical stylet allows one to navigate to the glottis without direct alignment of the airway axes. In the clinical scenario where ventilation has been established with an SGA of the LM variety, optical stylets have been used to facilitate intubation through this conduit. In an extreme emergency, an optical stylet can serve as a delivery device for a Melker 5.0-mm ID cricothyrotomy catheter. The rigid optical stylet allows one to confirm tracheal placement by either tactile detection or visualization of the tracheal rings as the stylet is advanced.

2 What distinguishes this device or technique from similar airway management methods?

The optical stylet is a modification of a tracheal tube intubating stylet to include imaging capability. It may be used alone or as an adjunct to a variety of other techniques that capable of creating adequate space in front of the larynx for endoscopic visualization. When employing conventional (or advanced) laryngoscopy, optical stylets add imaging from the point of view of the distal tracheal tube. Unlike flexible intubation scopes that serve as a mechanical guide for the tracheal tube, these devices serve as a visual guide and allow the intubation to be seen by the operator. Because they are rigid, the handling of these stylets is familiar to the traditional operator. As with all airway devices which incorporate optical elements, fluids in the airway have the potential to obscure visualization of the larynx.

Author Caveats

Proper device and patient preparation prevent a poor performance with optical stylet devices. Ample lubrication of the optical stylet eases the passage of the tracheal tube once the larynx is entered. On most devices, the proximal tracheal tube is mated with the optical stylet through an adjustable, 15-mm "tube stop," which can accommodate variable tracheal tube lengths. The tube stop position should be adjusted, so that the distal stylet is even with the midpoint of the tracheal tube's Murphy eye. With the Clarus Levitan optical stylet, a device with a fixed position tube stop, the tracheal tube position is adjusted with careful trimming of the length of the tracheal tube.

The optical stylet may be utilized alone or with the use of various aids to assist its transit to the larynx and trachea. Utilized alone, the optical stylet can be introduced in a midline approach with a firm jaw thrust to elevate the base of the tongue and epiglottis off of the posterior pharyngeal wall.

An optical stylet is often used as an adjunct to direct or video laryngoscopy. The optical stylet is introduced in the midline or by a retromolar approach with visual guidance of the stylet using the direct or video laryngoscope until the larynx is seen. It must be noted that the tip of the endoscope will magnify any adjustments made to the proximal end of the endoscope, so these movements must be slow and minor in magnitude.

As with other endoscopes, when anatomy cannot be recognized, slow withdrawal out of the airway is more helpful than continued advancement. Once anatomy is identified, the operator can once again steer toward the larynx.

When the larynx is identified, the tracheal tube–stylet combination is advanced between the vocal cords, and the tracheal tube is advanced off the stylet. If resistance to advancement occurs at this stage, the tracheal tube tip is lodging into the membranous space of the cricothyroid membrane, which is a natural consequence of the posterior–anterior course of the stylet. The optical stylet is slowly repositioned (with a caudad, forward tilt) to allow the tip of the tracheal tube and endoscope to align with the posterior-coursing direction of the trachea, and the tracheal tube is readvanced.

Recently, pairing of optical stylets with LM-type SGAs has been described. Two types of these airways, the LMA Classic Excel and the Air-Q, possess removable 15-mm connectors, which permit the passage of large lubricated tracheal tubes. The tracheal tube–optical stylet exits the SGAs at a position immediately posterior and superior to the laryngeal inlet. The specific technique to intubate the larynx involves an anterior lift and cephalad tilt of the stylet to advance the scope anteriorly and inferiorly into the larynx.

- Optical stylets are metal-reinforced, self-contained endoscopes that are often malleable to allow for a variety of shapes to guide tracheal intubation.
- Multiple intubating techniques are possible with these devices, as they can serve to deliver a tracheal airway tube as an adjunct to other devices.
- LM-type SGAs can serve as tracheal intubating conduits utilizing low-cost and durable fiberoptic endoscopes known as optical stylets.
- As an aid to creating a surgical airway, it is possible to utilize an optical stylet as a delivery device for a Melker 5.0-mm ID cricothyrotomy catheter.
- *See Figure 17.1 and* ***Video 17.1*** *for additional details.*

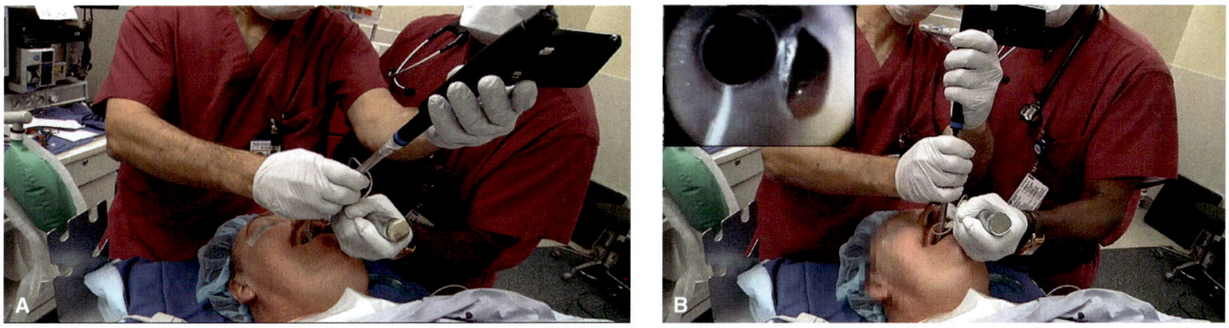

Figure 17.1. A, B: The Clarus video stylet being used combined with direct laryngoscopy.

Suggested Readings

Jagannathan N, Kho MF, Kozlowski RJ, Sohn LE, Siddiqui A, Wong DT. Retrospective audit of the air-Q intubating laryngeal airway as a conduit for tracheal intubation in pediatric patients with a difficult airway. *Paediatr Anaesth.* 2011;21(4):422–427.

Liem EB, Bjoraker DG, Graventstein D. New options for airway management: intubating fibreoptic stylets. *Br J Anaesth.* 2003; 91(3):408–418.

Paladino L, DuCanto J, Manoach S. Development of a rapid, safe, fiber-optic guided, single incision cricothyrotomy using a large ovine model: a pilot study. *Resuscitation.* 2009;80(9):1066–1069.

Setty H, Rawlings JL, Dubin S. Video RIFL: a rigid flexible laryngoscope to facilitate airway management. *J Clin Anesth.* 2010; 22(8):642–647.

18 Use of the Flexible Intubation Scope

P. Allan Klock Jr

1 Describe in detail the device or technique.

The flexible intubation scope (FIS) is a powerful tool for difficult airway management. Used properly, the scope has a high success rate even in patients with very challenging airways. FIS intubation has several attractive attributes:

- It can be used in all age groups.
- It can be used via an oral or nasal route.
- It can be used via a tracheostomy.
- It can be used when the patient is awake, sedated, or under general anesthesia.
- It can be used with controlled or spontaneous ventilation.
- The entire airway can be visualized.
- It can be used for diagnostic and therapeutic procedures.
- It can overcome intubation problems with the upper and lower airway.
- It works well in an anatomically distorted airway.
- Topical local anesthetics can be applied through the device when a working channel is present.
- Patient head and neck manipulation is often not necessary.
- The risk of dental damage and airway trauma is low.

The original FIS devices were fiberoptic bronchoscopes. These devices have an objective lens at the distal tip of an insertion cord, an eyepiece consisting of several lenses, and a coherent bundle of 10,000 to 30,000 glass fibers arranged to assemble an image at the eyepiece. The glass fibers produced a highly pixelated image, and the devices were expensive and fragile. Though the fiberoptic bronchoscope incorporated a light-carrying fiber bundle, a bulky external light source was often required.

The majority of FIS devices purchased currently are distal chip videoscopes that are either reusable or intended for single patient use. The reusable FIS is an expensive and relatively fragile device. Special equipment and trained personnel are needed to decontaminate, sterilize, and protect the FIS from damage. FIS devices should be stored with the insertion cord hanging vertically in a cabinet or protective tube to keep the cord from assuming a bent "memory shape" and to minimize the risk of damage. The ideal storage cart for a FIS contains a "locker" area that protects an unused clean scope from damage or contamination, a "ready" area where the scope is placed immediately before use, and a "soiled" area that both protects the scope from damage and prevents contamination of the cart. Some systems use protective single-use plastic tubes that travel with the FIS from cleaning to pre- and postpatient use, and back to the decontamination facility (Figure 18.1).

The basic parts of a FIS are the universal cord, which connects the scope to the light source and/or a video processor; the control section, also known as the handle; and the insertion cord, which contains the image transmission bundle, the light guide bundles, the working channel, and angulation wires to move the distal bending hinge of the scope in the sagittal plane. The working channel is used to suction secretions or blood, insufflate oxygen, administer local anesthetic or other drugs, and pass instruments such as biopsy forceps or a brush. Depending on the size of the scope, the diameter of the working channel may vary from 1.2 to 3.2 mm. Channels narrower than 2 mm usually do not suction well but are used to administer oxygen or local anesthetics.

One of the keys for successful FIS use is proper positioning of the airway manager, patient, and equipment. Ideally, the video display, if available, is positioned so that the operator is facing the patient when looking at the display. When using the FIS in a non-OR environment, patient–operator positioning should not be compromised (see Chapter 46: Out of the Operating Room Difficult Airway).

The insertion cord of the FIS is lubricated. Medical grade silicone spray, water-based surgical lubricant, or local anesthetic ointment may be used. The objective lens of the scope is warmed with sterile water or an antifog solution is applied to minimize fogging.

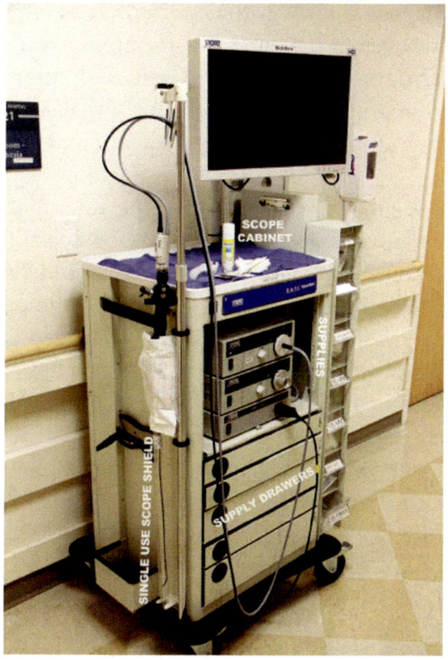

Figure 18.1. A dedicated flexible scope cart contains the electronics of the device as well as the required accessories. In many instances, the cart will double as the difficult intubation cart and contain many devices and accessories recommended by the American Society of Anesthesiologists, other societies and practice and personal preferences.

If the patient is supine, the table should be at a low position to allow the insertion cord to be as straight as possible. If the patient is sitting up, the operator should position himself or herself at the patient's side at a sufficient distance from the mouth to allow the insertion cord to be straight. If the insertion cord is not straight, rotation of the handle does not translate to the distal insertion cord. With gentle tension applied between the handle and the most distal part of the insertion cord, sufficient torsional rigidity improves FIS rotational control.

The intubation scope must be protected from biting. If an oral approach has been planned, a bite block or oral airway specifically designed for FIS intubation (eg, Ovassapian Airway, Teleflex Medical, Research Triangle Park, NC) may be inserted into the patient's mouth before introducing the scope. Compared to a bite block, intubating airway devices have the advantage of keeping the scope and tracheal tube in the midline, which improves the mechanics of the scope and aids passage of the tracheal tube through the vocal cords. These airways also create an imaging space in front of the FIS's objective lens.

The spontaneously breathing patient should receive supplemental oxygen via nasal cannula, face mask, or "blow-by" techniques while the airway is instrumented with a flexible scope. The patient's mouth is suctioned before scope insertion. Suctioning removes blood or secretions and confirms the absence of airway reflexes. Intubation of the awake patient is discussed in Chapter 11: Preparation for Awake Intubation.

If a nasal approach will be used, it may be helpful to use warm water to soften the tracheal tube. The tracheal tube should be lubricated and gently advanced into the patient's nose that has been appropriately prepared with a vasoconstrictor (eg, oxymetazoline or phenylephrine) and topical local anesthetics. When using a transnasal approach, it is important that the tube be advanced into the posterior nasopharynx or oropharynx before attempting to pass the scope through the vocal cords. This avoids the frustrating situation when the operator has successfully passed the scope through the vocal cords only to find that it is difficult or impossible to pass the tracheal tube through the nose.

There are three degrees of freedom under an operator's control during FIS intubation: depth of insertion, handle and insertion-cord rotation, and angulation of the distal-hinged segment. These variables interact in a complex manner that makes intubation with the FIS nonintuitive. Significant practice is often required before the user achieves sufficient skill. The FIS should be used regularly to maintain a high skill level.

One fundamental difference between intubation with a FIS and intubation with a bladed device (eg, direct or video laryngoscopy) is that the FIS does not create an open channel; rather, the scope is designed to navigate an already patent airway. If the patient is awake or sedated with a patent airway, the operator steers the scope through the open pharynx, hypopharynx, larynx, and proximal trachea. If the patient is anesthetized or deeply sedated, maneuvers to open the airway may be necessary, including positioning the patient with atlantoaxial extension, pulling the tongue out of the patient's mouth, or applying jaw thrust or anterior translation of the temporomandibular joint. For this reason, it is helpful to have high-quality assistance when attempting a flexible scope intubation in a patient under general anesthesia.

When initiating intubation, the FIS is inserted slowly and deliberately to identify the intended target through which the scope will pass. The control lever moves the hinged distal segment up or down in only one plane. The entire insertion cord and control section (ie, "handle") of the scope must be rotated in concert for the hinged distal segment to move in the desired direction. When viewing a video monitor, the operator must rotate the scope to bring the target in line with the vertical midline of the video image. Stated another way, when the target is identified, the scope handle and insertion cord must be rotated together to bring the target along the 12 o'clock to 6 o'clock axis. When the target is on this line, the control lever is moved to bring the target to the middle of the screen before the scope is slowly advanced into the airway. Adjustments are made to the scope via rotation and lever angulation to keep the target in the middle of the video display. When the vocal cords are identified, the operator aims for the anterior commissure of the cords. When the objective lens of the FIS is within 2 to 3 mm of the commissure, the tip of the scope is directed posteriorly, to bring it in line with the axis of the larynx. The scope is then advanced 5 to 7 cm into the trachea before the tracheal tube is advanced over the insertion cord and into position.

2 Where and when is this device or technique used in airway management?

FIS devices are used for elective or urgent situations to facilitate tracheal intubation. The American Society of Anesthesiologists Practice Guidelines for Management of the Difficult Airway does not include flexible scope intubation in the emergency pathway, also known as the "cannot-ventilate, cannot-intubate" scenario. Flexible scopes do not assist with lung ventilation. They are used to diagnose problems in the upper and lower airway and to assist the delivery of an endotracheal tube into the trachea.

3 What distinguishes this device or technique from similar airway management methods?

- A FIS device can steer around obstructions in an anatomically distorted airway. The scope causes minimal trauma to a tumor or friable tissues in the airway.
- Intubation with a FIS requires minimal force and is well suited for securing the airway in an awake or sedated patient whose airway is anesthetized with topical local anesthetics.
- Intubating the trachea while the patient is breathing spontaneously and maintaining airway patency is often the safest and most reliable way to care for a patient who is predicted to be difficult to intubate or ventilate with a face mask (see Chapter 11: Preparation for Awake Intubation).

Author Caveats

The FIS, although a powerful tool, has limitations. Because the device is flexible, gravity will pull it to the most dependent parts of the airway. Unfortunately, this is where blood, secretions, or, potentially, stomach contents will accumulate. The lens of the device is easily soiled, making it imperative that the airway be as dry as possible. Properly anesthetizing the airway requires some level of patient cooperation and may not be possible in all patients.

- FIS is uniquely useful tool for difficult airway management.
- FIS manipulation is nonintuitive and requires practice to achieve and maintain a high skill level.
- The FIS is expensive and fragile. Protocols must be developed to properly decontaminate and protect them.
- *See Figures 18.2 and 18.3 for additional details.*

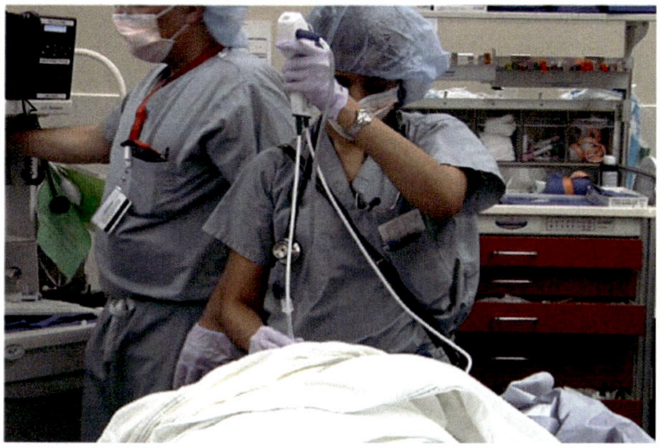

Figure 18.2. The flexible intubation scope is held in the dominant hand while keeping the insertion cord straight within the limitations of the patient's anatomy. *See* **_Video 18.1_** *for additional details.*

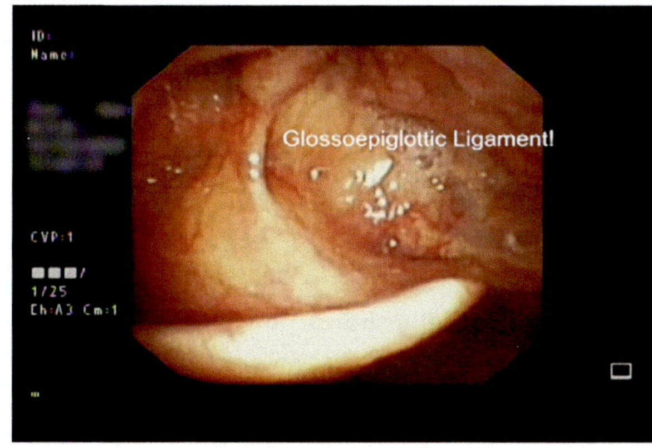

Figure 18.3. The flexible scope operator should endeavor to identify anatomic locations during the exam to ensure orientation. *See* **_Video 18.2_** *for additional details.*

Suggested Reading

Apfelbaum JL, Hagberg CA, Connis RT, et al. 2022 American Society of Anesthesiologists practice guidelines for management of the difficult airway. *Anesthesiology*. 2022;136(1):31–81.

19 Pitfalls in the Use of the Flexible Intubation Scope

P. Allan Klock Jr

1 Describe in detail the device or technique.

The flexible intubation scope (FIS) is a powerful tool for securing the airway of patients who present with a variety of challenging conditions. Despite this, a number of obstacles may hinder its effectiveness. This chapter discusses the most common of these situations and specific strategies to overcome them.

Skills in FIS use involve the complex mastery of hand–eye coordination and interpretation of a unique view of patient anatomy. Possibly more than any other airway management technique, training, and ongoing practice are needed to maintain mastery. Many expert airway managers incorporate the FIS into their routine practice as a means of maintaining a high skill level. A variety of practice mannequins, task trainers, cadaver preparations, and virtual-reality simulators are also available. Although simulation training is helpful, experts in the field agree that practice on live patients is uniquely instructive—recognition of altered anatomy, managing tissue movement, and bypassing obscuring secretions or blood are best learned in real patients.

The FIS is the most common instrument used in awake intubation. Keeping the patient cooperative, comfortable, and cough and gag reflex free are vital to success. These are discussed in Chapter 11: Preparation for Awake Intubation.

Fogging of the objective lens is a common problem during FIS intubation. When a room-temperature FIS is inserted into an airway containing warm, water vapor–saturated air, condensation will often occur. This problem can be overcome in one of two ways: (1) by applying chemical antifog agents to the lens immediately before use or (2) by gently warming the lens in water or saline. Both medical-grade antifog agents and warmed solutions are ubiquitous in the modern operating suite. Very hot liquids should not be used for this purpose to minimize the risk of patient injury and damage to the scope. The use of suction or insufflated oxygen via the scope's working channel can also be used to remove condensation. Lastly, touching the objective lens on the mucosa is often effective in defogging the lens, but may otherwise soil the lens.

Secretions in the airway may affect the ability to visualize structures, especially as the distal tip of the FIS will tend to seek a gravity-dependent position along with blood and saliva. In addition, if the FIS is being used in an awake patient, secretions will hinder the action of topically applied local anesthetics. An antisialogogue (eg, glycopyrrolate 0.2 mg) can be administered intramuscularly or intravenously 15 minutes before the application of topical anesthetics or intubation attempts. If this is inadequate, the airway can be dried by wrapping a gauze sponge around a tongue depressor and mechanically drying the mouth. Before inserting the FIS into the airway, a Yankauer suction device can be used to remove secretions or blood. If fluid or blood continues to collect in the airway, the Yankauer device can be left in the posterior pharynx lateral to the midline. This position serves the dual purpose of keeping the airway dry and creating a small channel for the fiberscope.

Unlike video laryngoscopes, the FIS has no mechanism to create a space in front of the objective lens or distal camera chip. An air space is required for the creation of an image; otherwise, only a pink or white field is seen as tissues collapse around the lens. A variety of maneuvers can facilitate this. Often, a simple chin lift or jaw-thrust maneuver translates the temporomandibular joint and lifts the anterior soft-tissue structures, creating an adequate space. Oral airways specifically designed for FIS-aided intubation, can be placed (eg, the Ovassapian airway from Teleflex Medical Research Triangle Park, NC). Moving the tongue anteriorly via gentle traction creates space in the posterior pharynx. Suction tubing can be applied to the tip of the tongue to remove it from the oropharynx. The tongue is then wrapped with gauze before firm but gentle traction is applied to hold it outside the mouth (Figure 19.1). The suction tubing should not touch the tongue for a prolonged time in order to minimize the risk of a blood blister or bruise.

An awake, spontaneously breathing patient can be asked to take a deep breath. With a deep inspiration, the patient will create a channel that can be navigated. The vocal cords will abduct and the operator may be able to see bubbles that indicate flowing air.

If the above conventional maneuvers fail, combination techniques using an supraglottic airway (SGA), laryngoscope, video laryngoscope, or retrograde wire have been described. The use of combination techniques is supported by the 2022 American Society of Anesthesiologists Practice Guidelines for Management of the Difficult Airway when difficulty is encountered with an individual technique.

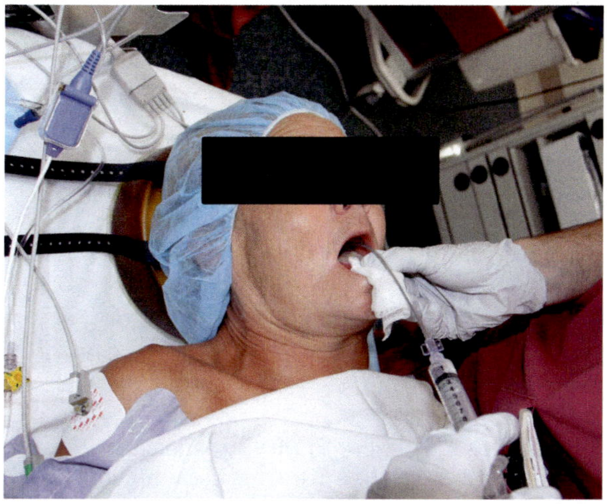

Figure 19.1. A gauze pad is carefully wrapped around the patient's tongue to facilitate topical anesthetic application. Not only does this maneuver help the clinician to expose the targeted anatomy, it will also prevent the patient from swallowing the local anesthetic when the laryngeal-tracheal analgesia is the intended goal.

An SGA designed to facilitate tracheal intubation (i-SGA), may be placed when the patient either has excellent topical anesthesia of the airway (in an awake intubation case) or is under general anesthesia. The i-SGA offers three distinct advantages: (1) it is a conduit to assist ventilation and oxygenation; (2) it opens the airway and creates a clear passage to the vocal cords; and (3) it creates a barrier that blocks oral secretions or blood (eg, from the bleeding nose or a tonsil bed) that would soil the airway and contaminate the scope's lens.

In 2001, Ferson et al. reported a series of 257 airway encounters in patients with difficult-to-manage airways. The focus of the study was the utility of the Fastrach laryngeal mask airway (LMA). One of the findings of the study was a 100% success rate in using a fiberscope through the Fastrach LMA (57 of 57 attempts), including seven patients in whom multiple attempts at blind intubation through the Fastrach LMA alone were unsuccessful.

A direct laryngoscope or video laryngoscope blade placed into the patient's mouth can be used to elevate the anterior airway structures, creating a channel for the FIS. This laryngoscopy-facilitated flexible scope intubation requires two skilled operators working in unison and does not assist with patient oxygenation or eliminate excessive secretions or blood. However, the screen of the videoscope can be used to guide the flexible scope operator when the flexible scope lens is soiled. A randomized clinical trial published in 2019 showed that the combination of FIS and video laryngoscope was more effective, faster, and caused less injury than using the video laryngoscope with a rigid stylet.

Last, the operator can deploy a wire from a retrograde intubation kit (Cook Medical, Bloomington, IN) through the cricothyroid membrane and out the mouth. The diameter of the wire in this kit is 0.038 inches (0.965 mm), which fits through the working channel of most intubating fiberscopes. The wire's 110-cm length allows it to be threaded into the working channel at the tip of the scope and out through the suction port in the handle. The scope (preloaded with an ETT) is then advanced over the wire, and into the airway. When the objective end of the FIS has passed through the vocal cords and the wire can be visualized entering the cricothyroid membrane, the wire is withdrawn, and the scope is inserted 4 to 6 cm before the ETT is advanced into the trachea.

- Practice and regular use are required to achieve and maintain proficiency with FIS.
- A key to success with an FIS for the awake, sedated, or general anesthesia patient is good airway preparation.
- Use of combination techniques to create an image space should be considered in all cases.
- *See Figure 19.2 and* ***Video 19.1*** *for additional details.*

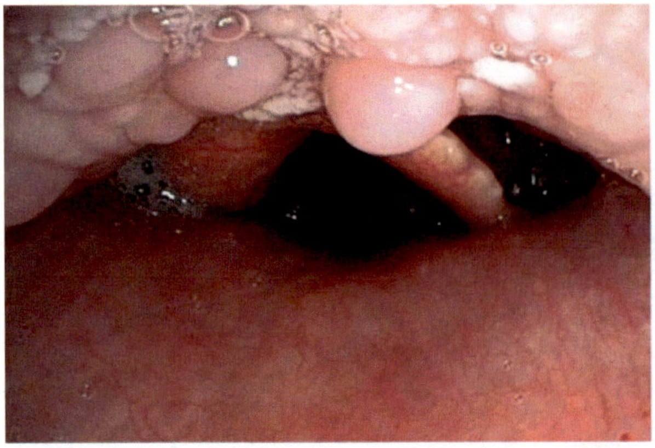

Figure 19.2. A variety of anatomic and pathologic structures may interfere with laryngoscopy. In general, the flexible scope is more capable of atraumatically moving past these structures as compared to rigid devices.

Suggested Readings

Apfelbaum JL, Hagberg CA, Connis RT, et al. 2022 American Society of Anesthesiologists practice guidelines for management of the difficult airway. *Anesthesiology*. 2022;136(1):31–81.

Ferson DZ, Rosenblatt WH, Johansen MJ, Osborn I, Ovassapian A. Use of the intubating LMA-Fastrach in 254 patients with difficult-to-manage airways. *Anesthesiology*. 2001;95:1175–1181.

Mazzinari G, Rovira L, Henao L, et al. Effect of dynamic versus stylet-guided intubation on first-attempt success in difficult airways undergoing glidescope laryngoscopy: a randomized controlled trial. *Anesth Analg*. 2019;128(6):1264–1271.

Hang-Up During Intubation with the FIS

20

P. Allan Klock Jr

Clinical Scenario: A patient with a known difficult airway is intubated with a flexible intubation scope (FIS) using an awake technique. The initial intubation attempts are complicated by patient discomfort and bleeding. On the third attempt, the FIS is passed into the larynx and the carina is visualized. A pre-threaded tracheal tube (TT) is advanced into the airway over the FIS. After passing the TT to 12 cm at the teeth, it will advance no further.

1 What are the anesthetic and airway management considerations for this case?

When the tracheal tube (TT) cannot be advanced into the larynx over a properly positioned FIS, the problem is referred to as a tube "hang-up." This is a particularly vexing problem for those managing the airway, and it commonly occurs during (50% to 67% of the time) FIS intubation attempts where a conventional TT is advanced over a 4-mm FIS. See figure 20.1 for an example of a TT hang-up.

The problem of TT hang-up is more likely to occur as the discrepancy increases between the external diameter of the FIS and the internal diameter of the TT. Initially, tube hang-up was attributed either to the arytenoids, interarytenoid muscle, vocal cords, or the tip of the epiglottis being entrapped in the cleft created between the two devices. However, a prospective observational study published in 2005 revealed that among tube hang-up events, which occurred in 24 of 45 (53%) study patients, impact with the right arytenoid was responsible in 19 of the 24 obstructions. Interarytenoid soft tissue entrapment occurred in the remaining 5 hang-ups. The epiglottis or vocal cords were not the cause of any hang-ups in this study.

2 How would you manage the airway in this case?

It is important that the intubating provider resists the urge to simply "push harder" on a TT that appears to be hung-up. Applying excessive force can lead to patient injury or push the FIS from the trachea into the esophagus. It is risky to induce general anesthesia in a patient with a difficult airway if tube hang-up is encountered during attempts at awake FIS intubation. Resolving the hang-up is more safely managed with the patient breathing spontaneously.

Knowing that the most common cause of TT hang-up is the impact of the bevel of the TT on the right arytenoid or interarytenoid space, hang-up can be overcome by withdrawing the tube 1 to 2 cm and rotating it 90 degrees counterclockwise (CCW) before reinsertion. This rotation brings the tip of the TT bevel from the 3 o'clock to the 12 o'clock position. With the tip of the TT in the midline with the bevel facing posteriorly, the leading part of the TT is aligned with the glottic opening. The tube is then gently readvanced over the FIS and into the trachea. The operator can also ask the patient to take a deep breath, which will abduct the vocal cords and make the glottic opening larger. If the TT does not advance after the initial 90 degrees CCW rotation, the TT can be withdrawn slightly and rotated CCW approximately 20 degrees to 45 degrees further (total rotation 110 degrees to 135 degrees) before reinsertion. The process of withdraw–rotate–reinsert can be repeated until the TT passes into the larynx.

Traditional polyvinylchloride (PVC) TTs have torsional laxity, which means that rotation at the proximal (near the breathing circuit attachment) end of the tube is not reliably transmitted to the distal tip of the TT. Repeated rotation and gentle reinsertion, referred to as "corkscrewing," may be especially helpful during intubation of patients with abnormal airway anatomy. If repeated attempts are unsuccessful, the flexible scope should be removed and alternative airway equipment should be used. Alternative options include minimizing the discrepancy between the outer diameter of the FIS and the inner diameter of the TT by placing a smaller TT over the flexible scope or using a FIS with a larger diameter. In addition, it may be helpful to use a second device to visualize the cause of the problem. A second FIS can be inserted via the nose or to the right of the primary FIS. A video laryngoscope can also be used for supraglottic visualization with the additional benefit of minimizing the curvature that the primary FIS needs to navigate. Using two modalities for airway management is known as a hybrid technique and is recommended in the ASA difficult airway algorithm in certain scenarios.

Prewarming a standard TT softens the plastic and can facilitate passage into the larynx. The softer TT will conform to the shape of the FIS, whereas a more rigid TT will deflect the scope from its original position. A softer tube will have less torsional rigidity, however, and may need to have more rotational displacement applied to the proximal end in order to affect proper CCW rotation of the bevel.

The anesthesia provider should always attempt to use the largest appropriate FIS available during initial attempts. A larger FIS reduces the diameter discrepancy between the scope and the TT tube. In addition, a FIS with a larger diameter provides better image quality and more rigidity. These characteristics of a larger FIS improve the probability of the TT passing into the larynx on initial attempts. Alternatively, if a larger-diameter FIS is not available, a smaller TT that minimizes the gap with the FIS should be considered. There are TTs that are specially designed to prevent TT hang-up, which are described further below.

3 What distinct airway device might be used in this case, and what are the special considerations?

Three particular TTs have been shown to reduce the incidence of tube hang-up during intubation with a flexible scope. The Parker Flex-Tip tube (Parker Medical, Highlands Ranch, CO) has a specially designed bevel that reduces the gap between the tube tip and the scope. One study showed this tube reduced the need for tube manipulation during intubation from 89% to 29%. Spiral wire-reinforced TTs have been shown to pass more easily into the larynx than conventional tubes. It has been suggested that the angle of the bevel and the softness of these tubes reduce the risk of hang-up. The TT designed for use with the Fastrach LMA (Teleflex, San Diego, CA) has a soft silicone tip with a medialized bevel that hugs the FIS as it is advanced into the airway. These TTs have also been shown to pass into the larynx more easily than wire-reinforced TTs.

- TT hang-up is a common problem that can be overcome by using appropriate tools and techniques.
- Use of the largest-diameter FIS available with the smallest TT (appropriate for the patient and surgical procedure) will minimize this problem.
- Using TTs with specially designed bevels further reduces the likelihood of tube hang-up.
- If tube hang-up is encountered in a patient who is breathing spontaneously, induction of general anesthesia should be avoided until after the trachea has been intubated.
- *See Figure 20.1 and* ***Video 20.1.***

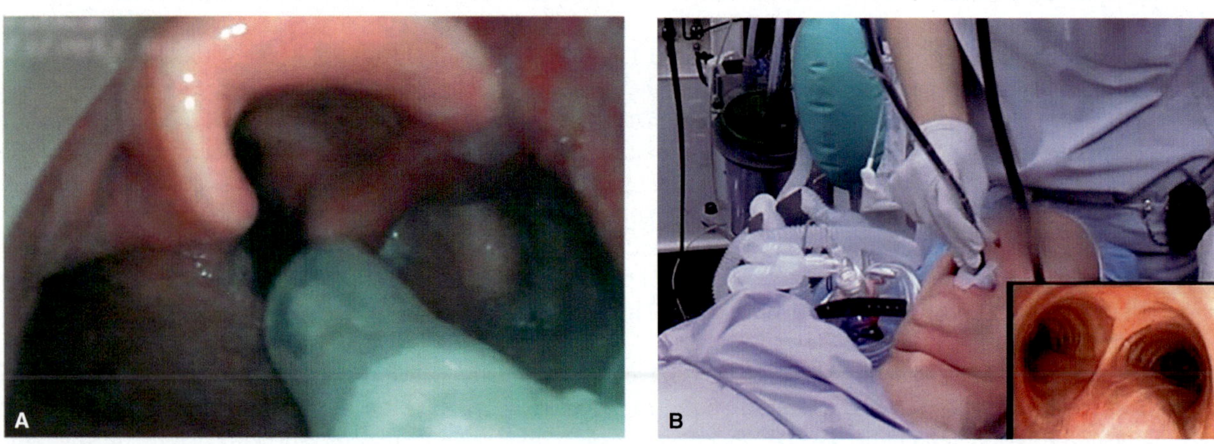

Figure 20.1. **A:** The cleft between the bevel of a tracheal tube (TT) and a flexible intubation scope is poised to entrap the right arytenoid complex, thwarting successful advancement into the larynx. **B:** Advancing the TT through the vocal cords and imaging the carina does not guarantee the TT will also freely pass to the same position due to hang-up. Planning FIS outer diameter and TT inner diameter concordance is required to smooth this transition.

Suggested Readings

Apfelbaum JL, Hagberg CA, Connis RT, et al. 2022 American Society of Anesthesiologists practice guidelines for management of the difficult airway. *Anesthesiology*. 2022;136:31–81.

Brull SJ, Wiklund R, Ferris C, Connelly NR, Ehrenwerth J, Silverman DG. Facilitation of fiberoptic orotracheal intubation with a flexible tracheal tube. *Anesth Analg*. 1996;78:746–748.

Johnson DM, From AM, Smith RB, From RP, Maktabi MA. Endoscopic study of mechanisms of failure of endotracheal tube advancement into the trachea during awake fiberoptic orotracheal intubation. *Anesthesiology*. 2005;102:910–914.

Kristensen MS. The Parker Flex-Tip tube versus a standard tube for fiberoptic orotracheal intubation: a randomized double blind study. *Anesthesiology*. 2003;98:354–358.

Maktabi MA, Hoffman H, Funk G, From RP. Laryngeal trauma during awake fiberoptic intubation. *Anesth Analg*. 2002;95:1112–1114.

21 Combined FIS and Video Laryngoscopy

Rainer Lenhardt

Clinical Scenario: A 45-year-old obese man presents for elective intra-abdominal surgery. He is noted to have an overbite and small oral aperture. After the induction of anesthesia, mask ventilation is easily accomplished, but attempts at direct and video laryngoscopy (VL) achieve no better than a Cormack and Lehane grade 3 view of the airway. A flexible intubation scope (FIS) is used by one operator, while another performs VL, which results in successful tracheal intubation.

1 What are the anesthetic and airway management considerations for this case?

In patients with a predicted or known difficult airway, the use of VL drastically improves the visualization compared with direct laryngoscopy. However, the anesthesia provider is occasionally unable to visualize the glottic opening using VL, resulting in a Cormack and Lehane grade 3 or 4 view of the airway.

A FIS may allow indirect visualization of the airway and can be used as a guide for insertion of an ETT in situations where a rigid device may fail. However, the use of a FIS for the purpose of tracheal intubation may be difficult without an adjunct device to assure an airspace proximal to the laryngeal opening. Combining the use of a FIS with a video laryngoscope may improve the success rate for intubation in some patients with predicted or unanticipated difficult airways.

2 How would you manage the airway in this case?

Different airway devices or a combination of devices can be used to manage the airway in the patient in the clinical scenario (Figure 21.1 and **Video 21.1**). Reusable or disposable video laryngoscope blades are available. Alternatively, a channeled scope (eg, Airtraq, Pentax Airway Scope) might be used to create a space for visualization. A patient with an overbite and narrow mouth opening should prompt the anesthesia provider to consider a combined device technique.

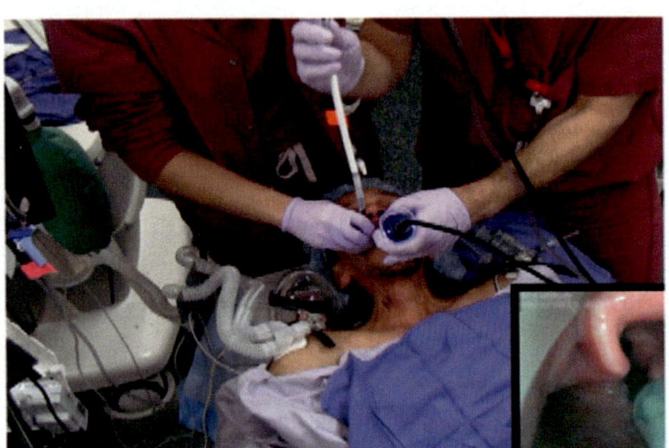

Figure 21.1. A patient with a difficult airway is being intubated with a flexible intubation scope while the video laryngoscope is used to create an image space and visualize the larynx.

During this combined intubation technique, a tracheal tube (TT) is loaded onto a FIS. A video laryngoscope is used to displace the tongue and pharyngeal tissues to create an airspace. The FIS, handled by a second operator, is then inserted through the mouth or nose. The course of the FIS can be observed on the video laryngoscope monitor as it is advanced toward the epiglottis. It is then directed beneath the epiglottis. The operator of the FIS then turns their attention to the FIS monitor or eyepiece. The operator drives the FIS through the glottis into the trachea and advances the FIS to the carina. The TT is advanced through the mouth and visualized on the video laryngoscope monitor. The tube is gently threaded past the vocal cords and into the larynx and trachea. Hang-up, which occurs in up to 10% of FIS intubations, can be mitigated by visual guidance using the video laryngoscope monitor and may be a distinct advantage of the combined technique. Once the distal TT reaches the midtrachea, its position is confirmed by visualization on the FIS monitor. In cases where distal TT position is critical, or there is likely to be movement of the TT with body positioning, the distance from the carina to TT bevel can be measured and adjusted as needed.

3 What distinct airway device might be used in this case, and what are the special considerations?

There are two common varieties of indirect laryngoscopes available: video laryngoscopes and channeled scopes. Use of the video laryngoscope combined with FIS is described above. Channeled scopes are characterized by a near 90-degree oral-to-pharyngeal blade angle with a right-lateral channel which holds a TT. The operator preloads the TT into the channel. When using a channeled device alone, the degree of freedom to maneuver the tube is greatly reduced. Therefore, the use of the FIS may be critical for rescuing tracheal intubation—the FIS can be used to complete the course from the channel scope to the larynx when difficulty with channel–tracheal alignment occurs.

Because the combined technique may be used in patients with difficult airways, it is important that the image quality and maneuverability of the FIS are optimal. Modern reusable bronchoscopes, as well as the latest generation of disposable FIS, typically fit these characteristics.

Although patient size should generally guide TT size, there are special considerations when using a FIS technique for intubation. Discrepancies between the inner diameter of the TT and the outer diameter of the FIS can lead to entrapment of tissues between the two.

An important consideration for combined video laryngoscope–FIS intubation is the requirement for a second operator. One operator inserts, positions, and stabilizes the video laryngoscope, while the other manipulates the FIS and inserts the TT. The second operator is not required to have advanced airway skills. An advanced airway manager can initially insert a video laryngoscope and establish its position. The video laryngoscope can then be handed off to a second operator (eg, nurse, respiratory therapist, etc.). The trained airway manager is then available to manipulate the FIS and insert the TT—actions that require more skill.

4 Are there special considerations for the emergence or the end of the case?

The patient who required advanced airway techniques for intubation should be considered high risk for airway failure at the time of emergence. The patient could fail extubation for reasons unrelated to the initial airway management (eg, residual muscle relaxation, fluid overload). Multiple attempts at laryngoscopy and tracheal intubation may render the upper airway injured, incompetent, or otherwise unable to compensate for minor alterations in physiology (eg, atelectasis). Reintubation, if necessary, is likely to be more difficult than the initial effort. Extubation precautions (full neuromuscular block reversal, fully awake emergence, use of an airway exchange catheter, etc.) should be practiced, and preparations for emergent reintubation should be made.

- Combining FIS with a video laryngoscope may improve the success rate during difficult intubations.
- Combining the use of a video laryngoscope with a FIS mitigates the risk of facing a prolonged apnea phase by minimizing intubation failure in the predicted difficult airway.
- Two providers are required to successfully perform this combined method for intubation.
- *See Figures 21.2 and 21.3 for additional details.*

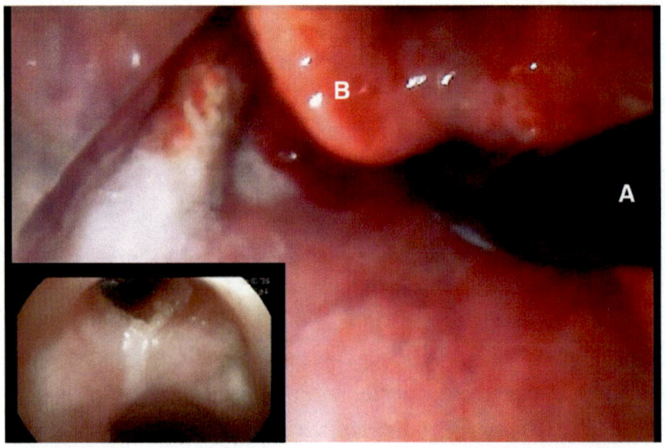

Figure 21.2. In a patient treated with radiation therapy, a flexible intubation scope (**A**) has been guided beneath the epiglottis (**B**) and a view of a tracheoesophageal fistula is obtained (*inset*). *See* **Video 21.2** *for additional details.*

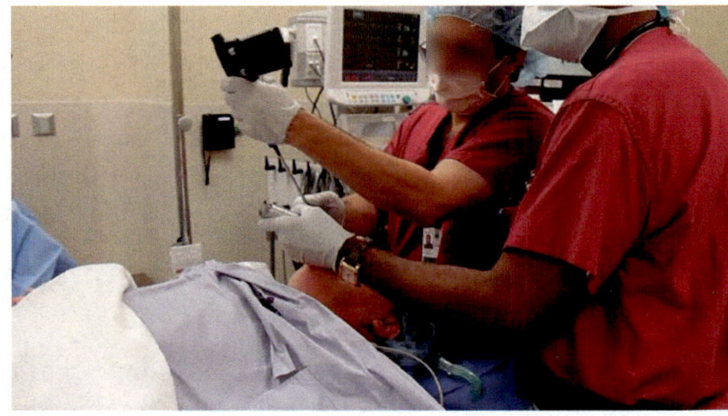

Figure 21.3. A Clarus Video-System is used in a combined technique with direct laryngoscopy. *See* **Video 21.2** *for additional details.*

Suggested Readings

Aziz MF, Dillman D, Fu R, Brambrink AM. Comparative effectiveness of the C-MAC video laryngoscope versus direct laryngoscopy in the setting of the predicted difficult airway. *Anesthesiology*. 2012;116:629–636.

Griesdale DEG, Liu D, McKinney J, Choi PT. Glidescope video-laryngoscopy versus direct laryngoscopy for endotracheal intubation: a systematic review and meta-analysis. *Can J Anaesth*. 2012;59:41–52.

Kim SM, Kim HJ. Successful advancement of endo- tracheal tube with combined fiberoptic bronchoscopy and video laryngoscopy in a patient with a huge goiter. *SAGE Open Med Case Rep*. 2020;8:2050313X20923232.

Lenhardt R, Burkhart MT, Brock GN, Kanchi-Kandadai S, Sharma R, Akça O. Is video laryngoscope-assisted flexible tracheoscope intubation feasible for patients with predicted difficult airway? A prospective, randomized clinical trial. *Anesth Analg*. 2014;118:1259–1265.

Mazzinari G, Rovira L, Henao L, et al. Effect of dynamic *versus* stylet-guided intubation on first-attempt success in difficult airways undergoing Glidescope laryngoscopy: A randomized controlled trial. *Anesth Analg*. 2019;128:1264–1271.

Optically Aided Intubation via an Intubating Supraglottic Airway

22

Lorraine J. Foley

Clinical Scenario: A 35-year-old woman presents with a history of difficult tracheal intubation. On physical examination, she has a short thyromental distance and a Mallampati III oropharyngeal score. She is overweight (body mass index of 29) and does not snore nor suffer from reflux.

1 What are the anesthetic and airway management considerations for this case?

What is unknown about this patient is the ability of past providers to manage her airway with face mask ventilation. Though awake intubation might be chosen for her management path, the use of intubating supralaryngeal airways could also be considered (see Chapter 1: Decision Making in the 2022 Difficult Airway Guidelines).

There are four commonly available intubating supraglottic airway (i-SGA) devices: the LMA-Fastrach (LMA North America, a Teleflex Company) consists of a mask attached to a rigid curved barrel with a handle. Within the mask is an epiglottic lifting bar. The Air-Q or Intubating Laryngeal Airway (Cook Gas, Saint Louis, MO) has a pliable, curved airway tube with a detachable proximal 15-mm connector and a laryngeal mask, but no epiglottic lifting bar. The Ambu Aura-I (Ambu, Glen Burnie, MD) also has a pliable, curved airway tube and mask, like Air-Q, but without the removable circuit connector. The Igel (Intersurgical Inc.) is wide-bore airway conduit with a soft noninflatable cuff designed to mirror the anatomy adjacent to the laryngeal inlet. Its barrel is less pliable than the Air-Q and Aura-I devices.

Success rates of blind intubation through these i-SGAs have been studied. The LMA-Fastrach intubation success rate after a second attempt was 89.5%, with an overall success rate of 96.5% after the fifth attempt in patients with airways difficult to manage. Comparison of blind tracheal intubation through the LMA-Fastrach and Air-Q showed success rates of 99% and 77%, respectively, after two attempts. Comparison of the Igel and LMA-Fastrach after the first attempt showed success rates of 69% and 74%, respectively. Intubation success with the Igel, Air-Q, and Aura-I can be improved with the use of a flexible optical guide.

For an elective surgical procedure in a patient with a known difficult intubation history, using any of the i-SGAs with optical intubation guidance would be appropriate. Graded views of the larynx via the various i-SGAs have been reported and may explain the failures with blind intubation. In adults, a Cormack and Lehane grade 1 vocal cord view was appreciated in only 37% of examinations through an LMA-Fastrach. In children with an in situ Air-Q or Aura-I, the following Cormack and Lehane grades were appreciated with a flexible intubating scope (FIS): grade 1, view 17% and 15%; grade 2, view 20% and 30%; and grade 3, view 35% and 35%, respectively. Intubation with the FIS was successful in all cases after a second attempt. In cases where the epiglottis was downfolded, the articulating capabilities of the FIS facilitated the intubation.

Apart from more successful blind intubation, LMA-Fastrach has advantages compared to the other three intubating supraglottic devices. The rigid handle and barrel allow increased in situ maneuverability, including side-to-side and anterior–posterior movement. A downfolded epiglottis can be repositioned with maneuvering.

2 How would you manage the airway in this case?

Assuming the patient does not have characteristics frankly consistent with a difficult mask ventilation, the author would place this patient under general anesthesia with muscle relaxation. An LMA-Fastrach would be placed after the induction of anesthesia. This i-SGA would be chosen because of its repositioning capabilities. With the use of a standard FIS or a Foley-Airway Stylet Tool (FAST) loaded with a tracheal tube (TT), the LMA-Fastrach would be maneuvered to optimize the optical view by lifting and rocking. This is the experience of the author with patients who have a short thyromental distance and a history of difficult intubation. The TT and optical device would then be advanced through the vocal cords. (See Figure 22.1 and **Video 22.1** for additional details.)

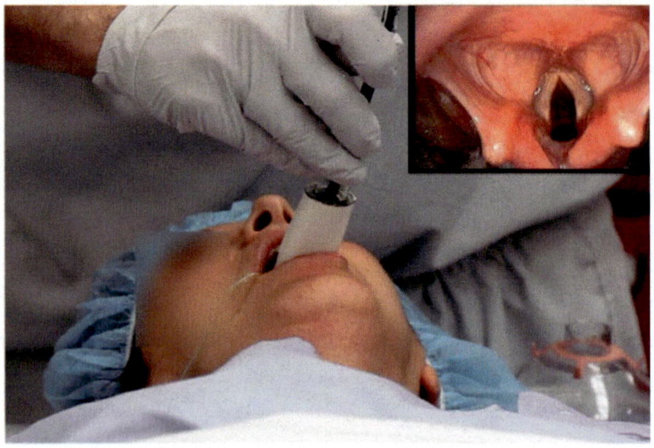

Figure 22.1. A flexible intubation scope is used to visualize the glottis through an Ambu Aura-i supraglottic device. Once the flexible scope is positioned in the trachea, a preloaded tracheal tube will be advanced over the scope.

3 What are the potential hazards and complications in regard to the airway?

In a patient with a known history of difficult tracheal intubation, inducing general anesthesia may risk a cannot intubate/cannot ventilate scenario. Kheterpal et al. found that the likelihood of a patient failing tracheal intubation, mask ventilation, and supraglottic airway (SGA) ventilation was 1 in 176,000 inductions.

Another option is to place an i-SGA with the patient awake and prepared with topical anesthesia (see Chapter 11: Preparation for Awake Intubation). Once the ventilation has been established with the SGA, general anesthesia is induced.

4 What distinct airway device might be used in this case, and what are the special considerations?

FIS is the most common optical aid for intubation through an i-SGA. The FIS can be steered (via an articulating joint) into the larynx. FIS may be used in any of the four i-SGAs described above. Though the FIS is passed into the larynx with image guidance, the passage of the TT is blind—the operator does not witness the TT as it is "rail-roaded" into position, which may be complicated by hang-up (see Chapters 18: Use of the Flexible Intubating Scope and 20: Hang-Up During Intubation with the Flexible Intubating Scope). The FAST, portable fiberoptic scope, has the advantage that both the distal scope and TT pass through the vocal cords together. Hang-up cannot occur. The disadvantage of the FAST is that there is no articulating mechanism—it is generally only used with the LMA-Fastrach whose handle allows maneuvering in situ.

The Air-Q intubating LMA has a curved airway conduit that can accommodate a TT-loaded optical stylet, such as the Clarus Video Optical Stylet or the Levitan Optical Stylet (both from Clarus Medical, Minneapolis, MN). Though these stylets do not have articulating portions, they are rigid and may be maneuvered within the intubating SGA in order to optimize laryngeal visualization. The Igel and LMA-Fastrach cannot accommodate a rigid optical stylet. At this time, there are no studies on this technique.

Another risk that may occur is oxygen desaturation during FIS intubation through the i-SGA due to an apneic patient. Continuous ventilation during intubation through the I-SGA can be done by placing a TT into the conduit of the i-SGA just before exiting the channel. The balloon of the TT is then inflated, and a blue bronchoscopy swivel adaptor is place on the TT and connected to the ventilator. The FIS will be place through the adaptor and intubated.

- All i-SGAs except the LMA-Fastrach require optical guidance to achieve a high intubation success rate.
- The LMA-Fastrach can be maneuvered in situ due to its rigid barrel and handle.
- Intubating supraglottic devices can be used during an awake intubation.
- The Air-Q can be used with a rigid optical stylet.
- *See Figure 22.2 for additional details.*

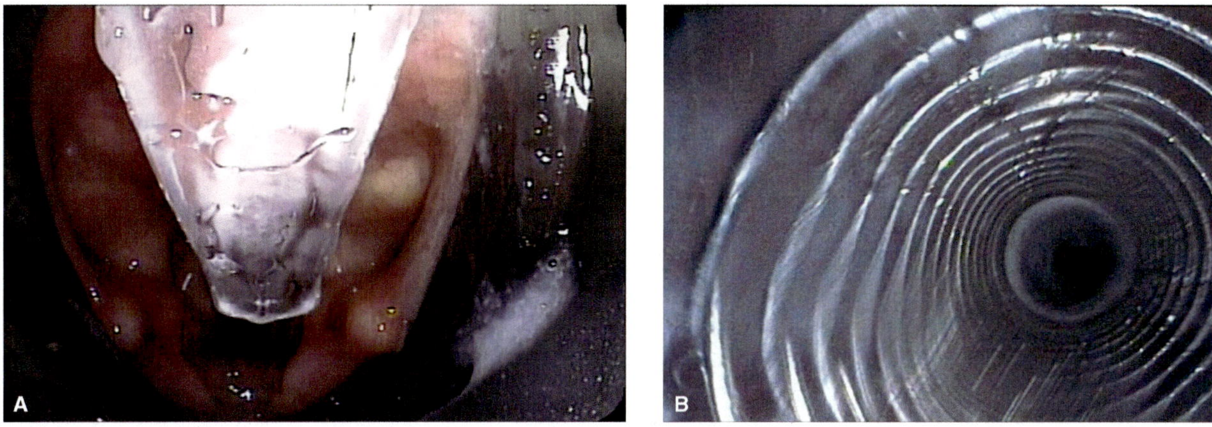

Figure 22.2. **A:** The epiglottic lifting bar of the single-use Fastrach LMA is situated against the laryngeal side of the epiglottis. The advancing tracheal tube will displace the epiglottic lifting bar and epiglottis. See **Video 22.2** for additional details. **B:** A wire-reinforced tracheal tube is advanced off the flexible intubation scope. See **Video 22.3** for additional details.

Suggested Readings

Ferson D, Rosenblatt W, Johansen M, Osborn I, Ovassapian A. Use of the intubating LMA-Fastrach in 254 patient with difficult-to-manage airways. *Anesthesiology*. 2001;95:1175–1181.

Gaitini L, Yanovski B, Mustafa S, Hagberg CA, Mora PC, Vaida SJ. A feasibility study using the VivaSight single lumen to intubate the trachea through the Fastrach laryngeal mask airway: a preliminary report of 50 cases. *Anesth Analg*. 2013;116:604–608.

Halwagi A, Massicotte N, Lailo A, et al. Tracheal intubation through the I-gel supraglottic airway versus the LMA Fastrach: a randomized controlled trial. *Anesth Analg*. 2012;114:152–156.

Heuer J, Crozier T, Neumann B, et al. The use of the Foley Airway Stylet Tool to guide tracheal intubations through an intubating laryngeal mask airway. *Minerva Anestesiol*. 2011;77:1037–1042.

Jagannathan N, Sohn L, Sawardekar A, et al. A randomized trial co-paring the Ambu Aura-I with the Air-Q intubating laryngeal airway as conduits for tracheal intubation in children. *Pediatric Anesth*. 2012;22:1197–1204.

Karim Y, Swanson D. Comparison of blind tracheal intubation through the intubating laryngeal mask airway (LMA Fastrach) and Air-Q. *Anesthesia*. 2011;66:185–190.

Kheterpal S, Healy D, Aziz MF, et al; Multicenter Perioperative Outcomes Group (MPOG) Perioperative Clinical Research Committee. Incidence, predictors, and outcome of difficult mask ventilation combined with difficult laryngoscopy: a report from the multicenter perioperative outcomes group. *Anesthesiology*. 2013;119(6):1360–1369.

Landsdalen HC, Berge M, Kristensen F, Guttormsen AB, Søfteland E. Continuous ventilation during intubation through a supraglottic airway device guided by fiberoptic bronchoscopy: a observational assessment. *Acta Anaesthesiol Scand*. 2017;61:23–30.

23 Oxylator Automatic Resuscitator

James C. DuCanto

Clinical Scenario: A 59-year-old woman with a history of super morbid obesity (body mass index 52 kg/m^2) presents for incision and drainage of an infected left hip wound following a left total hip arthroplasty. She has multiple additional medical comorbidities, including obstructive sleep apnea and chronic obstructive pulmonary disease. The patient is noted to have a room air SpO_2 of 72% in the preoperative holding area, and she is also febrile with a core temperature of 38.1 °C.

1 What are the anesthetic and airway management considerations for this case?

In addition to predicted difficulty with preoxygenation, ventilation following induction, and tracheal intubation, the patient is displaying signs and symptoms of early sepsis and respiratory failure. Prevention of hypoxemia, hypoventilation, and hemodynamic collapse during the induction of anesthesia should be the principal concern. Pressure-assisted preoxygenation (BiPAP) and continued ventilation with an automated pressure-limited resuscitator can help prevent hypoxemia and hypoventilation. Proper patient positioning during preoxygenation and induction is essential. Monitoring end-tidal oxygen concentration to ensure that the end-tidal oxygen concentration reaches 88% prior to induction is also crucial to ensure proper nitrogen washout and thorough preoxygenation prior to induction. Monitoring of the waveform capnography is important to gauge the effectiveness of mask ventilation following induction.

2 How would you manage the airway in this case?

An Oxylator HD Resuscitation Management System (Figure 23.1) is applied to the patient with a tight-fitting face mask to facilitate preoxygenation and preparation for induction and tracheal intubation. The Oxylator is initially set to the Inhalator mode, which provides 15 L/min of passive (nonpressurized) oxygen to the patient, as tight-fitting mask straps are applied to the mask from behind the patient's head. The Oxylator is then set to the Automatic mode, which pressurizes the patient's airway to a preset level based upon the setting of the Oxylator device. The Oxylator now provides preinduction, noninvasive respiratory support as a BiPAP unit, providing pressures of 15 cm H_2O inspiratory positive airway pressure (IPAP) and 2 to 4 cm H_2O expiratory positive airway pressure (EPAP). The patient tolerated this period of BiPAP-supported preoxygenation without complaint, and her SpO_2 levels rose to 98% prior to induction. General anesthesia was induced with propofol 50 mg and succinylcholine 80 mg. The patient was intubated on the first attempt by direct laryngoscopy with a 7.5-Mallinkrodt tracheal tube, to which the Oxylator was connected at a pressure-release setting

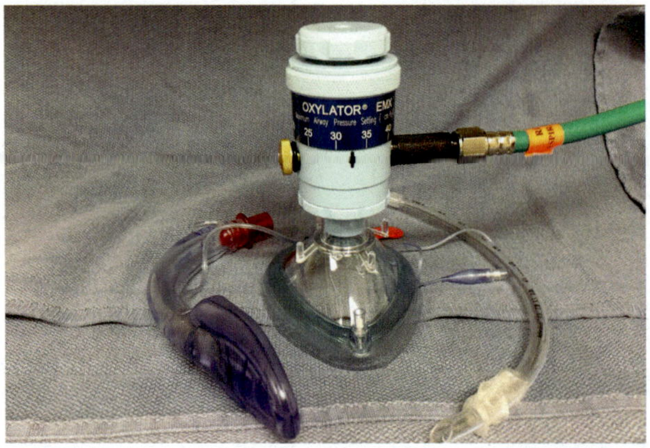

Figure 23.1. The Oxylator, tracheal tube, and super glottic airway.

of 30 cm H_2O. Bilateral breath sounds were confirmed, and the tracheal tube was connected to the anesthesia breathing circuit for the continuation of her anesthetic. At the conclusion of the surgical procedure, the patient was extubated after emergence from the anesthetic. The patient was found to be mildly hypoxic following extubation, and she required face mask ventilation with the Oxylator once again to improve her oxygen saturations. The patient was transferred to the intensive care unit utilizing the Oxylator as a transport BiPAP ventilation system and then placed on a formal BiPAP ventilator in the ICU with settings of IPAP 20 cm H_2O and EPAP 7 cm H_2O.

3 What are the potential hazards and complications in regard to the airway?

Specific hazards and complications in this case involve mishandling of the preinduction period of preoxygenation and ventilation of the patient following induction. If these two components of the patient's airway management are not handled well, hypoxemia is almost certain to occur during the airway management procedure. The thoroughness and efficiency of the preinduction–preoxygenation process are greatly enhanced with bilevel positive-pressure airway support, as the end-expiratory pressure combined with the peak inhaled airway pressure allows the pulmonary system to recruit active ventilation units in the patient's lung. Similarly, utilizing an automated resuscitator as a ventilation device maintains consistency of flow, airway pressures, and tidal volumes to maximize the efficiency of mask ventilation following induction.

- Assisting preoxygenation with bilevel-positive airway pressure accelerates nitrogen washout and prolongs the safe apnea time during airway management.
- The Oxylator serves as a rudimentary BiPAP system to deliver assisted ventilatory breaths to the patient while maintaining lung recruitment.
- The Oxylator can be utilized as a ventilation support device following tracheal extubation, should the patient require noninvasive ventilation postextubation.
- *See Figure 23.2 and* **Video 23.1** *for additional details.*

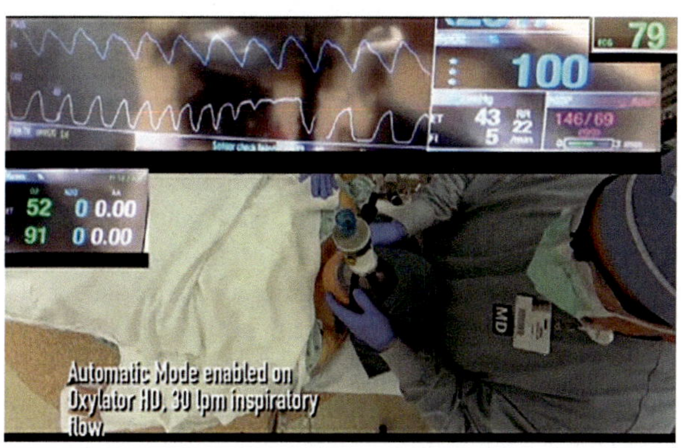

Figure 23.2. The chapter author uses the Oxylator for preoxygenation and induction of anesthesia.

Suggested Readings

El-Khatib MF, Kanazi G, Baraka AS. Noninvasive bilevel positive airway pressure for preoxygenation of the critically ill morbidly obese patient. *Can J Anesth.* 2007;54(9):744–747.

Vale H, Cattano D. Preoxygenation strategies and positioning tips. In: Hagberg CA, Artime CA, Daily WH, eds. *The Difficult Airway: A Practical Guide.* Oxford University Press; 2013:27–34.

Weingart S, Levitan R. Preoxygenation and prevention of desaturation during emergency airway management. *Ann Emerg Med.* 2012;59(3):165–175.

24 Total Intravenous Anesthesia

Jodi Sherman • Cliff Shelton

1 Describe in detail the device or technique.

The use of total intravenous anesthesia (TIVA) provides the anesthesiologist with the ability to easily titrate rapid-onset, short-acting medications. This makes TIVA the ideal choice of anesthetic for many ear–nose–throat (ENT) surgeries due to the often intensely stimulating but brief procedures and the lack of airway continuity in others (eg, tubeless field surgery). A potential drawback of TIVA is that plasma drug concentrations are estimated, not measured. This poses a risk of accidental awareness if intravenous access becomes compromised. The use of a processed electroencephalogram (pEEG)-based depth of anesthesia monitoring is therefore advocated, particularly when neuromuscular blocking drugs (NMBDs) are also being administered.

The most common hypnotic drug used for TIVA is propofol. The effective concentration to prevent movement in response to painful stimulus in 50% of patients (EC_{50}, a similar concept to minimum alveolar concentration) of propofol is 6 to 7 μg/mL. With the concomitant use of regional anesthesia or potent analgesics, the EC_{50} is substantially reduced. The predictable pharmacokinetics of propofol make it suitable for administration with a target-controlled infusion such as the Marsh, Schnider, or Eleveld models. If these models are not available, a manual infusion can be used. The "Bristol Regimen" is a manual infusion strategy for propofol TIVA comprising a loading dose of 1 mg/kg followed by 10 mg/kg/h for 10 minutes, 8 mg/kg/h for the next 10 minutes, and then 6 mg/kg/h thereafter. This model estimates an achieved plasma concentration of approximately 3 μg/mL, so this model should be used as part of a balanced anesthetic.

Propofol does not provide sufficient analgesia for surgical procedures, so it is typically combined with an IV opioid for a balanced anesthetic. Opioid selection should depend on the intensity and onset of surgical stimulation, length of procedure, anticipated level of postsurgical pain, and the postoperative care plan. Surgical procedures with intense stimulation, such as those involving rigid direct laryngoscopy (DL) and endoscopic sinus surgery, are best performed using an infusion of a highly potent, rapid-onset opioid. Remifentanil is 100 to 200 times more potent than morphine. It has a peak effect occurring at 1 to 2 minutes and a rapid recovery in 3 to 6 minutes, primarily due to metabolism by nonspecific esterases. Unlike other opioids, remifentanil does not accumulate with prolonged administration, making it especially desirable for long cases, procedures with minimal postoperative pain, and for ambulatory procedures. Like propofol, remifentanil can be administered using a target-controlled infusion (the Minto model), but because of its wide therapeutic range, a manual infusion can be used. Typical maintenance infusion rates range from 0.025 to 0.5 μg/kg/min. Alfentanil (0.5 to 3 μg/kg/min) is an alternative rapid-onset and short-acting opioid amenable to many ENT procedures. Alfentanil undergoes biotransformation in the liver, so it can accumulate unlike remifentanil. This must be taken into account if alfentanil is used in longer procedures. An alternative approach to opioid administration is by intermittent bolus (eg, of fentanyl or alfentanil), but this approach offers less ability to titrate than an infusion.

Dexmedetomidine is a selective α2-agonist with sedative, anxiolytic, and analgesic properties. It also does not cause respiratory depression. These drug properties make dexmedetomidine a good addition to a TIVA regimen. Dexmedetomidine reduces the EC_{50} of propofol and average opioid requirements in the intraoperative and early postoperative period. Its use can facilitate a smooth emergence from general anesthesia, including minimization of coughing. Dexmedetomidine is a sympatholytic, so it can cause hypotension and bradycardia. It should be avoided in patients with poor ventricular function, conduction abnormalities, shock, or hepatic impairment. Recommended rates range from 0.2 to 1.4 μg/kg/h. Boluses should be administered with caution, as large boluses can result in cardiac arrest. Peak effect occurs at 30 minutes without a loading dose or at 20 minutes with a loading dose (1 μg/kg over 10 minutes), and the half-life is 2 hours. Its effects are not quickly titratable, and so it is not well suited for surgeries of short duration.

In ENT cases that are intensely stimulating, continuous infusion of an NMBD can help negate the temptation to rely on anesthetic overdosing to prevent movement. Neuromuscular function must be carefully monitored with a peripheral nerve stimulator to avoid overdose, and neuromuscular recovery must be confirmed prior to emergence. In cases of short duration or when nerve testing by surgeons is required, NMBDs are not desirable. It is therefore common to administer a TIVA consisting of both remifentanil and propofol infusions, with the remifentanil at relatively high levels to prevent movement and avoid the need for maintenance muscle relaxation. If remifentanil dosing is maximized to the patient's tolerance, a lower level of propofol may be utilized to prevent delayed emergence.

2 Where or when is this device or technique used in airway management?

For surgeries that involve intermittent extubation or jet ventilation, TIVA is the desirable choice to smoothly control the depth of the anesthetic and avoid exposing the OR personnel unnecessarily to inhaled anesthetics. Procedures involving rigid DL or endoscopic sinus surgery are intensely stimulating but cause minimal postoperative pain, so a short-acting remifentanil infusion is ideal. A propofol maintenance infusion is helpful to decrease the risk of postoperative nausea and vomiting, which is of particular importance for upper airway surgeries and ear surgeries (near cranial nerve VIII that can affect equilibrium). For awake intubations, a low-dose remifentanil infusion is a helpful supplement to local anesthetic topicalization. A dexmedetomidine infusion can be added to remifentanil for awake intubations as it provides both anxiolysis as well as analgesia without respiratory suppression. Dexmedetomidine, however, can take 20 to 30 minutes to reach its peak effect, so it is insufficient without an adjunct infusion of remifentanil. For longer procedures, dexmedetomidine is also useful to prevent coughing and agitation on emergence.

3 What distinguishes this device or technique from similar airway management methods?

All inhaled anesthetics are potent greenhouse gases that are released directly to the environment unchanged through the scavenging system. In addition to avoiding occupational exposure during ENT procedures with a tubeless field, TIVA can reduce atmospheric pollution release stemming from clinical practice of using inhaled anesthetics (Figure 24.1).

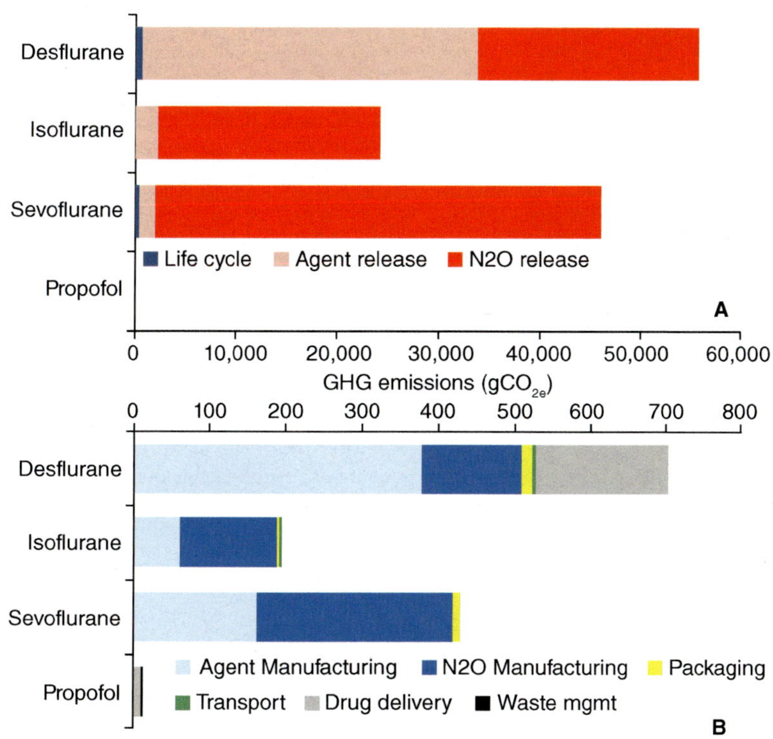

Figure 24.1. Life cycle greenhouse gas (GHG) emissions of anesthetics. **A:** Including waste anesthetic gas emissions of the halogenated drugs and nitrous oxide, and (**B**) excluding waste anesthetic gas emissions. (Reprinted with permission from Sherman J, Le C, Lamers V, Eckelman M. Life cycle greenhouse gas emissions of anesthetic drugs. *Anesth Analg*. 2012;114(5):1086–1090. Figure 1. Copyright © 2012 International Anesthesia Research Society.)

Author Caveats

With excellent communication with the surgical team and some experience, the timing of TIVA can be mastered regardless of the length of the procedure. Target-controlled infusions in combination with pEEG-based depth of anesthesia monitoring make titration more straightforward, but manual infusion regimens can still be successfully used. For longer surgeries, more lead time for weaning propofol is required to prevent emergence delays. To prevent coughing, it can be extremely helpful to wake patients up with a dexmedetomidine or very low-dose remifentanil infusion still infusing.

- TIVA is the preferred approach for maintenance anesthetic in procedures of the airway that require intermittent extubation for surgical exposure or jet ventilation.
- A potent short-acting opioid infusion is beneficial for procedures with intense surgical stimulation and minimal postoperative pain, such as rigid DL and nasal sinus surgery.
- TIVA techniques can significantly aid awake intubations.
- TIVA can overall reduce atmospheric pollution release stemming from the use of inhaled anesthetics, which are known potent greenhouse gases.
- *See Figure 24.2 for additional details.*

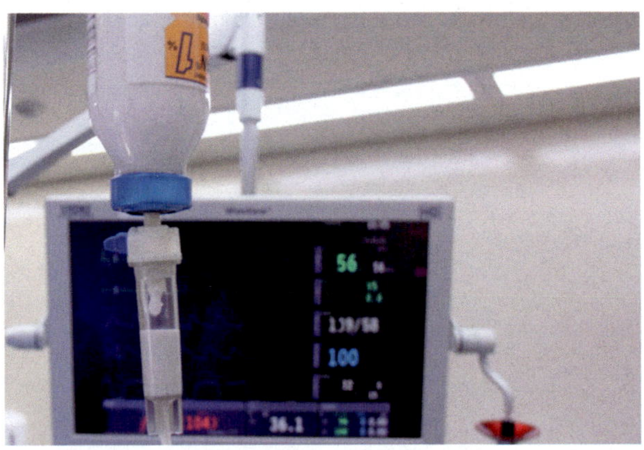

Figure 24.2. Total intravenous anesthesia.

Suggested Readings

Le Guen M, Liu N, Tounou F, et al. Dexmedetomidine reduces propofol and remifentanyl requirements during bispectral index-guided closed-loop anesthesia: a double-blind, placebo-controlled trial. *Anesth Analg*. 2014;118(5):946–955.

Nimmo AF, Absalom AR, Bagshaw O, et al. Guidelines for the safe practice of total intravenous anaesthesia. *Anaesthesia*. 2019; 74(2):211–224.

Sherman J, Le C, Lamers V, Eckelman M. Life cycle greenhouse gas emissions of anesthetic drugs. *Anesth Analg*. 2012; 114(5):1086–1090.

Intubation Without Muscle Relaxation

25

Adriana D. Oprea • Haitham Ibrahim

1 Describe in detail the device or technique.

Tracheal intubation without muscle relaxants can be achieved using conventional direct laryngoscopy, video laryngoscopy, or a flexible intubation scope.

Both laryngoscopy and tracheal intubation are very stimulating procedures, so an adequate anesthetic depth needs to be achieved in order to provide safe and optimal intubating conditions. If optimal conditions are not ensured, the attempts may be complicated by patient movement, soft tissue, dental, and laryngeal trauma, regurgitation and/or aspiration, and failure to intubate. In addition, failure to adequately blunt the hemodynamic effects of upper airway manipulation can lead to cardiovascular complications.

Multiple techniques to optimize intubating conditions for direct laryngoscopy have recently received attention. One of these techniques involves the use of inhalational agents alone (eg, sevoflurane) for the induction of anesthesia, followed by intubation or application of a laryngeal mask airway. While this is a well-described technique in the pediatric population, recent studies have confirmed that this technique also achieves excellent intubating conditions in adults. Older inhalational anesthetics have largely been replaced by sevoflurane in recent years. In the pediatric population, optimal intubating conditions require an end tidal concentration of sevoflurane of 2.7% to 2.8% when used in combination with O_2. When sevoflurane is used in conjunction with 60% N_2O, an end-tidal concentration of sevoflurane 1.6% to 2.2% is adequate. Even with the addition of N_2O, the timing of intubation should still be delayed by 3 minutes as compared with 60 seconds following the administration of succinylcholine.

In adults, an inhalational induction with sevoflurane at 8% concentration provides optimal intubating conditions. The concentration of sevoflurane required for intubation is higher than that required in children (3.4% vs 2.7%). Unfortunately, the high doses of sevoflurane required when used as a sole agent may cause hemodynamic instability in select patients, especially the elderly. If the patient is spontaneously breathing during the laryngoscopy attempts, the low blood-gas solubility of sevoflurane may cause the patient to emerge if the procedure is prolonged.

The time required to wait prior to intubation can be shortened with administration of intravenous sedatives adjuncts (eg, midazolam, fentanyl). The addition of narcotics to the sevoflurane technique has been studied. Fentanyl administration (at a dose of 4 µg/kg) decreases the concentration of sevoflurane necessary for intubation to less than 2%. Sevoflurane concentration requirements decrease similarly with the administration of remifentanil (bolus of 1 µg/kg followed by an infusion of 0.25 µg/kg/min).

Another alternative method to achieve intubation without muscle relaxants is a combined intravenous agent technique. Historically, intravenous thiopental was used at doses of 500 to 750 mg as a sole induction agent, but proved inadequate in many circumstances. In comparison to thiopental, propofol as the sole induction agent provides better jaw relaxation and cough suppression. When used alone, propofol should be used at doses 2.5 mg/kg and greater. Cardiovascular depression and hypotension may occur in some patients. The addition of opioid adjunct agents improves intubating conditions. Fentanyl (dosed at 3 µg/kg) administered 5 minutes before intubation blunts the hypertensive response to laryngoscopy. Alfentanil (10 to 50 µg/kg) and remifentanil (0.5 to 5 µg/kg) have quicker onset of action and can also be used in conjunction with propofol. When propofol is combined with a narcotic for induction, intubation should be timed to coincide with the peak effect of the drugs. While alfentanil and remifentanil have an onset of action similar to that of propofol, the delayed onset of action of fentanyl requires that the drug be administered in advance.

Alfentanil can be used as the primary induction agent (using doses as low as 10 µg/kg) when used in conjunction with other sedating medications (eg, benzodiazepines) or as the sole induction agent (using doses up to 50 µg/kg).

The use of remifentanil for intubation without muscle relaxation was recently investigated, and a dose of remifentanil of 1.4 µg/kg combined with propofol dosed at 1 mg/kg created acceptable conditions for intubation without the use of muscle relaxants. Remifentanil can also be used as part of a rapid sequence induction technique in conjunction with propofol for patients in which succinylcholine is contraindicated.

Intravenous lidocaine has also been studied as an adjunct induction medication. During a propofol induction, intravenous lidocaine given one minute prior to laryngoscopy can blunt the response to laryngoscopy and improve intubating conditions. When intravenous lidocaine is used in conjunction with opioids prior to propofol administration, it can decrease the dose of opioid necessary to improve intubating conditions. Intravenous lidocaine without opioid adjuncts should be administered at doses of 2 mg/kg in order to adequately suppress the cough reflex. Topical laryngotracheal lidocaine (administered 60 to 90 seconds prior to laryngoscopy) (See figure 25.1) during a propofol/alfentanil induction provides good intubating conditions, as well. Neither intravenous nor topical lidocaine, in addition to standard intravenous induction (including intravenous induction medication and a muscle relaxant) alters the pressor response to laryngoscopy.

Last, an intravenous induction agent (eg, propofol and thiopental, but not etomidate) in combination with dexmedetomidine 10 μg/kg provides adequate intubating conditions.

2 Where or when is this device or technique used in airway management?

This technique is useful for situations or patients in which muscle relaxants are contraindicated (allergy to nondepolarizing muscle relaxants, patients with neuromuscular disorders such as myasthenia gravis and muscle dystrophies, or patients with malignant hyperthermia, spinal cord injury, or burn injuries). In addition, this technique may prove useful during short procedures that require intubation but also require rapid emergence from anesthesia, such as many ENT procedures. This technique is also utilized for neurosurgical procedures which require neuromonitoring.

3 What distinguishes this device or technique from similar airway management methods?

The use of muscle relaxants for tracheal intubation provides optimal conditions for securing the airway. Muscle relaxants may help to place the patient in a true sniffing maneuver as well as help to relax the jaw musculature.

The position of the vocal cords during the laryngoscopy is affected by the use of muscle relaxants. While the muscle relaxant-sparing techniques described above add to the depth of anesthesia required for intubation, immobility of the vocal cords is not always achieved. Therefore, the timing of intubation attempts relative to the opening of the vocal cords and the skill of the anesthesiologist are paramount in ensuring a successful, atraumatic intubation. It has been observed that vocal cord trauma and sequelae are more frequent after intubation without muscle relaxants.

- A combination of agents including intravenous or inhalational anesthetics, opioids, sedating agents, and local anesthetics, should be used to achieve good intubating conditions.
- Intubating without muscle relaxants should be reserved for select groups of patients. Some examples include the pediatric population, adults undergoing procedures with neuromonitoring, or patients with other contraindications to muscle relaxant agents.
- Remifentanil or alfentanil have similar efficacy as adjunct agents when used for this technique, and are superior to fentanyl.
- *See Figure 25.1 and* ***Video 25.1*** *for additional details.*

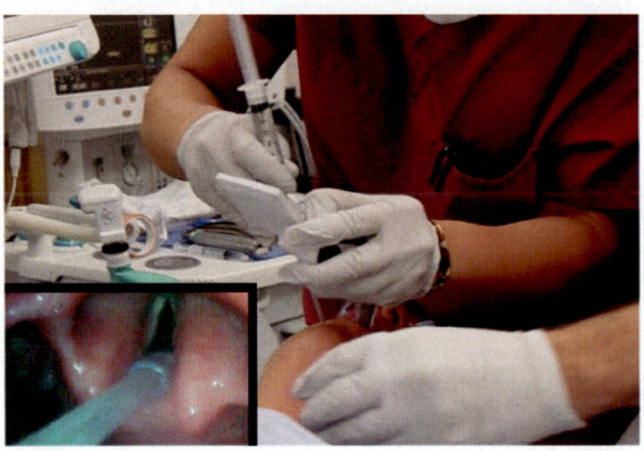

Figure 25.1. Local anesthetic is being applied during video laryngoscopy to aid in an intubation without muscle relaxant.

Suggested Readings

Bollucuoglu K, Hanci V, Yurtlu S, Okyay D, Ayoglu H, Turan IO. Comparison of propofol-dexmedetomidine, tiopental-dexmedetomidine and etomidate-dexmedetomidine combinations' effects on the tracheal intubation conditions without using muscle relaxants. *Bratisl Lek Listy*. 2013;114:514–518.

Goo EK, Oh AY, Cho SJ, Seo KS, Jeon YT. Optimal remifentanil dosage for intubation without muscle relaxants in elderly patients. *Drugs Aging*. 2012;29:905–909.

Lewis CB. Endotracheal intubation under thiopentone; an analysis of 200 cases. *Anaesthesia*. 1948;3:113–115.

Sneyd JR, O'Sullivan E. Tracheal intubation without neuromuscular blocking agents: is there any point? *Br J Anaesth*. 2010; 104:535–537.

Woods AW, Allam S. Tracheal intubation without the use of neuromuscular blocking agents. *Br J Anaesth*. 2005;94:150–158.

26 Inhalation Induction

Richard E. Galgon

Clinical Scenario: A 60-year-old man has a history of supraglottic cancer treated with supraglottic laryngectomy and radiation therapy. He now presents for direct laryngoscopy, esophagoscopy, and neck dissection for a newly discovered cervical mass. He has no gastroesophageal reflux disease (GERD) or respiratory symptoms and does not snore. Although he is edentulous, his oral aperture is less than 2 cm.

1 What are the anesthetic and airway management considerations for this case?

Head and neck cancer patients have complex clinical presentations. In some patients, restricted mouth opening (<2 cm) makes atraumatic airway instrumentation very difficult or impossible and limits the practitioner to specific devices and techniques. Significant tumor burden and/or a prior partial pharyngectomy may distort the upper airway anatomy. Preoperative irradiation may cause glottic and epiglottic edema, trismus, and immobile and friable pharyngeal and glottic tissues. The mobility of the cervical spine may be severely limited by previous surgery, cervical tumor expansion, and radiation fibrosis. Postradiation fibrosis of the neck makes subglottic invasive airway management very challenging. In these patients, percutaneous cricothyrotomy may fail and tracheotomy may require more time. A careful preoperative evaluation is necessary whenever these patients are encountered. In addition, prior CT and MRI images of the head and neck should be reviewed. If more information about the airway is needed, the patient should undergo a preoperative endoscopic airway evaluation. The patient's comorbidities should also be evaluated (alcohol and tobacco use, GERD, and metastasis to the liver, lung, and/or bones) as they may impact the functional capacity of the patient.

In this case, the patient's current clinical presentation indicates a intubation by direct or indirect laryngoscopy may be difficult but possible.

2 How would you manage the airway in this case?

The author's choice would be to preserve spontaneous ventilation until the airway is secured. A sevoflurane inhalational induction followed by nasotracheal flexible scope intubation would be pursued. Resources for airway manipulation in this patient should include access to a difficult airway cart, a capable assistant, and the surgeon available for immediate emergency intervention, if needed. The airway procedure should be explained to the patient, and sedation associated with inhalation induction should be carefully balanced against the risk of ventilatory depression that could compromise oxygenation and ventilation. Preinduction airway preparation, including airway topicalization, nasal vasoconstriction, and antisialagogue administration, can help to blunt hemodynamic perturbations and reduce secretion interference. As mentioned above, the goal of the intubation is to maintain spontaneous ventilation throughout the instrumentation and maintain hemodynamic stability.

Airway management starts following airway preparation with optimal positioning and preoxygenation with 100% FiO_2 (to increase the ETO_2 >90%). Anesthesia is induced with a "tidal breathing technique" with the patient breathing a mixture of sevoflurane 8% with 2 L/min oxygen and 3 L/min N_2O. The success of this technique relies on a good face mask seal and a cooperative patient. During the first minute of induction, transient apnea may be observable, usually induced by hypocapnia (excitement hyperventilation) or when the patient first loses consciousness. Loss of consciousness (unresponsiveness) and lid-lash reflex (in ~1 minute) is followed by pupil convergence (end of stage 2 of anesthesia), a drop in blood pressure, followed by a depth of anesthesia adequate for tracheal intubation (in ~4.7 minutes, stage 3). Once a steady pattern of respiration is established and adequate depth of general anesthesia is achieved, flexible scope intubation can proceed. The author's choice is to use a smaller outer diameter flexible video intubation scope (FIS) and a Parker Flex-Tip tube. If one contemplates removing the face mask after inhalation induction for apneic instrumentation, the anesthetic should be deepened beforehand and the carrier gases changed to 100% oxygen to increase the safe apneic period. An alternative approach would be to perform a wire-guided (Seldinger) technique, as described by Heier et al., which allows for continuous sevoflurane administration, oxygen delivery, and the application of CPAP through passage of the flexible scope and a wire into the trachea.

Contraindications to an inhalational induction are intolerance of a tight-fitting face mask, untreated gastroesophageal reflux disease (GERD), a full stomach, intracranial hypertension, malignant hyperthermia susceptibility, obesity/OSA, and snoring.

3 What are the potential hazards and complications in regard to the airway?

Respiratory complications are often induced by premature manipulation of the airway (eg, insertion of an oropharyngeal airway) or may be triggered by passive reflux. Partial obstruction may be relieved by a gentle chin lift. Cardiovascular diseases (QT prolongation, bradycardia, asystole, and tachycardia) and respiratory diseases (laryngospasm and cough) are potential complications of a sevoflurane induction. If airway obstruction occurs during an inhalational induction, the anesthesia provider has several options: (1) wake the patient by allowing inhaled agent redistribution, (2) attempt positive-pressure ventilation or CPAP application (see wire-guided technique mentioned above), (3) attempt intubation (video laryngoscope), or (4) allow the surgeon to proceed with an invasive airway. Mismatch between the outer diameter of the FIS and the inner diameter of the ETT can lead to "hang-up" on the arytenoids when the tube is advanced into the airway. Diameter matching and use of the Parker Flex tube help to reduce this occurrence. Finally, the patient with previous oral surgery and radiation therapy may be challenging to intubate with a flexible scope or video laryngoscopic technique due to abnormal and difficult-to-recognize anatomy with friable tissues that bleed easily.

4 What distinct airway device might be used in this case, and what are the special considerations?

Intubation in a patient who is breathing spontaneously can be accomplished with oral or nasal flexible scope technique, video laryngoscope, or tracheostomy under local anesthetic. Preparation for an awake flexible scope technique or tracheostomy in this patient may be challenging and unrewarding as the postradiation tissues are dry, edematous, and fibrotic, and the distorted anatomy makes nerve blocks and landmarks unreliable. A mouth opening ≥2 cm may allow insertion of an supraglottic airway that may be exchanged to an ETT using a FIS technique.

- Head and neck cancer patients with limited mouth opening, previous laryngectomy, and/or preoperative irradiation should have extensive clinical preoperative airway assessment followed by head CT and MRI and, if needed, preoperative nasal endoscopic airway evaluation.
- Inhalational induction is a time-consuming, elective technique that needs a fully cooperative patient and an experienced anesthesia provider.
- During an inhalation induction in a patient with a known difficult airway, it is paramount to have a difficult airway cart and additional experienced support personnel available.
- *See Figure 26.1 and* ***Video 26.1*** *for additional details.*

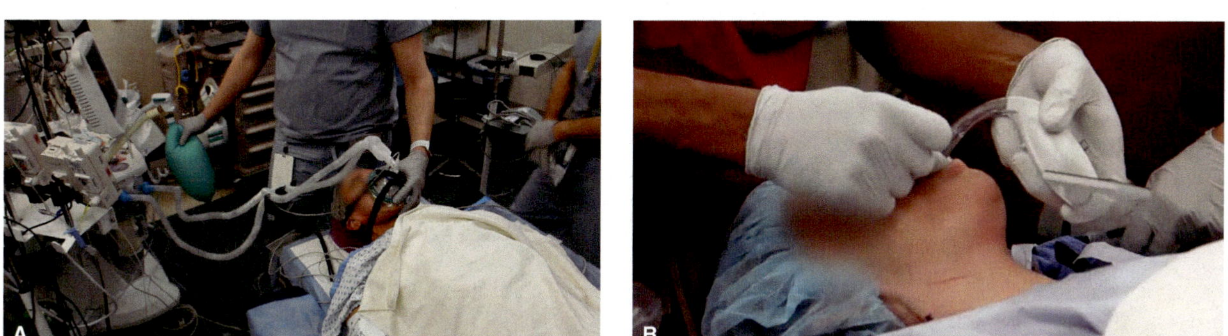

Figure 26.1. A: The patient is allowed to spontaneously breathe with a tight facemask seal, as the inhaled agent is introduced. Some clinicians employ a modest closure of the APL value to allow for constant circuit positive pressure during the induction. **B:** Once an adequate plane of anesthesia is reached with or without muscle relaxant, gentle laryngoscopy and intubation take place.

Suggested Readings

Heier JM, Schroeder KM, Galgon RE, Arndt GA. Wire-guided (Seldinger technique) intubation through a face mask in urgent, difficult and grossly distorted airways. *Saudi J Anaesth.* 2012;6(3):292–294.

McClelland SH, Hardman JG. Inhalational induction of anesthesia in adults: time for a breath of fresh air? *Anaesthesia.* 2007; 62:1087–1089.

Mishra S, Bhatnagar S, Jha RR, Singhal AK. Airway management of patients undergoing oral cancer surgery: a retrospective study. *Eur J Anaesthesiol.* 2005;22:510–514.

Muzi M, Robinson BJ, Ebert MD, O'Brien TJ. Induction of anesthesia and tracheal intubation with sevoflurane in adults. *Anesthesiology.* 1996;85(5):36–43.

Rosenblatt W, Ianus AI, Sukhupragarn W, Fickenscher A, Sasaki C. Preoperative endoscopic airway evaluation provides superior airway information and may reduce the use of unnecessary awake intubation. *Anesth Analg.* 2011;112:602–607.

Complications of Tracheal Intubation

27

Helga Komen

Clinical Scenario: A 49-year-old man with a history of alcoholism requires intubation in the intensive care unit (ICU) for recurrent seizures. The patient is 5′9″ tall and weighs 190 pounds. He is obtunded and a thorough airway exam is not possible. The patient appears to have a thyromental distance less than 3 fingerbreadths (6 cm) and a receding chin. A previous intubation record shows difficult facemask ventilation requiring the use of an oral airway. According to previous airway notes, the patient's mouth opening was 3 fingerbreadths, and the view of the glottis using a video laryngoscope was Cormack and Lehane grade IIb after cricoid pressure was applied. Considering the history, the ICU team decides to use a video laryngoscope with a hyperangulated blade. The team proceeds with rapid sequence induction and does not attempt ventilation. Laryngoscopy is performed by a trainee and the laryngoscope blade is repositioned twice in order to reach the vallecula. The view of the glottis is grade IIa and 7.5-mm internal diameter endotracheal tube (ETT) is placed. During the removal of the video laryngoscope's hyperangulated blade, a tear is noted in the palatoglossal arch as well as minimal bleeding. The ETT is secured, and mechanical ventilation is initiated.

1 What is the anesthetic management consideration for this case?

Patients in the ICU typically have complex medical histories. When creating an anesthetic plan, providers must consider present conditions and comorbidities. This patient has a history of alcoholism and recurrent seizures. It is probable that he has comorbidities related to the respiratory, digestive, and cardiovascular systems. The risk of desaturation, aspiration, and hemodynamic instability during the induction of anesthesia will shape the development of a plan. Patients should receive adequate preoxygenation to an expiratory oxygen level of over 90%. This may guarantee safe apnea time during intubation in the majority of patients. As this patient was obtunded, his active participation was not possible, so the patient was placed on 100% oxygen over a face mask to optimize his preinduction oxygen level. Desaturation during induction of anesthesia is a common event if the apnea time is prolonged or if the patient's functional residual capacity is low.

The aspiration risk depends on both the time of last oral intake as well as the functional status of the patient's digestive tract. This patient most likely has an increased risk of aspiration due to his history of alcoholism (eg, delayed gastric emptying, increased gastric acidity). The providers chose to perform rapid sequence induction to guarantee safety and minimize risk of aspiration. The suction device was readily available.

To guarantee hemodynamic stability during induction of anesthesia, providers dosed induction medications considering age, body weight, baseline blood pressure, and conditions of the patient, and had common vasoactive drugs available at the bedside, such as norepinephrine and phenylephrine. In case of failed intubation, sugammadex was readily available for swift reversal of neuromuscular blockade.

2 How would you manage the airway in this case?

It is essential to review previous airway management records, if available, to prepare appropriate equipment to ensure a safe and effective airway management plan. Prior records often describe airway exam details, types of past equipment used, vocal cord view, and any additional tools required (oral airway, bougie, etc.). Upon review of this patient's past anesthetic records, he required the use of an oral airway for adequate mask ventilation and was a grade IIb view upon video laryngoscopy with a Macintosh blade.

In formulating a future airway plan for this patient, it is essential to gather the equipment at bedside (video laryngoscope with hyperangulated blade, bougie, fiberoptic scope, supraglottic airway), provide adequate preoxygenation, position the patient, choose an appropriate mode of induction and induction drugs, and have the most experienced airway provider available (especially if supervising a trainee). Backup plans for failed airway attempts must also be considered.

3 What are the potential hazards/complications in regard to the airway?

Potential complications related to airway management are numerous and can happen during or after intubation. Anatomically, they may include upper and/or lower airway. It is extremely important to recognize a complication as soon as possible and treat accordingly.

The most common complications during laryngoscopy are facial soft tissue and dental injuries. Corneal abrasions and contusions, or lacerations of the lip can happen easily. Dental trauma compromises 30% to 40% of all anesthesia-related malpractice claims. In most cases, upper incisors are affected by the pressure of the laryngoscope blade against the tooth. In case of violation of dentition, the displaced tooth should be recovered and placed in saline for possible intervention.

Another potential hazard during airway management is cervical spine injury. It can occur if the patient has limited neck extension or if the patient comes with an unstable cervical spine. In these situations, the patient's head and neck must be kept in a neutral position. Fiberoptic technique is recommended to avoid manipulation of the neck.

Pharyngeal trauma is another complication of intubation and can be caused by pressure from the laryngoscope blade or by tube passage. It is more frequent when a video laryngoscope is used and the blade is introduced into the mouth without direct visualization, as that likely caused trauma to the palatoglossal arch in the clinical vignette. Other typical pharyngeal injuries include those of the soft palate and palatopharyngeal arch. It is essential to introduce all blades, video or otherwise, into the mouth under direct visualization and then rely on the video monitor to advance the blade past the base of the tongue.

Laryngeal trauma, however, is rare. It happens more frequently while using a flexible bronchoscope as a means to pass an endotracheal tube through the vocal cords. There is no direct view of the vocal cords during this time.

With difficult visualization of vocal cords during laryngoscopy comes the risk of esophageal intubation. This should be detected immediately by a lack of end-tidal CO_2 ($EtCO_2$).

Once the trachea is intubated, the ETT may be advanced too far into the airway resulting in bronchial intubation. It is important to auscultate the bilateral lung fields after each intubation to avoid this complication. The depth of the tube in females is most frequently 21 cm at the lips and in males 23 cm.

Rare, but serious complications of tracheal intubation involving lower airway are tracheal, bronchial and esophageal perforation. Tracheal perforation will more likely happen if the stylet protrudes from the ETT or when excessive force is used. Bronchial perforation may happen when a tube exchanger is used or during double-lumen tube placement. Airway perforation may result in subcutaneous emphysema, pneumomediastinum, or pneumothorax. Urgent chest drainage and surgical repair may be needed.

Once the patient is extubated, glottic edema can occur. Edema is a significant complication in the early postextubation period and is often a consequence of an oversized tube or prolonged prone positioning. Treatment includes intravenous steroids and elevated position of the head.

Postextubation vocal cord paralysis is another complication, often the result of an overinflated endotracheal cuff that injures the recurrent laryngeal nerve. In most instances, it resolves spontaneously.

Tracheoesophageal fistula and tracheal stenosis may also occur after intubation. They develop as a consequence of ischemia and necrosis of the tracheal mucosa. This happens when the ETT cuff is overinflated and exceeds the capillary perfusion pressure of the tracheal mucosa. It is important to check cuff pressure after intubation and periodically, during mechanical ventilation. The pressure should be between 20 and 30 mm Hg. Signs of tracheal stenosis are stridor and shortness of breath. Signs of tracheoesophageal fistula are coughing, difficulty breathing while ingesting, and vomiting.

- If available, airway management records should be reviewed during planning of tracheal intubation.
- The goal of an airway management plan is to ensure the first attempt success of tracheal intubation.
- Complications of tracheal intubation are relatively common, but typically minor and happen during the intubation process.
- *See Figure 27.1 and* ***Video 27.1*** *for additional details.*

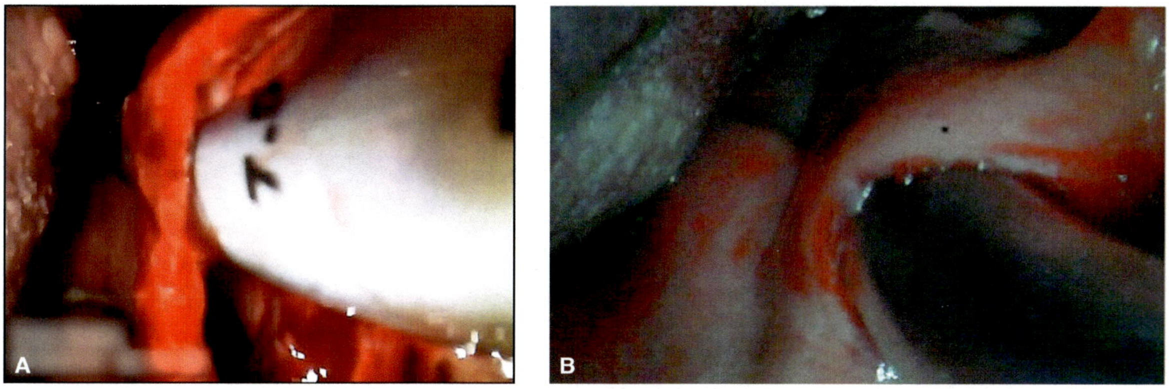

Figure 27.1. **A:** Traumatic pass of the tracheal tube through the palatoglossal arch during intubation with a video laryngoscopy. **B:** Example of complications of tracheal intubation. See also **Video 27.1**.

Suggested Readings

Brodsky MB, Akst LM, Jedlanek E, et al. Laryngeal injury and upper airway symptoms after endotracheal intubation during surgery: a systematic review and meta-analysis. *Anesth Analg.* 2021;132(4):1023–1032.

Hansel J, Rogers AM, Lewis SR, Cook TM, Smith AF. Videolaryngoscopy versus direct laryngoscopy for adults undergoing tracheal intubation. *Cochrane Database Syst Rev.* 2022;4(4):CD011136.

Joffe AM, Aziz MF, Posner KL, Duggan LV, Mincer SL, Domino KB. Management of difficult tracheal intubation: a closed claims analysis. *Anesthesiology.* 2019;131(4):818–829.

Liu J, Zhang X, Gong W, et al. Correlations between controlled endotracheal tube cuff pressure and postprocedural complications: a multicenter study. *Anesth Analg.* 2010;111(5):1133–1137.

28 The 2022 Difficult ASA Difficult Airway Infographic–Adult

William H. Rosenblatt

1 Describe in detail the device or technique.

The 2022 release of the American Society of Anesthesiologists (ASA) Guidelines for Management of the Difficult Airway introduced new tools for clinicians managing all patient airways. Whereas prior ASA airway management guidelines focused on patients receiving general anesthesia, and more specifically, where tracheal intubation was planned, the new guidelines consider plans for general, regional, and monitored anesthesia care (MAC). At the heart of these changes are the inclusion of a decision tree tool and an infographic (Figure 28.1) including this tool, an awake intubation pathway, and a "management after anesthetic induction" pathway. The phrase "anesthetic induction" or "induction of anesthesia" has become near synonymous with

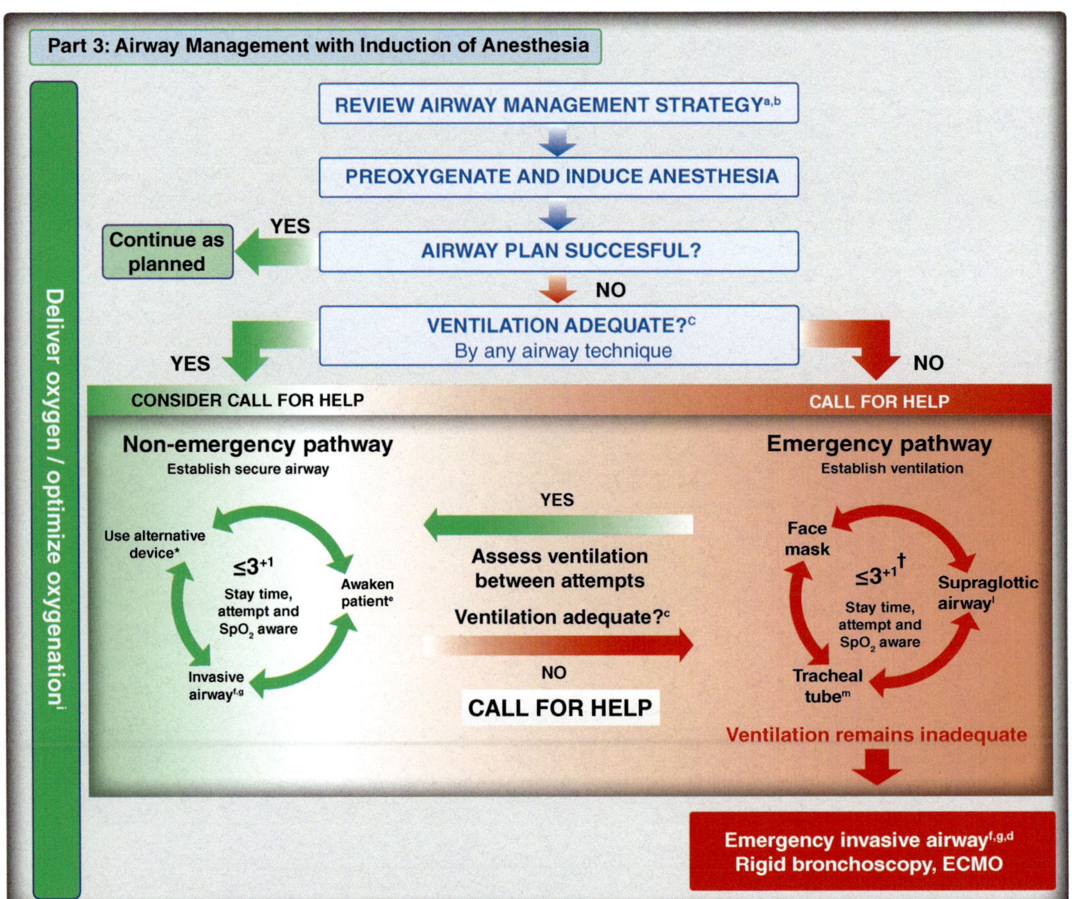

Figure 28.1. Adult Infographic, Part 3, of the American Society of Anesthesiologists Guidelines on Management of the Difficult Airway. (Reprinted with permission from Apfelbaum JL, Hagberg CA, Connis RT, et al. 2022 American Society of Anesthesiologists practice guidelines for management of the difficult airway. *Anesthesiology*. 2022;136(1):31–81. Copyright © 2021 The American Society of Anesthesiologists.)

the administration of a hypnotic agent that renders the patient unaware—this is a modern use of the term. The correct application of term "induction of anesthesia" is to any procedure that initiates or causes the anesthetic state (anesthesia meaning lack of sensation or lack of awareness). The new infographic includes pathways for care of the patient for whom a plan other than general anesthesia is implemented, but where that plan fails and manipulation and maintenance of the airway become necessary.

2 Where or when is the device used in airway management?

Part 3 of the infographic (Figure 28.1) is the airway management following induction of anesthesia pathway. This pathway is entered via the Decision Tree Tool (infographic part 1) after evaluation of the patient has revealed that, within the context of the clinician's experience and resources, their plan can be safely implemented. A review of the anesthetic and airway management plan is made, preferably with the entire group of clinicians caring for the patient. The elements of this review include anatomic risks, availability of resources (instruments and personnel), planned instrumentation, and contextual issues (eg, physical plant, space, and time considerations). All patients should receive preoxygenation in an effort to prolong an unintentional apneic period. Preoxygenation might be delivered via tight-fitting facemask, noninvasive positive pressure, or low or high-flow nasal cannula, depending on the plan.

Induction of anesthesia takes place and the clinician assesses the success of the management plan. The Infographic makes no effort to dictate the success or failure of the predetermined strategy—this is a clinical evaluation that is left to the managing clinician. Success might be an awake patient who has received minimal sedation and is undergoing a noninvasive and nonpainful procedure (eg, imaging), to a patient having a deep general anesthetic with invasive airway management. If the airway management plan is successful, the plan is continued. If the clinician deems that the plan is not successful, the adequacy of ventilation (as measured by detection of end-tidal CO_2) is assessed. "Ventilation" is the process of alveolar gas exchange, as assessed by the removal of CO_2. Sustained ventilation is the sine qua non of airway patency and alveolar gas exchange. Without alveolar gas exchange, oxygen cannot be supplied for metabolism. "Adequate" is a clinical judgment. The metabolic requirements of the patient must be maintained by the provision of oxygen. The clinician is charged with assessing that requirement, and clinically matching the ability to cause gas exchange.

If adequate ventilation has been achieved by any means (eg, face mask or supraglottic airway [SGA] ventilation, tracheal intubation, spontaneous ventilation), the nonemergency pathway is entered. The goal of this pathway is to provide a secure airway. This is achieved by one of three means: alternative means of airway control is attempted, the patient is allowed to return to their preinduction state or an invasive airway is performed (Table 28.1).

The question arises, how many attempts at laryngoscopy, SGA placement, and face mask ventilation should be used to secure an airway in the nonemergency pathway? The ASA guidelines, in its past iterations, has changed phrasing of the recommendation from "many" to "limit." Recent nonrandomized, prospective studies have informed the new infographic to recommend limiting attempts at each modality to 3 (though data for limiting facemask ventilation attempts is absent). Mort noted a significant increase in airway complications when greater than two attempts at direct laryngoscopy were used during intubation in an ICU setting. Other studies have found similar complications with three attempts, including when video laryngoscopy was employed. Likewise, decrease success rate at completing tracheal intubation occurred following three failed attempts at laryngoscopy. Similar data exist for SGA use. The goal of limiting attempts to equal or less than three for laryngoscopy and SGA placement is therefore twofold—first, to avoid fixating on a task with progressively less chance of success while expending safe apneic time; second, limiting airway trauma that might degrade the ability to continue adequate ventilation. One further attempt at airway management may be taken by a clinician with a higher level of skill than the primary operator.

Another often asked question is "when an attempt at one technique fails, what should I try next?" Given the differences in training and experience of clinicians, the variety of contexts in which care may be delivered, and the variability of equipment and skilled aid that may be available, a formula cannot be devised that will fit all scenarios. After a failed attempt at any technique of airway management, the next attempt will be dictated by the above factors as well as what is learned of the patient's airway during the prior attempts. For example, a failed direct laryngoscopy in an otherwise normal patient is likely due to lingual tonsil hyperplasia, and hyperangulated video laryngoscopy is likely to improve the view of the larynx. If, on the other hand, the clinician is not familiar with tracheal tube delivery around a hyperangulated blade, this might not be the best choice. Air

TABLE 28.1 Alternatives in Management in the Infographic Non-Emergency Pathway

Alternative Devices and Optimizations

Laryngoscopy and intubation
• Instrument
  • Direct laryngoscopy
  • Video laryngoscopy
    • Standard geometry blades
    • Hyperangulated blades
    • Channeled blades
  • Flexible laryngoscopy
  • Combined techniques
    • For example, rigid laryngoscopy/FIS[a] tube delivery
• Adjuncts and optimizations
  • Introducers
  • Rigid Stylets
  • Blade size
  • External laryngeal manipulation
Supraglottic airways
• First generation
• Second generation
• Size
• Design
• Combined techniques
  • For example, SGA and FIS tube delivery
Face mask ventilation adjuncts and optimizations
• Oral airway
• Nasal airway
• Mask size/design
• Two and three hand mask grip, VE grip
General optimizations
• Capable assistance
• Head and neck positioning
• Back elevated position
• Oxygenation throughout attempts
• Suction
• Muscle relaxants
• Consider other causes
  • Laryngospasm
  • Bronchospasm
  • Mass or foreign body

Awaken Patient
• Continue with awake intubation pathway • Postpone case: return with appropriate resource • Regional/infiltrative anesthesia • Elective invasive airway
Elective Invasive Airway
• In asleep or awake state • Continue upper airway ventilation throughout • Controlled conditions • Experienced provider as available

FIS: Flexible Intubation Scope.

leak during facemask ventilation in an individual with facial hair, is unlikely to be improved with the insertion of an oral airway, though SGA application may help.

Between attempts to secure the airway within the nonemergency pathway, ventilation should be reassessed. If at any point, ventilation becomes absent or inadequate, the emergency pathway is entered.

The goal of the emergency pathway is the establishment of adequate ventilation. This is achieved by cycling through the core techniques of airway management: facemask ventilation, SGA ventilation, and tracheal intubation. As with the nonemergent pathway, basic principles apply: limiting attempts at each core technique (three, plus one attempt for a clinician with more experience), assessing ventilation between attempts, and optimizing each attempt. The emergency pathway represents a more critical scenario—ventilation is not adequate and the patient is at risk of physiologic collapse and even death from the deprivation of oxygen. The Task Force recommends that the clinician stay aware of the number of attempts, contemplating the plateau of attempts with intubation and SGA ventilation, the passage of time, with the knowledge that limited oxygen reserves are being consumed, and the oxygen saturation that may herald the need to progress to an emergency invasive airway before the exhaustion of attempts. Yielding to the recommended number of attempts or a clinical appraisal of the exhaustion of safe apneic time encourages the clinician to progress to the emergency invasive airway pathway early, prior to a critical drop in the oxygen saturation. As discussed above, the literature indicates a futility in continuing with attempts at laryngoscopy and intubation. If attempts are continued into a period of plummeting oxygen saturation, the initiation of a surgical airway could also be futile. Severe physiologic compromise resulting from hypoxemia during the performance of an invasive airway may ensue. Early establishment of an invasive airway while oxygen reserves are sustaining the patient should result in a better outcome.

A controversial inclusion in the emergency pathway is the use of extracorporeal membrane oxygenation (ECMO) as a rescue modality. ECMO is a time and resource (human and equipment) intense procedure, and is unlikely to change patient outcome if instituted in a patient who is destined to experience severe oxyhemoglobin in a cannot intubate–cannot ventilate situation. The inclusion of ECMO in the pathway has two purposes. First, for the clinician who is casually reviewing the guidelines it is a prompt that ECMO may be a viable resource that would require preplanning. Second, in the clinical situation where ventilation is present, but inadequate, a patient may be maintained at marginal levels of oxygen saturation while ECMO resources are mustered.

The ASA Difficult Airway Infographic represents a departure from the traditional ASA Difficult Airway Algorithm. The utility of this tool will be judged over time, not only as a roadmap for airway management, but also as a cognitive aid during an airway crisis. Historically, the ASA Task Force on Management of the Difficult Airway reconvenes every decade to interpret the evidence-based literature and practice patterns. The infographic will undoubtedly undergo refinements in these cycles.

- The Adult Infographic provides a flexible, operator-centered algorithm for management of a failed airway plan.
- Adequate ventilation is the trigger evaluation for choosing between the nonemergent and emergent airway pathways.
- Attempts at laryngoscopy and SGA ventilation should be limited to three (each modality), with one more attempt by a more experienced clinician.
- ECMO can be considered in the patient with some, but not adequate gas exchange.
- *See Figure 28.2 and* ***Video 28.1*** *for additional details.*

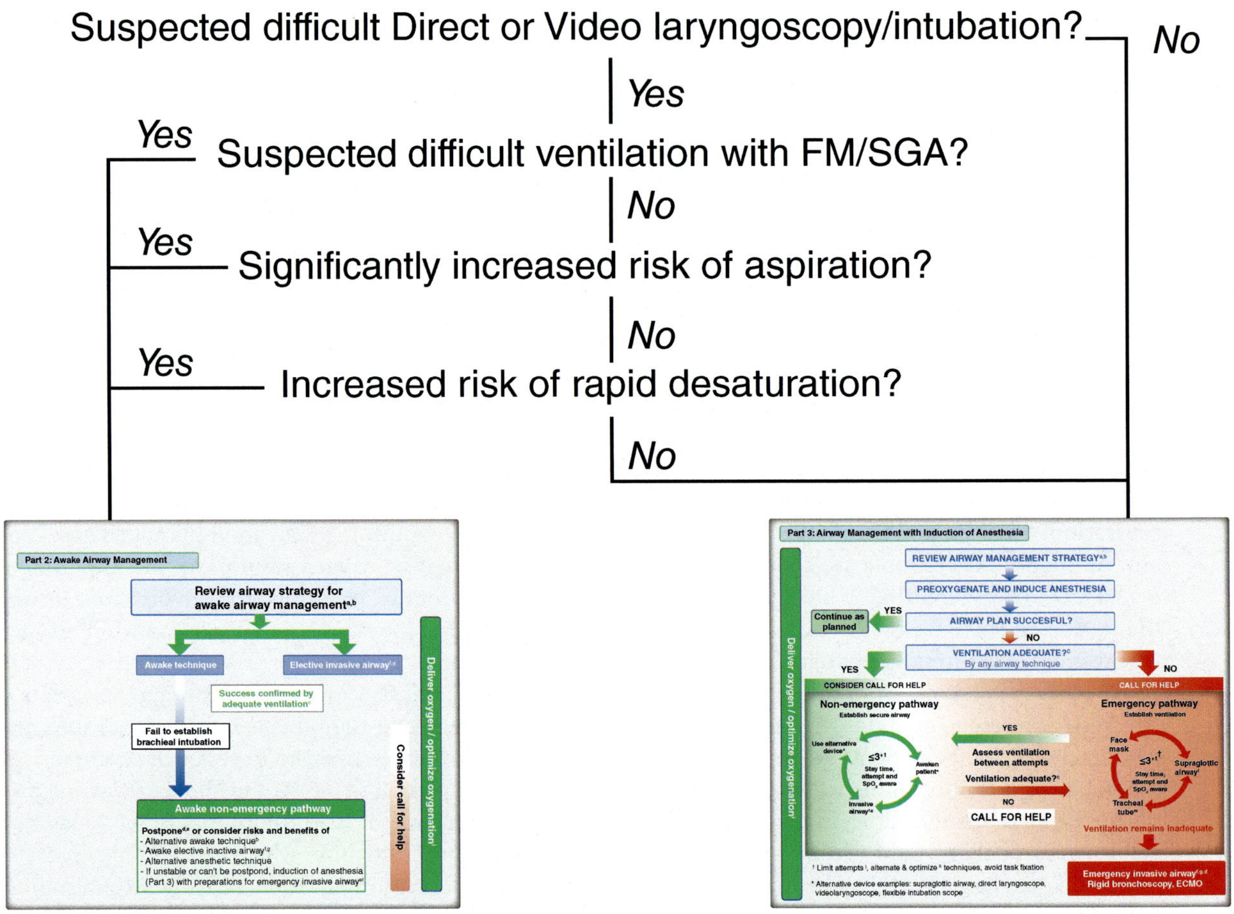

Figure 28.2. Factors included in Panel 1 of the ASA Difficult Airway Infographic aid the airway operator in choosing one of the two major management pathways, awake intubation or management after the induction of anesthesia. (Adapted with permission from Apfelbaum JL, Hagberg CA, Connis RT, et al. 2022 American Society of Anesthesiologists practice guidelines for management of the difficult airway. *Anesthesiology*. 2022;136(1):31–81. Copyright © 2021 The American Society of Anesthesiologists.)

Suggested Readings

Apfelbaum JL, Hagberg CA, Connis RT, et al. 2022 American Society of Anesthesiologists Practice Guidelines for Management of the Difficult Airway. *Anesthesiology*. 2021;136(1):31–81.

Goto T, Gibo K, Hagiwara Y, et al. Multiple failed intubation attempts are associated with decreased success rates on the first rescue intubation in the emergency department: a retrospective analysis of multicentre observational data. *Scand J Trauma Resusc Emerg Med*. 2015;23:5.

Jarvis JL, Barton D, Wang H. Defining the plateau point: When are further attempts futile in out-of-hospital advanced airway management? *Resuscitation*. 2018;130:57–60.

Kerslake D, Oglesby AJ, Di Rollo N, et al. Tracheal intubation in an urban emergency department in Scotland: a prospective, observational study of 3738 intubations. *Resuscitation*. 2015;89:20–24.

Mort TC. Emergency tracheal intubation: complications associated with repeated laryngoscopic attempts. *Anesth Analg*. 2004;99(2):607–613, table of contents.

The 2022 ASA Difficult Airway Infographic–Pediatric

29

Gabrielle Musci

1 Describe in detail the device or technique.

The 2022 update to the ASA guidelines for difficult airway management include, for the first time, a separate algorithm and infographic for pediatric patients (Figure 29.1). Specific pediatric concerns include the likelihood of an uncooperative patient and avoidance of using airway exchange catheters that can cause trauma in a small airway.

DIFFICULT AIRWAY INFOGRAPHIC: PEDIATRIC PATIENTS

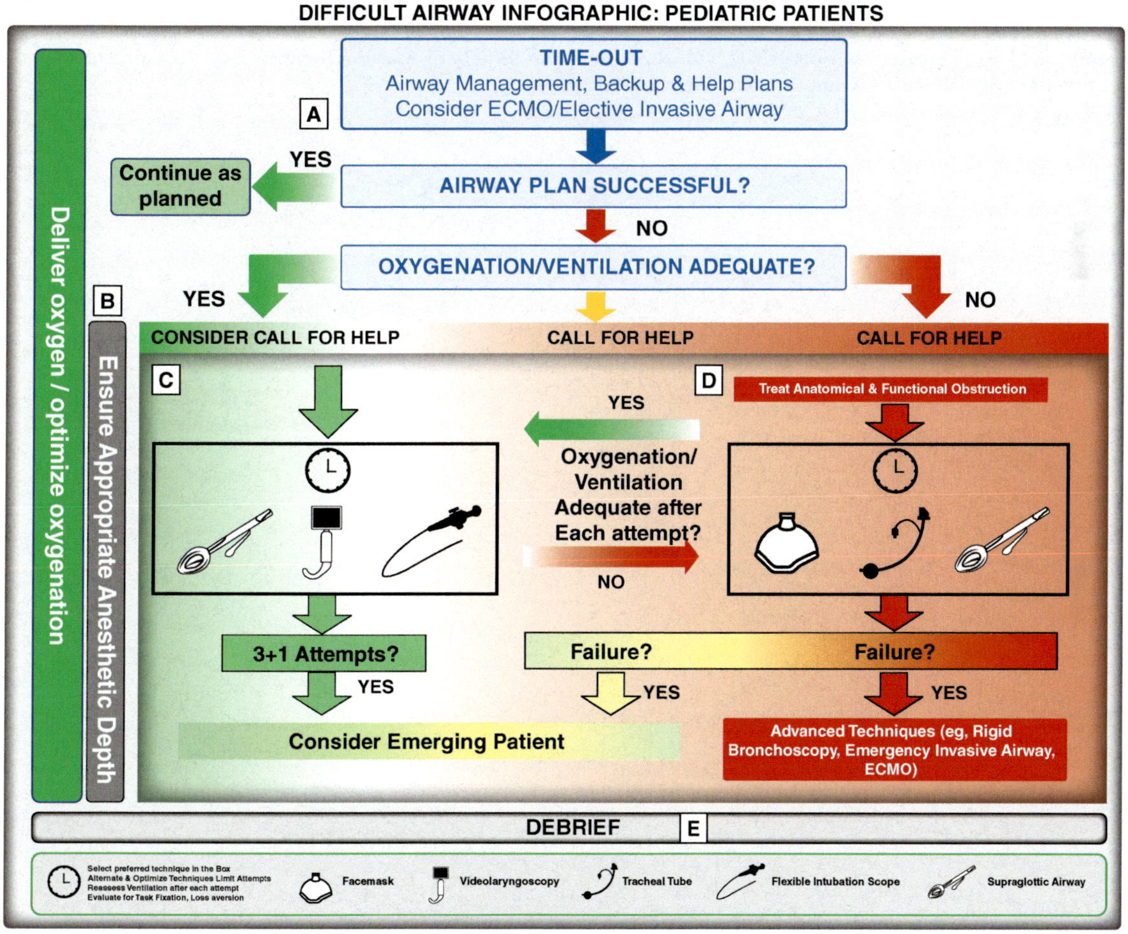

Figure 29.1. Difficult pediatric airway infographic. (Reprinted with permission from Apfelbaum JL, Hagberg CA, Connis RT, et al. 2022 American Society of Anesthesiologists practice guidelines for management of the difficult airway. *Anesthesiology*. 2022;136(1):31–81. Copyright © 2021 The American Society of Anesthesiologists.)

2 Where or when is this device or technique used in airway management?

As in the adult patient, the decision regarding airway management in a potential difficult airway must be made whether the intubation can be performed awake or after induction. However, pediatric patients prove more challenging since they will likely not tolerate an awake or lightly sedated intervention. When a difficult pediatric airway is anticipated, the importance of a time-out is emphasized and should include discussion of rescue airway techniques such as a surgical airway, ventilation via rigid bronchoscopy, or the initiation of ECMO.

After optimal positioning with an elevated head of the bed and a noninvasive oxygen source to enhance oxygenation, the care team may proceed with awake intubation via fiberoptic bronchoscopy, direct laryngoscopy, video laryngoscopy, or even a retrograde intubation with use of a wire. If initial attempts to secure the airway fail, then the team may need to halt airway manipulation, and the case may need to be postponed. If postponement is not an option, then the team should focus on oxygenation between attempts, consider placement of a supraglottic airway (to ventilate or for purposes of intubating), or rely on backup emergency methods.

The major differences between the adult and pediatric infographics echo the differences in guidelines as well as the typical challenges faced when anesthetizing a pediatric patient. Most children will need to proceed with postinduction intubation attempts. Preoxygenation is often difficult or impossible with an uncooperative patient; therefore, attempts to oxygenate throughout intubation attempts are highlighted. Finally, supraglottic airway use occurs earlier in the pediatric infographic than in its adult counterpart.

Important similarities between the pediatric and adult airway include optimization of oxygenation between attempts, limiting attempts, being aware of the passage of time, calling for help, and avoiding task fixation.

Suggested Readings

American Society of Anesthesiologists: Practice guidelines for management of the difficult airway: an updated report. *Anesthesiology.* 2013;118:251–270.

Apfelbaum JL, Hagberg CA, Connis RT, et al. 2022 American Society of Anesthesiologists Practice Guideline for Management of the Difficult Airway. *Anesthesiology*. 2022;136:31–81.

Unexpected Failed Direct Laryngoscopy

30

Jennifer E. Sainsbury

Clinical Scenario: An otherwise healthy patient presents for lower abdominal surgery. According to the patient, surgery under general anesthesia, 6 months earlier, was uneventful, though it was done elsewhere, and the records are unavailable. After induction of anesthesia, bag mask ventilation is easy, but direct laryngoscopy reveals a Cormack–Lehane grade III view that does not improve with external laryngeal pressure (backward upward rightward laryngeal pressure [BURP]) or head elevation (head elevation laryngoscopy position [HELP]). Blind intubation with an endotracheal tube introducer ("bougie") is unsuccessful.

1 How common is difficult laryngoscopy or intubation and can it be predicted?

This scenario is not uncommon (Figure 30.1 and **Video 30.1**). Despite performing bedside examination of the airway to predict ease of tracheal intubation, direct laryngoscopy can sometimes prove more difficult than expected. A large meta-analysis found that direct laryngoscopy resulted in a Cormack–Lehane grade III or IV view in 5.8% of patients without airway pathology. Among obese patients, this increased to 15.8% of patients. In a prospective study looking at an Intubation Difficulty Score (>5), at least moderate difficulty was encountered in 7.7% of patients, requiring two or more techniques in 9% of patients.

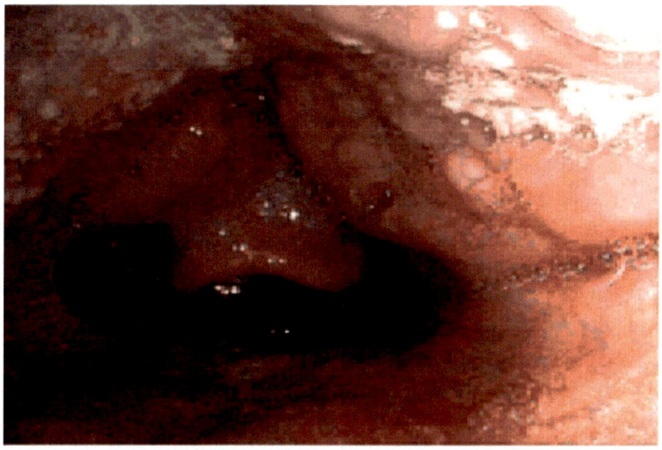

Figure 30.1. Case of unexpected failed direct laryngoscopy.

Bedside screening tests designed to predict a difficult tracheal intubation include the Mallampati oropharyngeal classification, thyromental distance, sternomental distance, mouth opening, upper lip bite test, mandibular protrusion, and composite scores such as the Wilson risk score. Individually, they yield poor to moderate sensitivity (20% to 62%) and moderate to fair specificity (82% to 97%). Until recently, it appeared that the most useful predictor was a combination of the Mallampati classification and thyromental distance (positive likelihood ratio 9.9; 95% CI 3.1 to 31.9). The Mallampati classification estimates the size of the tongue relative to the oral cavity and the likelihood that there is sufficient space to accommodate the tongue, laryngoscope, tracheal tube, and provide an unobstructed laryngeal view. Thyromental distance is an indicator of mandibular space, reflecting potential tongue displacement. A recent systematic review indicated that the "upper lip bite test" was the most predictive indicator of a potentially difficult intubation. The inability to bite the upper lip with the lower teeth (class 3) increased the probability of a difficult intubation from 10% to more than 60%.

These tests have been calibrated and validated for direct laryngoscopy and may not be applicable to other techniques. BURP and the HELP may increase laryngeal exposure. A tracheal introducer or "bougie" may facilitate blind intubation when laryngeal exposure cannot be obtained, however, recent guidelines advocate visualized tracheal intubation using video laryngoscopy in preference to a blind bougie technique (with its lower success and higher risk of airway trauma).

2 Does video laryngoscopy improve the laryngeal view and result in more successful intubations?

There is increasing evidence supporting a reduction in the incidence of intubation failure when using a video laryngoscope (VL) rather than a direct laryngoscope (DL), particularly in the context of a difficult airway. Video laryngoscopy has been demonstrated to produce superior laryngeal views. In a large study where the GlideScope (GVL) was used in 2004 of 71,570 attempted intubations, 81% of whom had features predictive of a difficult intubation by direct laryngoscopy, an overall success rate of 97% was observed. When used as the primary device in patients with and without predictors of difficult (direct) laryngoscopy, the success rates were 96% and 98%, respectively. When video laryngoscopy was used after failed direct laryngoscopy or flexible bronchoscopic intubation, the respective success rates were 94% ($n = 239$) and 8 of 10 cases. Many of the failures (35%) occurred despite good laryngeal exposure. Video laryngoscopy appears to provide better laryngeal exposure and reduce the number of laryngoscopies where the glottis cannot be seen, which therefore may reduce the incidence of laryngeal trauma, and consequently make tracheal intubation easier. It often proves successful in situations where the line-of-sight requirement of direct laryngoscopy fails. The hand–eye coordination necessary to deliver the tracheal tube to a glottis on a video display requires deliberate practice and may result in more prolonged intubation times.

Factors predicting difficult glideScope video laryngoscopy (GVL) intubation probably apply to other hyperangulated video laryngoscopes and include abnormal neck anatomy (thick neck, scars, radiation, or mass), thyromental distance <6 cm, reduced cervical extension, and prior experience with the selected device.

3 Do video laryngoscopes differ in laryngeal exposure and intubation success?

Direct and video laryngoscopy have the same goal—providing laryngeal exposure to enable tracheal intubation. Direct laryngoscopy achieves this by tongue displacement, mandibular protrusion, and occasionally the downward displacement of the larynx. Video laryngoscopy accomplishes this by positioning a lens, prism or video chip at the base of the tongue enabling a "look around the corner" without tissue compression or distraction. Some devices are more angulated, or hyperangulated, than others such as Verathon GVL, McGrath Series 5, and the Storz C-MAC D-blade. Others are configured like the Macintosh DL, for example, the Storz C-MAC Macintosh and McGrath Mac. Hyperangulated VLs are more likely to provide a laryngeal view when a line of sight is challenging, but they require the use of a stylet or tracheal tube introducer and practiced hand–eye coordination. Video laryngoscopes with channels (eg, Airtraq, Pentax AWS) offer a compromise. They provide good laryngeal exposure, may not require a stylet, the tracheal tube is housed within the blade, and are less demanding of hand–eye coordination. These advantages may be offset by a bulkier blade and the inability to independently manipulate the blade and tracheal tube. At this point, there is insufficient information to compare the clinical performance with devices; selection is largely a matter of preference, and outcomes depend upon prior practice under less demanding circumstances. It is important to bear in mind that many studies involve manikins, limited operator training, incomplete patient descriptions, inappropriate providers, and a variety of clinical outcomes, making it difficult to draw meaningful conclusions.

4 Our patient was easily bag mask ventilated. Direct laryngoscopy provided a Cormack–Lehane III view despite burp and head elevation. "Blind intubation" assisted by a "bougie" was unsuccessful. Where do we go from here?

Assuming that oxygenation was adequately maintained and the patient was not at increased risk of regurgitation and aspiration, it is important to select a technique that has a high probability of success in the operator's hands. Additional unsuccessful attempts are associated with significant complications and increase the probability of producing a cannot intubate/cannot oxygenate situation. A call for help would be appropriate, as would a request for a familiar alternative device. The options are many and include a supraglottic airway device (which may also be used as a conduit for tracheal intubation), a video laryngoscope, a video stylet, a flexible bronchoscope, or a combined approach of VL-assisted flexible bronchoscope. In a large, multicenter study, after failed direct laryngoscopy, 1619 rescue attempts were performed in 1427 out of 346,861 cases. Video laryngoscopy was the most frequently chosen rescue technique (69%) and had the highest success rate (92%) among the alternative techniques.

If a poor laryngeal view is obtained using a VL, a tracheal tube preloaded onto a flexible bronchoscope may provide better laryngeal exposure and serve as an introducer. Good laryngeal exposure is important, but is insufficient if difficulties are encountered directing the tracheal tube to the larynx. This can also be managed using a preloaded tracheal tube on a flexible bronchoscope.

If face mask ventilation or oxygenation had been challenging, the authors would recommend a supraglottic airway. It would also be prudent to ensure that the equipment and personnel are available for an emergency front-of-neck access, should this prove necessary.

In the situation described above, mask ventilation was easy. We would request a familiar video laryngoscope, and a stylet or "bougie" if appropriate for the device. If that device happened to be a hyperangulated VL, we recommend configuring a stylet in the shape of a "drooping J," lightly lubricating the superior surface of the blade, positioning it in the midline, and rotating it around the tongue base. A wider field of view, less anterior angulation of the laryngeal axis, and tracheal tube manipulation are more effectively achieved if the blade is not advanced deeply. With the distal portion of the blade parallel with the floor, taking care to avoid tilting the laryngeal axis upward, the blade is gently lifted vertically. Efforts to maximize laryngeal exposure impart unnecessary force and tend to result in anterior laryngeal rotation. The styletted tracheal tube should be introduced under direct vision, parallel and adjacent to the blade. Once past the soft tissues, the operator's attention is returned to the video monitor, and the tube is positioned proximal and dorsal to the arytenoid cartilages. Gentle elevation followed by very minimal tilting of the tracheal tube will generally result in successful placement. Once the tip of the tube is through the vocal folds, the stylet is partially withdrawn, and the tube is advanced. If resistance to tube advancement is encountered, gentle rotation of the tube will disengage it from the anterior tracheal wall.

The aforementioned technique provided good laryngeal exposure and easy tracheal intubation. A note was included in the anesthetic record indicating that bag mask ventilation had been easily achieved, direct laryngoscopy with a Macintosh laryngoscope provided a Cormack–Lehane III view despite BURP and HELP, but intubation with a GlideScope video laryngoscope resulted in a Cormack–Lehane I view and successful intubation. The authors recommend that the patient be provided with a difficult airway letter indicating the unsuccessful and successful strategies.

- When planning airway management, the airway provider should strive to achieve first-attempt success. This involves optimal positioning, appropriate equipment, and competent providers working in an atmosphere free from distractions.
- Never fail to prepare for failure.
- Each successive attempt at laryngoscopy and/or intubation increases the risk of complications, increasing the risk of converting a cannot intubate to a cannot oxygenate situation.
- Success with line-of-sight and indirect techniques have different risk profiles, demands different skills and success increases with practice.
- *See Figure 30.2 for additional details.*

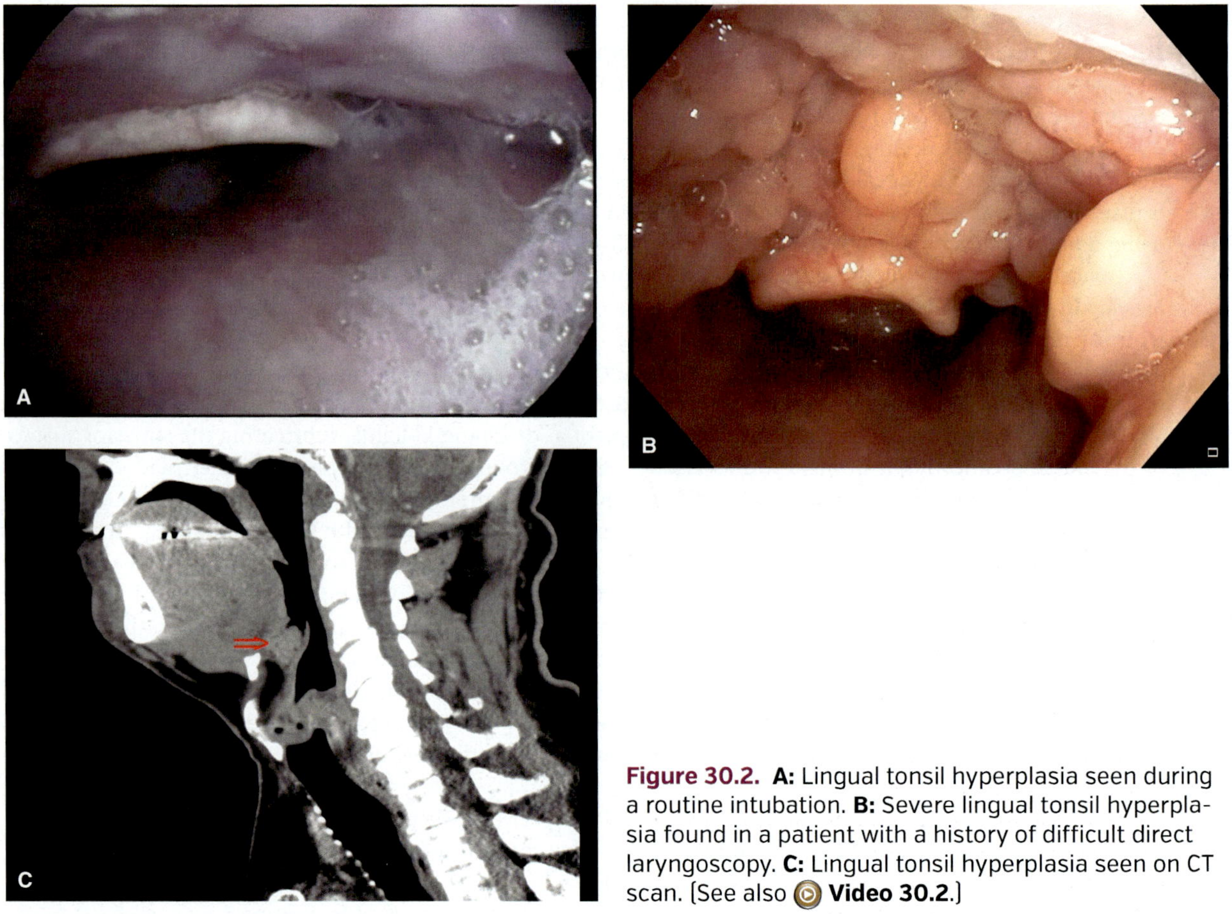

Figure 30.2. **A:** Lingual tonsil hyperplasia seen during a routine intubation. **B:** Severe lingual tonsil hyperplasia found in a patient with a history of difficult direct laryngoscopy. **C:** Lingual tonsil hyperplasia seen on CT scan. (See also **Video 30.2**.)

Suggested Readings

Adnet F, Racine SX, Borron SW, et al. A survey of tracheal intubation difficulty in the operating room: a prospective observational study. *Acta Anaesthesiol Scand.* 2001;45:327–332.

Aziz MF, Brambrink AM, Healy DW, et al. Success of intubation rescue techniques after failed direct laryngoscopy in adults: a retrospective comparative analysis from the multicenter perioperative outcomes group. *Anesthesiology.* 2016;125(4):656–666.

Aziz MF, Healy D, Kheterpal S, Fu RF, Dillman D, Brambrink A. Routine clinical practice effectiveness of the glidescope in difficult airway management: an analysis of 2,004 Glidescope intubations, complications, and failures from two institutions. *Anesthesiology.* 2011;114:34–41.

Cooper RM, Lee C. Role of rigid video laryngoscopy. In: Glick D, Cooper R, Ovassapian A, eds. *The Difficult Airway: An Atlas of Tools and Techniques for Clinical Management.* Springer; 2013: 77–111.

Cooper RM. Preparation for and management of "failed" laryngoscopy and/or intubation. *Anesthesiology.* 2019;130:833–849.

Detsky ME, Jivraj N, Adhikari NK, et al. Will this patient be difficult to intubate? The rational clinical examination systemic review. *JAMA.* 2019;321(5):493–503.

Jungbauer A, Schumann M, Brunkhorst V, Borgers A, Groeben H. Expected difficult tracheal intubation: a prospective comparison of direct laryngoscopy and video laryngoscopy in 200 patients. *Br J Anaesth.* 2009;102:546–550.

Levitan RM, Heitz JW, Sweeney M, Cooper RM. The complexities of tracheal intubation with direct laryngoscopy and alternative intubation devices. *Ann Emerg Med.* 2011;57:240–247.

Lewis SR, Butler AR, Parker J, Cook TM, Schofield-Robinson OJ, Smith AF. Videolaryngoscopy versus direct laryngoscopy for adult patients requiring tracheal intubation: a Cochrane Systematic Review. *Br J Anaesth.* 2017;119(3):369–383.

Mazzinari G, Rovira L, Henao L, et al. Effect of Dynamic versus stylet-guided intubation on first-attempt success in difficult airways undergoing Glidescope laryngoscopy: a randomized controlled trial. *Anesth Analg.* 2019;128:1264–1271.

Mihai R, Blair E, Kay H, Cook TM. A quantitative review and meta-analysis of performance of non-standard laryngoscopes and rigid fibreoptic intubation aids. *Anaesthesia.* 2008;63:745–760.

Shiga T, Wajima Z, Inoue T, Sakamoto A. Predicting difficult intubation in apparently normal patients: a meta-analysis of bedside screening test performance. *Anesthesiology.* 2005;103:429–437.

Sun DA, Warriner CB, Parsons DG, Klein R, Umedaly HS, Moult M. The GlideScope Video Laryngoscope: randomized clinical trial in 200 patients. *Br J Anaesth.* 2005;94:381–384.

Failed Direct Laryngotracheal Intubation Rescue

31

Kenneth N. Hiller • Neil S. Ballard • Carin A. Hagberg

Clinical Scenario: A 48-year-old woman presents for laparoscopic intra-abdominal surgery. She has a body mass index of 45 kg/m^2 and a neck circumference of 42 cm, with an otherwise normal airway examination. She is positioned on the OR table using a specialized obesity pillow to achieve external auditory meatus—sternal notch alignment. After induction of anesthesia and mask ventilation with an oral airway, direct laryngoscopy fails on two attempts. Mask ventilation remains easy between attempts. The patient's trachea is intubated with a channel-type video laryngoscope.

1 What are the anesthetic and airway management considerations for this case?

The preoperative airway physical examination reveals a significant nonreassuring finding, a thick neck, but is otherwise normal. A combination of increasing neck circumference and Mallampati score ≥3 has been associated with problematic intubation. It is recommended that neck circumference be routinely assessed during the preoperative airway evaluation, especially in obese patients.

The anesthetic and airway management considerations for this morbidly obese patient include risk of hypoxemia, pulmonary aspiration of gastric contents, a difficult airway (DA), and difficulty obtaining emergency invasive airway access. Deleterious respiratory physiologic changes in the morbidly obese patient include increase in airway resistance, oxygen consumption, and minute ventilation. Conversely, lung volumes, pulmonary compliance, chest wall compliance, and gas flows are reduced. Decreased expiratory reserve volume and functional residual capacity decline significantly following induction of anesthesia.

Several factors increase aspiration risk in the morbidly obese patient, including increased gastroesophageal reflux, reduced lower esophageal barrier pressure, and higher gastric volumes. Interestingly, recent literature suggests that gastric emptying is not impaired in obese patients and is not a primary factor in aspiration risk.

Pharyngeal obstruction resulting from "anatomical mismatch between the craniofacial bony enclosures and the amount of soft tissue" or physical obstruction from lingual tonsil hyperplasia, can increase the likelihood of experiencing difficulty with the airway in obese patients. Face mask ventilation, laryngoscopy, and emergency invasive airway access may prove more challenging. Preoperatively, attention should be paid to the recommendations of the American Society of Anesthesiologists' Practice Guidelines for Management of the Difficult Airway. The practitioner should consider awake intubation if the patient has multiple airway risk factors since alternative airway management plans will likely fail.

2 How would you manage the airway in this case?

In this scenario, direct laryngoscopy has failed twice, but face mask ventilation remains adequate. Thus, the nonemergent pathway of the DA algorithm should be followed. In such a situation, the authors would attempt video laryngoscopy (VL), and if unsuccessful, would place an intubating laryngeal mask airway (ILMA). VL has a high likelihood of success even in obese patients. ILMA placement is often successful since internal adipose tissue aligns the device along the midline with the glottis. It is important for the practitioner to oxygenate the patient in between intubation attempts and actively pursue opportunities to deliver supplemental oxygen throughout the process of DA management. Upon confirmation of adequate oxygenation and ventilation with an ILMA, a flexible intubating scope (FIS) can be used to place a tracheal tube. If an ILMA, such as the LMA Fastrach, is used, an FIS may not be necessary as this device is designed to be used as a blind technique. If unsuccessful, an FIS can be used. If an ILMA is not available, strong consideration should be given to the use of any immediately available supraglottic airway (SGA). Once an alternative SGA has been placed, an FIS loaded with an Aintree Intubation catheter (AIC) can be advanced into the trachea via the SGA. With the SGA and FIS withdrawn, an endotracheal tube of at least 7 mm internal diameter (ID) can be "railroaded" into the trachea over the well-lubricated AIC.

If unable to succeed with these alternative techniques, the authors would awaken the patient and perform an awake intubation.

3 What are the potential hazards and complications in regard to the airway?

Potential airway hazards inherent in the morbidly obese patient include precipitous oxygen desaturation, aspiration of gastric contents, and progressing difficulty with the airway, including loss of the airway. Proper positioning and preoxygenation, minimizing laryngoscopies, and early use of alternate airway devices may mitigate these dangers. Head-up positioning of 25 degrees (flexing the operating table at the hips) and nasal insufflation of oxygen after induction are simple maneuvers that have independently been shown to prolong the time of safe apnea.

Since multiple laryngoscopy attempts have been made in this patient, any further airway manipulation may result in a "cannot-intubate, cannot-ventilate" scenario. If this occurs, the practitioner should call for help. Emergency noninvasive airway ventilation via an SGA or emergency invasive airway access is recommended. Emergency invasive airway access includes jet ventilation and percutaneous or surgical airway. Difficulty in performing invasive techniques in morbidly obese patients is more likely than in nonobese patients if the neck circumference is high.

4 Are there special considerations for the emergence or end of the case?

Due to morbid obesity, the multiple airway manipulations, and likely iatrogenic airway trauma, the patient should be considered "at-risk" for extubation failure (see Chapter 44: Extubation of the Difficult Airway Patient). The practitioner should ensure that the patient is awake and responsive with adequate airway reflexes. Neuromuscular relaxation must be fully reversed. Although not foolproof, a cuff-leak test is recommended if airway edema or soiling is suspected. Administration of corticosteroids may reduce the likelihood of post-extubation stridor and reintubation.

The patient should be placed in a head-up position and preoxygenated. A staged extubation should be considered, with either an SGA or an airway exchange catheter. Postextubation, the patient should be positioned semi-upright. Early application of continuous positive airway pressure (CPAP) may be beneficial.

- Actively pursue opportunities to deliver supplemental oxygen throughout the process of DA management.
- Limit additional direct laryngoscopy attempts in "cannot-intubate, can-ventilate" scenarios.
- Consider using an alternative device, such as VL, or intubate via an SGA, during "cannot-intubate, can-ventilate" scenarios.
- *See Figures 31.1 and 31.2 for additional details.*

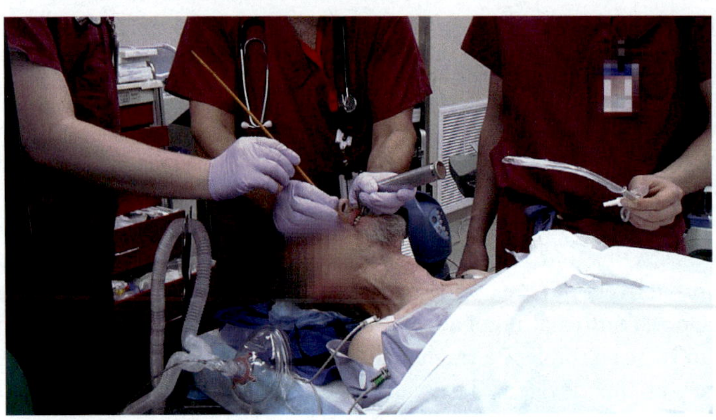

Figure 31.1. A bougie is used to facilitate intubation after a failed direct laryngoscopy. See **Video 31.1**.

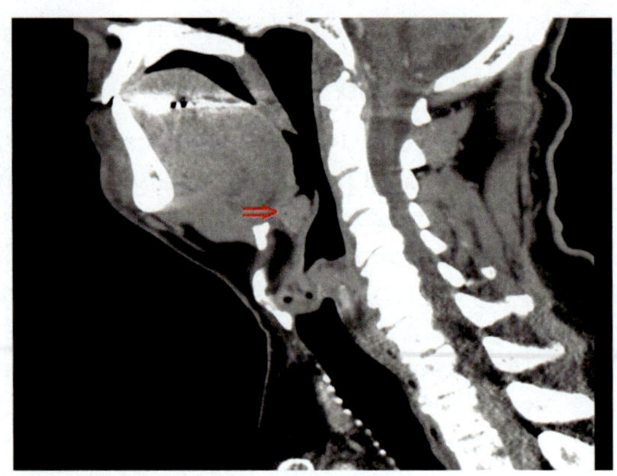

Figure 31.2. Incidental finding of lingual tonsil hyperplasia. See **Video 31.2**.

Suggested Readings

Apfelbaum JL, Hagberg CA, Connis RT, et al. 2022 American Society of Anesthesiologists Practice Guidelines for Management of the Difficult Airway. *Anesthesiology*. 2022;136(1):31–81.

Bein B, Scholz J. Anaesthesia for adults undergoing non-bariatric surgery. *Best Pract Res Clin Anaesthesiol*. 2011;25:37–51.

Buchholz V, Berkenstadt H, Goitein D, et al. Gastric emptying is not prolonged in obese patients. *Surg Obes Relat Dis*. 2013; 9(5):714–717.

Collins JS, Lemmens HJ, Brodsky JB, Brock-Utne JG, Levitan RM. Laryngoscopy and morbid obesity: a comparison of the "sniff" and "ramped" positions. *Obes Surg*. 2004;14(9):1171–1175.

de Leon A, Thorn SE, Wattwil M. High-resolution solid-state manometry of the upper and lower esophageal sphincters during anesthesia induction: a comparison between obese and non-obese patients. *Anesth Analg*. 2010;111:149–153.

Dixon BJ, Dixon JB, Carden JR et al. Preoxygenation is more effective in the 25 degrees head-up position than in the supine position in severely obese patients: a randomized controlled study. *Anesthesiology*. 2005;102(6):1110–1115; discussion 5A.

Gonzalez H, Minville V, Delanoue K, Mazerolles M, Concina D, Fourcade O. The importance of increased neck circumference to intubation difficulties in obese patients. *Anesth Analg*. 2008;106:1132–1136.

Kuriyama A, Umakoshi N, Sun R. Prophylactic corticosteroids for prevention of postextubation stridor and reintubation in adults: a systematic review and meta-analysis. *Chest*. 2017;151(5):1002–1010.

Moon TS, Tai K, Kim A, et al. Apneic oxygenation during prolonged laryngoscopy in obese patients: a randomized, double-blinded, controlled trial of nasal cannula oxygen administration. *Obes Surg*. 2019;29(12):3992–3999.

Neligan PJ, Malhotra G, Fraser M, et al. Continuous positive airway pressure via the Boussignac system immediately after extubation improves lung function in morbidly obese patients with obstructive sleep apnea undergoing laparoscopic bariatric surgery. *Anesthesiology*. 2009;110(4):878–884.

Turk M, Gravenstein D (2007): Aintree Intubation Catheter Technique in Unanticipated Difficult Intubation. Accessed January 21, 2002 from University of Florida Department of Anesthesiology, Center for Simulation, Advanced Learning and Technology, Virtual Anesthesia Machine Web site: http://vam.anest.ufl.edu/airwaydevice/aintree/index.html

Wong DT, Yang JJ, Mak HY, Jagannathan N. Use of intubation introducers through a supraglottic airway to facilitate tracheal intubation: a brief review. *Can J Anaesth*. 2012;59(7):704–715.

32 Stylet-Like Adjuncts to Laryngoscopy and Intubation

James C. DuCanto • Yen Chow

Clinical Scenario: A 45-year-old presenting for general anesthesia has an unanticipated difficult tracheal intubation (UDTI) with both direct and video laryngoscopies.

1 What are the anesthetic and airway management considerations for this case?

The incidence of a difficult laryngoscopy or intubation varies from 1.5% to 13%, and failed intubation has been identified as one of the anesthesia-related causes of death or permanent brain damage. In the management of UDTI, the anesthesia provider should follow the principles of the American Society of Anesthesiologists Difficult Airway Guidelines and prioritize the maintenance of ventilation and oxygenation, and seek additional resources including personnel (see Chapter 31: Failed Direct Laryngotracheal Intubation Rescue).

The causes of UDTI have at their root the inability to position the patient adequately to align the oral, hypopharyngeal, and laryngeal axes as well as the inability to displace the tongue and other tissues of the hypopharynx to permit either direct line-of-sight visualization or visualization of the airway structures with a laryngoscope (direct, video, or otherwise). Prevalent causes of UDTI include initial improper patient positioning (especially with morbidly obese patients), large tongue relative to oral cavity, lingual tonsil hypertrophy, limited mouth opening, and limitations in neck extension (see Chapters 30: Unexpected Failed Direct Laryngoscopy and 33: Optimizing Positioning for Direct Laryngoscopy).

When the laryngeal view is poor, use of a tracheal tube introducer with an angled distal tip can allow the anesthesia provider to negotiate a tracheal tube into the larynx and trachea without visualization. Tracheal tube introducers are commonly known as "bougies." The technique was originally described by Sir Robert Macintosh using a urinary "gum elastic bougie" and later popularized with the Eschmann tracheal tube introducer.

Passage of a bougie through the laryngeal inlet in cases of laryngeal pathology (distorted by swelling, infection, or tumor) is considerably more effective than with a tracheal tube due to its small diameter and intrinsic rigidity.

2 How would you manage the airway in this case?

If face mask ventilation is adequate, a repeat attempt at optimized direct or video laryngoscopy with the plan to use bougie-aided intubation is a reasonable follow-up maneuver. An attempt is made to place the bougie into the larynx and trachea, with partial visualization (modified Cormack–Lehane grade IIb) or without visualization (grade III or IV). Blind insertion of the bougie into the larynx and trachea is possible if the angled tip of the bougie can be negotiated along the posterior surface of the epiglottis in the midline. Once the distal bougie is beyond sight, noting markings on the shaft helps to keep the angulated tip oriented anteriorly. Entry of the bougie into the trachea is often accompanied with tactile feedback along the bougie's shaft as its angulated tip passes over the cartilaginous rings and intermembranous spaces of the trachea, producing "clicks," as it were. If clicks are not elicited, the bougie should be advanced gently to a maximum distance of 45 cm, or until distal holdup occurs, indicating contact with the narrowing bronchial tree. If clicks, holdup, or coughing (from tracheal irritation of the catheter) does not occur, it is likely that the bougie is not in the trachea, and thus is within the esophagus. Removal of the bougie is warranted with a return to mask ventilation between each intubation attempt.

Following successful tracheal placement of the bougie, a lubricated tracheal tube of appropriate size is passed over the catheter and into the trachea (often referred to as "railroading"). The smallest, clinically adequate tracheal tube should be chosen to reduce hang-up (see Chapter 20: Hang-Up During Intubation with the Flexible Intubation Scope). Tracheal tube passage over the bougie may be facilitated by keeping the airway axes aligned and by using a laryngoscope to anteriorize the soft tissues of the upper airway. Hang-up may occur when the tracheal tube bevel impinges on the right aryepiglottic fold, and will often be relieved by a 90-degree counterclockwise rotation.

Should the technique of bougie-aided intubation prove unsuccessful, a flexible intubation scope (FIS) or optical stylet can be substituted for the bougie during direct or video laryngoscopy in order to visually guide the intubation (see Chapters 17: Optical Stylets and 21: Combined Flexible Intubation Scope and Video Laryngoscopy).

3 What are the potential hazards and complications in regard to the airway?

Pitfalls in the use of the intubation bougie include the potential for tracheal abrasion, perforation of a bronchus if inserted too deeply (and/or with excessive force), as well as the potential to create a false passage in the piriform fossa.

4 What are the specific equipment?

A variety of tracheal tube introducers are available. As mentioned, the classic Eschmann tracheal tube introducer is a semimalleable, solid, resin-coated woven polyester device. Also available are hollow lumen introducers (eg, Frova Tracheal Tube Introducer, Cook Critical Care, Bloomington, IN) that may be fitted with a rigid stylet, and can accommodate jet ventilation and resuscitation bag adaptors. There are a variety of tracheal tube introducers with mechanical control components that alter the shape of the distal tip to navigate the oropharyngeal and hypopharyngeal curves such as the Flexible Tip Bougie and the Total Control Introducer.

5 Are there special considerations for the emergence or the end of the case?

Any patient can present a risk for respiratory failure at the time of emergence and extubation. Widely circulated criteria for tracheal extubation are available and are applied whenever possible. Despite the achievement of these criteria, the patient in whom tracheal intubation was unexpectedly difficult should be extubated with extra caution. Not only will the same anatomic parameters interfere with efforts to reintubate, but also it is likely that the initial manipulation of the airway resulted in local trauma and edema, which may confound efforts further (see Chapter 44: Extubation of the Difficult Airway Patient).

- In the management of UDTI, maintenance of ventilation and oxygenation takes precedence over the insertion of a tracheal tube.
- Blind insertion of the bougie into the larynx and trachea is possible if the angled tip of the bougie can be negotiated along the posterior surface of the epiglottis in the midline.
- Tactile detection of bougie contact with the tracheal rings is a more specific than sensitive indicator of successful placement into the trachea.
- Overzealous and forceful insertion of a bougie can result in upper airway, tracheal, and bronchial trauma.
- *See Figures 32.1 and 32.2.*

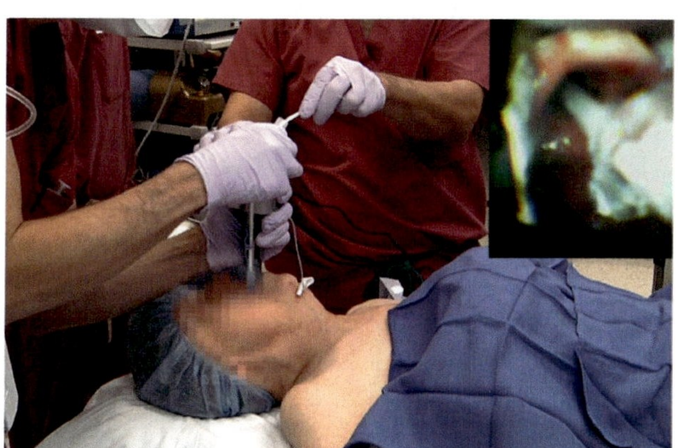

Figure 32.1. A bougie like device is used to intubate a patient through a channel scope device. Bougie and tracheal tube are seen entering the larynx (*inset*). See **Video 32.1**.

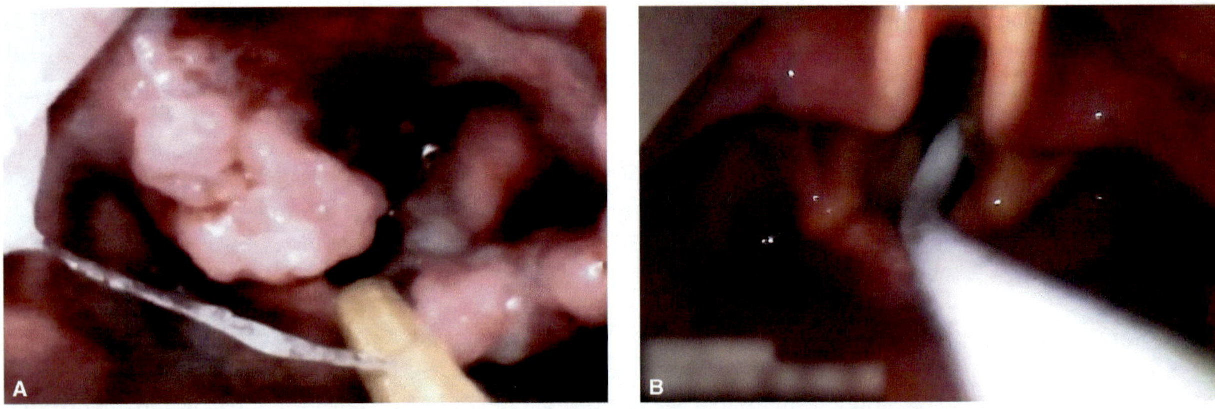

Figure 32.2. **A:** A tracheal tube introducer is introduced into the larynx of a patient with papillomatosis [**Video 32.2**]. **B:** The coude tip of a tracheal tube introducer is seen within the larynx [**Video 32.3**].

Suggested Readings

Cattano D, Melnikov V, Khalil Y, Sridhar S, Hagberg CA. An evaluation of the rapid airway management positioner in obese patients undergoing gastric bypass or laparoscopic gastric banding surgery. *Obes Surg*. 2010;20:1436–1441.

El-Ganzouri AR, McCarthy RJ, Tuman KJ, Tanck EN, Ivankovich AD. Preoperative airway assessment: predictive value of a multivariate risk index. *Anesth Analg*. 1996;82(6):1197–1204.

El-Orbany MI, Salem MR, Joseph NJ. The Eschmann tracheal tube introducer is not gum, elastic, or a bougie. *Anesthesiology*. 2004;101:1240.

Henderson JJ, Popat MT, Latto IP, Pearce AC; Difficult Airway Society. Difficult Airway Society guidelines for the management of the unanticipated difficult intubation. *Anaesthesia*. 2004;59(7):675–694.

Nurfadilah M, Jaafar Z, et al. The performance of the Flexible Tip Bougie™ in intubating simulated difficult airway model. *Frontiers in Medicine*. 2021;8:677626.

Randell T. Prediction of difficult intubation. *Acta Anaesthesiol Scand*. 1996;40(8 Pt 2):1016–1023.

Optimizing Positioning for Direct Laryngoscopy

33

Michael Ancuta

1 Describe in detail the device or technique.

In 1944, Bannister and Macbeth recommended Ivan Magill's "sniffing position" (Sniffing Position) for glottic exposure when using a straight laryngoscope blade, and suggested adding further elevation of the head when using a curved Macintosh laryngoscope blade. They believed that neck flexion combined with head extension aligned the oral, pharyngeal, and laryngeal axes (Three Axes Alignment Theory [TAAT]), thus allowing a direct line of vision to the glottis. Since that time, the sniffing position has become the standard head position for direct laryngoscopy (DL). More recently, explanations and theories other than the TAAT have been used to explain the advantages of this position during DL.

However, the advantage of the sniffing position for DL has not been universally accepted. Adnet et al. were unable to demonstrate axes alignment in the sniffing position using radiographs during tracheal intubation. Another study by this group claimed no significant advantages of the sniffing position compared to simple head extension for tracheal intubation. Interestingly, this latter study did find an advantage of the sniffing position in patients with obesity and those with limited ability to extend their neck, two important subgroups of patients with the potential for difficulty during DL. These "negative" studies have stimulated heated debate among anesthesiologists who have challenged their results. The studies have been criticized since the degree of neck flexion, the amount of head extension, the avoidance of neuromuscular agents for paralysis, and even the nonperformance of laryngoscopy in some subjects do not reflect actual clinical situations. Even the potential for bias has been raised because all these studies were not blinded.

To achieve a proper sniffing position, the patient's head should be elevated so that the angle of neck flexion over the chest is 35 degrees. The height of the head support to achieve this degree of flexion will depend on the individual's head and neck anatomy and the size of their chest. For most normal-weight patients with normal airways, the height of head elevation needed for optimal exposure is 7.0 to 9.0 cm. However, the actual degree of neck flexion and head elevation that gives the best view during DL will differ for individual patients. The endpoint for proper sniffing position is achieved when an imaginary horizontal line can be drawn from the sternum to the patient's external auditory meatus. For many patients with limited head and neck mobility, or for those with a less-than-optimal view with the head elevated to this degree, further elevation of the head improves the Cormack–Lehane view during DL. More recent studies have shown that 25-degree backup positioning can improve glottic visualization and efficacy of preoxygenation in comparison to supine positioning.

It is important to use a noncompressible head support. When pillows and blankets are used, the weight of the head will cause these supports to sag, resulting in a decrease in head elevation, attainment of only partial sniffing position, and a compromised view during DL. In addition, simply elevating the head in obese patients will not achieve the sniffing position. Padding or special elevation devices placed under the upper back, shoulders, head, and neck must be used to achieve a "ramped" or head-elevated laryngoscopy position (HELP) in obese patients. Adjustable inflatable pillow devices allow head elevation to be adjusted in real time, allowing for optimal positioning for each particular patient. Again, horizontal alignment between the sternum and the ear is the goal.

Head elevation alone will not produce the sniffing position. Sniffing position requires not just neck flexion from raising the head, but also head extension at the atlanto-occipital joint. For patients with limited ability to extend their neck, true sniffing position may not be achievable and visualization by DL may be suboptimal.

The consensus from the medical literature and clinical experience is that conventional sniffing position provides the best laryngeal view during DL. The degree of head elevation and the amount of neck flexion will vary from patient to patient.

- Optimal positioning for DL results from a horizontal alignment between the sternum and the external auditory meatus.
- The actual degree of neck flexion and head elevation that gives the best view during DL will differ for individual patients.
- Obtaining the optimal laryngoscopy position should be done with noncompressible head support. Adjustable inflatable pillow device allows real-time optimization of head position during DL.
- *See Figures 33.1 and 33.2 for additional details.*

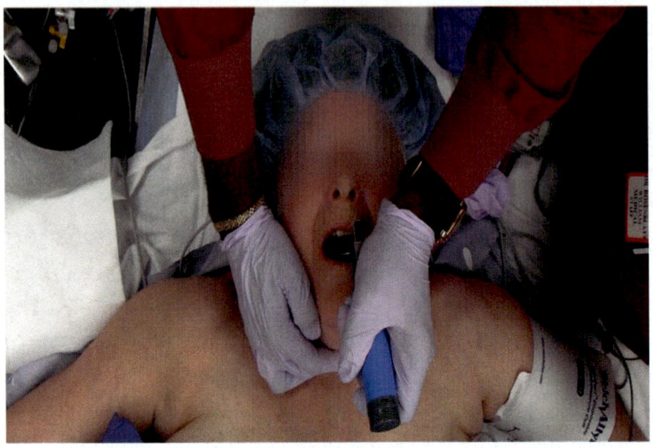

Figure 33.1. Positioning is a key factor in first-pass success when using direct laryngoscopy. See **Video 33.1**.

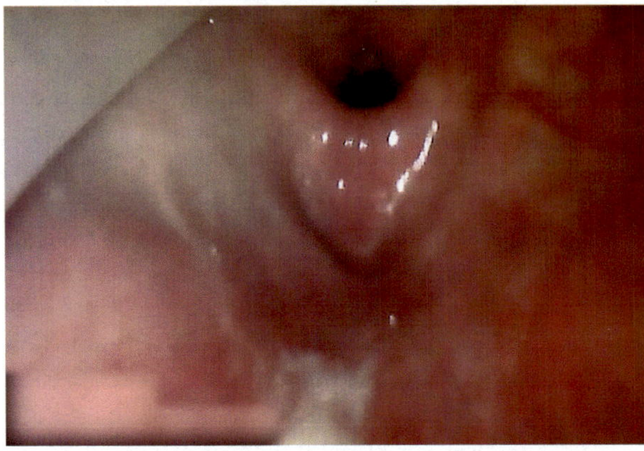

Figure 33.2. Poor laryngoscopic technique which can be complicated by poor positioning may result in errors such as the visualization of the esophageal inlet. See **Video 33.2**.

Acknowledgment

We gratefully acknowledge the contributions of previous edition author, Jay B. Brodsky, as portions of those chapters have been retained in this revision.

Suggested Readings

Adnet F, Baillard C, Borron SW, et al. Randomized study comparing the "sniffing position" with simple head extension for laryngoscopic view in elective surgical patients. *Anesthesiology*. 2001;95:836–841.

Al-Jadidi AM, Khan RM, Sharma PK, Kaul N. Dynamic optimization of the sniff position during laryngoscopy using a pressure infusion bag. *Anaesthesia*. 2012;67:677–678.

Collins JS, Lemmens HJ, Brodsky JB, et al. Laryngoscopy and morbid obesity: a comparison of the "sniff" and "ramped" positions. *Obes Surg*. 2004;14:1171–1175.

Dixon BJ, Dixon JB, Carden JR, et al. Preoxygenation is more effective in the 25 degrees head-up position than in the supine position in severely obese patients: a randomized controlled study. *Anesthesiology*. 2005;102(6):1110–1115; discussion 5A.

El-Orbany M, Woehlck H, Salem MR. Head and neck position for direct laryngoscopy. *Anesth Analg*. 2011;113:103–109.

Lee BJ, Kang JM, Kim DO. Laryngeal exposure during laryngoscopy is better in the 25 degrees back-up position than in the supine position. *Br J Anaesth*. 2007;99:581–586.

Levitan RM, Mechem CC, Ochroch EA, Shofer FS, Hollander JE. Head-elevated laryngoscopy position: Improving laryngeal exposure during laryngoscopy by increasing head elevation. *Ann Emerg Med*. 2003;41:322–330.

Schmitt HJ, Mang H. Head and neck elevation beyond the sniffing position improved laryngeal view in cases of difficult direct laryngoscopy. *J Clin Anesth*. 2002;14:335–338.

Preinduction Determination of Cannot Ventilate by Face Mask

34

Ramneek Maan

Clinical Scenario: An elderly man presents with profuse bleeding following a Mohs procedure on the bridge of his nose. He requires urgent hemostatic control and skin flap coverage. His nose is covered by a large, blood-soaked bandage, and he has been kept NPO. There is no evidence of internal bleeding. The patient has a history of ischemic cardiomyopathy, with a recent ejection fraction of 30%. He is being treated for unstable angina with oral nitrates and clopidogrel. The bleeding has persisted for over 6 hours, and the exact volume of the blood loss is unknown.

1 What are the anesthetic and airway management considerations for this case?

The anesthesia face mask is the most widely used device for both preoxygenation prior to the induction of anesthesia and for preintubation positive-pressure ventilation. Although rare, there may be clinical situations where the use of the anesthesia face mask is not feasible or contraindicated. In the current case, the patient requires control of the airway without the use of a face mask, which requires an airtight seal over the bridge of the nose. Given the patient's significant heart disease and potential intravascular volume depletion, a stable hemodynamic approach to the induction of anesthesia is essential. An awake intubation technique may be considered; however, it could lead to increased blood pressure during laryngoscopy that could exacerbate bleeding. However, this risk can be mitigated through the aggressive use of airway analgesia, sedation, and antihypertensive therapy. In addition, there is a risk of aspiration of gastric contents if the patient has swallowed blood.

2 How would you manage the airway in this case?

Several approaches to airway management may be considered in this case. The author would opt for a second-generation supraglottic airway (2nd SGA) for the initial control of the airway. Compared to tracheal intubation, the placement of an SGA requires a less profound depth of anesthesia. In addition, the gastric drain of a 2nd SGA can channel any regurgitated gastric contents (eg, swallowed blood) away from the airway. Once intravascular volume has been stabilized with fluid replacement and preoxygenation has been achieved with a loose-fitting face mask (due to the nasal lesion and large bandage), an intravenous induction is achieved, and a 2nd SGA is placed at the loss of consciousness. After 2nd-SGA ventilation is established, muscle relaxants may be administered, and the patient brought to an anesthetic plane adequate for tracheal intubation. At this time, a gastric tube may be inserted through the gastric drain and stomach contents aspirated. When neuromuscular relaxation and a stable anesthetic state are attained, the 2nd SGA is removed, and tracheal intubation is performed using the method chosen by the operator.

3 What are the potential hazards and complications regarding the airway?

There are several hazards to consider during the airway management of this patient. First, at any point during airway management, including before induction of anesthesia, the patient may be at risk of aspiration of gastric contents, particularly if there has been occult ingestion of large volumes of blood. Since an air-tight face mask fit cannot be achieved prior to the induction of anesthesia, complete preoxygenation is compromised, and rapid oxyhemoglobin desaturation may occur if the airway remains uncontrolled at any juncture. Failure to successfully place the 2nd SGA may necessitate immediate direct or indirect laryngoscopy and intubation before a stable anesthetic state is established. In addition, laryngoscopy and intubation may be complicated by the presence of blood in the upper airway. Rescue laryngoscopy and intubation could require a rapid and possibly uncontrolled deepening of the anesthetic level, potentially compromising the patient's hemodynamic state.

4 Are there special considerations for the emergence or the end of the case?

Persistent hemorrhage in or around the airway should alert the anesthesiologist to the possibility of inadequate hemostasis. If there is suspicion of ongoing hemorrhage, it is imperative to engage in a discussion with the surgeon regarding the necessity of continuing tracheal intubation. If adequate hemostasis has been achieved, retained blood in the upper airway or passively swallowed blood remains a concern; thus, meticulous suctioning of the stomach and throat should precede extubation. Given that the surgical procedures in this case were distanced from the airway, the risk of airway edema or direct trauma compromising airway patency after extubation is minimal. Nonetheless, ensuring a full return of neuromuscular function is critical, not only to promote adequate airway patency, but also to afford maximal protection against blood aspiration. Due to the highly vascularized area of surgery, measures must be implemented to prevent coughing during emergence. Ideally, the patient should be awake, spontaneously breathing, and responsive to commands at the time of extubation. Should airway failure occur after extubation, face mask ventilation will likely remain contraindicated and possibly unachievable. Therefore, the clinician should be prepared for either 2nd-SGA rescue or immediate tracheal intubation.

- Routine preoxygenation is likely to be suboptimal or impossible in cases where an anesthesia face mask is contraindicated.
- In situations where an anesthesia face mask is contraindicated or likely to fail, immediate use of an SGA should be considered as an alternative.
- In the setting of bleeding around the face and airway, constant vigilance is required regarding the possibility of blood aspiration, subsequent regurgitation, and pulmonary aspiration.
- In patients at risk of having hemorrhagic complications around the head and neck, emergence and tracheal extubation precautions should be taken.
- *See Figures 34.1 and 34.2 for additional details.*

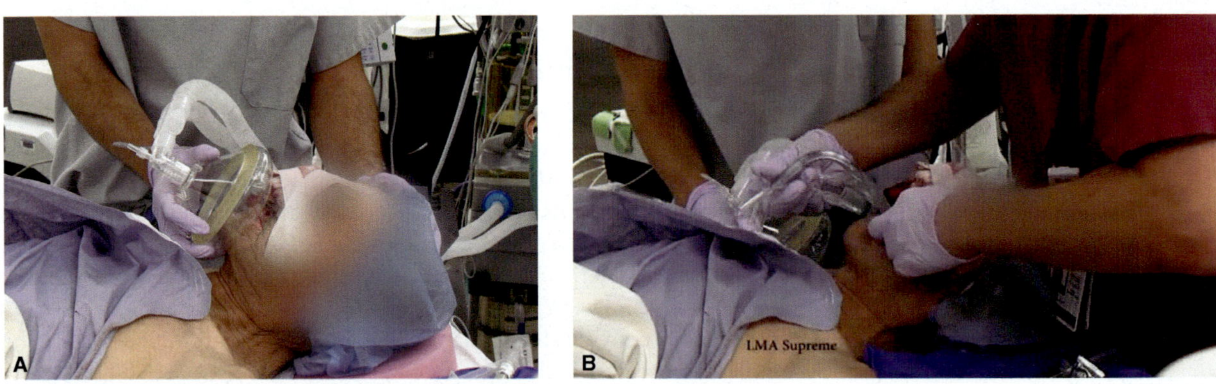

Figure 34.1. **A:** Before induction of anesthesia, the patient is preoxygenated with an anesthesia facemask. See **Video 34.1**. **B:** After induction of anesthesia, a supraglottic airway is used to ventilate the patient.

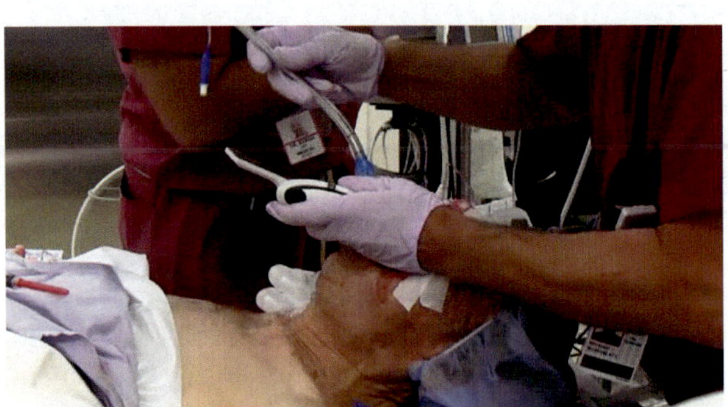

Figure 34.2. When the patient was ready for tracheal intubation, the supraglottic airway is removed and a video laryngoscope is used to complete the intubation.

Suggested Readings

Garcia-Marcinkiewicz AG, Lee LK, Haydar B, et al. Difficult or impossible facemask ventilation in children with difficult tracheal intubation: a retrospective analysis of the PeDI registry. *Br J Anaesth*. 2023;130.

Hagberg CA. Current concepts in the management of the difficult airway. *Anesthesiology News*. 2013;39:10.

Kheterpal S, Martin L, Shanks A, Tremper KK. Prediction and outcomes of impossible mask ventilation: a review of 50,000 anesthetics. *Anesthesiology*. 2009;110(4):891–897.

35 Preinduction Determination of Should Not Ventilate by Face Mask

Sonia Vaida • Arne Budde

Clinical Scenario: A 22-year-old woman has a cerebrospinal fluid (CSF) leak after transsphenoidal surgery for a pituitary tumor. The surgeon has requested that positive-pressure ventilation via face mask be avoided.

1 What are the anesthetic and airway management considerations for this case?

Patients with a known or suspected skull base defect are at risk for the development of pneumocephalus with positive-pressure mask ventilation (PPMV). In these patients, mask ventilation is contraindicated during the induction of anesthesia, including situations where intubation or supraglottic ventilation fails. In addition, mask ventilation will need to be avoided at the end of the procedure, at the time of emergence and extubation.

Transsphenoidal surgery for pituitary tumor removal can result in a communication between the nasal cavity and the intracranial cavity due to the defect of the bony skull structures, and subsequent spontaneous pneumocephalus can occur. Pneumocephalus is manifested by headaches, impaired mental status, and seizures. PPMV can aggravate an existing pneumocephalus with the forceful addition of more air into the cranium through the bony defect. The resulting mass effect of a tension pneumocephalus can become a life-threatening emergency.

After transsphenoidal surgery, nasal intubation is contraindicated for at least 2 weeks postoperatively due to the bony defect and consequent risk of cranial vault penetration by the tracheal tube.

An increased risk for difficult mask ventilation and laryngoscopy must be considered in a patient who has presented for pituitary surgery, especially if the underlying pathology is manifest as acromegaly (prognathism due to mandibular bone proliferation, enlarged tongue, upper airway soft tissue hypertrophy, obstructive sleep apnea) or Cushing disease (obesity, obstructive sleep apnea). A patient with an infected graft post-transsphenoidal pituitary tumor resection may present with trismus.

2 How would you manage the airway in this case?

Mask ventilation as well as nasal intubation should be completely avoided in this patient's case. Planning the airway management will initially require an assessment of the patient's ability to cooperate during an awake intubation, and the likelihood of successful insertion and ventilation with a supraglottic airway (SGA) device. The patient should be fasted, and risk factors for gastric content aspiration should be considered. Based on this evaluation, several possible airway management options exist: awake intubation, induction of anesthesia with a spontaneously breathing patient, or asleep intubation using rapid sequence induction (RSI).

For increased safety, an awake intubation technique may be preferred. Sedation should be limited, keeping in mind that mask ventilation is not an option should the patient become apneic (see Chapter 11: Preparation for Awake Intubation). If the patient has trismus due to an infected graft, the preparation for awake intubation may be difficult. Despite this, careful preparation should result in a patient who can undergo awake intubation. Alternatively, if access to the upper airway is not possible, tracheotomy or cricothyrotomy performed under local anesthesia could be considered.

If awake intubation is not considered mandatory for patient safety, there are several other options for management.

A variety of SGA devices can be used as an alternative to mask ventilation primarily to control the airway, followed by exchange with a tracheal tube for definitive airway control (see Chapter 84: Aintree Catheter Use for Supraglottic Airway to Endotracheal Tube Conversion). Several techniques have been described to facilitate tracheal intubation through an SGA device, such as blind or flexible intubating scope (FIS)-guided intubation or intubation facilitated by intubation introducers. Intubating SGA devices, such as the LMA-Fastrach, Aura-I, and AirQ, have the advantage of being both effective ventilatory devices and conduits for a blind

(LMA-Fastrach) or an FIS-guided intubation. If deemed necessary, these devices can be inserted in the awake patient, followed by the induction of anesthesia. The SGA device can then be changed to a tracheal tube with or without the maintenance of spontaneous ventilation. Positive-pressure ventilation through an SGA device does not completely eliminate the risk of pneumocephalus.

Finally, if there does not appear to be any likely difficulty with routine tracheal intubation, and the only concern is the avoidance of mask ventilation, RSI without mask ventilation can be used.

3 What are the potential hazards and complications in regard to the airway?

Loss of airway control and oxygenation in a situation where PPMV cannot or should not be used can be catastrophic. The equipment and personnel to perform a surgical airway should be readily available.

Pneumocephalus can occur even with small defects in the bony skull and can be exacerbated by PPMV, leading to tension pneumocephalus. Tension pneumocephalus is a serious complication associated with major neurologic morbidity and mortality. Vulnerability to PPMV-induced pneumocephalus can last as long as 6 weeks postoperatively.

4 Are there special considerations for the emergence or the end of the case?

The patient must be breathing spontaneously at the time of extubation. The anesthesiologist should strive for a quiet emergence, avoiding bucking, straining, and coughing, all which can increase intracranial pressure. A deep extubation technique can be pursued, but it must be kept in mind that mask ventilation will be contraindicated if the patient cannot support ventilation on his or her own. The Bailey maneuver (see Chapter 38: The Bailey Maneuver), where the patient is transitioned from the tracheal tube to an SGA device, can also be used if the clinician is practiced in this technique, trismus does not hinder access to the airway and the patient is not at risk of gastric content aspiration.

In the postoperative period, no device that could possibly create end-expiratory pressure or continuous positive airway pressure (CPAP) should be used. Oxygen administration through a nasal cannula should be avoided.

- PPMV can cause or worsen pneumocephalus.
- An SGA device can be used as an alternative to mask ventilation, but pneumocephalus has been reported with positive-pressure ventilation with this technique.
- Awake intubation may be the safest approach to secure the airway. Regardless of the technique chosen, a backup plan including a surgical airway should be ready to be implemented.
- Concerns regarding the avoidance of mask ventilation continue during emergence and extubation.
- *See Figure 35.1 and* ***Video 35.1*** *for additional details.*

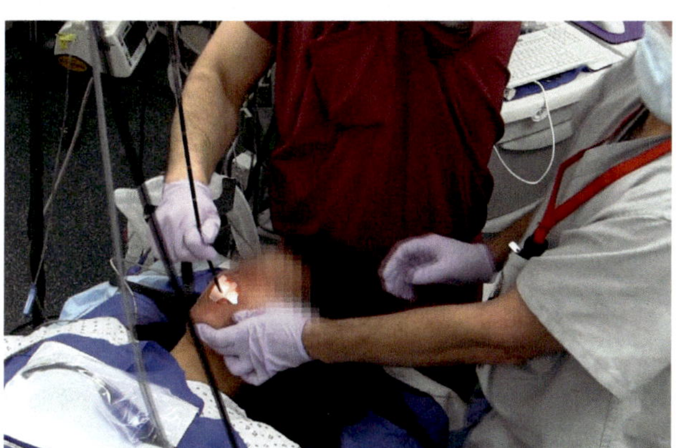

Figure 35.1. A patient with a frontal cranial cerebrospinal fluid leak has been induced under general anesthesia and is being intubated without mask ventilation. (See **Video 35.1.**)

Suggested Readings

Esfahani K, Dunn LK. Anesthetic management during transsphenoidal pituitary surgery. *Curr Opin Anaesthesiol*. 2021; 34:575–581.

Gurajala I, Azharuddin M, Gopinath R. General anaesthesia with laryngeal mask airway may cause recurrence of pneumocephalus in a patient with head injury. *Br J Anaesth*. 2013;111:675–676.

Kopelovich JC, de la Garza GO, Greenlee JD, et al. Pneumocephalus with BiPAP use after transsphenoidal surgery. *J Clin Anesth*. 2012;24:415–418.

Nemergut EC, Dumont AS, Barry UT, et al. Perioperative management of patients undergoing transsphenoidal pituitary surgery. *Anesth Analg*. 2005;101:1170–1181.

Rosenblatt W. The airway approach algorithm: a decision tree for organizing preoperative airway information. *J Clin Anesth*. 2004;16:312–316.

Melker Emergency Cricothyrotomy

36

Rainer Lenhardt

1 Where or when is this device or technique used in airway management?

Airway obstruction represents a sudden medical emergency and can be encountered during several scenarios, such as neck trauma, pharyngeal and laryngeal bleeding, neck tumors, foreign bodies, and airway edema. In most cases, patients will be mask ventilated and emergently intubated. However, occasionally, the practitioner is unable to mask ventilate or to intubate the patient's trachea. When the insertion of a supraglottic airway (SGA) also fails, cricothyrotomy is indicated as a last resort in a life-threatening situation. Depending on the environment, there are two methods of rapid airway rescue commonly employed by anesthesiologists: needle cricothyrotomy or Seldinger cricothyrotomy. In most hospitals, there is at least one Seldinger cricothyrotomy kit available.

2 Describe in detail the device or technique.

When the decision to proceed with emergency invasive airway access is made, the patient's airway is positioned with the head and neck extended to provide maximum access to the cricothyroid membrane. The thyroid cartilage is grasped with thumb and middle finger of the operator's nondominant hand. The cricoid cartilage is located and the cricothyroid membrane is felt with the index finger. After cursory cleansing with an antiseptic solution, a vertical 1- to 2-cm midline incision is made through the skin only with the included scalpel. The hollow needle–syringe assembly is used to puncture the subcutaneous tissues and cricothyroid membrane in the midline, at a 45-degree caudal angle. By using constant syringe–plunger retraction, air is aspirated as the needle enters the larynx. Many authors recommend puncturing the cricothyroid membrane at a 90-degree angle until air is aspirated, and only then, assuming the 45-degree angle in order to reduce the risk of posterior wall puncture (see Chapter 51: Translaryngeal Ventilation and Complications). The flexible end of the included, short guidewire is introduced 15 to 20 cm into the needle. The needle is removed, leaving the guidewire in place. The preassembled Melker catheter/dilator is advanced over the guidewire. If time allows, the distal end of the dilator is lubricated. Significant resistance is appreciated as the dilator abuts the cricothyroid membrane and is then forcefully thrust through it. Difficult insertion through the membrane may be facilitated by extending the skin incision, or passing the scalpel blade through the cricothyroid membrane, using the wire as a guide. The catheter/dilator assembly is inserted until the flange comes to rest on either side of the scalpel incision. The dilator and guidewire are removed, leaving the flanged catheter in place. The cuff of the catheter is inflated with about 10 cc of air, and an oxygen delivery/ventilation system (eg, resuscitation bag, anesthesia circuit) is attached. The Melker catheter's position is confirmed by the detection of end-tidal CO_2, low ventilation pressures, chest rise, and auscultated breath sounds. Last, the catheter is fixed to the neck with sutures or another fixation method.

3 What distinguishes this device or technique from similar airway management methods?

The Melker emergency cricothyrotomy kit comes equipped with a guidewire and a preassembled catheter/dilator. After needle insertion into the trachea, a guidewire is used to lead the catheter/dilator combination into the trachea per the Seldinger technique. Once in place, the catheter's cuff can be inflated and the patient has a secured airway. The adaptor of the catheter allows the patient to be connected to a standard ventilator, resuscitation bag, or anesthesia circuit. This is in contrast to a simple needle cricothyrotomy, in which a needle is loaded with a catheter. On insertion of the needle and identification of the trachea, the catheter is inserted without the use of a guidewire. In an emergency, a simple needle cricothyrotomy may speed up the process and allow for faster oxygenation with minimal bleeding. However, the lumen of a needle cricothyrotomy is narrow and oxygenation may be inadequate, unless a transtracheal jet ventilation (TTJV) device and a high-pressure oxygen source are readily available. In addition, TTJV requires supraglottic patency to allow gas egression, which may not be adequate in emergency airway obstruction.

Author Caveats

The above-described procedure is not without major risks. First, identification of the cricothyroid membrane may be difficult, particularly in patients with short and thick necks. There is a chance that a false lumen may be created that will result in failure to oxygenate the patient due to extratracheal catheter placement. Second, the cricothyroid membrane is surrounded by adjacent structures and cricothyroid arteries that are easily injured. Major bleeding may occur when cutting the skin or during insertion of the catheter/dilator assembly. Bleeding may result in major aspiration, inhibiting meaningful ventilation of the patient. Third, laceration of the thyroid and injury of the larynx or the vocal cords may ensue. However, given the urgency of establishing adequate oxygenation of the patient, the benefit of using a Melker emergency cricothyroid kit by far outweighs the potential complications.

After successful insertion of a breathing catheter, a surgical airway should be obtained in the OR under controlled conditions and as soon as possible. This will prevent delayed complications such as formation of fistulae, scarring or tracheal stenosis, and tracheomalacia.

- Airway obstruction represents a sudden medical emergency that must be treated immediately.
- Needle cricothyrotomy or Seldinger cricothyrotomy can be used to reopen an obstructed airway.
- The Melker emergency cricothyrotomy kit has a complete set of tools to perform a cricothyrotomy successfully.
- In case of life-threatening airway obstruction, the benefit of using a Melker kit by far outweighs the potential complications.
- *See Figures 36.1 and 36.2 for additional details.*

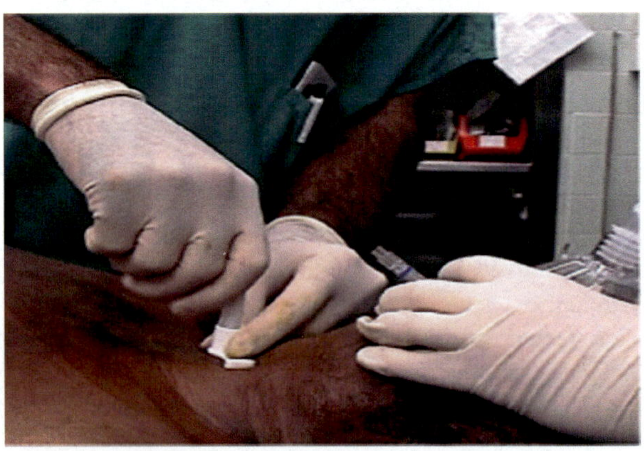

Figure 36.1. The Melker catheter has been placed into the neck and the operator is about to remove the airway obturator. (See **Video 36.1.**)

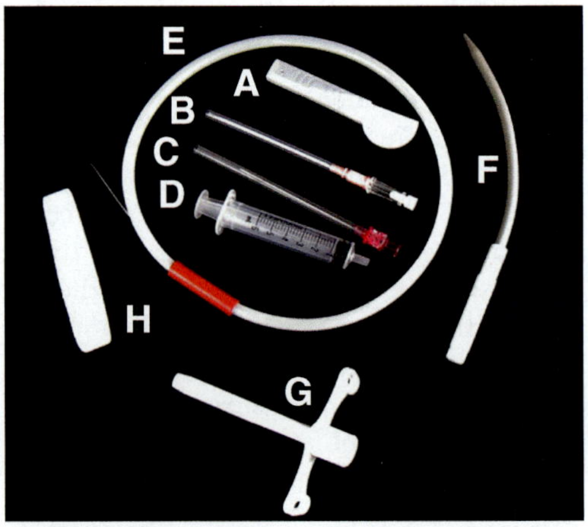

Figure 36.2. Components of the Melker Emergency Cricothyrotomy Kit. *A*, scalpel blade; *B*, 20-g cannula over the needle catheter; *C*, stainless steel needle; *D*, syringe for air aspiration; *E*, wire; *F*, obturator; *G*, airway catheter; *H*, neck tie.

Suggested Readings

Heymans F, Feigl G, Graber S, Courvoisier DS, Weber KM, Dulguerov P. Emergency cricothyrotomy performed by surgical airway-naive medical personnel: a randomized crossover study in cadavers comparing three commonly used techniques. *Anesthesiology*. 2016;125:295–303.

Law JA, Broemling N, Cooper RM, et al. The difficult airway with recommendations for management—part 1—difficult tracheal intubation encountered in an unconscious/induced patient. *Can J Anesth*. 2013;60:1089–1118.

Melker JS, Gabrielli A. Melker cricothyrotomy kit: an alternative to the surgical technique. *Ann Otol Rhinol*. 2005;114(7):525–529.

Metterlein T, Frommer M, Ginzkey C, et al. A randomized trial comparing two cuffed emergency cricothyrotomy devices using a wire-guided and a catheter-over-needle technique. *J Emerg Med*. 2011;41(3):326–332.

Deep Extubation

37

Richard E. Galgon

Clinical Scenario: A 68-year-old man on clopidogrel for recently placed cardiac stents is undergoing neck dissection for squamous cell carcinoma under general endotracheal anesthesia. His cardiologist recommended the continuation of perioperative antiplatelet therapy. The surgeon is concerned about postoperative bleeding and hematoma formation. In response, you elect to do a deep extubation technique.

1 What are the anesthetic and airway management considerations for this case?

For this patient, undergoing a neck dissection and treated with clopidogrel, extubation is a high-risk event for bleeding or cardiac ischemia triggered by hypertension, tachycardia, and/or dysrhythmias from coughing and straining on the tracheal tube or hypoxia from breath-holding. These risks can be reduced with a deep extubation technique when a patient presents with a straightforward, nondifficult airway, and no increased aspiration risk, as is the case for this patient. It is generally accepted that deep extubation is contraindicated in cases of cervical spine surgery, known or predicted difficult airway, increased pulmonary aspiration risk, or increased risk for upper airway obstruction from neck pathology or obesity/obstructive sleep apnea.

2 How would you manage the airway in this case?

Prior to initiating emergence in this case, ensure the surgical stimulation is complete, thoroughly suction the oropharynx, fully reverse any neuromuscular blockade, and reestablish spontaneous ventilation with 100% oxygen filling the anesthesia circuit to provide adequate extubation preoxygenation. This author would then position the patient in a supine, semi-upright position to facilitate diaphragmatic expansion, increase functional residual capacity, and reduce airway/postsurgical edema. Importantly, ensure pharmacologic agents and equipment are immediately available to address any postextubation upper airway obstruction, laryngospasm, or reintubation need.

In contradistinction to the routine/awake extubation, endotracheal tube removal during deep extubation will occur with the patient in a deep (surgical) plane of anesthesia (ie, the patient is nonresponsive to commands and tactile simulation, has no gag reflex, and should tolerate the insertion of an oral or nasopharyngeal airway and suctioning of the oropharynx). There is no clear requisite for the inhalational anesthetic agent concentration that is needed to proceed with safe deep extubation. Studies in adult and pediatric patients have targeted end-tidal inhalational anesthetic agent concentrations at the time of extubation that correspond respectively to a minimum alveolar concentration (MAC) of 1.0 to 1.5. However, the concomitant effects of other administered pharmacologic agents (eg, narcotic medications, systemic or topical lidocaine, propofol, or dexmedetomidine) lower the MAC requirement.

When ready to proceed with deep extubation, an adequate tidal volume (~3 mL/kg or greater), respiratory rate (10 to 20 bpm), and oxygenation status (Pa_{O_2} >90) should be present. Extubation and airway manipulation in stage 2 of anesthesia, where divergent pupils, irregular respiratory patterns, and excitement exist, should be avoided, as this phase is associated with laryngospasm, coughing, straining, aspiration, and hypoxia. Careful deflation and reinflation of the tracheal tube cuff prior to removal should not elicit cough or a change in the respiratory patterns. Once these criteria are met, the endotracheal tube can be gently removed. The author's preference is to support the postextubation airway with head/neck positioning, a gentle chin lift/head extension, and insertion of an oral or nasopharyngeal airway if needed. Alternatively, a continuous positive airway pressure (CPAP) circuit using a full-face or nasal mask can be applied. Note, in the current case, nasopharyngeal airways would be contraindicated due to the increased bleeding risk while on anticoagulation. Postextubation supplemental oxygen and monitoring (oxygen saturation and end-tidal carbon dioxide if available) should be applied during transport to the recovery room.

3 What are the potential hazards and complications in regard to the airway?

The potential complications of deep extubation include airway obstruction and aspiration of gastric contents. Even with a nondifficult airway patient, postextubation obstruction is possible. The anesthesia provider must be prepared to recognize and treat it in a timely manner. While complete airway obstruction is an acute event and immediately threatens the patient's life, hypoventilation generated by a partial airway obstruction may be insidious and masked by the increased oxygen FIO_2. The incidence of respiratory complications has been found to be greater after deep extubation, regardless of the type of operation.

In the context of complete obstruction, the author chooses minimally stimulating ventilation techniques: positive-pressure face mask ventilation with an oral or nasopharyngeal airway, then intravenous induction (eg, propofol) followed by supraglottic airway device (SAD) placement. Emergence with a correctly positioned SGA should be nonstimulating. Administer a paralytic agent (10% to 20% of intubation dose) for suspected persistent laryngospasm. Reintubation may be necessary, particularly if negative pressure pulmonary edema results.

Treatment with clopidogrel places this patient in a high-risk category that will need close supervision even beyond the first couple of hours. Periodic checks (breathing, deglutition, wound examination, and blood pressure control) are paramount for this patient's safety. The availability of qualified personnel in the recovery room, during transport, and in the ICU, who understand the associated risks and are capable of managing airway complications, have to be considered. Prophylactic treatment of postoperative nausea and vomiting should be routine. Deep extubation should be used only after careful consideration of the risk/benefit ratio.

4 What distinct airway device might be used in this case, and what are the special considerations?

The main concern after a deep extubation is the possibility of airway obstruction. This presents as a partial obstruction (easily treated with an oral or nasopharyngeal airway, head/neck repositioning, or a gentle chin lift) or complete obstruction (requiring invasive instrumentation). Deep extubation is traditionally contraindicated in patients with difficult airways (or at high risk for difficult reintubation or face mask ventilation). Nevertheless, it can be attempted after securing the airway with an airway exchange catheter ("staged or reversible extubation") (see Chapter 44: Extubation of the Difficult Airway Patient). Another technique that effectively reduces coughing and bucking and the cardiovascular response during extubation is to replace the tracheal tube with a SAD in deep anesthetic plane (the Bailey maneuver) (see Chapter 38: The Bailey Maneuver). Catanno and Rane have described a method for ventilation through an extraglottic tracheal tube as a technique for deep extubation and airway control, but this method has not been formally studied.

After a lengthy neck dissection, an "easy" airway may become "difficult," and this may reveal itself only with a failed deep extubation attempt. The anesthesia provider needs a plan to address this critical situation and have personnel and specific devices ready to use (eg, SADs, video laryngoscopes, etc.). Airway management relevant to deep extubation may be challenging and should be carried out by experienced practitioners on selected patients in an optimal environment.

- Extubation should always proceed according to a preformulated strategy that considers the surgery, the patient, and the skills and preferences of the anesthesia provider.
- Prior to deep extubation, the surgical stimulation should be completed.
- Failed deep extubation is a critical situation in need for immediate intervention, and as such this type of extubation should be carried out by an experienced anesthesia provider, on a selected population, in an optimal environment.
- *See Figures 37.1 and 37.2 for additional details.*

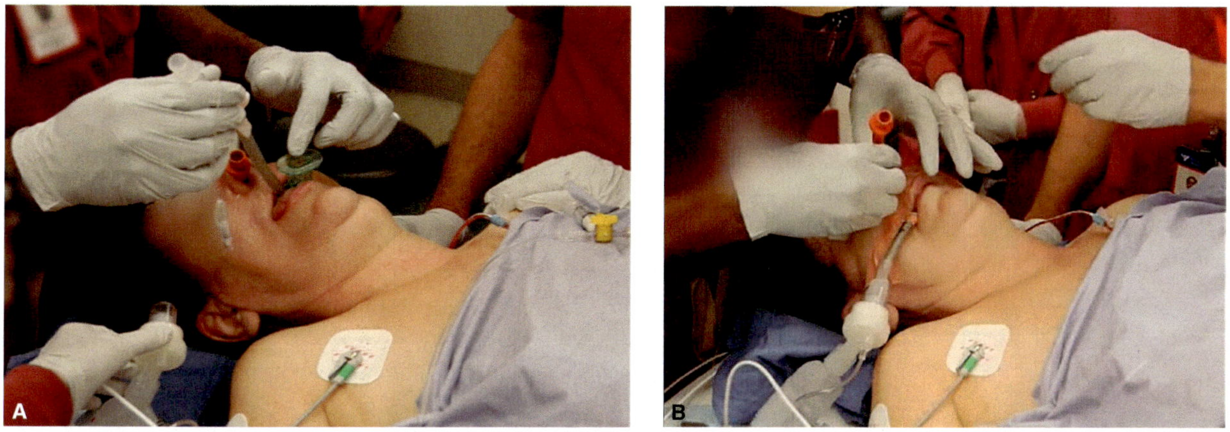

Figure 37.1. **A:** Nasal and oral airways have been placed without evidence of patient arousal. Extubation will now take place. See **Video 37.1**. **B:** In the first stage of a graded deep extubation, a nasal airway is placed.

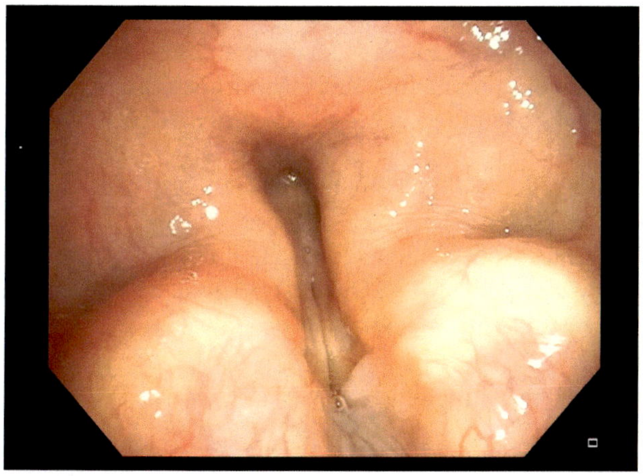

Figure 37.2. Avoiding laryngospasm (as seen here) is a key component of deep extubation. See **Video 37.2**.

Acknowledgment

We gratefully acknowledge the contributions of previous edition author, Adrian A. Matioc, as portions of those chapters have been retained in this revision.

Suggested Readings

Cattano D, Rane M. Ventilation through an extraglottic tracheal tube: a technique for deep extubation and airway control. *Br J Anaesth*. 2017;118(6):959–960.

Daley MD, Norman PH, Coveler LA. Tracheal extubation of adult surgical patients while deeply anesthetized: a survey of United States anesthesiologists. *J Clin Anesth*. 1999;11:445–452.

Juang J, Cordoba M, Ciaramella A, et al. Incidence of airway complications associated with deep extubation in adults. *BMC Anesthesiology*. 2020;30:274.

Koo C, Lee SY, Chung SH, Ryu J. Deep vs. awake extubation and LMA removal in terms of airway complications in pediatric patients undergoing anesthesia: a systematic review and meta-analysis. *J Clin Med*. 2018;7:353.

Mort TC. Continuous airway access for the difficult extubation: the efficacy of the airway exchange catheter. *Anesth Analg*. 2007;105:1357–1362.

Wong TH, Weber G, Abramowicz AE. Smooth extubation and smooth emergence techniques: a narrative review. *Anesthesiol Res Pract*. 2021;2021:8883257.

38 The Bailey Maneuver

Ann Marie Melookaran Iliff

Clinical Scenario: A 32-year-old female with severe reactive airway disease and obstructive sleep apnea (OSA) is scheduled for a nasal sinus procedure. She has a history of multiple ICU admissions her severe reactive airway disease.

1 What are the anesthetic and airway management considerations for this case?

This patient who has both reactive airway disease and obstructive sleep apnea undergoing an airway surgery may lead to conflicted management goals. A tailored plan for emergence, such as use of the Bailey maneuver, can be used to address the risks associated with airway surgery for each disease process.

Bronchospasm can be triggered by manipulation of the airway, especially in a patient with a history of reactive airway disease. Tracheal intubation and extubation are potent stimuli for bronchospasm. Bronchospasm can also be triggered by the administration of dry gases, aspiration of blood and surgical debris, and the removal of inhaled anesthetics at the end of the case.

Deep extubation is commonly employed as a technique to reduce the potential for bronchospasm, coughing, Valsalva-like straining, and a hyperdynamic response during emergence in these patients. Conversely, deep extubation may be contraindicated in patients with significant OSA, those who are at risk for gastric contents aspiration, patients with difficult airways, and others. The patient with OSA may experience irreversible airway obstruction when extubated in the anesthetized state during both spontaneous and positive-pressure ventilation.

An airway adjunct (eg, oral–pharyngeal airway, nasal airway, supraglottic airway [SGA]) may be required to overcome this obstruction.

The Bailey maneuver was initially described as an alternative to primary tracheal extubation in otolaryngologic surgery. An in situ tracheal tube is replaced with an SGA in a deeply anesthetized patient. The maneuver is used to assist with airway protection and provides a smooth, nonstimulating emergence from anesthesia in a fasting patient. Though the LMA is not meant to protect the airway from the regurgitated gastric contents, aspiration of blood and debris from upper airway surgery may be reduced.

2 How would you manage the airway in this case?

To employ the Bailey maneuver, the clinician should ensure that the patient is in a plane of anesthesia deep enough to blunt airway reflexes. Reactivity to oropharyngeal suctioning should be suppressed with the deepening of the anesthetic plane using inhaled or intravenous agents. Although the maneuver can be performed during spontaneous ventilation, an apneic state (without neuromuscular relaxation) ensures a deeper level of anesthesia. A fully deflated and lubricated LMA is inserted with continuous pressure against the hard palate. During insertion, the in situ tracheal tube is kept in an anterior position. The LMA is inserted to its usual depth, appreciated by increased resistance as the distal LMA comes to rest behind the cricoid cartilage. The presence of the tracheal tube reduces the risk of epiglottic downfolding during insertion. After the LMA is inflated, the tracheal tube cuff is deflated, and the tube is removed. The LMA is tested for patency by ventilating through the LMA, and the patient is then allowed to emerge from anesthesia. The LMA is removed when the patient meets appropriate removal criteria.

3 What are the surgical considerations that impact anesthetic management?

An emergence with minimal airway reactivity, normal to low venous compartment pressure, and the absence of a hyperdynamic state are desirable conditions at the end of otolaryngologic procedures. Valsalva-like straining by an intubated patient raises the central venous pressure and can lead to bleeding at a highly vascularized surgical site. Hypertension can result in severe arterial bleeding in the fresh surgical field. Similarly, increases in intracranial pressure may be detrimental to the integrity of a recently resected arteriovenous malformation bed or cerebrospinal fluid leak.

Concurrently, surgery of the upper airway or nasal sinuses may produce surgical debris or minor bleeding which soil the upper airway, so practicing deep extubation may result in lower airway aspiration of these remains. Although many techniques for yielding a smooth anesthetic emergence have been described, the Bailey maneuver has the added advantage of improved protection of the lower airway. In addition, the use of an SGA provides the ability to administer oxygen and positive-pressure ventilation after the removal of the tracheal tube, prevents obstruction, and provides airway protection until the patient's protective reflexes have returned.

4 What distinct airway device is used in this case, and what are the special considerations?

The Bailey maneuver was initially described using the LMA Classic. Subsequently, it has been described using alternative SGAs, but a low-profile device may be easier to insert than some larger devices due to the in situ tracheal tube. Second-generation SGAs, although often recommended in situations where there may be increased gastric contents (eg, swallowed surgical debris), may be difficult to insert behind the in situ tracheal tube.

- The Bailey maneuver is used to facilitate smooth, nonstimulating emergence in a deeply anesthetized patient to avoid coughing and straining.
- The Bailey maneuver overcomes airway obstruction after deep extubation in at-risk patients.
- The presence of an SGA may offer some protection from the aspiration of surgical debris and blood in the deep extubation patient, though it is not ideal for patients with high risk of aspiration.
- *See Figure 38.1 and* ***Video 38.1*** *for additional details.*

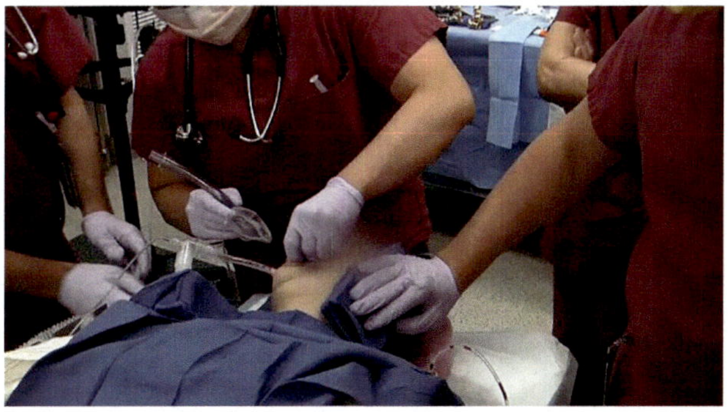

Figure 38.1. Prior to the patients emergence from general anesthesia, a supraglottic airway is placed behind the in-situ tracheal tube.

Suggested Readings

Modir H, Moshiri E, Yazdi B, Mohammadbeigi A, Modir A. Comparing the efficacy and safety of laryngeal mask airway, streamlined liner of the pharyngeal airway and I-gel following tracheal extubation. *Med Gas Res.* 2018;7(4):241–246.

Parotto M, Cooper RM, Behringer EC. Extubation of the challenging or difficult airway. *Curr Anesthesiol Rep.* 2020;10:1–7.

Verghese C. Laryngeal mask airway devices: three maneuvers for any clinical situation. *Anesthesiol News Guide Airway Manag.* 2010:15–16.

39 Nasal to Oral Tube Exchange

Neil S. Ballard • Kenneth N. Hiller • Carin A. Hagberg

Clinical Scenario: A patient in the intensive care unit has been intubated through the right naris for 5 days. She has developed fever and opacification (on CT) of the right maxillary sinus. The intensive care team has asked for an exchange of the endotracheal tube (ETT) to an oral position.

1 What are the anesthetic and airway management considerations for this case?

The airway management considerations for this intubated intensive care patient include the necessity of mechanical ventilatory support, the risk of aspiration, and the possibility of a difficult nasal to oral ETT exchange. During any airway exchange, the patient is potentially at risk for oxygen desaturation and loss of control of the airway.

Before initiating the exchange, prepyloric tube feeds should be held for an appropriate period of time, and the stomach should be decompressed and suctioned prior to any airway manipulation. The bed should be placed in a head-up position, and the patient should be ventilated with 100% oxygen before the exchange to increase oxygen reserves. The oropharynx should be suctioned thoroughly to improve visibility. All equipment necessary for the ETT exchange and backup airway management should be immediately available at the bedside.

2 How would you manage the airway in this case?

The authors recommend performing either direct laryngoscopy (DL) or video laryngoscopy (VL) in combination with an airway exchange catheter (AEC) through the existing nasal ETT to manage the airway in this case. An advantage of VL is that any assistants will be able to visualize the airway during the procedure.

First, if a nasogastric tube is present, it should be suctioned to empty gastric contents. In addition, the patient should be preoxygenated with 100% oxygen for approximately 10 minutes prior to the airway exchange. A double-swivel bronchoscopy adaptor, which will allow placement of an AEC during continuous ventilation, should be placed on the indwelling nasal ETT. An AEC is inserted through the bronchoscope adaptor and into the lumen of the preexisting nasal ETT to a depth of 28 cm at the naris. If oral intubation fails for any reason, the AEC will be maintained for immediate nasal reintubation and also offers the possibility of oxygenation and ventilation.

Following thorough suctioning of the oral cavity, either DL or VL can be performed. Pressure can be applied over the thyroid cartilage to facilitate the view of the airway structures. If visualization is adequate, the preexisting ETT cuff is deflated, and the nasal ETT is withdrawn over the AEC until its tip is in the hypopharynx. A styletted ETT or an intubation catheter along with an ETT can then be inserted into the trachea. If there are any difficulties with either of these techniques, a second operator may insert an flexible intubating scope (FIS) preloaded with an ETT into the oropharynx. The first operator can then manually guide it under the epiglottis while performing laryngoscopy, until the glottic opening is visualized via the FIS. The FIS is passed through the glottis and further advanced by the second operator to a position just above the carina. Subsequently, the new oral ETT is advanced over the FIS by the second operator. With the airway secure at this point, the first operator may remove the laryngoscope. When proper position of the new oral ETT is confirmed by endoscopy, capnography, and/or auscultation of bilateral breath sounds, the nasal ETT and AEC are removed.

An alternative to the intraoral technique described above is using a FIS and an intubating airway instead of DL or VL.

3 What are the potential hazards and complications in regard to the airway?

Potential complications of the exchange procedure include loss of a secure airway, aspiration, and difficulty adequately oxygenating/ventilating patients requiring greater mechanical support. Visualizing the airway throughout the exchange procedure, decompressing the stomach, and adequately preoxygenating the patient minimize these risks. If any assistants are involved, a preprocedure "huddle" should be performed so that all present understand the intended plan and the backup strategies.

4 What distinct airway device might be used in this case, and what are the special considerations?

This technique involves distinct airway devices including a bronchoscopy adaptor, AEC, and possibly, two indirect visualization devices (VL and FIS). Using these devices ensures optimal safety and maintains mechanical support. AECs must be employed carefully as they pose the risk of tracheobronchial penetration, tissue laceration, malposition, or barotrauma. Additionally, the use of a Parker Flex Tip Tube (Parker Medical) could be considered for use to facilitate ETT advancement over the FIS and into the trachea. This tube was designed for increased ease of passage over an intubation stylet or FIS.

- Prepyloric tube feeds should be held and the stomach decompressed/suctioned prior to an ETT exchange.
- An AEC inserted through the preexisting nasal ETT with continued mechanical ventilation provides additional safety during the exchange.
- Visualizing the airway throughout the ETT exchange is recommended.
- *See Figures 39.1 and 39.2 for additional details.*

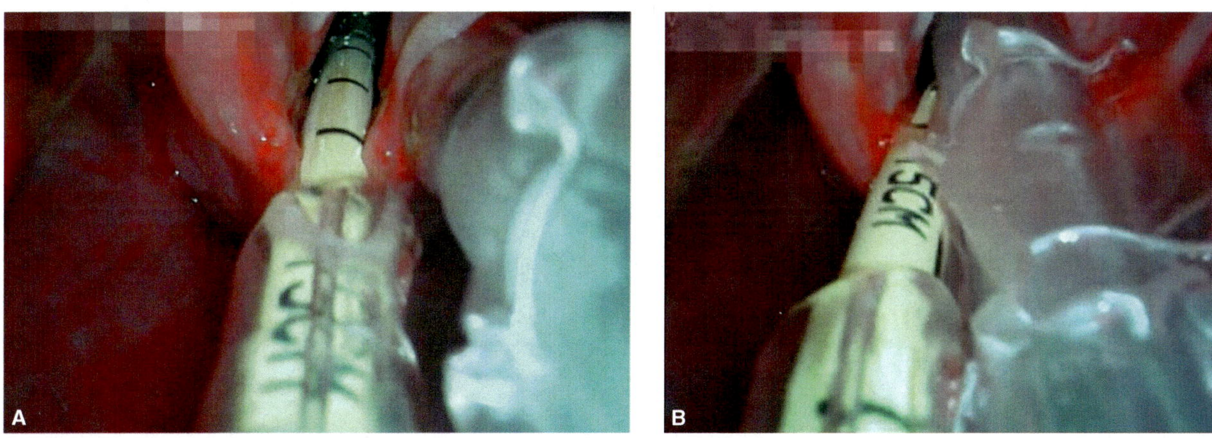

Figure 39.1. A: The nasotracheal tube (with an inserted exchange catheter) is retreated from the airway. An orally placed tube can be seen on the right of the larynx. See **Video 39.1**. **B:** A video laryngoscope is used to visualize the larynx in a patient who has a nasotracheal intubation.

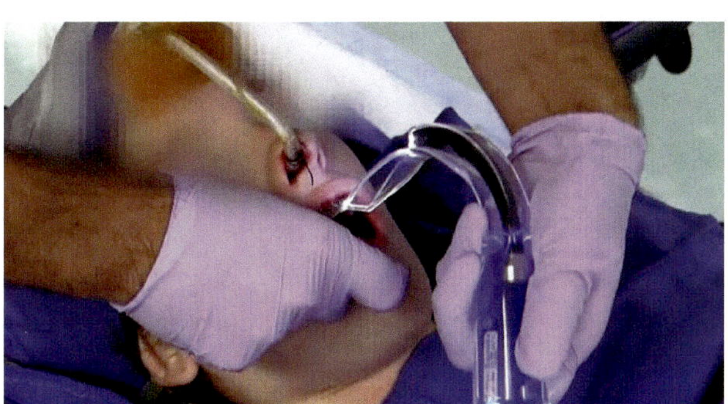

Figure 39.2. The orally placed tracheal tube is guided into the larynx.

Suggested Readings

Hung KC, Chen JY, Feng IJ, et al. Efficacy and airway complications of Parker Flex-Tip tubes and standard endotracheal tubes during airway manipulation: a meta-analysis and trial sequential analysis. *Eur J Anaesthesiol.* 2021;38(8):813–824.

Kaplan MB, Ward D, Hagberg CA, et al. Seeing is believing: the importance of video laryngoscopy in teaching and in managing the difficult airway. *Surg Endosc.* 2006;20(suppl 2):S479–S483.

McLean S, Lanam CR, Benedict W, Kirkpatrick N, Kheterpal S, Ramachandran SK. Airway exchange failure and complications with the use of the Cook Airway Exchange Catheter®: a single center cohort study of 1177 patients. *Anesth Analg.* 2013; 117(6):1325–1327.

Mort TC, Braffett BH. Conventional versus video laryngoscopy for tracheal tube exchange: glottic visualization, success rates, complications, and rescue alternatives in the high-risk difficult airway patient. *Anesth Analg.* 2015;121(2):440–448.

Intraoperative Oral to Nasal Tracheal Tube Exchange

40

Kenneth N. Hiller • Neil S. Ballard • Carin A. Hagberg

Clinical Scenario: A 19-year-old boy with facial dysmorphism is undergoing a Le Fort 1 osteotomy for midfacial advancement. He was initially intubated orally for a rhinoplasty prior to the Le Fort. The surgical team is now requesting nasal intubation.

1 What are the anesthetic and airway management considerations for this case?

Le Fort fractures, first described in 1901, are facial fractures involving the maxillary bone in the horizontal (type 1), pyramidal (type 2), or transverse (type 3) plane. They may be of traumatic origin, or, as illustrated here, surgically created. Le Fort 1 maxillary fractures extend horizontally from the nasal septum to the pyriform rim and typically extend bilaterally. Although intubation for this procedure may be performed orally or nasally, nasal intubation allows unfettered surgical access for this midface repair. Facial dysmorphism can increase the likelihood of turbinate-impeded endotracheal tube (ETT) passage during nasal intubation. The presence of blood (from either the initial injury or the nasal surgery) can contaminate the airway and can make FIS use difficult or impossible. When performing nasal intubation, the right naris is usually chosen for easier passage of an ETT past the nasal turbinates.

2 How would you manage the airway in this case?

In this case, the authors' preference is to use a flexible intubating scope (FIS) and airway exchange catheter (AEC) approach. Conventional flexible scope-aided intubation is a well-established procedure for both tracheal intubation and airway exchange procedures in patients with difficult airways. Using a FIS to facilitate this exchange provides optimal control over the airway. Nasal preparation should begin with application of a topical vasoconstrictor followed by the slow, steady insertion of a lubricated nasopharyngeal airway. The airway can then be removed and replaced with a nasal RAE ETT that has been softened with warm water. A FIS can then be inserted into the nasal RAE ETT and the end of the scope guided into the trachea. An AEC is then placed via the existing oral ETT and the oral ETT removed, leaving the AEC and FIS in the airway. The nasal RAE ETT is then threaded over the FIS. Once proper ETT placement is confirmed, the AEC can be removed. If ETT placement becomes problematic, the AEC can be used to safely replace the oral ETT to secure the airway. If replacement of the ETT over the AEC is hindered, oxygen may be insufflated via the AEC. The surgical team should be prepared for a surgical airway prior to the exchange procedure.

In order to decrease trauma during the FIS-facilitated nasal intubation, a smaller-sized ETT is typically chosen (as compared to a FIS-directed oral intubation). In addition, special maneuvers can facilitate ETT passage over the FIS, for example, turning the ETT 90 degrees counterclockwise upon glottic approach, using the smallest, clinically adequate ETT which threads onto the flexible scope, and/or using a specially designed ETT tip (eg, Parker Flex-Tip tube). In addition, combining direct laryngoscopy or video laryngoscopy with FIS intubation may increase the success rate of ETT exchange under difficult conditions. The laryngoscope accomplishes the displacement of pharyngeal tissue that is not possible with the FIS alone. Even if the glottic opening is not visualized, the FIS can be diverted under the epiglottis using this technique, with or without laryngeal manipulation.

If difficulty is encountered during advancement of the nasal RAE ETT through the nasal cavity, the distal end may first be telescoped into a red rubber catheter (RRC) to facilitate the ETT's passage past the turbinates. The RRC is advanced through the naris and then recovered in the oropharynx. Gentle traction is then applied to the RRC as the nasal RAE ETT is advanced from above. Once the tip of the nasal RAE ETT has made the turn into the oropharynx, the RRC is then detached and discarded. Alternatively, a nasogastric tube may be advanced through the naris and the nasal RAE ETT "railroaded" over it; this may increase the likelihood that the nasal RAE ETT passes below the inferior turbinate.

If a FIS is not available or visualization is inadequate, direct or video laryngoscopy could be performed and the nasal ETT advanced with Magill forceps assistance, although this technique risks ETT cuff laceration. Temporarily inflating the cuff may direct the ETT tip more anteriorly toward the glottic opening. Use of an AEC through the oral ETT should still be performed with either of these techniques.

3 What are the potential hazards and complications in regard to the airway?

ETT exchange involves inherent risks, especially in the presence of a difficult airway, soiling and edema from prior surgical manipulation, and/or poor pulmonary gas exchange in which uninterrupted mechanical oxygenation and ventilatory support is required. The procedure described previously mitigates the inherent dangers of inadvertent extubation/reintubation in "at-risk" patients. The AEC can provide both oxygenation (manually, by insufflation, or by jet ventilation) and the ability to reinsert an oral ETT should nasal intubation fail (eg, accidental removal of the flexible scope from the larynx during ETT advancement, unresolvable hang-up). Prior to using an AEC for either oxygenation/ventilation or reintubation, confirmation of proper tracheal positioning should be performed (eg, via capnography, auscultation, chest radiography).

Failure to strictly adhere to a few straightforward concepts of a properly placed AEC can result in life-threatening barotrauma. This risk can be reduced by avoiding excessive AEC insertion depth (suggested depth of insertion is 24 to 26 cm orally or 27 to 30 cm nasally), using minimal effective inflation pressure, and using a short inspiratory/long expiratory time to ensure chest fall to the neutral position prior to further inflation should oxygen insufflation be required.

Additional complications include hypoxia during airway management, unintended esophageal placement, tracheobronchial penetration, lung laceration, dislodgement, and failure of reintubation.

4 Are there special considerations for the emergence or the end of the case?

There are special considerations for emergence and extubation in this patient who has been both intubated and subsequently reintubated. The provider should take precautions concerning the presence of edema and/or blood. Although not foolproof, a cuff leak test or visualization of the vocal cords (by direct, indirect, or FIS techniques) could be performed prior to extubation to ensure lack of edema and airway competence. If the clinician is concerned, extubation can be postponed or an AEC can be placed via the nasal ETT prior to its removal, leaving the AEC in place should reintubation become necessary. Planning for emergence and extubation is a critical portion of the anesthetic management, especially in patients with difficult airways or "at-risk" for extubation failure.

- Nasal intubation provides unfettered access for a Le Fort 1 midface repair.
- A FIS/AEC oral to nasal ETT exchange approach provides optimal control and safety.
- An improperly positioned AEC can result in life-threatening barotrauma.
- *See Figure 40.1 and* ***Video 40.1*** *for additional details.*

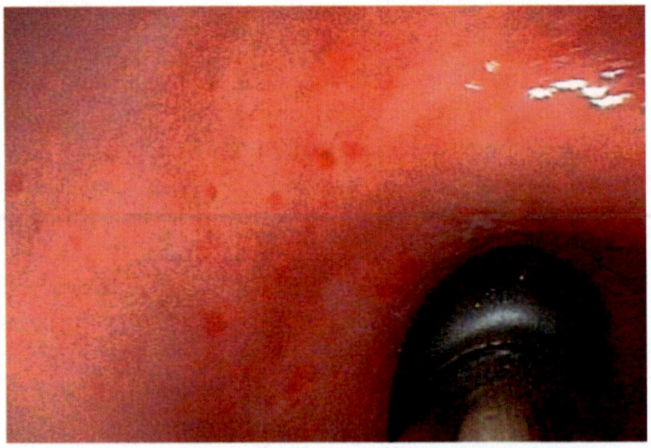

Figure 40.1. Using a flexible intubation scope passed through the nose, the cuff of the orally placed tracheal tube is seen in the trachea. The oral tube will be removed over an exchange catheter, and a new tracheal tube advanced over the flexible intubation scope.

Suggested Readings

Cavallone LF, Vannucci A. Extubation of the difficult airway and extubation failure. *Anesth Analg.* 2013;116:368–383.

Lim CW, Min SW, Kim CS, Chang JE, Park JE, Hwang JY. The use of a nasogastric tube to facilitate nasotracheal intubation: a randomised controlled trial. *Anaesthesia.* 2014;69(6):591–597.

McLean S, Lanam CR, Benedict W, Kirkpatrick N, Kheterpal S, Ramachandran SK. Airway exchange failure and complications with the use of the Cook Airway Exchange Catheter®: a single center cohort study of 1177 patients. *Anesth Analg.* 2013; 117(6):1325–1327.

Pinsky J, Hagberg CA. Combined airway management techniques. In: Hagberg CA, Artime CA, Daily WH, eds. *The Difficult Airway: A Practical Guide.* Oxford University Press; 2013:143–153.

Prior S, Heaton J, Jatana KR, Rashid RG. Parker flex-tip and standard-tip endotracheal tubes: a comparison during nasotracheal intubation. *Anesth Prog.* 2010;57(1):18–24.

41 Upper Airway Surgery with a Supraglottic Airway

Terrence Feldheim • James Turnbull • Anil Patel

Clinical Scenario: A 25-year-old otherwise healthy woman presents for functional endoscopic sinus surgery. Because of a bad experience with postoperative throat pain, she requests not to be intubated.

1 What are the anesthetic and airway management considerations for this case?

The use of the laryngeal mask airway (LMA) for nasal surgery has gained popularity with the advent of the flexible LMA (FLMA) in 1990. These new prototypes retained the identical cuffs of their predecessors but replaced the compressible silicone shaft with a longer, narrower, flexible compression-resistant shaft. This design modification offers several advantages:

- **Resistance to kinking and compression:** The flexometallic shaft is significantly more resistant to kinking or compression compared to its silicone counterpart. This allows for secure taping of the device to the chin, well away from the nasal surgical site.
- **Minimized cuff displacement:** The flaccid nature of the flexometallic shaft reduces the transmission of force to the cuff, thereby minimizing the risk of cuff displacement during surgical manipulation.

These features of the FLMA contribute to its superiority over traditional tracheal intubation for nasal surgery:

- **Reduced airway instrumentation:** The FLMA requires less airway instrumentation than tracheal intubation, decreasing the risk of airway or laryngeal trauma and postoperative sore throat.
- **Lower anesthetic requirements:** The FLMA often requires lower anesthetic doses compared to tracheal intubation, leading to a smoother and quicker emergence from anesthesia.
- **Smoother emergence:** The ease of removal and the absence of laryngeal irritation contribute to a smoother emergence from anesthesia.

The literature has demonstrated superior protection of the lower airway from blood and surgical debris afforded by LMA placement during upper airway surgery, as compared to the tracheal tube.

Kaplan and colleagues showed significantly less contamination of the FLMA compared with a tracheal tube in patients undergoing nasal surgery, with blood often observed pooling above the cuff in the intubated group.

This was confirmed by Karaaslan et al. in a fiberoptic evaluation of the airway postseptoplasty, which showed less blood leakage detected in both anatomic areas in the LMA-S group than in the endotracheal tube (ETT) group.

Surgical bleeding leading to ingestion of blood may lead to stomach irritation. The advent of the gastric port in second-generation LMAs provides an added benefit for gastric venting.

2 How would you manage the airway in this case?

The primary decision regarding airway management is whether to use an FLMA or caudad-facing preshaped Ring, Adair, and Elwyn (RAE) tracheal tube. In our institution, contraindications to FLMA use include full stomach, uncontrolled gastroesophageal reflux disease, morbid obesity, and those with peak inspiratory pressures over 20 cm H_2O. In the above case, our standard technique is to perform an intravenous induction followed by insertion of a well-lubricated size 4 FLMA. For men, we would generally use a size 5 FLMA. The cuff of the FLMA should be fully deflated with smoothed edges and a slight dorsal upturn at the tip. Difficulty with insertion and high-conversion rate to ETT are frequently described. However, most issues can be overcome by ensuring an adequate depth of anesthesia and using the correct insertion technique. The classic insertion technique involves using the index finger to guide the dorsum of the FLMA cuff along the curvature of the palatopharyngeal arch. A jaw thrust may facilitate easy passage.

Once inserted, we ensure the FLMA cuff pressure is within the recommended range (<60 cm H_2O), and carefully check for a leak at an inflation pressure of 20 cm H_2O. This should be repeated with the head in flexion, extension, and lateral rotation—the head is often manipulated by the surgeon during the procedure. Careful leak testing with the head in different positions prior to starting surgery should help avoid any difficulties. We then insert a throat pack and prepare the nose with a mixture of local anesthetic and vasoconstrictor. The patient is managed with controlled ventilation. Maintenance anesthesia can be with either intravenous or inhalational anesthetic, and if required to provide a quiet surgical field, a short-acting, nondepolarizing muscle relaxant is administered. The use of remifentanil has been described, and it is used in our institution if blood pressure control is difficult. A study comparing FLMA with ETT insertion found those with an FLMA required a lower rate of remifentanil infusion and had less blood loss.

3 What are the surgical considerations that impact anesthetic management?

The primary surgical considerations are adequate access and a quiet surgical field. With the shaft taped to the chin, the FLMA causes no impediment to surgical access. We connect flexible extension tubing to the FLMA before the filter, thus removing caudal traction and any hindrance to surgery. Blood pressure control is important to minimize blood loss and provide a quiet surgical field. Usually, a 15-degree head-up tilt and adequate pain relief are sufficient. If the blood pressure remains difficult to control, either a remifentanil infusion or intravenous β-blockers may be required. Care must be taken when removing surgical drapes at the end of all types of ear, nose, and throat (ENT) and upper body surgery, including nasal, ear, throat, and eye surgeries, as the drapes are frequently stuck to the FLMA or adjacent tubing.

4 Are there special considerations for the emergence or the end of the case?

Extubation following nasal surgery presents a significant clinical challenge. When a tracheal tube is inserted, a critical decision arises: should the patient be extubated under deep anesthesia or after regaining full consciousness and reflexes?

Deep extubation:

- **Risk of airway contamination:** Blood pooling above the tracheal tube cuff poses a significant risk of airway contamination if the patient is extubated while still deeply sedated and with diminished reflexes.

Awake extubation:

- **Potential for complications:** Awake extubation, while reducing the risk of aspiration, can trigger excessive coughing, straining, and sympathetic stimulation. These responses can exacerbate surgical bleeding and lead to further airway complications.

The optimal approach to extubation following nasal surgery requires careful consideration of the individual patient's condition, the extent of surgical bleeding, and the anticipated airway response.

Webster and colleagues looked at this problem in a randomized study of 114 patients for elective nasal surgery. Three trial groups were used: FLMA and awake extubation, ETT with deep extubation, and ETT with awake extubation. No throat packs were used in any group. The FLMA group had a significantly lower incidence of coughing, oxygen desaturation, and laryngospasm compared to both ETT groups. This study, as well as our own experience of over 10,000 nasal procedures, suggests the FLMA provides better airway protection and a smoother emergence compared to an ETT.

Caution must be used when using throat packs. Throat pack insertion and removal is part of the pre- and postsurgery checklist in our hospital and is the responsibility of both the surgeon and anesthesiologist. Gentle direct laryngoscopy and suctioning of blood from the pharynx should be performed following throat pack removal. Flexion of the neck at this point is important as it encourages drainage of pooled blood from the nose. The FLMA should be left in situ during emergence to provide continuous airway protection and maintain cardiovascular stability. The cuff should remain inflated during removal to allow the FLMA cuff to carry blood, surgical debris, and secretions out of the airway.

- The FLMA can be used safely and effectively for the majority of nasal surgeries.
- Studies have shown that the FLMA provides equivalent or better protection against blood and debris in the pharynx compared with a tracheal tube.
- The FLMA provides unobstructed surgical access and enables better blood pressure control with lower anesthetic requirements.
- Muscle relaxants and/or opioid infusions may be used to provide a still surgical field.
- *See Figures 41.1 and 41.2 for additional details.*

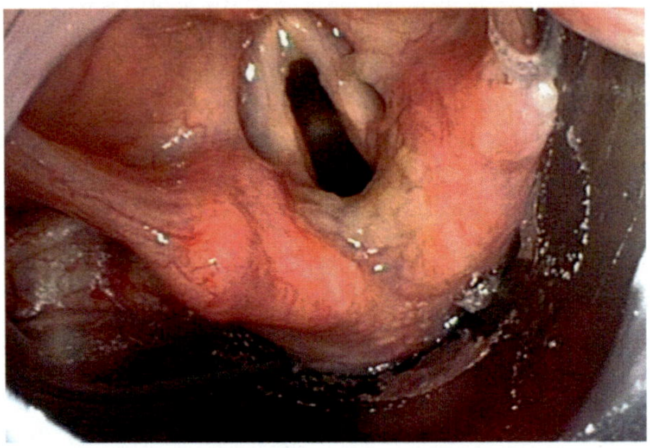

Figure 41.1. The view of the larynx from the barrel of a well-placed LMA Unique. See **Video 41.1**.

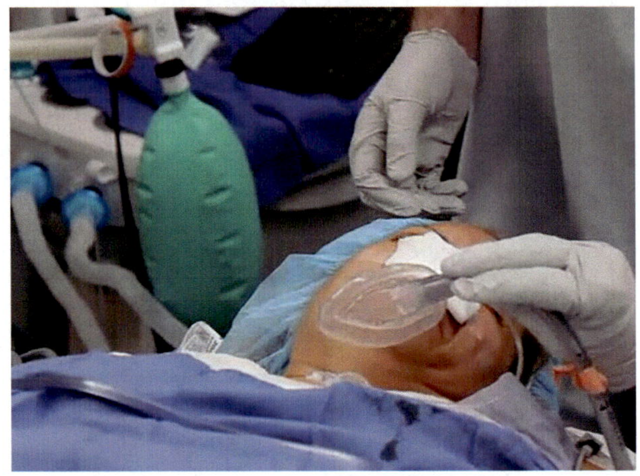

Figure 41.2. As the LMA Flexible is removed, the laryngeal side is shown blood free.

Suggested Readings

Alexander CA. A modified intavent laryngeal mask for ENT and dental anaesthesia. *Anaesthesia*. 1990;45(10):892–893.

Atef A, Fawaz A. Comparison of laryngeal mask with endotracheal tube for anesthesia in endoscopic sinus surgery. *Am J Rhinol*. 2008;22(6):653–657.

Brain AI. The laryngeal mask—a new concept in airway management. *Br J Anaesth*. 1983;55(8):801–805.

Kaplan A, Crosby GJ, Bhattacharyya N. Airway protection and the laryngeal mask airway in sinus and nasal surgery. *Laryngoscope*. 2004;114(4):652–655.

Karaaslan E, Akbas S, Ozkan AS, Colak C, Begec B. A comparison of laryngeal mask airway-supreme and endotracheal tube use with respect to airway protection in patients undergoing septoplasty: a randomized, single-blind, controlled clinical trial. *BMC Anesthesiol*. 2021;21:5.

Webster AC, Morley-Forster PK, Janzen V, et al. Anesthesia for intranasal surgery: a comparison between tracheal intubation and the flexible reinforced laryngeal mask airway. *Anesth Analg*. 1999;88(2):421–425.

Williams PJ, Thompsett C, Bailey PM. Comparison of the reinforced laryngeal mask airway and tracheal intubation for nasal surgery. *Anaesthesia*. 1995;50(11):987–989.

Supraglottic Airway to Tracheal Tube Exchange

42

David T. Wong • Narasimhan Jagannathan

Clinical Scenario: After a failed attempt at video laryngoscopy and a difficult mask ventilation, the airway of an obese, bearded male patient is rescued successfully with a supraglottic airway (SGA). The patient is being anesthetized for upper abdominal surgery. His past medical history is notable for gastroesophageal reflux.

1 What are the anesthetic and airway management considerations for this case?

Obesity is associated with difficult mask ventilation, difficult SGA insertion and maintenance, difficult landmarking of the cricothyroid membrane, and the propensity for obstructive sleep apnea. The presence of a beard is also a predictor of difficult mask ventilation. Although there are reports of using an SGA for ventilation during upper abdominal surgery, most clinicians consider tracheal intubation the preferred method of airway control in patients undergoing upper abdominal surgery. This patient's obesity further influences the need for conversion to tracheal intubation.

2 How would you manage the airway in this case?

After the airway is rescued with an SGA, the clinician has several options of how to proceed. The patient could emerge from anesthesia prior to proceeding with an awake intubation technique. The anesthetic could be performed with the in situ SGA. In addition, the SGA could be removed prior to using an alternative intubation technique, and finally the SGA could be used as a conduit for intubation. Abandoning further attempts at intubation and awakening the patient should continually be considered even as the clinician proceeds with further attempts to intubate. Morbidity increases as the number of intubation attempts increases. As stated before, removing the SGA and employing an alternative intubating instrument, such as FIS may be considered. However, in a patient who has already proven to be difficult to both intubate and ventilate, many clinicians would prefer to use the SGA as a conduit for intubation, thereby minimizing further airway manipulation and trauma.

Due to the inner diameter limitation and the length of the SGA (eg, the LMA-Unique™ or LMA Supreme™), direct insertion of an adequately sized adult tracheal tube (TT) through its lumen is generally not recommended. There are three well-described techniques for LMA to TT exchange using a TT introducer—either an (1) Aintree Intubation Catheter, (2) guidewire, or (3) gum elastic bougie (GEB).

1. The Aintree Intubation Catheter is a hollow catheter with an inner diameter of 4.7 mm, allowing internal passage of a pediatric FIS. The intubation scope/Aintree complex is passed through the SGA and into the trachea. The FIS and the SGA are then removed, leaving the Aintree catheter in situ. A TT is then inserted over the Aintree, which serves as a guide to the tracheal position.
2. The second option involves inserting the FIS directly through the SGA and into the trachea. A guidewire is then passed through the working channel of the scope. The wire is retained as the FIS and SGA are removed and is used to pass a TT. Hang-up may occur during this technique because of the large discrepancy in size between the guidewire and even a small TT. An airway exchange catheter may be used to overcome this discrepancy and reduce the chances of this hang-up.
3. A third technique, preferred by the author, involves the placement of a GEB under FIS guidance. Unlike the Aintree catheter, the GEB is a ubiquitous device. Although blind bougie insertion through the SGA has been described, it has a low success rate. Preparation for intubation involves lubricating both a pediatric FIS and GEB. Generally, two operators are required to advance the scope and GEB in tandem. Once the bougie has been advanced through the glottis to 2 to 3 cm above the carina, the intubation scope and SGA are removed and a TT is inserted into position over the GEB. Using the smallest TT that is clinically adequate for the patient will reduce the incidence of hang-up.

Whenever feasible, ventilation and oxygenation should be continued during the Aintree and GEB intubation procedures. This can be achieved with the use of a variety of bronchoscope ports interposed between the SGA and the anesthesia circuit. Whereas the Aintree/flexible scope technique will require a single-port adaptor, a dual instrument port (eg, Arndt or Cohen BB ports) will be needed for the GEB technique.

If the attempt to intubate using the SGA as a conduit is unsuccessful and three or more total intubating attempts have been performed, this author recommends allowing the patient to wake up with plans of rescheduling the surgical procedure for a later date. Likewise, should airway manipulation cause deterioration to a "cannot-intubate, cannot-ventilate" situation, front of neck access (FONA) may be needed and should always be anticipated during management of the difficult airway.

3 Are there special considerations for the emergence or the end of the case?

Because of the initial difficulties with tracheal intubation and difficult mask ventilation, caution should be exercised at the time of emergence and extubation. This is further complicated by the patient's obesity. The anesthesia provider should ensure the availability of the appropriate equipment and personnel in anticipation of extubation failure. The patient should be fully awake and following commands, neuromuscular blockade should be fully reversed, and all other standard extubation criteria should be met. Depending on how many attempts at intubation were performed, the anesthesia provider might consider performing an airway leak test prior to extubation. It may also be reasonable to extubate the airway after placement of an airway exchange catheter and/or provide CPAP immediately postextubation.

- Obese patients are at risk for difficult airway management and perioperative rapid oxygen desaturation.
- If intubating attempts are unsuccessful, priority should be the maintenance of ventilation and oxygenation.
- A rescue SGA can be utilized as an intubating conduit.
- A bougie in parallel with a pediatric FIS or an Aintree catheter over a pediatric FIS can be used to facilitate tracheal intubation through an SGA.
- *See Figures 42.1 and 42.2 for additional details.*

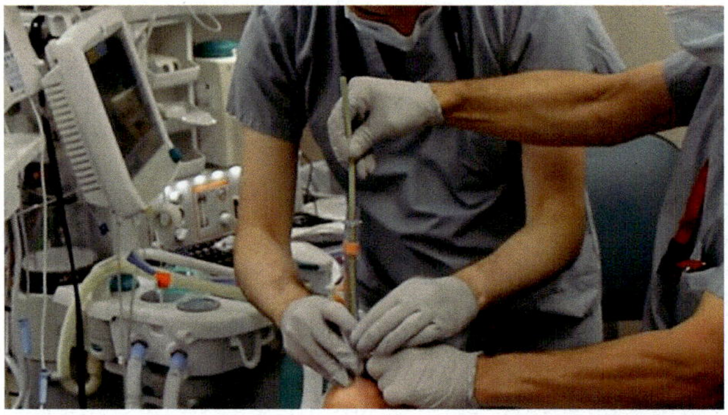

Figure 42.1. A tracheal tube introducer has been placed into the proximal end of a supraglottic airway.

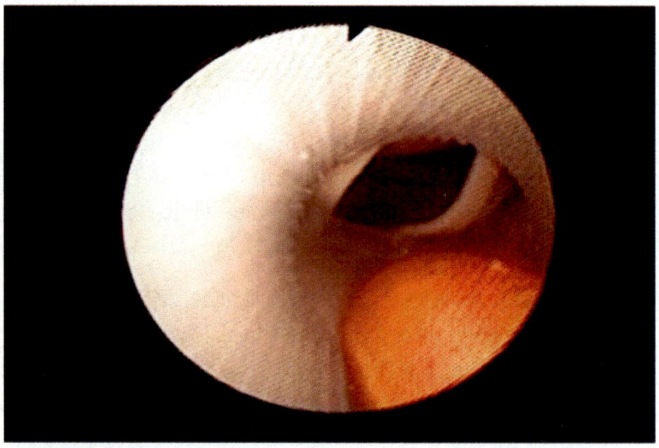

Figure 42.2. A gum elastic bougie is seen approaching the aperture bars of the supraglottic airway as it is aimed toward the larynx. Once seen to be in place in the mid trachea, the supraglottic airway will be removed and a tracheal tube advanced over the gum elastic bougie. See **Video 42.1**.

Suggested Readings

Apfelbaum JL, Hagberg CA, Connis RT, et al. 2022 American Society of Anesthesiologists Practice Guidelines for Management of the Difficult Airway. *Anesthesiology*. 2022;136(1):31–81.

Doyle DJ, Zura A, Ramachandran M, et al. Airway management in a 980-lb patient: use of the Aintree intubation catheter. *J Clin Anesth*. 2007;19(5):367–369.

Law JA, Duggan LV, Asselin M, et al. Canadian Airway Focus Group updated consensus-based recommendations for management of the difficult airway: part 1. Difficult airway management encountered in an unconscious patient. *Can J Anaesth*. 2021;68(9):1373–404.

Wong DT, Yang JJ, Mak HY, Jagannathan N. Use of intubation introducers through a supraglottic airway to facilitate tracheal intubation: a brief review. *Can J Anaesth*. 2012;59(7):704–715.

43 Combitube to Tracheal Tube Exchange

Kenneth N. Hiller • Neil S. Ballard • Carin A. Hagberg

Clinical Scenario: A 40-year-old appearing unidentified man is brought into the emergency department after a motor vehicle accident. At the scene, paramedics were unable to intubate him by direct laryngoscopy (DL). A Combitube was placed (esophageal position) in the field. Prior to being sent for diagnostic imaging, you are asked to exchange the Combitube for a tracheal tube.

1 What are the anesthetic and airway management considerations for this case?

The primary anesthetic considerations for this case, in order of priority, are maintaining the airway, managing aspiration risk, and observing cervical spine precautions. The esophageal–tracheal Combitube (ETC) was placed because paramedics could not intubate in the field, and a soiled and/or traumatized airway is likely to be encountered during further airway manipulation.

The plan should include several key components. First, to the extent possible, one should determine why the patient's airway was deemed difficult. A paramedic's assessment of a "difficult airway" may not equate to a "difficult airway" as defined by an experienced airway manager, such as an anesthesia provider. Second, the ETC should not be removed until the airway is secured in another fashion. Third, one should anticipate the loss of a secure airway while performing the exchange and have an appropriate backup plan(s) ready for implementation. Finally, one should consider the merits of direct versus indirect techniques, nasal versus oral approaches, and the use of muscle relaxants. The mechanism of injury and the likelihood of occult injuries may influence the use of specific medications to facilitate intubation.

The challenge of visualization around an inflated ETC oropharyngeal cuff must be balanced against the problems associated with interrupting ventilation with cuff deflation.

The conversion could be managed by DL or video laryngoscopy (VL) by deflating the large oropharyngeal cuff and interrupting ventilation. VL may be used as the initial technique or used if DL fails to provide an adequate view of the glottis. A flexible intubation scope (FIS) can be used either alone, or in combination with DL or VL. A bougie or intubating catheter could also be used in conjunction with these techniques. Neither VL nor FIS requires a linear view for intubation, which eliminates the need for neck extension and the sniffing position. This may be beneficial in the patient with a known or suspected cervical spine injury. There is no universal consensus on which intubation modality should be used in these patients. The modality depends on practitioner familiarity and experience and the clinical situation at hand.

FIS-aided exchange can be performed nasally or orally with little deflation of the oropharyngeal cuff and with or without muscle relaxant. A nasal approach facilitates passage of the FIS posterior to the oropharyngeal cuff, although it might still necessitate slight (~1 cm) withdrawal of the ETC. Partial deflation of the oropharyngeal cuff to "just sealing" preserves oxygenation and ventilation during FIS passage. Maintenance of pharyngeal tone and spontaneous movement of the laryngeal structures during spontaneous ventilation facilitates identification of the epiglottis and the larynx.

If the ETC was placed in the trachea (approximately 5% chance), a simple tube exchange could be performed with the aid of an airway exchange catheter. Regardless of the technique, the exchange should occur under DL, VL, or FIS visualization. Lack of predictable continuity between extraglottic devices and the glottic opening discourages blind techniques.

Gastric suctioning and decompression should be performed prior to the exchange. Cervical spine precautions should be exercised throughout the procedure, if indicated.

2 How would you manage the airway in this case?

Esophageal positioning of the ETC should be confirmed before making the exchange. A bag valve mask (BVM) or anesthesia circuit attached to the proximal end of the blue (number 1) lumen should result in bilateral chest movement, breath sounds, absence of gastric insufflation, and end-tidal CO_2 when cardiac output is present.

Passage of either a small nasogastric tube or the suction catheter that accompanies the ETC kit through the clear (number 2) lumen should be used to decompress and empty the stomach.

When esophageal placement cannot be confirmed, the BVM or circuit should be attached to the number 2 lumen. The ETC is in the tracheal position if bilateral breath sounds and chest rise are present without gastric insufflation.

For exchange of an ETC in the esophageal position, the authors' preference is to use VL with or without a bougie. If there is a possible cervical spine injury, cervical spine precautions should be maintained. The anterior portion of the cervical collar may be removed, if necessary, while maintaining in-line stabilization.

The oropharyngeal cuff should be deflated while VL is performed. Laryngoscopic view may be improved with careful pressure on the thyroid cartilage. Upon adequate glottic visualization, the trachea should be intubated. If necessary, a bougie can be placed into the trachea under visualization and an ETT advanced over it while VL is maintained. The distal ETC cuff is then deflated and the ETC is removed.

3 What are the potential hazards and complications in regard to the airway?

Potential hazards of exchanging an ETC for an ETT include aspiration of gastric contents, airway soiling, oxygen desaturation, and loss of the airway. Some patients may not tolerate even brief disruptions of oxygenation and/or ventilation. If the techniques described above are unsuccessful, a surgical airway may be required and can be performed with the ETC in place. Many of these considerations will also apply to other nonlaryngeal mask airways, such as the EasyTube and the King LT. Anesthesia providers should familiarize themselves with these nonlaryngeal mask airways that they may encounter during their practice.

4 Are there special considerations regarding the eventual extubation of this patient?

Initial intubation attempts failed in this patient. Airway edema and trauma should be presumed, potentially impacting airway competency. If DL or VL was performed during the exchange procedure, the laryngeal view should be documented to aid clinicians in making extubation decisions.

- Do not remove an extraglottic airway until a secure airway or conduit is in place.
- Esophageal ETC position should be confirmed prior to formulating an exchange plan.
- Gastric suctioning and decompression of an ETC in the esophageal position should be done prior to its exchange.
- A nasal approach employing a FIS, partial deflation of the pharyngeal cuff, and maintenance of spontaneous ventilation facilitates the exchange of an esophageal ETC for an ETT while maintaining oxygenation/ventilation.
- *See Figures 43.1 and 43.2 for additional details.*

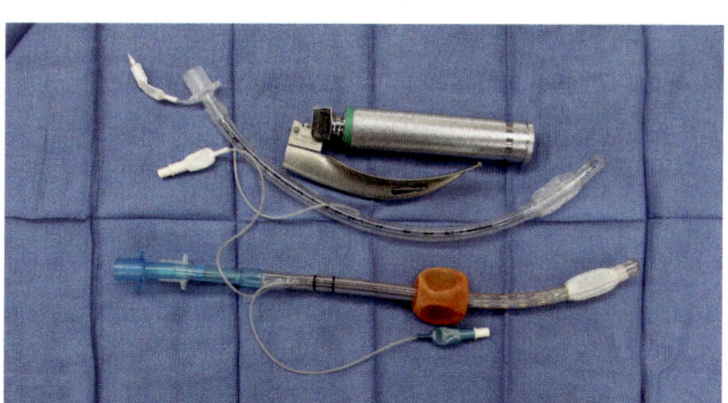

Figure 43.1. The esophageal-tracheal Combitube.

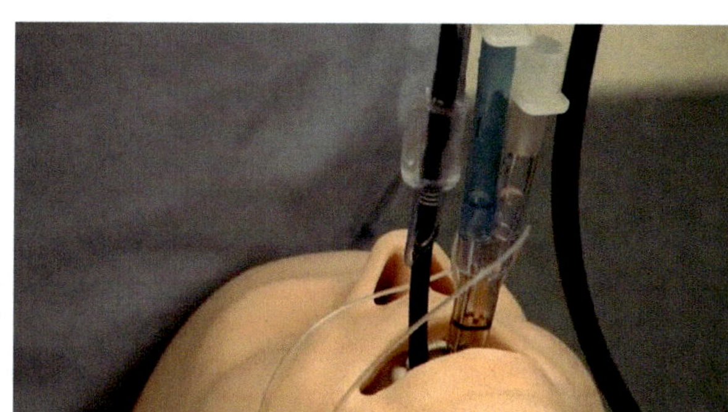

Figure 43.2. A flexible intubation scope (FIS) has been loaded with a single-lumen tracheal tube. The FIS will be advanced anterior to the Combitube (with cuffs deflated) and into the larynx. Once ventilation with the tracheal tube has been assured, the Combitube will be removed. See **Video 43.1**.

Suggested Readings

Dodd KW, Kornas RL, Klein LR, Reardon RF, Driver BE. Endotracheal intubation with the King Laryngeal Tube™ in situ using video laryngoscopy and a bougie: a retrospective case series and cadaveric crossover study. *J Emerg Med.* 2017;52(4):403–408.

Lam NC, Hagberg CA, Bassili LM. Use of the video laryngoscopy for Combitube exchange in a difficult airway. *J Clin Anaesth.* 2009;21:294–296.

Ostermayer DG, Gausche-Hill M. Supraglottic airways: the history and current state of prehospital airway adjuncts. *Prehosp Emerg Care.* 2014;18(1):106–115.

Robitaille A. Airway management in the patient with potential cervical spine instability: continuing professional development. *Can J Anaesth.* 2011;58(12):1125–1139.

Subramanian A, Garcia-Marcinkiewicz AG, Brown DR, Brown MJ, Diedrich DA. Definitive airway management of patients presenting with a pre-hospital inserted King LT(S)-D laryngeal tube airway: a historical cohort study. *Can J Anaesth.* 2016;63(3):275–282.

Extubation of the Difficult Airway Patient

44

Richard M. Cooper

Clinical Scenario: A 65-year-old man who previously underwent a mandibular resection and a microvascular free flap (fibula) reconstruction presents 6 months later for direct laryngoscopy and biopsy of a new lesion. The patient underwent an awake orotracheal intubation for the procedure, and he is now intubated with a 6.5 internal diameter tracheal tube (TT).

1 What are the airway management considerations for emergence?

This patient's airway is significantly distorted as a result of his prior head and neck surgery. Access may be restricted by limited mouth opening and reduced cervical extension (from the neck dissection and radiotherapy). There may be swelling, bleeding, induration, and pain prior to the procedure, and this current procedure may have induced further bleeding and/or edema. The patient also likely had a previous tracheotomy, which can lead to subsequent circumferential subglottic airway narrowing.

When preparing to extubate any patient, there are two essential considerations: (i) what is the likelihood of the patient tolerating extubation and (ii) if reintubation is required, how likely can this be achieved safely. Extubation success depends on adequate oxygenation, ventilation, airway patency, ability to clear secretions, and recovery of airway reflexes. The latter depends on the ease of accessing the airway under the prevailing situational and physiologic challenges.

2 How would you manage the airway in this case?

Likelihood of successful extubation depends on the factors mentioned above, which should be carefully considered in each patient. A "cuff-leak test" should be also performed, though its value is uncertain. The mouth should be cleared of secretions prior to performing this test. The TT cuff is slowly deflated, the TT is occluded, and an audible leak is assessed during exhalation. Its absence is nonreassuring, but its presence does not guarantee that extubation will be successful.

A visual airway assessment may help identify potential difficulties. The value of performing this with a tracheal tube in situ is limited, although seeing airway swelling or bleeding should prompt concern. Likewise, the inability to see the airway is worrisome. Whenever possible, this should be done with indirect (video) laryngoscopy or flexible bronchoscopy.

In this patient, the pharynx was carefully suctioned, and an audible leak was demonstrated when the cuff was deflated. The patient was allowed to resume spontaneous ventilation and emerge to full consciousness. When these conditions were met, a suitably sized airway exchange catheter (AEC) was introduced through the existing tracheal tube, aligning the distance markings of the two devices. This places the distal end of the AEC in the mid-trachea. The tracheal tube was carefully withdrawn over the AEC. The latter was secured to the maxilla and mandible, at an appropriate depth. The AEC was well tolerated by the patient. Intolerance of the AEC, demonstrated through coughing or straining, should prompt suspicion of catheter migration.

The AEC can be used to monitor end-tidal CO_2. Rarely, if life-threatening hypoxemia cannot be corrected by facemask supplementation or high-flow nasal oxygen, low-flow oxygen insufflation (1 to 2 L/min) through the AEC or jet ventilation may be required. Fatal barotrauma has been reported from insufflation and jet ventilation. The risks of hypoxemia and barotrauma must be weighed against the immediate need for ventilation. If insufflation or jet ventilation is attempted, every effort should be made to provide an open airway and minimize the duration of this intervention.

If reintubation is required, visualized advancement of the tracheal tube over the AEC by indirect laryngoscopy offers several advantages. The laryngoscope blade retracts the tongue and may provide a view of translaryngeal passage and immediate confirmation, avoiding tracheal tube impingement on the arytenoids or the posterior commissure. The use of an AEC significantly reduces the risk of multiple reintubation attempts, arterial oxygen desaturation, hemodynamic disturbances, and esophageal intubation.

Less-severe degrees of airway compromise may permit more conservative strategies. These include high-flow nasal oxygen or CPAP, elevation of the head of the bed, corticosteroid administration, inhalation of racemic epinephrine, and/or providing oxygenation with an admixture of helium and oxygen.

An alternative approach to extubation is the "Bailey maneuver," which is described in a separate chapter. This method can be considered in patients with less distorted airways in which rapid airway access is possible and the major postextubation concerns relate to oxygenation, ventilation, or airway patency (rather than access).

3 What distinct airway device might be used in this case, and what are the special considerations?

A variety of commercial AECs are available including the Cook Airway Exchange Catheter and Arndt Staged Extubation Set (Cook Medical, Bloomington, IN) or the Endotracheal Ventilation Catheter (12 Fr, outer diameter [OD] 4.0 mm, CardioMed Supplies, Ontario, Canada). The Cook devices are available in a range of diameters (8 Fr to 19 Fr) and lengths. To facilitate reintubation, the catheter must be sufficiently rigid, and its OD should minimize the gap between the inner diameter and OD of the tracheal tube and AEC, respectively. *It is important to point out that the Cook AEC has not been approved to remain in situ. This use, though commonly performed, is considered "off-label."*

4 How long should an exchange catheter be left in place?

One study showed that approximately half of the reintubations were performed after 2 hours, but most before 4 hours. Accordingly, it is prudent to resist the temptation to remove the AEC prematurely. A "Staged Extubation Set" (Cook Medical) leaves an Amplatz guidewire rather than an AEC in the trachea, though, as of this writing, this device has not been approved for use in North America. The Arndt Exchange Catheter Set (Cook) makes use of an Amplatz guidewire which is positioned bronchoscopically, followed by removal of the original tracheal tube and the immediate advancement of an AEC over the guidewire. The replacement tracheal tube is then "railroaded" over the AEC. Ensuring the appropriate depth and secure fixation can increase the tolerance of the device. Local anesthetics instilled into the trachea are almost never required for this maneuver.

- Emergent reintubation is almost always more difficult than elective intubation.
- Extubation of the difficult airway involves advance planning, preparation, and a backup plan to secure the airway.
- Visualized tube exchange offers numerous advantages over blind advancement.
- The use of an AEC can reduce morbidity during reintubation attempts.
- Placing an AEC too deeply increases intolerance and other serious complications.
- *See Figures 44.1 to 44.3 for additional details.*

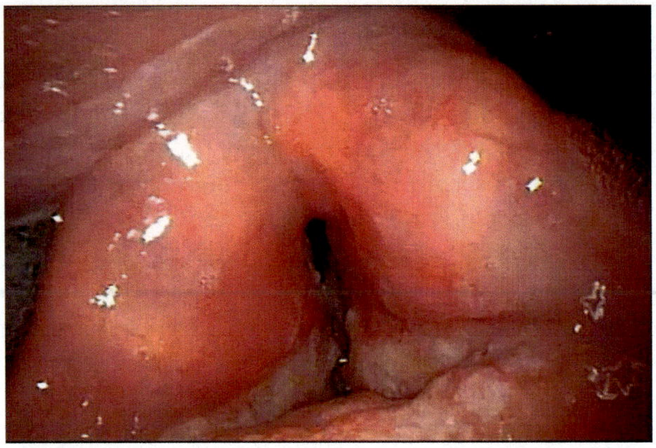

Figure 44.1. Prior to intubation, the patient's larynx was noted to be affected by radiation treatments and there is a risk of extubation failure. See **Video 44.1**.

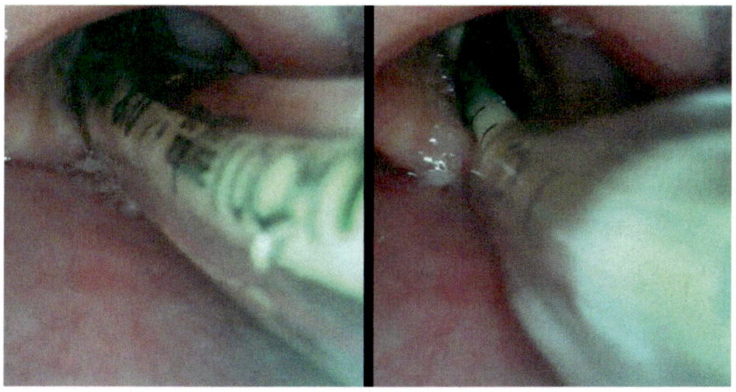

Figure 44.2. When the patient was ready for extubation, a Cook Airway Exchange Catheter was placed to a level above the carina (**left**) and the tracheal tube removed (**right**). See **Video 44.2**.

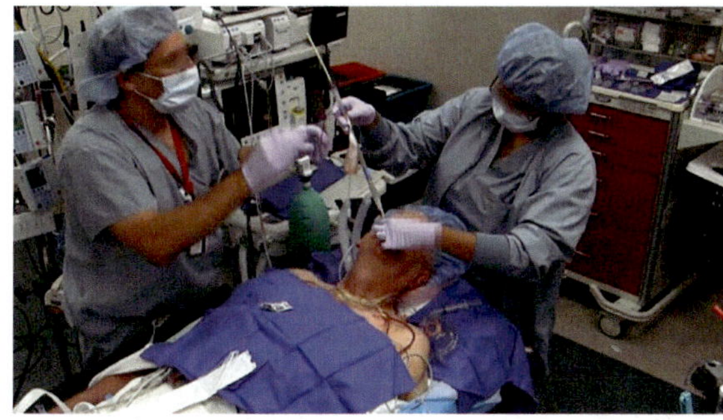

Figure 44.3. As the tracheal tube is removed, the exchange catheter is left in situ.

Suggested Readings

Cooper RM, Parotto M. Extubation and reintubation of the difficult airway. In: Hagberg C, ed. *Benumof and Hagberg's Airway Management*. 5th ed. Elsevier-Saunders; 2022.

Duggan LV, Law JA, Murphy MF. Brief review: supplementing oxygen through an airway exchange catheter: efficacy, complications, and recommendations. *Can J Anaesth*. 2011;58:560–568.

Mort TC. Continuous airway access for the difficult extubation: the efficacy of the airway exchange catheter. *Anesth Analg*. 2007;105:1357–1362.

Mort TC. Tracheal tube exchange: feasibility of continuous glottic viewing with advanced laryngoscopy assistance. *Anesth Analg*. 2009;108:1228–1231.

Popat M, Mitchell V, Dravid R, Patel A, Swampillai C, Higgs A. Difficult Airway Society Guidelines for the management of tracheal extubation. *Anaesthesia*. 2012;67:318–340.

45 Extubation in the Nonoperating Room, Non-ICU Environment

Jessica L. Feinleib • Andres De Lima Arboleda

Clinical Scenario: A 65-year-old morbidly obese woman, with body mass index of 48, was intubated for an upper endoscopy procedure in the gastroenterology suite. She has Barrett esophagus, and has limited neck extension secondary to a remote fusion after a motor vehicle accident. The patient is ready for extubation.

1 What are the anesthetic and airway management considerations for this case?

Surveys reveal that extubation outside the operating room (OR) results in more mishaps than previously appreciated. Results from the Fourth National Audit Project of the Royal College of Anaesthetists (NAP4) demonstrated that one-third of major airway complications (unanticipated or prolonged ICU admission, emergency surgical airway, brain damage, or death) occurred with extubation or the removal of a supraglottic airway (SGA). The 2022 American Society of Anesthesiologists Practice Guidelines for Management of Difficult Airway include a section on extubation of the difficult airway. The different recommendations include:

1. Having a preformulated strategy for extubation and subsequent airway management.
2. Clinical assessment of the patient's readiness for extubation.
3. Assessment of potential benefit in the short-term use of an airway exchange catheter or supraglottic airway in case an expedited reintubation is needed.
4. Implementation of supplemental oxygen throughout the extubation process.
5. Assessment of clinical factors that may adversely impact ventilation following extubation.

At least one-quarter of all NAP4-analyzed events transpired in emergency departments (EDs) or ICUs. The ED events were twice as likely to lead to death or brain damage as events in the OR. There is currently little data on the incidence of untoward events occurring with the extubation of the known difficult airway patient in a remote location. The combined elements of a difficult airway and a difficult environment will enhance the likelihood of complications. Of the several strategies employed to mitigate these risks, a few may be provided by institutional policies. Flagging known difficult airway patients, establishing protocol for tracheal extubation, and combining these with airway simulation training for staff may lessen the risk of poor outcomes.

2 How would you manage the airway in this case?

Preliminary discussions with consulting services to determine the need for extubation on completion of the procedure are especially pertinent for difficult airway patients. If the patient's airway is anticipated to critically worsen during the perioperative period, or if reintubation will be required in the near term, then a recommendation for continued intubation may be most prudent.

A difficult airway trolley should be brought to the site of extubation. The remote location's staff should be briefed on what assistance they can offer. If available, the institutional difficult airway team should be notified, otherwise discussions with relevant services about the possible need for emergent surgical airway access are recommended. If, during these discussions, it becomes clear that the risk of remote extubation of the patient is overly burdensome, then a viable alternative is to transport the patient, while intubated, to the OR or other appropriate environment for extubation.

Bringing the patient to an awake, cooperative state, with full neuromuscular function, improves safety. Emerging evidence confirms that residual neuromuscular blockade is associated with an increased risk of postoperative pulmonary complications following emergence from anesthesia and extubation. Practice guidelines from the American Society of Anesthesiologists recommend quantitative neuromuscular monitoring at the adductor pollicis to confirm the recovery of a train-of-four (TOF) ratio greater than 0.9 prior to extubation. Pharmacologic reversal of neuromuscular blockade, either with sugammadex or neostigmine as clinically appropriate, is recommended in all instances in which there is residual blockade.

Remote locations often lack design features that optimize access to the airway and infrequently have the adjustable procedure tables that are found in the OR. However, efforts to position the patient to provide optimal access should be aggressively sought. Raising the patient's upper body 25 degrees or greater will further improve pulmonary physiology. Transferring the patient to a different bed or location prior to emergence may be needed for this reason. Testing for a cuff leak may help predict the occurrence of airway obstruction after extubation. While the lack of a leak is a concerning finding and should prompt a reevaluation of the extubation plan, the presence of one should be interpreted carefully as it does not rule out obstruction following extubation.

The use of noninvasive positive-pressure ventilation (NIPPV) immediately after extubation has been shown to have pleiotropic and long-lasting effects. Immediate application of NIPPV after extubation of bariatric surgical patients, more effectively reverses losses in functional residual capacity over 24 hours than delayed application of NIPPV. In addition, a study of NIPPV after laparotomy demonstrated a reduction in reintubation rate from 10% to 1% and was associated with an 80% reduction of pneumonia and a 70% reduction of infection occurrences. Portable devices operated by a standard flowmeter are available (see Chapter 58: Preoperative Continuous Positive Airway Pressure). Moreover, the application of high-flow nasal cannula has been demonstrated to be at least noninferior to NIPPV in reducing reintubation rates, following high-risk extubation patients in the ICU environment. Although most of the data comes from critically ill patients, the increasing availability of portable high flow nasal cannula (HFNC) devices makes this tool a valuable option for anesthesiologists practicing in remote locations.

The use of airway exchange catheters (AECs) during extubation has been highly touted as a means to increase safety during extubation by two functions. First, the tube exchanger can be used to provide oxygenation. Second, the AEC can be used to guide reintubation. In a study by Mort et al., 92% of 51 difficult airway patients with a tube exchange catheter and a failed extubation were reintubated successfully.

3 What are the potential hazards and complications in regard to the airway?

The greatest hazard of extubating the difficult airway patient is loss of the airway. Even the use of an AEC does not ensure success in normal airways. The use of AECs has been associated with 14% intubation failure rate and a 1.5% pneumothorax rate. Other alternatives, such as a supraglottic airway device or the use of NIPPV or HFNC (as discussed previously) should be considered.

4 Are there special considerations for the emergence or the end of the case?

An institutional difficult airway extubation protocol is a useful tool. These documents allow for multiservice consensus building about the safe management of these patients before a particular patient is considered. Unambiguous policies decrease unfounded assumptions and reduce errors made due to poor planning. That being said, a policy does not nullify the importance of open communication between services discussing specific patients.

- Institutional policies and teams can help formalize and streamline remote extubation practice.
- Remote anesthetizing locations should have immediate access to all backup airway management equipment provided in the OR.
- Optimization of patient positioning, testing for cuff-leak, and assurance of neuromuscular blockade reversal should occur when evaluating readiness for extubation.
- Extubating high-risk patients to NIPPV or HFNC should be considered to increase success rates.
- Transporting an intubated patient to a familiar environment is a preferable alternative to struggling with inadequate equipment and staff during extubation.
- In scenarios in which difficulty is encountered, the patient and/or responsible person should be informed of the difficulty to provide guidance for future delivery of care. Documentation of difficulty encountered should be included in the medical record to facilitate future delivery of care.
- *See Figure 45.1 for additional details.*

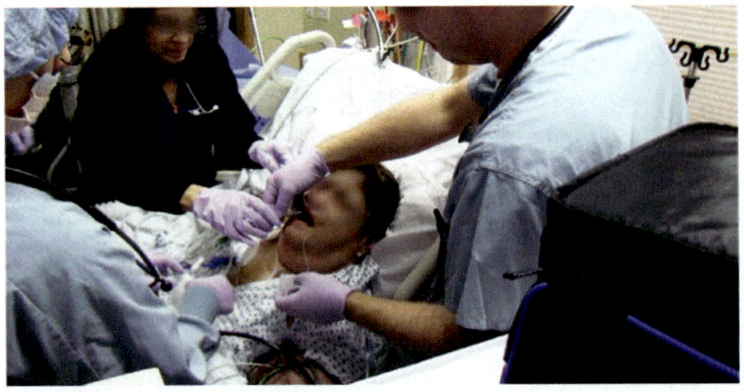

Figure 45.1. A patient is extubated in a NORA environment.

Suggested Readings

Apfelbaum JL, Hagberg CA, Connis RT, et al. 2022 American Society of Anesthesiologists practice guidelines for management of the difficult airway. *Anesthesiology*. 2022;136(1):31–81.

Cook TM, Woodall N, Frerk C; Fourth National Audit Project. Major complications of airway management in the UK: results of the Fourth National Audit Project of the Royal College of Anaesthetists and the Difficult Airway Society. Part 1: Anaesthesia. *Br J Anaesth*. 2011;106(5):617–631.

Cooper RM, O'Sulivan E, Popat M, Behringer E, Hagberg CA. Difficult Airway Society guidelines for the management of tracheal extubation. *Anesthesia*. 2013;68(2):217.

Hernandez G, Paredes I, Moran F, et al. Effect of postextubation noninvasive ventilation with active humidification vs high-flow nasal cannula on reintubation in patients at very high risk for extubation failure: a randomized trial. *Intensive Care Med*. 2022;48(12):1751–1759.

Thilen SR, Weigel WA, Todd MM, et al. 2023 American Society of Anesthesiologists Practice guidelines for monitoring and antagonism of neuromuscular blockade: a Report by the American Society of Anesthesiologists Task Force on Neuromuscular Blockade. *Anesthesiology*. 2023;138(1):13–41.

Out of the Operating Room Difficult Airway

46

Lauren C. Berkow

Clinical Scenario: You are called to an emergent intubation in a location out of the operating room (OR).

1 What are the anesthetic/airway management considerations for this case?

Patients requiring emergent airway management outside of the OR present many challenges. Oftentimes, the patient's airway history is unknown or unavailable, and the condition of the patient and urgency to secure the airway may prevent a thorough airway examination. Space and access to the patient are often limited. Infectious status may also be unknown, so additional personal protective equipment may be required during airway management.

These patients may be hemodynamically unstable and difficult to preoxygenate. Poor pulmonary reserve may lead to rapid desaturation during airway management, and anesthetic agents may cause significant hypotension. Some of these patients have recently failed extubation, so significant laryngeal edema may be present, which makes glottic visualization more difficult.

2 How would you manage the airway in this case?

When planning airway management for these patients, there are several important questions to consider.

1. Will the patient be difficult to mask ventilate?
2. Will supraglottic airway (SGA) placement be difficult?
3. Will the patient be difficult to intubate?
4. What resources might I need to manage the patient?
5. Are those resources readily available?

The last two questions are especially important because advanced airway equipment and additional personnel may not be immediately available outside of the OR setting. If difficulty with airway management is anticipated, ensure the necessary equipment is available at your location before proceeding. Also, consider whether managing the patient's airway in the OR is a safer option, assuming that the patient is stable for transport. Airway management in the OR setting provides more space and easier access to equipment and trained personnel.

When managing a patient's airway outside of the OR suite, the anesthesia provider should strive to maintain the same level of care that is provided in the OR. This includes standard American Society of Anesthesiologists (ASA) monitoring including pulse oximetry and capnography. Oxygen, suction, adequate intravenous access, and medications for sedation and hemodynamic control should also be available. Most importantly, a variety of airway tools and devices must be immediately available. They may be transported in a "code bag" or provided in an intubation "cart" or "box." At minimum, laryngoscope blades and handles, oral and nasal airways, endotracheal tubes, stylets and intubating bougies, and SGAs must be available.

If time permits, preoxygenation with 100% oxygen should precede attempts at airway management. A clear airway plan with at least one backup plan should be formulated and clearly stated to all personnel in the room. For patients at risk for desaturation, consider perioxygenation during airway management via high-flow nasal cannula or other similar devices.

A recent study of intubations in the emergency department found an increased success rate using video laryngoscopy compared to direct laryngoscopy. While video laryngoscopy may not be immediately available outside the OR, if difficulty is anticipated and time permits, adjunct airway devices such as a video laryngoscope or FIS should be brought to the bedside. Video laryngoscopes as well as FISs are now available in compact, battery-operated, and even disposable versions, making them easily portable. An emergency difficult airway cart should be developed for use both inside and outside the OR and should include video laryngoscopes, FISs, rigid intubating scopes, adjuncts, and equipment necessary to perform a surgical airway.

When feasible, a team approach to off-floor difficult airway patient management is critical—remote locations may be difficult to locate by a "stat" consultant so planning ahead is necessary. Several hospitals have created multidisciplinary difficult airway teams to manage these types of patients. The Fourth National Audit Project of the Royal College of Anaesthetists et al. (NAP4) demonstrated that many difficult airway situations occur during evenings or weekends, so 24/7 coverage should be considered, if feasible. This report also recommended the use of capnography for all intubations, the creation of multiple backup airway plans, and team training using simulation. The NAP4 report as well as the ASA Difficult Airway Task Force also recommend the use of standardized airway equipment carts. Standardization of equipment, personnel, and training has been shown to reduce the need for an emergent surgical airway.

Finally, patients requiring emergent intubation are at much higher risk of complications, including hypoxia, hypotension, aspiration, and cardiac arrest. The incidence of difficult laryngoscopy, multiple intubation attempts, and need for a surgical airway are all higher in these patients.

- Intubation performed outside of the OR may be more challenging, so be prepared with multiple plans to secure the airway.
- Consider perioxygenation during airway management for patients at risk for desaturation.
- Anticipate a higher incidence of difficulty with airway management and the need for alternate airway devices.
- Consider recruiting additional skilled personnel as well as multidisciplinary inputs when managing these patients.
- *See Figure 46.1 for additional details.*

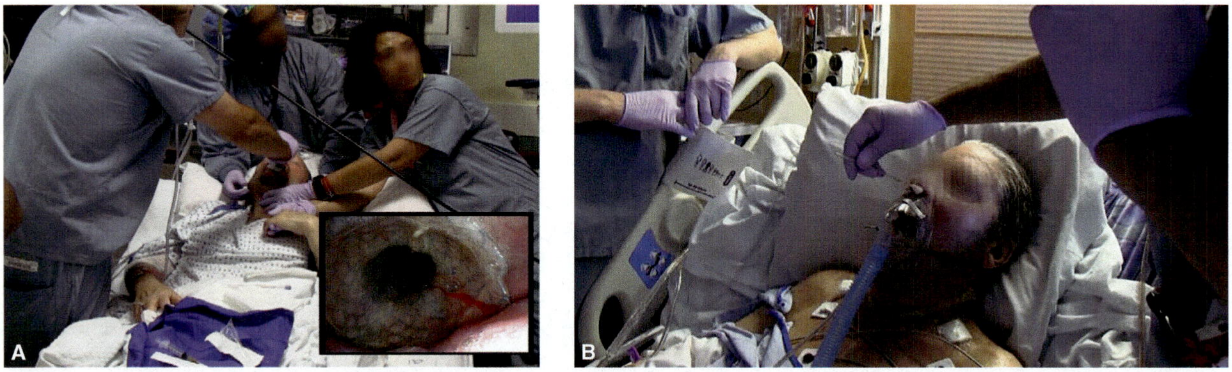

Figure 46.1. **A:** A patient with a tracheal stent requires advanced airway management including awake intubation in a crowded gastroenterology endoscopy suite. See **Video 46.1**. **B:** Advanced airway management may be required in a variety of nonoperating room environments, including the ICU. Here, an intensive care patient is prepared for awake intubation.

Suggested Readings

Berkow LC, Greenberg RS, Kan KH, et al. Need for emergency surgical airway reduced by a comprehensive difficult airway program. *Anesth Analg*. 2009;109:1860–1869.

Cook T, Behringer EC, Benger J. Airway management outside the operating room: hazardous and incompletely studied. *Curr Opin Anesthesiol*. 2012;25:461–469.

Cook TM, Woodall N, Harper J, Benger J; Fourth National Audit Project. Major complications of airway management in the UK: Results of Fourth National Audit Project of the Royal College of Anaesthetists and the Difficult Airway Society. Part 2: Intensive Care and Emergency Departments. *Br J Anaesth*. 2011;106:632–642.

Kornas RL, Owyang CG' Sakles JC, Foley LJ, Mosier JM; Society for Airway Management's Special Projects Committee. Evaluation and management of the physiologically difficult airway: consensus recommendations from society for airway management. *Anesth Analg*. 2021;132(2):395–405.

Endotracheal Tube Exchange in the ICU

47

Thomas C. Mort • F. Luke Aldo

Clinical Scenario: A 72-year-old male with laryngeal cancer has been urgently intubated with an 8.0-mm spiral wire–reinforced endotracheal tube (ETT) which is now partially obstructed due to the patient "biting" the tube. A large-caliber (19-Fr) airway exchange catheter (AEC) will not pass through the deformed ETT.

1 What are the anesthetic and airway management considerations for this case?

ETT exchange is conceptually simple, but it is not always a simple procedure as hypoxemia, esophageal intubation, and loss of airway can easily occur. An understanding of potential failures and complications are imperative. The emergent and elective need for an ETT exchange varies (Table 47.1).

TABLE 47.1 Common Reasons to Exchange ETT

1. Upsizing ETT diameter to allow therapeutic/diagnostic bronchoscopy
2. Change location (nasal vs oral)
3. ETT dysfunction (pilot balloon assembly, kink, sidewall damage, luminal narrowing from excessive biofilm/secretions)
4. Cuff failure (perforation, tear)
5. Change ETT type (double lumen tube [DLT] for single lumen ETT, for example)

ETT, endotracheal tube.

The method of ETT exchange chosen should be based on the airway status and potential for difficulty, availability of equipment and skilled personnel, and the team's experience and judgment. A key principle of ETT exchange is maintaining continuous airway access throughout the procedure. In straightforward situations, visual access via laryngoscopy, preferably video laryngoscopy (VL), may suffice for ETT removal and reintubation. However, airway trauma, secretions, edema, body habitus, or difficult airway anatomy combined with limited cardiopulmonary reserve may hinder exchange efforts. Continuous airway access is best maintained by an AEC, which is carefully inserted via the in situ ETT to an appropriate depth (based on matching the black depth marks on both the ETT and AEC).

A member of the airway team should be assigned to maintain the AEC position, given the possibility of proximal or distal AEC migration that can occur with removal of the old ETT or passing of the new ETT. Once the old ETT is removed, the AEC maintains access to the airway. Its position can be reconfirmed under continuous VL viewing. The new ETT is passed over the AEC and guided into the trachea. Again, visualization and AEC techniques are best practiced simultaneously. Patient participation is not required during ETT exchange, and some patients may benefit from additional sedation/analgesia. Neuromuscular relaxation may be useful in high-risk patients and those who resist oropharyngeal manipulations despite sedation. When using an AEC, simultaneous laryngoscopy helps to provide an unobstructed path for ETT passage, as well as allow visualization. Direct laryngoscopy (DL) offers limited visualization. However, VL is superior for visualizing the airway during an ETT exchange. FIS-guided ETT passage is possible when the airway is not overburdened by secretions and/or edema. Adjunct laryngoscopy (DL or VL) may assist with FIS navigation.

2 How would you manage the airway in this case?

Preoxygenation, optimal patient positioning (such as ramping the obese patient), and ETT/oropharyngeal suctioning are essential steps to perform prior to the exchange. Enteral feeds should be discontinued 2 to 4 hours prior, if possible, and any in situ nasogastric tube should be suctioned. The patient should be sedated as necessary to a cooperative state to prevent patient interference with the procedure. The risks and benefits of using neuromuscular blocking agents should be carefully considered. Neuromuscular blockade should only be used after an initial diagnostic laryngoscopy confirms the ETT is at least partially through the vocal cords. If the ETT is supraglottic, paralysis could rapidly lead to a disastrous scenario. This initial or "pre-exchange" diagnostic laryngoscopy should ideally be performed with a VL. VL optimizes assessment of the airway status and assists with the exchange strategy. Laryngoscopy may uncover partial or complete tracheal extubation masquerading as a "cuff leak." Blind advancement of an AEC without doing an initial diagnostic laryngoscopy could lead to AEC placement into the esophagus or damage to the oropharynx if the tip of the ETT is lying within the oropharynx.

It is imperative to assign tasks to team members during the exchange: (1) laryngoscopist, (2) AEC stabilizer, (3) ETT remover/advancer). Skilled airway personnel should be present, including a surgical team if marked difficulty is anticipated. All airway equipment and suction should be at the bedside. The exchange plan and contingencies for failure should be outlined.

In the current scenario, the crimped lumen of the reinforced ETT precludes the use of a large-caliber AEC. It is best to minimize the "gap" between the ETT and the AEC.

In this case, the 19 Fr could not be advanced due to luminal deformity. However, an alternative option is to advance a smaller caliber, 11 Fr or 14 Fr, AEC if possible. Following ETT removal, a lubricated Aintree catheter (Cook) may be placed over the AEC to provide support to the AEC and minimize the "gap." Access may also be maintained by passing an AEC (difficult to perform), intubation bougie, or preloaded FIS into the larynx alongside the ETT after cuff deflation. Adjunct laryngoscopy, preferably VL, offers both visualization and tissue displacement to facilitate exchange. Once the distal end of the FIS or AEC is assuredly at the mid-tracheal level or below, the indwelling ETT is removed. A new ETT is then inserted into the airway. ETT tip impingement on the arytenoid/vocal cord is remedied by gentle ETT retraction (1 to 2 cm) then counter clockwise (CCW) rotation followed by readvancement. The FIS or AEC is removed. Double gloving is recommended for personnel working with lubricated devices (easily remove the outer glove when it becomes slippery).

3 What are the potential hazards and complications in regard to the airway?

Most ETT exchanges are planned in an elective or urgent time frame where the patient is being managed with an airway which is faulty but adequate for the moment (eg, ruptured ETT cuff, obstructed by secretions, etc.). In this situation where the airway is partially functional, the risk of exchanging a marginal airway to a failed airway must be weighed. The preexisting airway pathology may add to the exchange difficulty; bleeding, necrotic tumor debris, friability, secretions, edema, airway obstruction upon removal of the ETT, and limited working space may exist in the airway. ETT tip hang-up on airway structures along its route to the trachea may occur. A mismatching size of the ETT and AEC or FIS is often the cause of this.

The risk of frictional dragging of the AEC or FIS out of the larynx during ETT removal is significant. The smaller-diameter AECs (11 Fr, 14 Fr) have less longitudinal strength and may be prone to dislocation and impair ETT advancement due to their pliability. They should be avoided, if possible, or augmented by Aintree placement as a "jacket" if adaptable to the clinical situation.

Adequate preoxygenation and a well-planned, rapidly executed airway exchange will ideally eliminate the need for supplemental oxygen delivery during the procedure. Clearing the airway of secretions will reduce exposure of the trachea to soilage and other potential sources of infection during the unprotected phase of the exchange. Some high-risk exchanges may be best performed in the OR.

4 What distinct airway device might be used in this case, and what are the special considerations?

A VL and the standard contents of a difficult airway cart, including a FIS should be immediately available. In addition, maintaining continuous airway access during the exchange via an AEC is recommended in nearly all cases.

- Attempt to visualize the larynx during ETT exchange.
- Adjunct laryngoscopy can be used during parallel FIS insertion.
- Ensure the availability of alternative airway equipment and surgical backup at the bedside.
- Consider performing the exchange in the OR if the patient is deemed high risk.
- Assign specific tasks (laryngoscopist, AEC holder, ETT remover/advancer) to team members.
- Match AEC, FIS, and ETT size based on longitudinal strength to reduce tip hang-up and ETT wobble during advancement (minimize the gap).
- *See Figure 47.1 and* ***Video 47.1*** *for additional details.*

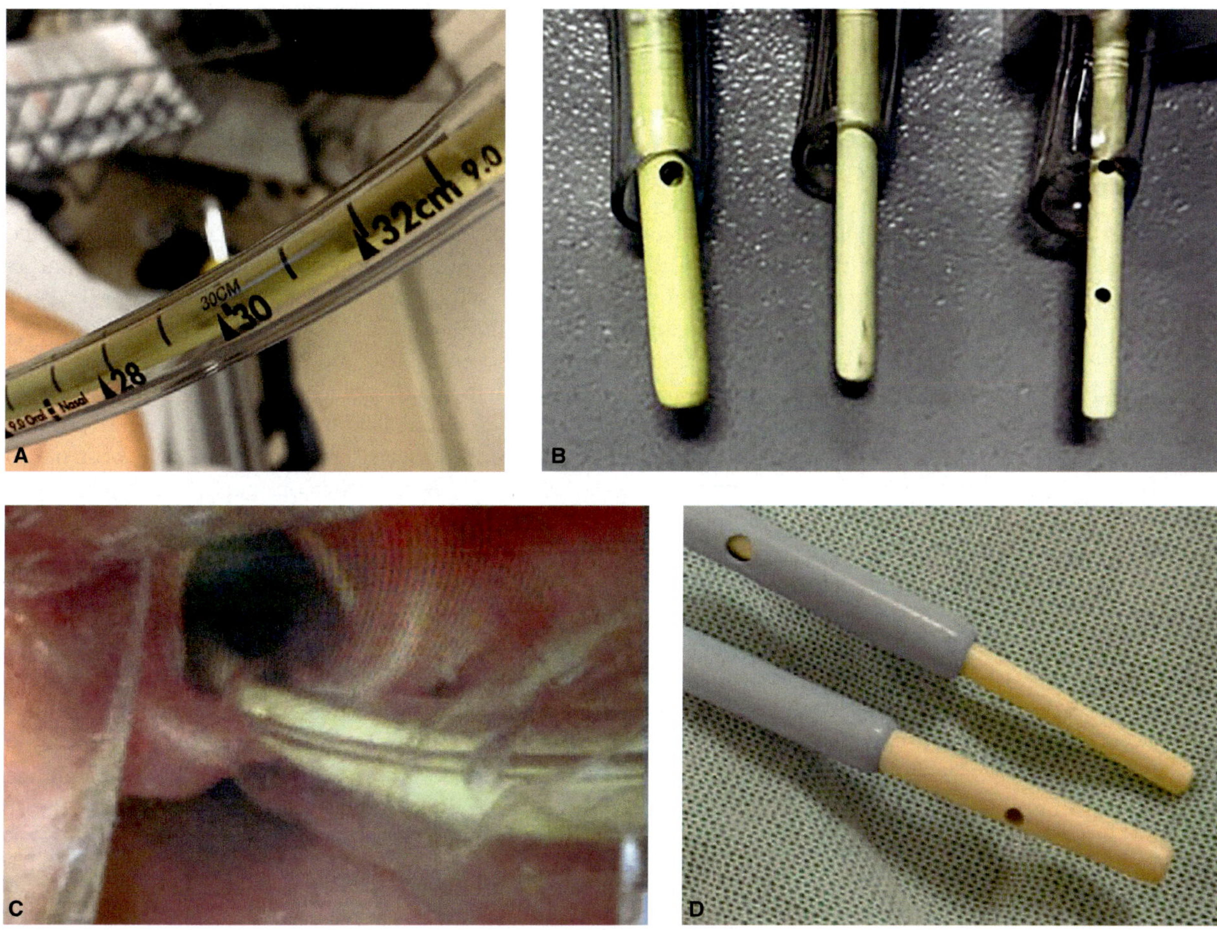

Figure 47.1. **A:** The airway exchange catheter (AEC) depth markings can be advanced to match those of the endotracheal tube (ETT). **B:** 19-Fr, 14-Fr, 11-Fr AEC in an 8.0-mm ETT (L→R). Note the significant "gap." **C:** 14-Fr AEC positioned in the posterior glottis. Bevel impingement inhibited forward advancement. Corrective measures included retraction of the ETT (1 to 2 cm), followed by ETT rotation CCW, then smooth advancement. **D:** Aintree Catheter acting as a "jacket" over the 14-Fr (lower) and 11-Fr (upper) AEC to minimize the gap, reducing both "wobble" and ETT bevel impingement.

Suggested Readings

Harris K, Chalhoub M, Maroun R, Elsayegh D. Endotracheal tube exchangers: should we look for safer alternatives? *Heart Lung*. 2012;41(1):67–69.

McLean S, Lanam CR, Benedict W, Kirkpatrick N, Kheterpal S, Ramachandran SK. Airway exchange failure and complications with the use of the Cook Airway Exchange Catheter®: a single center cohort study of 1177 patients. *Anesth Analg*. 2013; 117(6):1325–1327.

Mort TC. Tracheal tube exchange: feasibility of continuous glottic viewing with advanced laryngoscopy assistance. *Anesth Analg*. 2009;108(4):1228–1231.

Mort TC, Braffett BH. Conventional versus video laryngoscopy for tracheal tube exchange: glottic visualization, success rates, complications, and rescue alternatives in the high-risk difficult airway patient. *Anesth Analg*. 2015;121(2):440–448.

48 Reintubation in the ICU Patient with Unexpected Postextubation Stridor

Thomas C. Mort • F. Luke Aldo

Clinical Scenario: A 72-year-old male is being readied for his third trial of extubation following 12 days of mechanical ventilatory support in the ICU. He is nonobese and his prior tracheal intubations (DL-VC grade 2a view, video laryngoscopy (VL) full view; one attempt each) were documented as uncomplicated. Ten minutes postextubation, he has hoarseness on phonation and mild biphasic stridor. He develops subsequent increased work of breathing, tachycardia, worsening stridor, and perspiration.

1 What are the anesthetic and airway management considerations for this case?

Postextubation "stridorous" (PES) noise may have a variety of etiologies. Stridor, typically a high-pitched, musical sound, results from turbulent airflow and suggests airway narrowing or obstruction. This is in contrast to "stertor" which is a lower-pitched, noisy "snoring' type of breathing that typically emanates from the nose, nasopharynx, soft palate or oropharynx, or the supraglottic region.

Stridor is a symptom, not a diagnosis per se. This "noise" should command immediate medical attention to establish its etiology and render therapy. Moreover, patient effort will influence the pitch and intensity of airway noise thus, changes, for example, reduced stridor, may be influenced by a tiring patient. Stridor may be classified as inspiratory, expiratory, or biphasic. Generally, inspiratory stridor suggests airway obstruction above the glottis while an expiratory stridor suggests subglottic or lower trachea obstruction. A biphasic stridor suggests a glottic or subglottic lesion. PES in the ICU occurs in 10% to 15% of planned extubations and up to 33% of unplanned, "self"-extubations.

Attempts at reintubation may be more difficult due to the etiology causing the stridor, for example, edema, anatomical distortion, narrowing, swelling, or foreign body. Securing the airway may be fraught with hemodynamic and airway-related perturbations. Laryngoscopy (preferably video assisted), naso/oropharyngoscopy, or bronchoscopy may provide evidence of the etiology and the level of the pathology (supraglottic, glottic, subglottic, or a combination). Bronchospasm may mimic stridor and vice versa, or they may coexist. Vocal cord (VC) edema, granulations, ulcerations, and VC immobility or arytenoid dislocation may contribute to PES, especially in the setting of recent head and neck surgery, upper endoscopic procedures, or other airway interventions. Periglottic edema or unrecognized orohypopharyngeal edema and/or hematoma with airway encroachment may present as PES. Subglottic granulations, swelling, and/or mucosal ischemia/necrosis from excessive tracheal tube (TT) cuff pressure or traumatic ETT passage may lead to PES. Other causes include excessive intravenous volume administration, prolonged supine or prone positions, or interruption of the venous drainage of the head/neck from deep vein thrombosis or central venous access. Uncommonly, patient anxiety may lead to VC dysfunction. It is typically misdiagnosed as asthma in ~80% of cases, and this can further cloud the etiology of stridor.

2 How would you manage the airway in this case?

Following rapid review of the patient's history and current systemic, surgical, and airway concerns, the degree of airway flow obstruction and its impact on the patient's safety should be evaluated. The airway should be secured emergently if rapid deterioration is apparent. It is prudent to assume that airway management may be difficult even if the previous intubation was straightforward. Contingency plans should be made for an emergent surgical airway, ensuring the presence of capable personnel prior to any airway manipulation. Routine and difficult airway equipment should be brought to the bedside. Awake intubation should be considered if previous airway interventions in this patient required advanced devices/techniques or if a rapid airway assessment suggests difficulty with ventilation, laryngoscopy, and/or intubation. An awake approach, if time permits, may allow simultaneous diagnostic evaluation if this had not been previously performed. If there is low concern for difficult intubation, a rapid sequence intubation technique may be chosen. The degree of patient preparation and the specific induction approach are personal choices based on experience, judgment, and the skill set of the airway team. To date, evidence-based research has not concluded that either a rapid sequence or induction with paralysis is superior for the rapidly deteriorating patient with stridor.

If a PES patient presents with a relatively stable status, several noninvasive interventions may be prescribed. Inhaled racemic epinephrine may reduce tissue edema, reducing stridor and respiratory work. The response is rapid if airway edema is the culprit for the stridor. Heliox (Helium-oxygen blend) is a low-density gas blend that may improve airflow past an obstruction rapidly. Using Heliox precludes the use of 100% oxygen since it is routinely administered in a 70/30 or 60/40 (Heliox/O_2) ratio. Steroid or diuretic administration may also aid in reducing airway edema, but these interventions both take longer to produce clinical results. Cautious use of anxiolytics to combat anxiety may be indicated, particularly in patients with paradoxical VC motion or dysfunction, where anxiety or other psychogenic factors may be causing PES. Forced inspiration and expiration worsen airflow, so tachypnea may worsen symptoms by increasing turbulent flow across the obstruction.

The stable patient with PES provides an opportunity for a more thorough investigation. Bedside nasopharyngoscopy requires minimal patient preparation and the information derived may allow for more targeted therapies (eg, optimize head elevation, diuresis to promote negative fluid balance, steroid trial, otolaryngology consult, foreign body discovery, reintubation, surgical airway access, reoperation, etc.).

3 What are the potential hazards and complications in regard to the airway?

Investigating the cause of PES is important, but some patients may require immediate life-saving therapy without further investigation. The airway team must remain flexible in adapting to a variety of PES etiologies. Likewise, it is dangerous to assume that a previously "easy" airway can be secured in the same way when PES is a concern. The clinician must be prepared to deploy advanced airway adjuncts and instrumentation supported by contingencies for a surgical airway. Awake intubation and maintaining spontaneous ventilation during reintubation should be considered. If an awake/aware approach is employed, the sitting and head-up positions may be more advantageous for the patient and the airway team.

4 Are there special considerations for reemergence?

Planned reextubation of the patient with a history of PES should be approached expectantly. Preparation for removal of the TT should be directed by the findings, if any, from the evaluation of the stridor, and should begin well in advance of extubation. Preextubation VL to evaluate the glottic/supraglottic anatomy may be useful in certain clinical scenarios. Likewise, flexible endoscopy may be informative. Head of bed elevation, careful attention to fluid balance, reversal of anticoagulation, and steroid, bronchodilator, or vasoconstrictor administration should be considered when appropriate. A leak test, although not sensitive, may provide some reassurance for the absence of significant airway edema. However, a negative leak test should not be relied upon as the sole indicator that the airway is "okay" or "safe." Use of an airway exchange catheter (AEC) to maintain airway access postextubation can be considered, especially in the patient who was a previous difficult intubation. However, if subglottic narrowing is the culprit, an indwelling AEC may further reduce the cross-sectional area of the airway. Last, some patients may require elective surgical intervention such as posterior cordotomy, tracheostomy, or tracheal dilatation in cases of moderate or severe subglottic scarring or stenosis.

- In a patient with postextubation stridor, a careful and rapid search for its etiology is reasonable if the patient is stable.
- Assume difficult mask ventilation, visualization, and intubation in the stridorous patient even if prior airway management was uncomplicated.
- A subglottic source may require immediate access to smaller caliber ETT or surgical access.
- *See Figures 48.1 and 48.2 for additional details.*

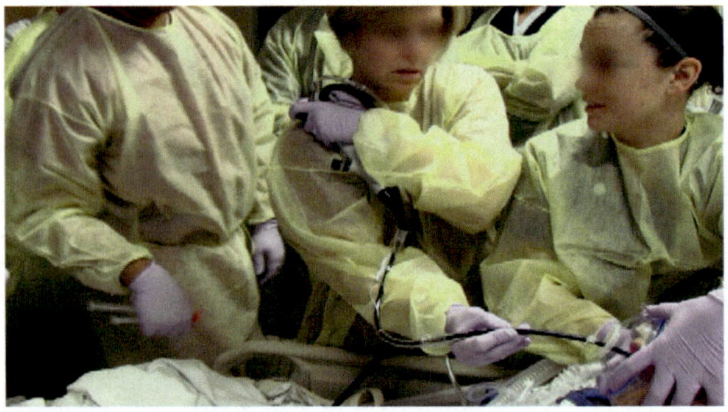

Figure 48.1. A patient in an ICU setting undergoes emergent reintubation. See **Video 48.1**.

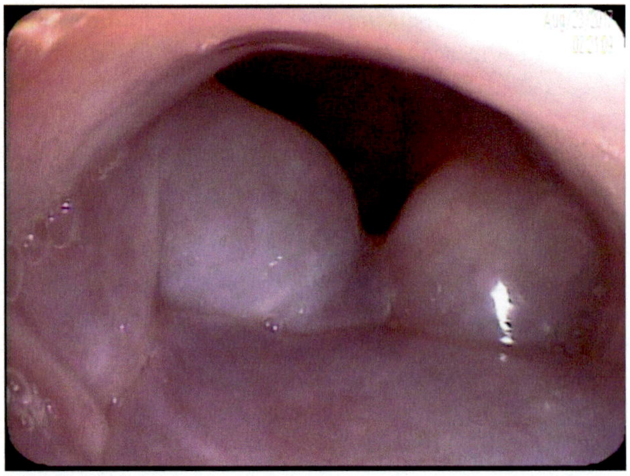

Figure 48.2. Urgent examination of a self-extubated ICU patient with stridor reveals Reinke edema. See **Video 48.2**.

Suggested Readings

Apfelbaum JL, Hagberg CA, Connis RT, et al. 2022 American Society of Anesthesiologists Practice Guidelines for Management of the difficult airway. *Anesthesiology*. 2022;136(1):31–81.

Cavallone LF, Vannucci A. Extubation of the difficult airway and extubation failure. *Anesth Analg*. 2013;116(2):368–383.

Cooper RM, O'Sullivan E, Popat M, Behringer E, Hagberg CA. Difficult Airway Society guidelines for the management of tracheal extubation. *Anaesthesia*. 2013;68:217.

Difficult Airway Society Extubation Guidelines Group; Popat M, Mitchell V, Dravid R, Patel A, Swampillai C, Higgs A. Difficult Airway Society Guidelines for the management of tracheal extubation. *Anaesthesia*. 2012;67:318–340.

Rosenblatt W, Ianus AI, Sukhupragarn W, Fickenscher A, Sasaki C. Preoperative endoscopic airway examination (PEAE) provides superior airway information and may reduce the use of unnecessary awake intubation. *Anesth Analg*. 2011;112(3):602–607.

Partial Extubation Masquerading as Cuff Leak

49

Thomas C. Mort • F. Luke Aldo

Clinical Scenario: An intubated patient in the ICU has an audible air leak that has been worsening over the past 24 hours. The "leak" temporarily resolves with the addition of air to the pilot balloon but recurs soon thereafter. The endotracheal tube (ETT) is secured at 25-cm depth, and the pilot balloon is inflated and appears undamaged and intact. The patient's oxygen saturation is 90% on 50% FiO_2.

1 What are the anesthetic and airway management considerations for this case?

Self-extubation describes the accidental removal of an ETT by either the patient or a non–patient-initiated action (eg, repositioning). Most commonly, the ETT exits the trachea completely, resulting in an airway management emergency. Alternatively, cephalad migration of the ETT, with full or partial herniation of the ETT cuff-tip above the vocal cords, may present with a confusing clinical picture (Table 49.1). Partial extubation demands a concise diagnosis coupled with a sound strategic plan to resecure the airway. Partial extubation typically presents with an audible air leak during positive-pressure ventilation. The depth of the ETT may appear appropriate with little correlation to ETT tip position within the airway. For example, the ETT may be 24 cm at the lip, but the ETT actually bows inside the oropharynx and the ETT tip/cuff may be at or above the glottic opening. Other leak etiologies include the ETT tip/cuff lying at the carinal bifurcation, the cuff abutting the underside of the glottis, a tracheal wall–ETT incongruency (tracheomalacia), a fistulous communication (TE fistula), or misplacement of a nasogastric tube (NGT) or esophageal temperature probe in the trachea. Each of these situations may lead to an "air leak." Overall, the most common leak is due to an incompetent or damaged ETT cuff or pilot balloon. Of the remaining leaks, partial or complete herniation of the ETT cuff is the most common etiology for an air leak in a mechanically ventilated ICU patient. A continuous $ETCO_2$ reading does not rule out partial or complete extubation.

TABLE 49.1 ETT Cuff-Tip Complex Dislocation (Partial or Complete Extubation)

Class 1. Cuff within glottis
Class 2. Cuff above glottis, ETT tip within glottis
Class 3. Cuff-tip above glottis (complete extubation)

ETT, endotracheal tube.

Each leak etiology may require a unique remedy. Improper assessment of the leak may lead to an incorrect therapy. Proper pilot balloon function (staying inflated) in the presence of a leak strongly suggests partial or complete extubation. The air leak may be continuous or intermittent and may vary with the patient's body, head, or neck position. The leak may compromise ventilation and oxygenation and also increase the risk of aspiration. Partial displacement can rapidly deteriorate to complete extubation.

El-Orbany and Salem reviewed ETT cuff leaks and their causes, consequences, and management. They suggest that an airway assessment with a fiberoptic scope (FIS), video laryngoscopy (VL), or direct laryngoscopy (DL) is essential. Each may be useful for diagnostic and therapeutic measures, though DL has limited success compared to FIS and VL. FIS use led to an 80% reduction in multiple attempts to reintubate. The need for a rescue device and incidence of hypoxemia and bradycardia were also reduced. The FIS provided excellent diagnostic and therapeutic conditions. Advancement of a thermosoftened ETT lying supraglottically (class 2 or 3) may be difficult to accurately advance due to excessive softening, leading to ETT malpositioning or esophageal placement. Replacement with a new styletted ETT is the best management option. Class 3 extubation was notably problematic due to difficult glottic visualization from a confined hypopharyngeal space, secretions, periglottic edema, luminal kinking, luminal biofilm accumulation, and ETT-tip impingement/abutment. In these cases, the Murphy eye may be the sole portal for ventilation and oxygen delivery.

A serpentine curvature or "bowing/arching" configuration of the displaced ETT is common. ETT cuff-tip displacement into the supraglottic area may allow excessive cuff inflation (eg, 25 to 125 mL of air) without the commensurate rise in measured cuff pressure.

2 How would you manage the airway in this case?

There is little formal guidance in the literature regarding the management of a cuff leak or air leak. Diagnostic investigation to uncover its etiology is key. An audible leak coupled with an inflated pilot balloon should create suspicion that partial or complete extubation exists. End-tidal CO_2 detection or the maintenance of oxygen saturation does not eliminate the possibility of extubation. Prior to any ETT manipulation, the patient should be placed on 100% oxygen. Injecting lidocaine into the ETT may improve patient tolerance of airway manipulation. It is ideal to maintain spontaneous ventilation efforts. A FIS equipped with a swivel adapter allows for continuous oxygen delivery during the ETT examination. Secretions may hinder visualization, so access to a working suction channel is crucial. ETT tip impingement may limit visualization, so it may be necessary to carefully withdraw the ETT in order to identify laryngeal or tracheal anatomy. Ideally, laryngeal structures, tracheal rings, or carina should be identified before concluding that the ETT remains in the larynx. Transglottic passage of the FIS into the trachea should allow ETT advancement to the proper depth. VL imaging of a partially extubated ETT is far superior to that achieved with DL. However, advancement of the partially extubated ETT may prove challenging due to softening of the ETT, as mentioned before. Use of an AEC through the indwelling ETT to assist reintubation should be done cautiously and only after ETT visualization via FIS or VL.

3 What are the potential hazards and complications in regard to the airway?

No evidence-based data exist to support or refute any specific management approach. Blind advancement of a suspected herniated ETT is discouraged. Blind placement of an AEC/bougie to assist with ETT advancement could result in tissue injury or loss of the airway (class 3). Likewise, laryngoscopy-managed class 3 extubations are best managed with placement of a new styletted ETT, as mentioned before. Misdiagnosis of the air leak etiology can lead to devastating consequences. A backup rescue plan and immediate access to advanced airway equipment is imperative.

4 What distinct airway device might be used in this case, and what are the special considerations?

The clinician should be equipped with accessory rescue devices, including VL and FIS, and immediate access to a difficult airway cart as suggested by the ASA Difficult Airway Task Force. Less experienced clinicians or trainees should be discouraged from managing these cases without proper backup or supervision.

- Unrecognized partial or complete tracheal extubation are the leading causes of an air leak in the ICU (followed by cuff malfunction/perforation).
- Blind advancement of the malpositioned ETT should be strongly discouraged.
- Diagnostic followed by therapeutic intervention with a FIS or VL is strongly recommended.
- Blind AEC passage through an unrecognized displaced ETT may result in trauma or esophageal placement.
- *See Figures 49.1 to 49.3 for additional details.*

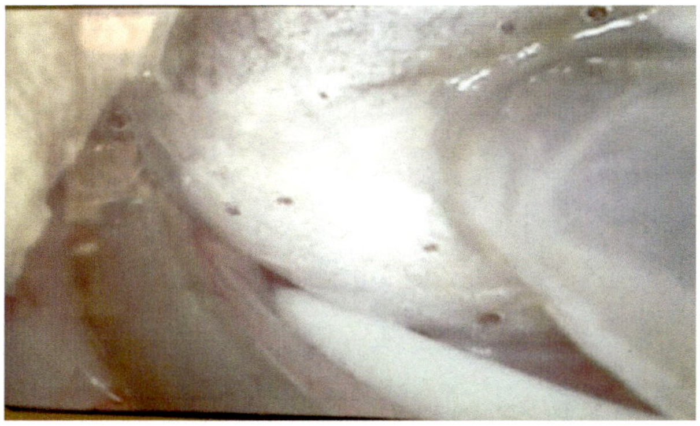

Figure 49.1. Class 3 extubation: VL view of complete extubation. The ETT cuff is hyperinflated in the hypopharynx abutting against the base of the tongue. The feeding tube and NGT are visible posterior to the cuff. See **Video 49.1**.

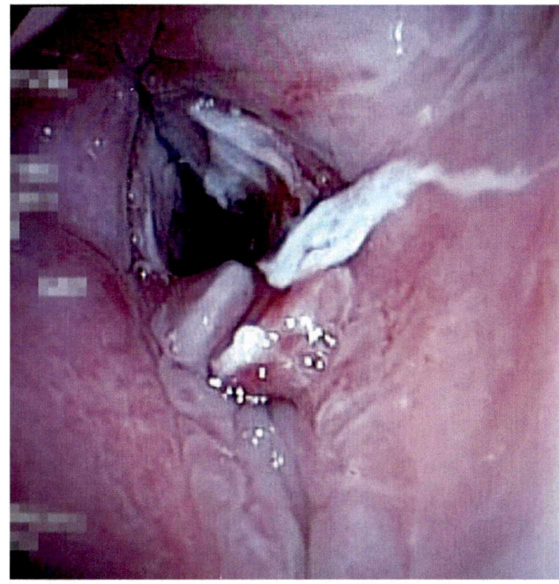

Figure 49.2. Class 3 extubation (view via FB, intermittent leak, pilot cuff intact, ETT depth at 25 cm, 65 mL of air removed from cuff, reintubated via FB).

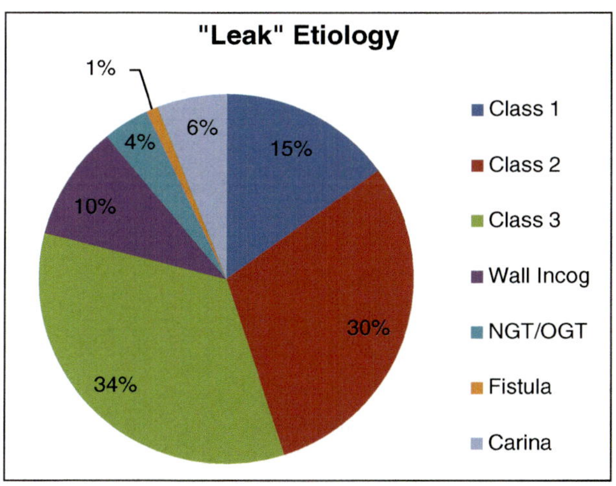

Figure 49.3. "Leak" etiology in 1010 ICU patients (excluding cuff dysfunction).

Suggested Readings

El-Orbany M, Salem MR. Endotracheal tube cuff leaks: causes, consequences and management. *Anesth Analg.* 2013:117; 428–434.

Kearl RA, Hooper RG. Massive airway leaks: an analysis of the role of endotracheal tubes. *Crit Care Med.* 1993;21:518–521.

Sultan P, Carvalho B, Rose BO, Cregg R. Endotracheal tube cuff pressure monitoring: a review of the evidence. *J Perioper Pract.* 2011;21:379–386.

50 Difficult Extubation in the ICU

Akhil Khosla • Elizabeth C. Behringer

Clinical Scenario: A 67-year-old man being treated for congestive heart failure in the medical intensive care unit (MICU) is being weaned from mechanical ventilator support. His initial intubation was reportedly difficult. The MICU attending has requested your assistance with extubation.

1 What are the anesthetic/airway management considerations for elective extubation of a patient with a known difficult airway?

Reintubation of the critically ill patient remains a rather common event with up to 25% of extubated ICU patients eventually requiring reintubation. Extubation failure is generally defined as the need for reintubation during the first 48 to 72 hours after extubation. Extubation failure has been associated with poor outcomes including increased procedural complications compared to the initial intubation, hypotension, hypoxia, longer duration of mechanical ventilation, increased tracheostomy rates, longer length of stay, and increased mortality. Preventing extubation failure and assessing a patient's readiness for extubation remains a multifactorial, multilayered process. A spontaneous breathing trial (SBT) can be completed either using a T-piece or pressure support ventilation to assess readiness for extubation. A positive rapid shallow breathing index (RSBI), defined as the respiratory rate divided by the tidal volume in liters, of less than 105 may predict successful extubation, whereas values greater than 105 may predict patients at higher risk of failed extubation.

This patient's acute and chronic medical problems place him at increased risk of rapid deterioration in the event of extubation failure. The patient's other medical conditions should be optimized to ensure readiness for successful extubation. Since the patient is a known "difficult airway" additional measures of investigation are warranted. Preextubation considerations in intubated ICU patients should include:

- *Review of the most recent chest imaging:* looking for current endotracheal tube position as well as evidence of significant pulmonary abnormalities.
- *Review of current ventilator settings:* Ventilator requirements should be modest. Ideally, FiO_2 40% or less and a PEEP of 5. The patient should be observed for an unlabored respiratory pattern, as well as ensuring adequate respiratory rates, tidal volume, and minute ventilation (ideally <10 L) during an SBT. The results of prior SBTs and the RSBI should be noted.
- *Review of current hemodynamic status:* Current vital signs, point-of-care ultrasound findings, advanced hemodynamic monitoring (if available), and volume status should be reviewed. Ideally, patients will be on minimal vasopressors prior to extubation and have a euvolemic to hypovolemic volume status.
- *Review of adequacy of pulmonary toilet:* Is the patient requiring frequent endotracheal suctioning (eg, more than every 2 hours)? Does the patient have an adequate cough?
- *Investigation for the presence of glottic edema:* In a known difficult airway patient who required multiple laryngoscopic attempts prior to successful intubation, assessing the glottis for edema with the endotracheal tube in situ is a mandatory part of extubation evaluation. Methods include a cuff leak assessment or glottic visualization utilizing video laryngoscopy or a flexible intubation scope. Review of the patient's prior intubation records can provide guidance on what techniques and equipment will be required in the event the patient needs to be reintubated.
- *Mental status:* Ensure the patient has an improving or stable mental status.
- *Cause of respiratory failure or need for intubation addressed:* The underlying cause of the patient's respiratory failure or need for intubation should be addressed prior to extubation to prevent recurrent episodes of respiratory failure.

Mort's excellent review of strategies for extubation in critically ill patients includes a preextubation checklist. Components of the process of extubation include the following basics:

- Assess/assure complete neuromuscular block reversal.
- Assess/assure normothermia.
- Perform orotracheal suction to assure that oral cavity is free from secretions or blood, which may be inadvertently aspirated periextubation.
- Ensure the patient is NPO.
- Preoxygenate prior to the extubation.
- If pulmonary toilet is performed immediately before extubation, ensure preoxygenation occurs again.
- Sit the patient up as tolerated.
- Examine the mouth for foreign bodies prior to the extubation in certain patient populations (eg, loose teeth in trauma patients).
- A difficult airway cart should be proximal to the patient's bed or room.
- If there is a significant risk that a surgical airway could be needed, the appropriate consultant should be involved and available.

There are multiple clinical variables that can help predict which critically ill patients may require reintubation. A higher Simplified Acute Physiology Score II, secretion burden, minute ventilation, and number of previously failed SBTs, as well as lower oxygenation and diastolic blood pressures have been identified as risk factors for failed extubation.

2 What are your strategies for extubation of this patient?

If possible, a discussion with the previous intubating team should be sought to better understand why securing the airway was considered difficult. This allows the team to prepare a strategy for potential reintubation if needed. Given this patient's history of heart failure, extubation to noninvasive ventilation (NIV) would be a reasonable choice to help prevent the need for reintubation. Reliable and adequate intravenous access should be maintained in the event the patient requires urgent reintubation. In addition, plans for reintubation should be shared with all care team members prior to extubation, and the patient's code status should be confirmed. Rescue strategies require the ability to adequately and efficiently ascertain the development of respiratory compromise by available ICU staff. Plans and preparation should include consideration of a "reversible" extubation strategy utilizing an airway exchange catheter (AEC).

Mort et al. published an important study of the efficacy of the AEC in difficult extubations. When an AEC was used, 92% of patients were successfully reintubated over the catheter (87% first-attempt success rate). In four patients, the AEC was inadvertently removed from the larynx. When an AEC was not in situ, 70% of patients required three or more attempts with laryngoscopy plus accessory device/technique. Four patients required urgent surgical airway access. Complications of reintubation were more common in the non-AEC group. Oxygen desaturation occurred in 90%, esophageal intubation in 18%, and bradycardia in 14% of this group of patients. Although AECs can be a valuable tool in assisting with a difficult airway, they have been associated with complications including airway injury, pneumothorax/barotrauma, and loss of the airway.

Oxygenation and ventilation strategies post extubation should be assessed and readily available at bedside. The use of prophylactic NIV and high-flow nasal cannula (HFNC) devices rather than conventional oxygen therapy in the postextubation phase has proven to be useful in preventing reintubation. This effect is most pronounced in patients who are considered high risk for reintubation (eg, hypercapnia, moderate-to-severe obstructive airways disease, body mass index >30, heart failure, etc.). However, some studies support that the routine use of HFNC is associated with reduced extubation failure even in the low-risk patient population.

3 What distinct airway devices might be used in this case, and are there any other special considerations for management?

An AEC is a hollow, semirigid polyurethane tube that is available in a number of lengths and diameters. An AEC with the diameter that will most closely fit a preferred reintubation tracheal tube should be used. When inserted through the existing endotracheal tube, it can be aligned with the length markings of the in situ tube. It may be connected to an anesthesia circuit or jet ventilator for emergency oxygenation. Once inserted, the in situ endotracheal tube can be removed and the AEC left in place and secured to the face. Oxygen supplementation via facemask or nasal cannula can ensue with the AEC in situ. The patient can then be assessed serially for strength, ventilatory capacity, cough, and general ability to tolerate and maintain a patent airway. Should the patient require reintubation, the AEC can serve as a reintubation conduit. If the patient tolerates the AEC and is deemed stable postextubation, the AEC can then be removed at the clinician's discretion. Intolerance of an AEC (eg, coughing) is typically due to overinsertion. Using the length markings, the AEC should be inserted to the same depth chosen for a tracheal tube.

Several malpositions of an AEC have been reported including accidental extubation of the AEC or malposition into the esophagus or a mainstem bronchus. A properly placed AEC can be bent behind the glottis during tracheal tube insertion. Use of video laryngoscopy during tracheal tube reinsertion over an AEC can be helpful.

- ICU patients should be medically optimized prior to extubation. This includes an SBT and an assessment of hemodynamic stability, adequate cough, minimal secretion burden, and adequate mental status.
- A reintubation plan should be formulated and shared with the care team prior to extubation. This includes a review of prior intubation attempts to understand what difficulties may have been previously encountered and what equipment may be required for reintubation.
- An AEC could be considered as an airway adjunct for patients with a known or suspected difficult anatomic airway with a high risk of requiring reintubation.
- *See Figure 50.1 and* ▶ ***Video 50.1*** *for additional details.*

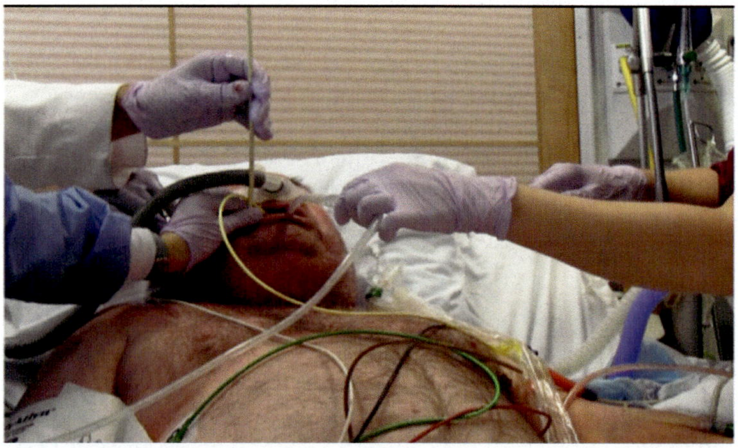

Figure 50.1. A critical patient in the ICU is extubated with an airway exchange catheter left in situ. Noninvasive nasal ventilation is in use.

Acknowledgments

We gratefully acknowledge the contributions of previous edition author, Asher Emanuel, as portions of those chapters have been retained in this revision.

Suggested Readings

Difficult Airway Society Extubation Guidelines Group; Popat M, Mitchell V, Dravid R, Patel A, Swampillai C, Higgs A. Difficult Airway Society Guidelines for the management of tracheal extubation. *Anaesthesia*. 2012;67(3):318–340.

Hernández G, Paredes I, Moran F, et al. Effect of postextubation noninvasive ventilation with active humidification vs high-flow nasal cannula on reintubation in patients at very high risk for extubation failure: a randomized trial. *Intensive Care Med*. 2022;48(12):1751–1759.

Hryciw BN, Hryciw N, Tran A, et al. Predictors of noninvasive ventilation failure in the post-extubation period: a systematic review and meta-analysis. *Crit Care Med*. 2023;51(7):872–880.

Miu T, Joffe AM, Yanez ND, et al. Predictors of reintubation in critically ill patients. *Respir Care*. 2014;59(2):178–185.

Mort TC. Continuous airway access for the difficult extubation: the efficacy of the airway exchange catheter. *Anesth Analg*. 2007;105(5):1357–1362.

Translaryngeal Ventilation and Complications

51

Michiel de Wolf • Ankie Hamaekers

Clinical Scenario: Following a three-level anterior cervical spine fusion, a 67-year-old man experiences complete airway obstruction after extubation at the end of the procedure. Video laryngoscopy reveals swollen supraglottic tissue, and the larynx cannot be identified. Ventilation through a supraglottic airway (SGA) and bag mask ventilation both fail. A 14-gauge transtracheal cannula is inserted through the cricothyroid membrane (CTM) and ventilation with Ventrain (connected to an oxygen cylinder) is started. The oxygen saturation improves rapidly. After stabilization, the patient is intubated via an intubating SGA with the use of a flexible bronchoscope.

1 What are the anesthetic/airway management considerations for this case?

Surgery on the anterior cervical spine is associated with an increased risk of postoperative airway complications and reintubation. Overflexion of the cervical spine and severe prevertebral soft tissue swelling due to hematoma or edema are the most common causes of upper airway obstruction, potentially impeding mask ventilation and reintubation. Essential steps in the management of the obstructed airway are: (1) clearing the airway (positioning, jaw thrust, two-person mask ventilation, and insertion of an oro- or nasopharyngeal airway); (2) ensuring adequate anesthetic depth and administration of a neuromuscular relaxant; and (3) early insertion of an SGA if intubation and/or mask ventilation fail. When maximal efforts at noninvasive techniques fail to relieve severe hypoxemia, immediate percutaneous emergency airway access must be performed to prevent hypoxic brain injury and death.

2 How would you manage the airway in this case?

In an emergency situation, the CTM is the preferred route for percutaneous access to the trachea. The membrane between the cricoid and thyroid cartilages lies superficially and can be identified by palpation. A cannula can be passed through this membrane into the trachea with a minimal risk of hemorrhage. The circumferential cricoid cartilage is partially resistant to compression, and its posterior lamina lies behind the CTM, minimizing the risk of posterior wall injury. International guidelines recommend railroading a cuffed 6.0-mm endotracheal tube over a bougie through the CTM using a stab and twist technique. Placement of a small-bore (inner diameter [ID] ≤2 mm) cannula can be done instead, but only by clinicians who have the proper equipment and expertise to oxygenate through these cannulas. Although it is often suggested that in an emergency situation, any type of available narrow-bore cannula is suitable, an intravenous catheter is not designed for this purpose and has a high risk of kinking. Therefore, it is strongly recommended to use a kink-resistant transtracheal cannula such as the Ravussin (VBM Medizintechnik GmbH, Sulz, Germany) or Cricath (Ventinova, Eindhoven, The Netherlands) cannulas. The steps of narrow-bore cannula insertion through the CTM are:

1. Have an assistant continue attempts to oxygenate the patient (through face mask or SGA).
2. Attach a 5- or 10-mL syringe, partially filled with saline or lidocaine 2%, to a kink-resistant narrow-bore cannula.
3. Position the patient (head and neck extended).
4. Immobilize the larynx between the thumb and middle finger of the nondominant hand. Palpate the CTM with the index finger.
5. Puncture the CTM in the midline while aspirating with the syringe.
6. Confirm needle placement in the trachea by aspiration; there should be no resistance to aspiration of air, seen as bubbles in the saline. Occasionally, tissue or blood can block the needle and prevent aspiration of air. If you are convinced the needle is in the trachea, a small volume of saline can be injected through the needle to clear it.
7. Advance the cannula in a caudal direction over the needle; remove the needle only when the cannula is fully inserted.

8. Attach the syringe to the cannula and aspirate air to confirm correct placement. Capnography may also be used to confirm tracheal placement.
9. Delegate one person to hold the cannula in position.

Although insertion of a narrow-bore cannula through the CTM is fast and minimally invasive, ventilation through this cannula requires careful attention and specialized equipment. A high-pressure gas source is needed to achieve adequate tidal volumes for swift reoxygenation. A standard anesthetic circuit or self-inflating bag-valve system cannot provide effective ventilation through a narrow-bore cannula. Several types of ventilators are available: (1) pressure-controlled devices such as automated (primarily used for elective airway surgery) or hand-triggered jet ventilators; (2) flow-controlled devices without expiratory control, such as Enk Oxygen Flow Modulator (Cook Medical, Bloomington, IN, USA) and Rapid-O2 (Meditech Systems Ltd., Shaftesbury, UK); and (3) flow-controlled device with expiratory ventilation assistance as Ventrain (Ventinova Medical, Eindhoven, Netherlands) (Figure 51.1). Self-assembled devices, like a three-way stopcock, should NOT be used.

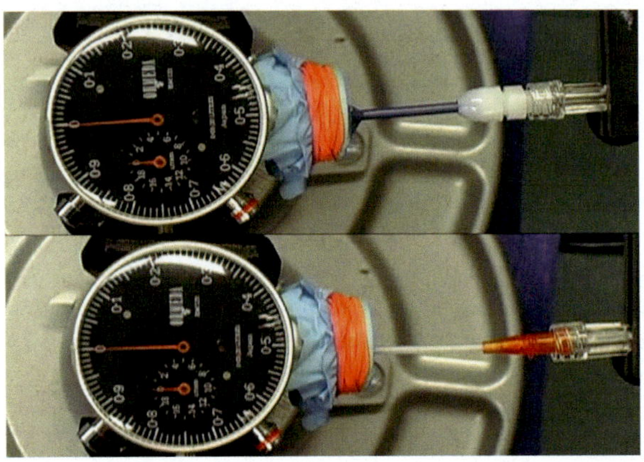

Figure 51.1. Flow testing of angio- versus dedicated translaryngeal catheters demonstrates the flow and antikinking capabilities of the latter. **Upper:** 15-gauge cannula-over-needle angiocath. **Lower:** Cook translaryngeal catheter.

With manual pressure-controlled jet ventilation, driving pressure is set at 1 bar using a short inspiratory/long expiratory time. Before connecting the ventilator to the cannula, correct intratracheal placement needs to be confirmed by aspiration of air or capnography. Before commencing insufflation, it is vital to ensure an open upper airway for the egress of gas. The driving pressure can be gradually increased until chest expansion is achieved. Watch the chest movements closely to ensure complete expiration prior to the next injection of oxygen and adjust the frequency (typically between 6 and 10 injections per minute) when necessary. In emergency situations, jet ventilation carries a high risk of hyperinflation and barotrauma and might better be substituted by a flow-controlled technique.

With flow-controlled injectors, the inspiratory tidal volume can be easily calculated: 2 seconds of insufflation at a flow of 15 L/min will result in a volume of 500 mL. Although Enk Oxygen Flow Modulator and Rapid-O2 provide a low resistance to expiratory flow, the driving force for expiration is the elastic recoil of lungs and chest. This means expiration needs to be considerably prolonged in the case of upper airway obstruction (at least 30 seconds for 500 mL through a 14-Ga cannula). With Ventrain, expiration is expedited through the cannula by creation of subatmospheric pressure proximal to the cannula. Even with an occluded upper airway, it is possible to achieve complete expiration of the injected tidal volume in a similar time as inspiration. In contrast to other methods where ventilation is contraindicated or expiration must be considerably prolonged, ventilation and oxygenation are optimized when ventilating with Ventrain. Readers are encouraged to learn what equipment is available for use at their institutions and how to utilize this equipment safely.

3 What are the potential hazards/complications in regard to the airway?

Cannula insertion and subsequent high-pressure ventilation have a high success rate and low morbidity in elective cases. Under stressful and challenging conditions, however, successful placement and ventilation can be more difficult and potentially hazardous. Complications can be divided into two categories: those associated with insertion of the narrow-bore cannula and those due to subsequent ventilation.

Failure to identify the CTM occurs frequently and is the principal cause of failed cannula insertion. In an elective setting, ultrasound can be used to identify the CTM. Additional complications are dislodgement of the cannula and obstruction of the cannula due to kinking. Hematomas, lesions of the posterior wall, and vocal cord injuries are fortunately rare complications. Although high pressures are used to overcome high resistance to flow of the cannula, pressures in the patient's airways should be considerably lower. If, however, incorrect settings are used or expiration is not complete before a new inspiration is started, ventilation-related complications such as barotrauma, subcutaneous emphysema, pneumothorax, pneumomediastinum, and circulatory arrest due to impaired venous return can occur. Expertise and appropriate use of equipment help to limit the risk of severe complications associated with narrow-bore cricothyroidotomy.

4 Are there special considerations for the emergence or the end of the case?

A narrow-bore cricothyroidotomy should be considered a temporary airway until a more secure airway is established. The nonhumidified oxygen causes drying of the tracheal mucosa, and the lungs are not protected against aspiration of secretions, gastric contents, or blood. Also, tidal volumes and airway pressures cannot be monitored continuously. A new attempt at tracheal intubation may be aided by bubbles emerging from the larynx during insufflation of air into the trachea. Postoperatively, the cricothyroidotomy cannula can be left in position for use in case of further airway problems following extubation.

- When maximal efforts at noninvasive techniques fail to relieve severe hypoxemia in a cannot intubate, cannot ventilate situation, immediate percutaneous emergency airway access must be performed.
- Placement of a narrow-bore cricothyroidotomy cannula is only useful if designated (usually hand-held) equipment is readily available for oxygenation and ventilation.
- When ventilating through a cannula, constant vigilance is vital to prevent barotrauma.
- *See Figure 51.2 and* ***Video 51.1*** *for additional details.*

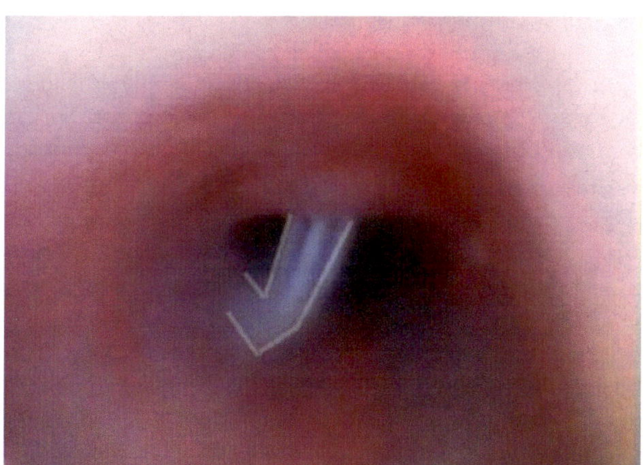

Figure 51.2. A translaryngeal placed angiocatheter is seen to kink in situ (outline added).

Suggested Readings

Duggan LV, Ballantyne SB, Law JA, Morris IR, Murphy MF, Griesdale DE. Transtracheal jet ventilation in the 'can't intubate can't oxygenate' emergency: a systematic review. *Br J Anaesth*. 2016;117(Suppl 1):i28–i38.

Frerk C, Mitchell VS, McNarry F, et al; Difficult Airway Society Intubation Guidelines Working Group. Difficult Airway Society 2015 guidelines for management of unanticipated difficult intubation in adults. *Br J Anaesth*. 2015;115(6):827–848.

Hamaekers A, Henderson J. Equipment and strategies for emergency tracheal access in the adult patient. *Anaesthesia*. 2011; 66(Suppl 2):65–80.

Lohse R, Wagner N, Kristensen MS. Palpation versus ultrasonography for identifying the cricothyroid membrane in case of a laterally deviated larynx: a randomized trial. *Anesth Analg*. 2024;139(1):195–200.

Paxian M, Preussler NP, Reinz T, Schlueter A, Gottschall R. Transtracheal ventilation with a novel ejector-based device (Ventrain) in open, partly obstructed, or totally closed upper airways in pigs. *Br J Anaesth*. 2015;115(2):308–316.

52 The Voice Professional

Ann Marie Melookaran Iliff

1 Describe in detail the device or technique.

When providing anesthetic care to voice professionals or any patient with concerns regarding their voice, special consideration can be given to the pre-, intra-, and postoperative management to mitigate the risk of voice complications. Common surgeries that can lead to voice complications can include airway and neck surgeries such as thyroidectomy, carotid endarterectomy, and anterior cervical spine surgery as well as thoracic or mediastinal surgery. Airway management plans for these patients should be designed to prevent mechanical damage to the larynx.

A detailed discussion with the patient prior to the day of surgery should include topics such as the anesthetic requirements for surgery, alternative approaches, pre- and postoperative planning, management of expectations, as well as possible postoperative outcomes and voice complications. An enumeration of their concerns should be sought and documented. The surgeon should also discuss with the patient any potential effects to the voice due to both the surgical procedure and its anesthetic requirements.

Dysphonia, hematoma, edema, discomfort, and other issues have been concerns linked to intubation and general anesthesia, which can be detrimental to patients who are dependent on their voice for their livelihood. Prevention of trauma during laryngoscopy, intubation, anesthetic maintenance, emergence, and extubation is the primary goal to minimize voice complications. Opportunities for infiltrative or regional anesthesia should always be sought.

Initial airway management should be focused on optimizing intubation conditions so that a tracheal tube can be placed atraumatically on the first attempt by an experienced provider. The most common causes of postintubation complications are secondary to abrasion of the vocal cords or trauma during placement of the tracheal tube. Vocal cord trauma has also been attributed to patient's movement under general anesthesia with tracheal intubation. Small-diameter tracheal tubes and use of minimal tracheal tube cuff pressures reduce mucosal trauma. Intermittent measurement of cuff pressures during surgery can also be helpful. Nitrous oxide should be avoided to prevent tracheal cuff overinflation, and sevoflurane may be appropriate as it is the least irritating halogenated agent. Deep levels of anesthesia should be used to prevent coughing or swallowing, thus reducing frictional interaction between the laryngeal structures and the tracheal tube. Neuromuscular relaxation further prevents mechanical trauma during maintenance of anesthesia but may be contraindicated or even contrary to the goal of voice preservation (eg, neuromonitoring during thyroid surgery). The tracheal tube should be securely fixed in place to prevent movement and irritation of the laryngeal mucosa. Extubation of the larynx while the patient is in a deep plane of anesthesia may reduce the risk of damage during emergence.

In one study, 6.2% of patients had severe larynx and vocal cord lesions after tracheal intubation and 4.5% developed hematomas of the vocal cords. Bilateral vocal cord paralysis after intubation with a double lumen endotracheal tube (DLT) has been reported. A study on 130 patients did not show a difference in vocal cord complications between use of a DLT and a bronchial blocker, the latter was preferred by the authors. Avoidance of both tracheal intubation and supraglottic airways should always be considered if possible. The incidence of postoperative sore throat after general anesthesia is 14.4% to 50% after tracheal intubation and 5.8% to 34% after laryngeal mask airway use.

Most cases of hoarseness or sore throat resolve spontaneously within 72 hours without any treatment, but lasting symptoms may be due to more serious damage, including hematomas or laceration, granulation formation, or arytenoid dislocation.

Prophylaxis for prevention of irritation and edema can be beneficial in these patients. Preoperative treatment to increase gastric pH (eg, proton-pump inhibitor [PPI] therapy) and intraoperative steroids (eg, dexamethasone) to reduce edema should be considered along with prophylactic antiemetics. Occasionally, 1 week of PPI therapy postoperatively is prescribed.

Deep extubation or maneuvers with alternative airways before airway reflexes have returned can help smooth emergence. Postoperatively, the patient should be kept in an upright position and well hydrated. Antiemetics, continued PPI therapy, and voice rest versus speech/voice therapy recommendations are variable based on provider preference.

2 Where or when is this device or technique used in airway management?

Professional voice users include but are not limited to singers, actors, politicians, teachers, and clergy members. They depend on vocal endurance and quality for their livelihood. Postsurgical voice morbidity can have devastating consequences to this patient population, and it is important to have a plan in place to minimize the risk of a voice complication. In particular, attention should be paid to techniques of airway manipulation and maintenance and emergence of anesthesia. In these populations, preoperative discussions are key. Patients should be assured that precautions will be exercised and that most often, voice-related complications are minor and transient.

3 What distinguishes this device of technique from similar airway management methods?

Voice complications in the postoperative period can be a consequence of the surgical procedure (especially when undergoing airway or neck surgery) or a result of procedures during anesthetic care. Though often unavoidable in the delivery of an appropriate anesthetic, the anesthesiologist must use every precaution for this specific patient population and focus on preservation of voice and minimizing the risk of voice complications. Adequate planning, preparation, and prophylaxis throughout the perioperative period can decrease the likelihood of voice complications.

- Discuss anesthetic options, risks, and postoperative expectations with the patient who has voice concerns.
- Facilitate the best conditions for intubation on the first attempt with smaller tracheal tubes to prevent mechanical trauma.
- Neuromuscular relaxation and maintaining a deep level of anesthetic to prevent coughing or swallowing against the endotracheal tube are beneficial.
- Pre- and postoperative PPI, intraoperative steroid, antiemetics, and hydration therapy should be considered.
- *See Figure 52.1 and* ***Video 52.1*** *for additional details.*

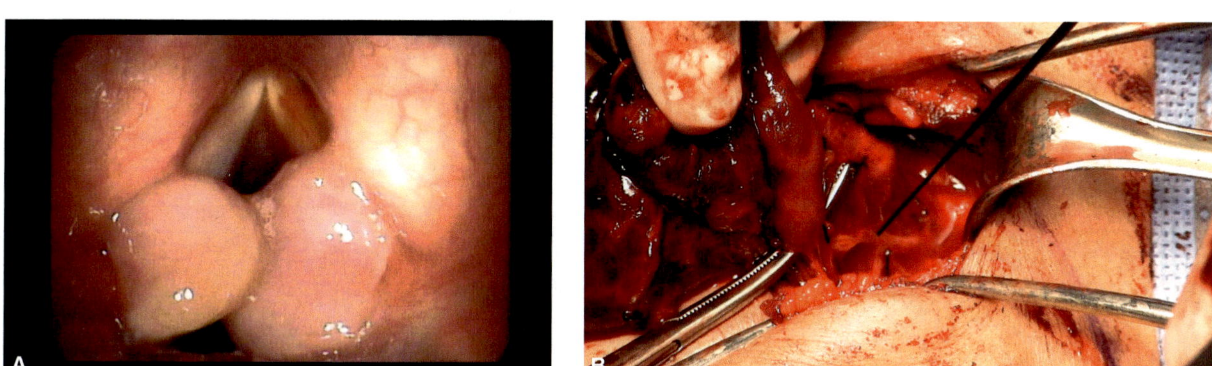

Figure 52.1. **A:** Bilateral vocal cord granulations following tracheal intubation. **B:** During thyroid surgery, the recurrent laryngeal nerve is carefully identified.

Acknowledgment

We gratefully acknowledge the contributions of previous edition author, Nwanmegha Young, as portions of those chapters have been retained in this revision.

Suggested Readings

Kosarek L, Busch E, Abbas A, Falterman J, Nossaman BD. Effective use of bronchial blockers in lung isolation surgery: an analysis of 130 cases. *Ochsner J.* 2013;13(3):389–393.

McHardy FE, Chung F. Postoperative sore throat: cause, prevention and treatment. *Anaesthesia.* 1999;54(5):444–453.

Meacham RK, Schindler J. Anesthesia care for the professional singer. *Anesthesiol Clin.* 2015;33(2):347–356.

Teng SE, Booth JR, Fritz MA, Groves MW, Postma GN. Airway management in singers: a cross-sectional survey. *J Voice.* 2023;37(5):772–778.

Airway Management Strategies for Asleep/Awake/Asleep Craniotomies

53

Katherine Herrera • Irene Osborn

Clinical Scenario: A 62-year-old male presents for resection of a tumor in the left temporal lobe and will require intraoperative speech testing. He had one seizure related to the tumor, and he reports no other medical problems aside from moderate obstructive sleep apnea.

1 What are the anesthetic and airway management considerations for this case?

The "awake" craniotomy has evolved to now an "asleep/awake/asleep" craniotomy. This approach is better tolerated by the patient and helps to avoid some associated complications such as hypercarbia, nausea, patient intolerance, or intraoperative seizures. This procedure demands a balance of pharmacologic administration, timing, and skill. The patient is maintained under general anesthesia with controlled ventilation for the most stimulating portions of the procedure (eg, headframe application and scalp pinning, scalp incision, dural opening, and closure) but is awake during cortical mapping and testing. Most lesions amenable to this technique are in the temporal or parietal regions, so the supine position is often used with head fixation to prevent head movement.

At the beginning of the procedure, the patient undergoes induction of general anesthesia with securement of the airway. Local anesthetic is injected at the pinning sites prior to placement of the headframe, and a scalp block is often performed to reduce incisional discomfort during the later, midcraniotomy awake stage. After surgical exposure, the patient is awakened and the airway device is removed. The patient must then be awake enough to cooperate with cortical mapping and neurologic testing. Following the awake resection of the tumor, a deeper plane of anesthesia is subsequently induced again (airway device can be reinserted or not) and the surgical procedure is completed.

Airway management for these procedures is complicated in a number of respects. First, application of the headframe and positioning for surgical exposure must be balanced with the anesthesiologist's access to the airway as well as patient comfort during the awake portion of the procedure. Second, the anesthesiologist must plan airway and pharmacologic management to provide a smooth transition from the asleep to the awake state, not only during the intraoperative emergence, but also at the end of the case. This is often achieved with the use of a supraglottic airway (SGA). Positioning and head fixation make access to the airway for laryngoscopy (direct or indirect) very difficult. Coughing and increases in intracranial pressure associated with tracheal intubation should be avoided. Despite this, rapid tracheal intubation may be needed in an emergency due hyperventilation and/or airway protection in the event of seizures, apnea, or other compromising events. Finally, planned reinsertion of the SGA for the postmapping resection and surgical closure must be achieved smoothly despite compromised access to the head of the patient.

2 How would you manage the airway in this case?

Preoperative discussion with the patient revealed anxiety about the procedure including being conscious for portions of the surgery. The patient should receive a full explanation of the entire anesthesia plan for the surgery, emphasizing that the patient will be deeply sedated during the most painful portions of the procedure.

Given the patient's history of obstructive sleep apnea, there is particular concern about airway obstruction during deep sedation which could lead to hypercarbia and/or hypoxemia. An SGA device would be an appropriate choice to support adequate ventilation and oxygenation during the sedated portions of the procedure.

3 What are the surgical considerations that impact anesthetic management?

No patient head movement should occur during surgical opening and particularly during surgical planning with the use of a neuronavigation system. Once the procedure begins, the surgeon may encounter brain swelling and request additional ventilation as well as administration of diuretics. General anesthesia with the use of an airway device supports these conditions.

During the awake portion, it is imperative that coughing, straining, and bucking be avoided. The patient must be cooperative and responsive for neurologic testing. Communication between anesthesiologist and surgeon is essential throughout this portion of the procedure.

Patient positioning ideally should give the surgeon access to the operative location while also allowing the anesthesiologist access to the airway for placement and removal of the chosen airway device. It is also essential to avoid excessive neck flexion, which can compromise breathing and could affect intracranial dynamics.

4 What are the potential hazards and complications in regard to the airway?

The most significant hazard in these procedures is difficult access to the patient's airway. Once the patient's head is fixed in a headframe, there can be no further head movements.

Throughout the entire procedure, there is always a potential risk of losing the airway in the event of a seizure or apnea due to sedation or other causes. It is important to avoid light anesthesia during the surgical opening to prevent laryngospasm and other unwanted airway responses. During the awake phase, patients may suffer nausea and/or vomiting due to anesthetic agents or surgical stimulation.

The anesthetic regimen can include intravenous agents and/or low-dose volatile anesthesia. Brain monitors such as bispectral index (BIS) or Sedline can help to predict anesthetic depth and timing of awakening.

5 What alternative airway devices might be used in this case?

The literature best supports using a supraglottic device for airway control during awake craniotomies. There are case reports and other small studies describing the efficacy of second-generation devices such as the LMA Supreme which allows for easy insertion, ventilation at higher pressures, and a gastric port. The LMA Supreme allows for placement in a variety of patient positions, and the intra-airway position of this SGA can be confirmed. The gastric port must be at the upper esophageal sphincter to provide protection in the event of regurgitation. In addition, positive pressure ventilation may be performed at higher peak pressures as compared to most first-generation SGAs. This is needed to ensure adequate minute ventilation or hyperventilation, if needed.

Another described technique is the use of bilateral nasal trumpets which when placed gently into the nasopharynx, can help to maintain the airway under deep sedation. This technique can be used for patients with potential for airway obstruction and inability to tolerate SGAs. The nasal trumpets can remain in place throughout the entire procedure.

High-flow nasal oxygenation (HFNO) has recently been described as a useful technique for supplemental oxygenation during awake craniotomies. This technique provides humidified oxygen which maintains airway patency and may be used in place of an SGA in patients with adequate chest compliance. Intravenous sedation can be safely provided with careful titration of agents and capnography monitoring.

6 Are there special considerations for the emergence at the end of the case?

A smooth emergence from anesthesia is important. Emergence can begin after the headframe is removed, and the patient may resume spontaneous ventilation as the head wrap dressing is being applied. Appropriate analgesics should be titrated to the patient's respiratory rate. Once the patient begins to respond to commands and starts swallowing, the SGA can be removed (**Video 53.1**).

- The asleep/awake/asleep craniotomy technique improves patient tolerance during intracranial procedures that require intraoperative patient participation.
- Second-generation SGAs are an appropriate choice for airway management during these procedures.
- Head fixation and patient positioning can compromise patient ventilation during these craniotomies.
- It is important to avoid coughing, bucking, and straining during all phases of the procedure.
- HFNO is another alternative to an SGA in select patients.
- *See Figure 53.1 and* ***Video 53.1*** *for additional details.*

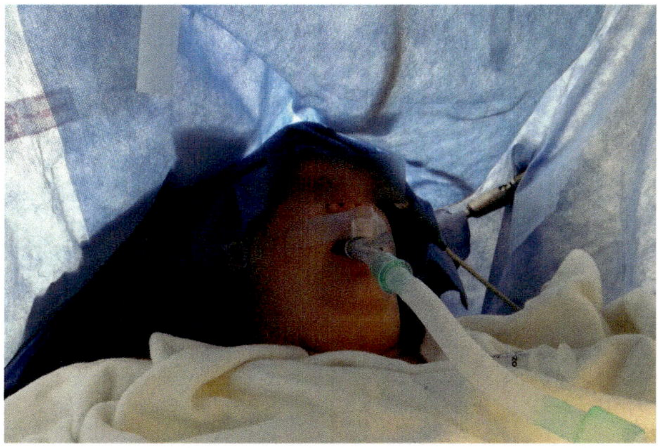

Figure 53.1. A patient undergoing craniotomy with a supraglottic airway (SGA) in place. The SGA can be removed and reinserted during the asleep/awake/asleep sequence.

Acknowledgment

We gratefully acknowledge the contributions of previous edition author, Douglas Wetmore, as portions of those chapters have been retained in this revision.

Suggested Readings

Lobo FA, Wagemakers M, Absalom AR. Anaesthesia for awake craniotomy. *Br J Anaesthesia.* 2016;116(6):740–744.

Sarang A, Dinsmore J. Anaesthesia for awake craniotomy–evolution of a technique that facilitates awake neurological testing. *Br J Anaesth.* 2003;90(2):161–165.

Sivasankar C, Schlichter RA, Baranov D, Kofke WA. Awake craniotomy: a new airway approach. *Anesth Analg.* 2016;122(2):509–511.

Yi P, Li Q, Yang Z, Cao L, Hu X, Gu H. High-flow nasal cannula improves clinical efficacy of airway management in patients undergoing awake craniotomy. *BMC Anesthesiol.* 2020;20(1):156.

54 Positioning of the Morbidly Obese Patient

Michael Ancuta • Jay B. Brodsky

Clinical Scenario: A 40-year-old woman presents for cystoscopy under local anesthesia in a lithotomy position. The surgeon is asking for "light sedation." She weighs 450 lb and is 5′4″ tall. She has a history of obstructive sleep apnea (OSA) and uses continuous positive airway pressure (CPAP) device at home. In the supine position, her oxygen saturation is 89%.

1 What are the anesthetic and airway management considerations for this case?

Increasing numbers of overweight, obese, and morbidly obese patients are now presenting for every type of surgical procedure. Many of the usual options for anesthesia that would be appropriate for normal-weight patients are not safe for these obese patients. In addition, the presence of OSA further complicates the management of these patients.

Although a cystoscopy in the lithotomy position under local anesthesia would be an appropriate choice for many patients, it is not safe for this patient. Total lung volume and functional residual capacity (FRC) decrease in direct proportion to increasing weight. These changes occur in the sitting position, but become even more pronounced when an obese patient lies flat. The presence of altered pulmonary physiology is clearly demonstrated in this patient.

Placement of a morbidly obese patient in either the lithotomy or the Trendelenburg position increases intra-abdominal pressure with additional compression of the lungs, which in turn reduces chest wall compliance. Venous return to the heart is also increased in these positions and results in an increase in both cardiac output and pulmonary blood flow. A morbidly obese patient should never be allowed to breathe without assistance (either awake or anesthetized), undergoing a procedure while in either the lithotomy or the Trendelenburg position. Positive-pressure ventilation with an ETT is necessary to compensate for the markedly decreased lung volume.

The presence of OSA in this patient is a further contraindication for management under "light sedation." Although OSA can be present in patients of any weight, it is extremely common in patients with morbid obesity. As many as 70% of morbidly obese patients in some series presenting for bariatric surgery have been found to have OSA. A patient with OSA is very sensitive to the effects of opioids and sedatives, and in the absence of an ETT, even "light" levels of sedation can lead to airway obstruction and hypoxemia.

2 How would you manage the airway in this case?

Even though the scheduled cystoscopy procedure is minimally invasive and can probably be accomplished quickly, this patient needs a general anesthetic with controlled or assisted ventilation via an ETT. Morbidly obese patients should never be allowed to lie supine, even for the induction of general anesthesia. Obese patients should be placed in the "head elevated laryngoscopy position" (HELP) once they are moved from their gurney to the operating table. This position can be achieved with pillows or with specially designed commercial elevation devices. In this position, their upper body and head are "ramped" or elevated so that an imaginary horizontal line connects their sternum to their ear. In more recent studies, reverse Trendelenburg positioning with CPAP support during the preoxygenation period is shown to reduce time to achieve adequate preoxygenation and increase the safe nonhypoxic apnea after induction as compared to ramped position, only allowing for better intubating conditions. Following adequate preoxygenation, anesthesia is induced, and the patient is muscle relaxed for tracheal intubation. After the tracheal tube is placed, general anesthesia is administered, and the obese patient should be ventilated with controlled or assisted ventilation. The great majority of morbidly obese patients can have the tracheal tube successfully placed by conventional direct laryngoscopy. Although mask ventilation is often difficult in an obese patient, obesity or BMI itself is not a risk factor for a difficult laryngoscopy. The presence of OSA has also been associated in some studies with intubation difficulties, but since so many morbidly obese patients have OSA and the majority of these patients are not difficult to intubate, other risk factors are probably more important. The major predictors for a difficult laryngoscopy in the extremely obese patient are a modified Mallampati score of 3 or 4, and a neck circumference >60 cm. If intubation difficulty is anticipated or experienced, tracheal intubation with a flexible intubating scope (FIS) has historically been the best choice. More recently, video laryngoscopes have been used successfully for tracheal intubation in obese patients considered at risk for difficulty with direct laryngoscopy.

Unless it is an extremely short procedure, the patient should not be allowed to breathe spontaneously (when either awake or asleep) in a supine, lithotomy, or Trendelenburg position. During the procedure, sedatives and long-acting opioids should be avoided; if that is not possible, they should be kept to a minimum. The risks to this patient of postoperative hypoventilation and the potential for airway obstruction are real, and analgesic alternatives that do not depress airway reflexes and ventilation are preferred to opioid agents. Acetaminophen has been demonstrated to be an acceptable analgesic in obese and OSA patients.

3 Are there special considerations for the emergence or the end of the case?

At the completion of surgery, this patient should be taken out of the lithotomy position and again placed with the head and upper body elevated in preparation for emergence from anesthesia and tracheal extubation. If muscle relaxants were used, paralysis must be completely reversed with return of function before the patient's trachea is extubated. For patients with OSA, an oral airway and/or a nasal trumpet should be placed before extubation to avoid sudden airway obstruction when the tracheal tube is removed. During transfer from the OR to the postanesthesia care unit (PACU) and while in the PACU recovering from anesthesia, the patient should remain in a semiupright sitting position and receive supplemental oxygen by face mask or nasal prongs. Patients with OSA should be instructed to bring their CPAP device to the hospital, and CPAP should be applied if any signs of obstruction are observed. If a patient does not have, or did not bring their own CPAP mask, the commercially available Boussignac mask is a practical alternative (see Chapter 58: Preoperative Continuous Positive Airway Pressure).

Author Caveat

Greater numbers of obese patients are having surgery at ambulatory surgery centers. Obesity itself is not a contraindication for performing interventional procedures on an outpatient basis. The presence of serious medical comorbidities, especially OSA with carbon dioxide retention, is probably the most important reason not to do these cases at stand-alone facilities. Outpatient centers must have a "difficult airway" cart containing a variety of adjuncts (eg, bougies, video laryngoscopes, a FIS) to help if an airway problem occurs. A second physician or nurse must be identified preoperatively and be readily available to assist with airway management if help is needed. Following surgery, the patient with OSA, who has received any opioids, should be observed in the PACU for up to 3 hours before being discharged home.

- Total lung volume and FRC decrease in direct proportion to increasing weight; these effects are augmented when the patient is placed in the supine position.
- Anesthetized morbidly obese patients should never be allowed to breathe without assistance.
- An ETT should be the default airway in morbidly obese patients undergoing surgical procedures.
- *See Figure 54.1 and* **Video 54.1** *for additional details.*

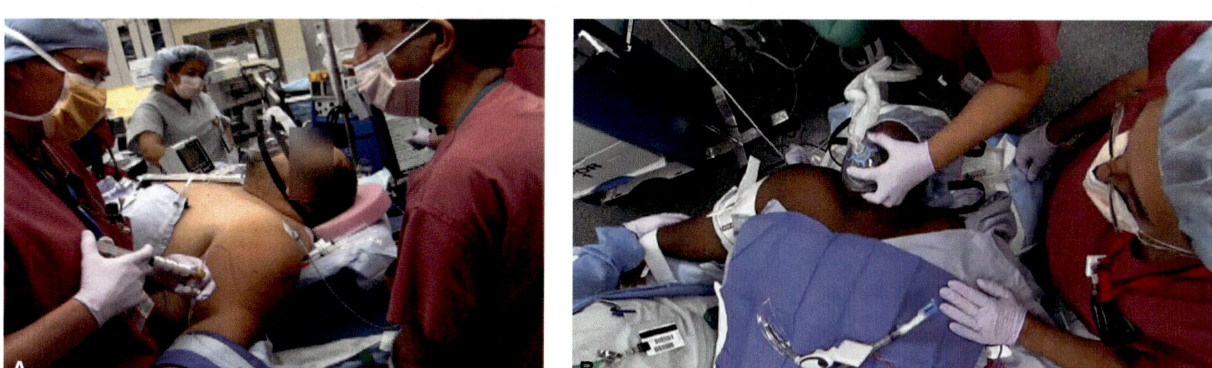

Figure 54.1. A: Back elevated positioning of a morbidly obese patient. **B:** A morbidly obese patient in a back elevation position is mask ventilated.

Suggested Readings

Brodsky JB, Lemmens HJ, Brock-Utne JG, Vierra M, Saidman LJ. Morbid obesity and tracheal intubation. *Anesth Analg.* 2002; 94:732–736.

Couture EJ, Carrier-Boucher A, Provencher S, Tanoubi I, Marceau S, Bussières JS. Effect of reverse Trendelenburg position and positive pressure ventilation on safe non-hypoxic apnea period in obese, a randomized-control trial. *BMC Anesthesiol.* 2023;23(1):198.

Nightingale CE, Cousins J, Fox WT, Kennedy N, Margarson MP, Shearer E. Comment on fourth national audit project from the Society of Bariatric Anaesthetists. *Brit J Anaesth.* 2011;107:272–273.

Pelosi P, Croci M, Ravagnan I, et al. Respiratory system mechanics in sedated, paralyzed, morbidly obese patients. *J Appl Physiol.* 1997;82:811–818.

Wong DT, Adly E, Ip HY, Thapar S, Maxted GR, Chung FF. A comparison between the Boussignac™ continuous positive airway pressure mask and the venturi mask in terms of improvement in the $PaO_2/F(I)O_2$ ratio in morbidly obese patients undergoing bariatric surgery: a randomized controlled trial. *Can J Anaesth.* 2011;58:532–539.

Obstructive Sleep Apnea Surgery

55

David T. Wong

Clinical Scenario: An obese man is scheduled for surgery to correct obstructive sleep apnea (OSA). His airway examination is within normal limits for a predicted nondifficult airway, and he has no gastroesophageal reflux.

1 What are the anesthetic and airway management considerations for this case?

Patients with *OSA* are prone to upper airway obstruction, especially during sleep or sedation. There is a fixed component of obstruction from excessively bulky tissue in the pharyngeal inlet (oropharynx and hypopharynx) and a dynamic component from negative inspiratory forces and positioning. OSA has been associated with difficult mask ventilation and difficult intubation with direct laryngoscopy. Medically, OSA is associated with hypertension, coronary artery disease, restrictive lung disease, pulmonary hypertension, diabetes, and gastroesophageal reflux. About 70% to 80% of patients who present with OSA are obese, with a roughly 2:1 preponderance in men compared to women. Physiologically, *obesity* is associated with reduced functional residual capacity, decreased respiratory compliance, increased oxygen consumption, and rapid oxygen desaturation upon apnea. Airway management concerns associated with obesity include difficult mask ventilation, difficult supraglottic airway (SGA) insertion or maintenance, difficult landmarking of cricothyroid membrane, and propensity for OSA.

Due to his OSA, this patient has an increased risk of rapid oxygen desaturation in the perioperative period. Preoperatively, he should receive adequate preoxygenation. Intraoperatively, recruitment maneuvers and PEEP can help optimize oxygenation. Airway management following the induction of anesthesia is a reasonable approach for patients with no significant clinical indicators of a difficult airway. A video laryngoscope, flexible intubating scope (FIS), intubating SGA, and surgical airway equipment should be readily available, however.

2 How would you manage the airway in this case?

A primary intubation plan with alternative plans should be considered. All airway equipment potentially needed should be immediately available. Preoxygenation is best accomplished with a tight-sealing face mask in a semisitting position until end-tidal O_2 is ≥90%. Low-flow nasal prongs or high-flow nasal oxygenation should be provided for apneic oxygenation during intubation attempts. In this patient with a relatively normal airway exam and low risk for aspiration, intubation would follow the induction of anesthesia. The decision to use an oral or nasal tracheal tube is made in consultation with the surgical team. Video laryngoscopy would be the preferred choice of instrumentation by the author. If video laryngoscopy is unsuccessful, bag mask ventilation should be performed between further intubation attempts. Alternative intubation techniques such as combined video laryngoscopy and FIS should be attempted. After successful tracheal intubation, ventilation management should include PEEP and intermittent recruitment maneuvers to reduce atelectasis.

3 What are the surgical considerations that impact anesthetic management?

Prior to any surgery for OSA, the surgeon has performed a thorough evaluation of the patient's airway, including awake flexible nasopharyngoscopy or drug-induced sleep endoscopy, in an effort to identify the area and degree of obstruction. Surgical treatment for OSA may involve a variety of methods, including uvulopalatopharyngoplasty, maxillomandibular advancement, radiofrequency ablation, or tracheostomy. Discussion with the surgeon is important to understand the planned procedure and the appropriate airway management.

Intraoperatively, the surgeon will ideally have an unobstructed view and access to the oropharyngeal tissue for surgical resection. A nasal–tracheal intubation is often preferred as it provides better surgical access unless nasal surgery needs to be performed also. If an orotracheal tube is placed, it should be secured in the midline, and consideration should be given to the use of a flexible, wire-reinforced tube to prevent compression by surgical instrumentation. An SGA is generally not considered appropriate during OSA surgery due to limited surgical access and possible dislodgement. There should be a clear discussion with the surgeon regarding the preference for airway management prior to proceeding with the induction of anesthesia.

Preemptive extubation planning is essential. As blood may accumulate in the hypopharynx, it is important to suction the pharynx prior to emergence, rinse the nasal cavities with irrigation, and maintain sufficient endotracheal tube cuff pressure to reduce the possibility of aspiration. The surgeon may request minimal coughing during emergence to reduce the possibility of the disruption of sutures. Though extubation in the deeply anesthetized state is possible, this technique places the patient at increased risk of aspiration and laryngospasm. Strategies to minimize coughing during emergence include the use of a low-dose remifentanil infusion, intravenous lidocaine, or bridging to an SGA. Postoperatively, these patients are prone to upper airway obstruction from pharyngolaryngeal edema, bleeding, pharyngeal collapse from loss of muscle tone secondary to OSA, residual muscle relaxant, anesthetics, sedative drugs, and narcotic analgesia. Multimodal analgesia options can help in reducing the risk of opioid-induced ventilatory depression.

4 Are there special considerations for the emergence or the end of the case?

This patient is at increased risk of postoperative hypoxemia and airway obstruction. To improve postoperative oxygenation, recruitment maneuvers should be performed prior to emergence with the maintenance of PEEP using a pressure support mode ventilation and FIO_2 of 1.0 until the time of extubation. Muscle relaxant should be fully reversed, the pharynx dry, and the patient placed in a semisitting position. For the patient who had a difficult intubation, careful extubation precautions should be exercised. Finally, for patients with high FIO_2 requirements or those who were treated with a CPAP device preoperatively, CPAP should be utilized in the postanesthesia care unit (PACU) and the surgical ward. For some, immediate CPAP at the time of extubation may be appropriate. In the postoperative period, nonnarcotic analgesics should be prioritized over opioids. The PACU team should be vigilant for signs of airway obstruction, and equipment and personnel for reintubation should be immediately available. Patients who were difficult to intubate, have high FIO_2 and analgesic requirements, or surgical concerns regarding bleeding or edema should be admitted to an intensive care or step-down unit. Postoperative inpatient monitoring should be considered for patients with high apnea–hypopnea index, morbid obesity, obstructive episodes in the PACU, or other significant comorbidities.

- Patient who present for OSA surgery are prone to hypoxemia during anesthesia induction, so optimal preoxygenation and apneic oxygenation should be provided.
- A primary intubation plan as well as alternative plans should be carefully contemplated.
- Due to a shared airway intraoperatively, the surgeon and anesthesiologist should discuss the planned surgical procedure, optimal tracheal tube type, and location prior to proceeding.
- Postoperatively, these patients are prone to hypoxemia and upper airway obstruction.
- *See Figure 55.1 and* ***Video 55.1*** *for additional details.*

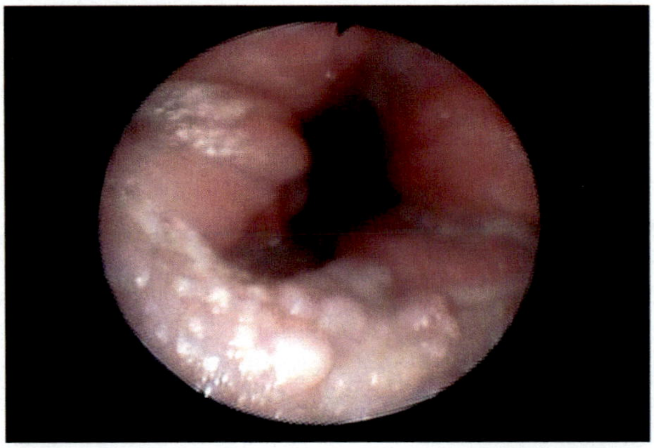

Figure 55.1. Crowding of tissue in the pharynx of a severe obstructive sleep apnea patient.

Acknowledgment

We gratefully acknowledge the contributions of previous edition author, Brian W. Rotenberg, as portions of those chapters have been retained in this revision.

Suggested Readings

Kandasamy T, Wright ED, Fuller J, Rotenberg BW. The incidence of early post-operative complications following uvulopalatopharyngoplasty: identification of predictive risk factors. *J Otolaryngol Head Neck Surg.* 2013;42(1):15.

Murphy C, Wong DT. Airway management and oxygenation in obese patients. *Can J Anaesth.* 2013;60(9):929–945.

Nagappa M, Wong DT, Cozowicz C, Ramachandran SK, Memtsoudis SG, Chung F. Is obstructive sleep apnea associated with difficult airway? Evidence from a systematic review and meta-analysis of prospective and retrospective cohort studies. *PLoS One.* 2018;13(10):e0204904.

Seet E, Nagappa M, Wong DT. Airway management in surgical patients with obstructive sleep apnea. *Anesth Analg.* 2021;132(5):1321–1327.

Spence EA, Rajaleelan W, Wong J, Chung F, Wong DT. The effectiveness of high-flow nasal oxygen during the intraoperative period: a systematic review and meta-analysis. *Anesth Analg.* 2020;131(4):1102–1110.

56 Drug-Induced Sleep Endoscopy

Darpan Kayastha

Describe in detail the technique

Obstructive sleep–related breathing disorders encompass a broad array of abnormalities ranging from benign snoring to upper airway resistance syndrome (UARS) and obstructive sleep apnea (OSA). These entities vary only in their severities of apnea/hypopnea events, reductions in nocturnal blood oxygen saturation, arousals from sleep, and daytime hypersomnolence. As an increasingly pervasive disease among the modern epidemic of metabolic syndrome, untreated OSA has well-established associations with increased cardiovascular and all-cause mortality, neurocognitive dysfunction, psychiatric disturbance, and several comorbid conditions, including hypertension, insulin resistance, and gastroesophageal reflux disease. Depending on the relative contributions of anatomic collapse and central neurologic dysfunction, OSA can be characterized as obstructive, central, or mixed in etiology. Irrespective of cause, the gold standard for diagnosis and classification is nocturnal polysomnography (PSG), a multimodal study that monitors key neurophysiologic parameters during sleep. Analyzing these parameters, such as number of apnea, hypopnea, or respiratory effort–related arousal (RERA) events during sleep, also allows for the grading of disease severity (eg, apnea–hypopnea index [AHI] of <5 is normal, 5 to 15 is mild, 15 to 30 is moderate, and >30 is severe).

In OSA, obstruction results from the interplay of anatomic factors such as body habitus and craniofacial structure, loss of neuromuscular tone during low arousal states, and single- or multilevel upper airway collapse, all of which contribute to a loss of pharyngeal patency and resultant hypoventilation and physiologic stress. Excessive fat deposition in obesity can further narrow the pharyngeal airway and restrict lung volumes and ventilation. As such, weight loss is commonly prescribed as a conservative first step in treatment. Continuous positive airway pressure (CPAP) works through pneumatic stenting of the pharynx and remains the first-line treatment for moderate to severe OSA, though compliance with therapy remains a challenge for many patients. Oral appliances are a second-line adjunct with higher rates of adherence but less therapeutic benefit. For patients with refractory or severe disease, surgical treatments may be offered.

Comprehensive aerodigestive examination, stratification (eg, Mallampati, Friedman, and/or Fujita classifications), and fiberoptic nasopharyngoscopy are essential for identifying each individual patient's particular pattern of collapse and for crafting a surgical protocol that addresses these sites of obstruction. While most patients have some combination of retropalatal and retrolingual collapse, there may be contributions from nasal obstruction, adenotonsillar hypertrophy, microretrognathia, glossoptosis, epiglottic retroflexion, glottic restriction, and more. The Müller maneuver involves forced inhalation against a closed glottis while the nose and mouth are closed and can be invoked during awake nasopharyngoscopy to obtain a more dynamic view of the sites of collapse. Given the limitations of an awake evaluation, however, most surgeons perform a preoperative evaluation with drug-induced sleep endoscopy (DISE) in which nasopharyngoscopy is performed during pharmacologically induced sleep (eg, with propofol or dexmedetomidine and midazolam) in order to evaluate airway dynamics and patterns of obstruction during simulated natural sleep. One standardized schema for describing obstruction is the VOTE (velum, oropharyngeal, tongue base, epiglottis) classification, which attempts to describe the pattern of collapse at four levels: velum (anterior–posterior or concentric), oropharynx (lateral or concentric), tongue base (extent of anterior–posterior collapse), and epiglottis (extent of retroflexion).

What distinguishes this technique from similar airway management methods?

Prior studies have established propofol as a short-acting agent that does not influence AHI but may affect sleep architecture by shortening the length of rapid eye movement (REM) sleep. Use of benzodiazepines, in contrast, may more accurately replicate natural sleep architecture. Regardless of the choice of anesthetics, DISE demands adequate sedation for pharyngeal muscle relaxation and transient obstruction without complete depression of respiratory drive. Use of a bispectral index (BIS) monitoring system can allow for proper anesthetic titration to achieve this narrow therapeutic window. Target-controlled infusion (TCI) of propofol to a concentration of 1 to 3 μg/mL, although slightly more time consuming, has proven to be superior to intermittent bolus delivery due to improved control of sedation level. In general, minimizing the delivery of opioids and fraction of inspired oxygen (FIO_2) can help avoid complete depression of respiratory drive. Despite the overall safety of this procedure, communication between the anesthesia and surgical teams is essential, and emergency airway adjuncts should be immediately available (eg, video laryngoscope, flexible intubation scope [FIS], nasal trumpets, and supraglottic airways).

- DISE is an important method for evaluating level of obstruction in patients with OSA.
- Midazolam and propofol can be used alone or in concert for induction and maintenance.
- TCI of propofol and BIS monitoring are becoming the favored modality.
- *See Figure 56.1 as well as* ***Videos 56.1*** *and* ***56.2*** *for additional details.*

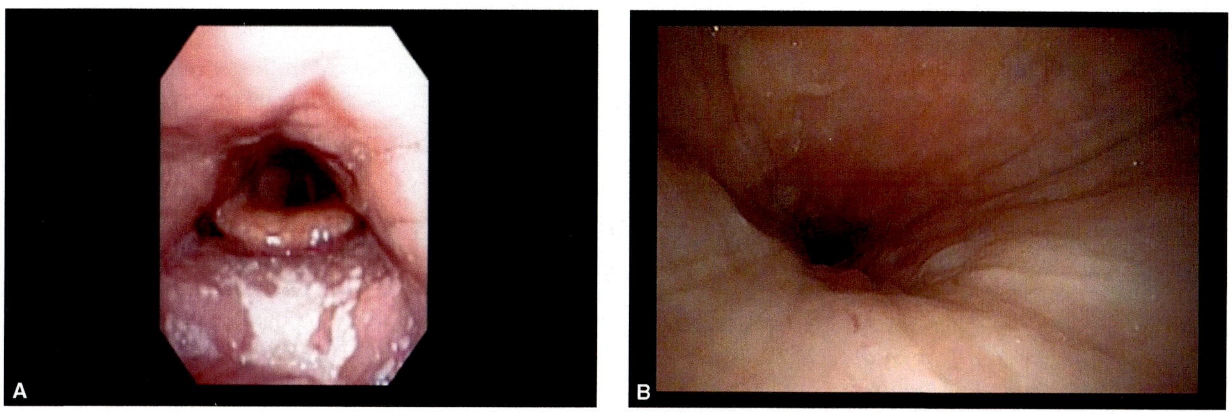

Figure 56.1. **A, B:** The hypopharynx of a patient with obstructive sleep apnea demonstrates tissue crowding.

Acknowledgments

We gratefully acknowledge the contributions of previous edition authors, Kenneth Bagwell, Christopher Schutt, and Mark Bianchi, as portions of those chapters have been retained in this revision.

Suggested Readings

Abbasi A, Gupta SS, Sabharwal N, et al. A comprehensive review of obstructive sleep apnea. *Sleep Sci.* 2021;14(2):142–154.

Carrasco-Llatas M, Matarredona-Quiles S, De Vito A, Chong KB, Vicini C. Drug-induced sleep endoscopy: technique, indications, tips and pitfalls. *Healthcare (Basel).* 2019;7(3):93.

Traxdorf M, Tschaikowsky K, Scherl C, Bauer J, Iro H, Angerer F. Drug-induced sleep endoscopy (DISE) with target controlled infusion (TCI) and bispectral analysis in obstructive sleep apnea. *J Vis Exp.* 2016;(118):54739.

57 Severe Obstructive Sleep Apnea in a Pregnant Patient

Anna M. Weyand • Ashutosh Wali

Clinical Scenario: A 26-year-old primiparous patient presents for cesarean delivery. She is morbidly obese and has severe obstructive sleep apnea (OSA). She uses continuous positive airway pressure (CPAP) device at night.

1 What are the anesthetic and airway management considerations for this case?

While the safety of anesthetic care of pregnant women in the United States continues to improve, anesthetic complications are still the tenth leading cause of maternal mortality. Management of the parturient requires the anesthesiologist to have a thorough knowledge of the physiologic changes that occur during pregnancy, labor, and delivery. The incidence of fatal failed intubation is 13 times higher in the obstetric population than in nonpregnant patients. A thorough airway evaluation should be completed with particular attention paid to Mallampati score, protruding incisors, receding mandible, length of neck, and the presence of facial edema. Mallampati score tends to increase throughout pregnancy as a result of weight gain as well as fatty infiltration and edema of the pharyngeal tissues. During labor and delivery (whether vaginal or surgical), the Mallampati score can further increase due to the administration of intravenous fluids and the bearing down efforts of the patient. The edematous pharyngeal tissues are accompanied by hyperemic nasal mucosa, which renders nasal intubation hazardous. Finally, the increased weight and engorged breast tissue found in pregnant patients may further complicate airway management, including insertion of a regular-sized laryngoscope handle.

This case is further complicated by the patient's morbid obesity, which places her at a significantly higher risk for complications associated with pregnancy such as preeclampsia, diabetes, and gestational hypertension as well as increasing her risk for airway complications, including pulmonary aspiration and failed tracheal intubation. Obesity has been shown to be a major risk factor for maternal mortality, and the analysis of the closed claims database finds that obese patients have a 4.5-fold increase in damaging respiratory events compared to nonobese parturients.

Neuraxial anesthesia is typically used for cesarean delivery in the absence of contraindications because general anesthesia is more commonly associated with a higher maternal morbidity/mortality, and patients commonly prefer to remain awake for the birth of their children. Nevertheless, equipment for tracheal intubation and airway rescue should be immediately available for all parturients during cesarean sections. This is particularly true for obese patients, as these patients have a higher rate of failed epidural anesthesia due to increased difficulty of epidural placement and a high incidence of movement of the epidural catheter in the subcutaneous fat.

2 How would you manage the airway in this case?

Assuming no contraindication to neuraxial anesthesia, oxygenation can be supplemented initially via nasal cannula. Due to the increased oxygen consumption and reduced functional residual capacity in pregnancy, a nonrebreather facemask or CPAP may be necessary. The anesthesiologist should be prepared for an emergent tracheal intubation at any point during the surgery. The patient should be optimally positioned with a ramp under the shoulders and head/neck at the outset of surgery, as repositioning may be exceedingly difficult during the procedure. A video laryngoscope and a regular short-handled laryngoscope should be immediately available. Airway rescue devices such as a second-generation supraglottic airway (SGA) and a cricothyrotomy kit should also be available.

The type of rescue device that is most useful depends largely on the expertise and experience of the anesthesiologist. Video laryngoscopes and optical stylets have all been used successfully in parturients. SGAs such as the laryngeal mask airway (LMA), i-Gel, or laryngeal tube are important adjuncts and may be lifesaving. These devices may also be used as a temporizing measure and a bridge to a definitive airway control, although

LMA and i-Gel have been successfully used for entire cesarean sections with no reports of pulmonary aspiration. Regardless of the device(s) chosen, ready availability and thorough familiarity with the American Society of Anesthesiologists' difficult airway algorithm is essential.

The presence of OSA in this patient underscores the necessity of a thorough airway evaluation and proper positioning prior to the start of the procedure. Sedation should be avoided, if possible, given the exaggerated response that many patients with OSA exhibit after exposure to opioids and benzodiazepines. Patients who are on home CPAP should be instructed to bring their CPAP machines with them to the hospital for postoperative use.

If neuraxial anesthesia is contraindicated (due to coagulopathy, ongoing excessive hemorrhage, overlying skin infection, pulmonary hypertension, severe thrombocytopenia, or an uncooperative patient) or fails prior to the beginning of the procedure, general anesthesia will be the next step.

Awake orotracheal intubation should be considered if a difficult airway is anticipated. Nasal intubation should be avoided. If induction of general anesthesia is deemed safe, ensure that a functional suction unit is ready and an assistant is available to apply cricoid pressure (CP). The parturient should be administered gastrointestinal prophylaxis, placed in a ramped position, optimally preoxygenated to a target EtO_2 >90, induced using rapid sequence and CP, and the trachea intubated orally using a video laryngoscope (if available) for first pass success. If laryngoscopy is suboptimal, consider transiently releasing CP during tracheal intubation. Tracheal extubation should be carried out in the fully awake patient in the head-up or left lateral position. Postoperatively, the parturient may need oxygen supplementation with a nasal cannula, nonrebreather facemask, or CPAP.

3 What are the surgical considerations that impact anesthetic management?

Although this is a primary cesarean section and, thus, not associated with a risk of increased blood loss or extended operative time typical of repeat cesarean delivery, the patient's morbid obesity independently increases these risks. Two large-bore intravenous catheters should be placed. An invasive arterial catheter should be considered in morbidly obese patients to facilitate optimal blood pressure monitoring and frequent blood sampling in the event of major blood loss.

In addition, a neuraxial technique with the option for re-dosing should be considered, such as a combined spinal–epidural (CSE), dural puncture epidural (DPE), continuous epidural, or continuous spinal. The catheter technique allows for extending surgical anesthesia time in patients with morbid truncal obesity in whom access to hysterotomy/cesarean delivery may be delayed, and surgical closure of all abdominal layers may take additional time.

4 What are the potential hazards and complications regarding the airway?

Pregnancy-associated physiologic derangements of the respiratory system, including decreased functional residual capacity, increased oxygen consumption, and a cephalad displacement of the diaphragm, render the parturient more susceptible to hypoxic events and airway catastrophe. Due to pregnancy-induced delayed gastric emptying, decreased lower esophageal sphincter tone, and altered angle of the gastroesophageal junction, pregnant patients are particularly susceptible to pulmonary aspiration of regurgitated gastric contents.

- Parturients are at high risk of difficult intubation.
- Obese parturients are at increased risk for both pregnancy and airway complications.
- Patients with OSA are vulnerable to airway obstruction with typical doses of sedative agents.
- While neuraxial anesthesia remains the technique of choice for cesarean delivery, the anesthesiologist must be prepared to intubate the patient's trachea emergently.
- Preparation includes proper positioning and the availability of rescue devices.
- *See Figure 57.1 for additional details.*

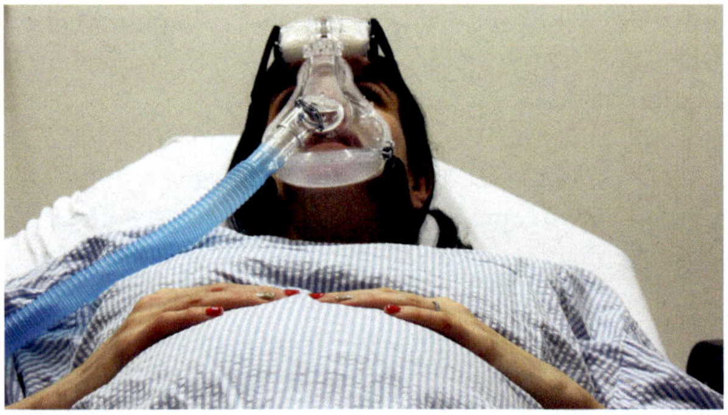

Figure 57.1. Due to prepartum conditions or the onset of physiologic and anatomic changes during pregnancy, some parturients will present with snoring or frank obstructive sleep apnea.

Suggested Readings

2022 American Society of Anesthesiologists Practice Guidelines for Management of the Difficult Airway. *Anesthesiology*. 2022; 136:31–81.

Ankichetty SP, Angle P, Joselyn AS, Chinnappa V, Halpern S. Anesthetic considerations of parturients with obesity and obstructive sleep apnea. *J Anaesthesiol Clin Pharmacol*. 2012;28(4):436–443.

Mushambi MC, Kinsella SM, Popat M, et al. Obstetric Anaesthetists' Association and Difficult Airway Society guidelines for the management of difficult and failed tracheal intubation in obstetrics. *Anaesthesia*. 2015;70(11):1286–1306.

Patel S, Wali A. Airway management of the obstetric patient. *Curr Anesthesiol Rep*. 2020;10(Dec).

Preoperative Continuous Positive Airway Pressure

58

Adriana D. Oprea • Haitham Ibrahim

Clinical Scenario: A morbidly obese, 60-year-old male presents for a gastrectomy. He snores loudly, has daytime somnolence, and his partner believes that he "stops breathing at night." He has refused to undergo a sleep study in the past. In the preoperative holding area, his oxygen saturation on room air is 91%.

1 What are the anesthetic/airway management considerations for this case?

Obstructive sleep apnea (OSA) is a common condition associated with relaxation of the pharyngeal tissues during sleep leading to diminished (hypopnea) or total cessation of airflow (apnea). OSA leads to hypoxia, hypercapnia, altered sleeping pattern, daytime drowsiness, and an increased risk of hypertension, diabetes, and cardiovascular diseases. While only 2% to 4% of the general population is affected, up to 70% of bariatric surgery patients carry a diagnosis of OSA.

OSA is formally diagnosed with polysomnography and is classified based on the apnea–hypopnea index (AHI) into mild (AHI 5 to 15), moderate (AHI 15 to 30), or severe (AHI >30). Many patients remain undiagnosed prior to presenting to the operating room for a variety of surgical procedures.

In patients at risk for OSA, the diagnosis is suspected based on subjective complaints (snoring, observed pauses during sleep, daytime sleepiness, morning headaches, restless sleep, morning confusion, intellectual impairment, or personality changes). Physical characteristics can corroborate with the symptoms and make the diagnosis more likely (obesity, male gender, females undergoing menopause). In addition, craniofacial abnormalities (retro- or micrognathia, presence of large tonsils nearly touching or touching in the midline, macroglossia, long soft palate, anatomical nasal obstruction) and an increased neck circumference (17 inches in men, 16 inches in women) are independent risk factors for OSA.

When patients present to the operating room without a formal diagnosis of OSA, a simple questionnaire ("STOP BANG") in addition to the features described above can be used as a screening tool to make a presumptive diagnosis (Table 58.1).

TABLE 58.1 The STOP BANG Questionnaire

S	Do you SNORE loudly (louder than talking or loud enough to be heard through closed doors)?
T	Do you often feel TIRED, fatigued, or sleepy during daytime?
O	Has anyone OBSERVED you stop breathing during your sleep?
P	Do you have or are you being treated for high blood PRESSURE?
B	BMI more than 35 kg/m^2?
A	AGE over 50 y old?
N	NECK circumference >15.75 inches (40 cm)?
G	Male GENDER? ≥3 yes answers: High risk for OSA <3 yes answers: Low risk for OSA

Adapted with permission from Dr. Frances Chung and University Health Network. www.stop-bang.ca

Patients with OSA pose unique anesthetic challenges to the clinician. In addition to a higher risk of difficult mask ventilation and tracheal intubation, there may be preexisting cardiovascular consequences of severe, untreated OSA. Chronic hypoxia and hypercapnia can lead to pulmonary hypertension, arrhythmias (especially atrial fibrillation), and right ventricular hypertrophy and failure. Postoperatively, these patients are at increased risk of respiratory failure, pneumonia, acute respiratory distress syndrome, and the need for postoperative reintubation and mechanical ventilation.

2 How would you manage the airway in this case?

The presence of OSA will affect the airway management in all phases of anesthetic care. Preoperatively, patients with OSA should be optimized for surgery with weight loss, continuous positive airway pressure (CPAP) therapy, or placement of a mandibular advancement device. In patients with moderate to severe OSA, autotitrated CPAP overnight that was used three nights preoperatively and five nights postoperatively has been linked to a significant reduction in the AHI score and improvement of oxygen saturation.

The benefits of using perioperative CPAP are not limited to patients with OSA. A recent meta-analysis showed that CPAP use in conjunction with supplemental oxygen in abdominal surgery patients was associated with a decreased rate of postoperative pulmonary complications, endotracheal intubations, and pneumonia when compared to supplemental oxygen alone.

In patients with a high likelihood of OSA and a STOP BANG score >3, optimization is limited to improving oxygenation in the brief period from preoperative anesthetic assessment to surgery. While supplemental O_2 is a usually accepted method of improving oxygenation, this may not be effective in morbidly obese patients. Better results can be obtained with high-flow nasal cannula or positive pressure systems (CPAP, BiPAP, or NIPPV) as mentioned above. While some of the latter methods may require a formal mask fitting, preoperative CPAP can be achieved either through a tightly fitted face mask attached to a portable oxygenation/ventilation circuit or by the use of a dedicated, oxygen flow meter powered CPAP system (eg, the Boussignac CPAP device, Vygon, United Kingdom). These methods may improve the O_2 saturation preoperatively and prolong the safe-apneic period during anesthetic induction. Unlike long-term preoperative CPAP, however, they have no effect on the long-term complications associated with OSA.

Preoperative sedation should be administered with caution, given the possibility of complete airway obstruction in these patients. For patients undergoing awake intubation, supplemental oxygen should be provided through a nasal cannula. In patients who will be intubated after anesthetic induction, preinduction CPAP at 5 to 10 mm Hg improves the safe apneic period through increasing the functional residual capacity. With the Boussignac CPAP system, the positive end expiratory pressure is adjusted via the oxygen flow (15 L O_2 for 5 mm Hg to 25 L O_2 for 10 mm Hg). Positioning the patient's torso in a semirecumbent position with the head in a sniffing position improves the chances of successful mask ventilation and intubation. In all cases, emergency airway rescue tools should be readily available.

3 What are the surgical considerations that impact anesthetic management?

Surgical considerations that impact anesthetic management are related to the site of the surgery. When appropriate, regional anesthetic techniques should be considered, thus avoiding manipulation of the airway. In this case, positioning of the patient and the duration of the surgical procedure should be taken into account. The patient will need to tolerate the surgical position, and the use of sedative agents will be limited by OSA. In addition, the effects of the regional anesthetic on respiration should be considered, and the anesthesiologist will need to have unobstructed access to the airway for the duration of the procedure.

Unless a laparoscopic surgical approach is chosen for the patient in this case, epidural analgesia in addition to general anesthesia would be an optimal choice for this patient. While a pure neuraxial technique may have detrimental effects on respiration due to the dermatomal level that needs to be achieved for a gastrectomy (higher than T7), the combined approach of neuraxial and general anesthesia would limit the amount of narcotic (and consequent respiratory depressant effects) required with a general anesthetic technique alone, thus facilitating extubation and safe postoperative care.

4 Are there special considerations for the emergence or the end of the case?

Careful extubation precautions should be exercised at the end of all surgical procedures in patients with OSA. Patients who fail tracheal extubation may be more difficult to reintubate. Immediately after removal of the tracheal tube, patients with OSA can be successfully transitioned to a portable CPAP system as long as their mental status is intact and they are initiating spontaneous breaths. Postoperative CPAP has been shown to prevent reintubation in the immediate postoperative period and can be used as needed until the patient can successfully maintain their preanesthetic oxygen saturation level.

Another airway adjunct that can be used during extubation of OSA patients is the nasopharyngeal airway device. It can maintain the patency of the airway, and is well tolerated by awake patients compared to oral airways.

Multiple studies have shown that the use of nasal trumpet after extubation in OSA patients significantly decreases their postoperative AHI and their lowest oxygen saturation recorded.

Patients with OSA have increased sensitivity to narcotics, and respiratory problems may not manifest for up to 16 hours after the surgical procedure. Even in patients undergoing regional techniques, narcotics cannot always be completely omitted.

It is preferable for patients with severe OSA undergoing oral surgical procedures or surgeries associated with major fluid shifts to remain intubated until upper airway edema, superimposed on an already redundant soft tissue, improves.

- Many patients with OSA symptoms do not carry a formal diagnosis.
- Measures such as preoperative CPAP can be administered immediately before surgery.
- Careful extubation precautions should be exercised.
- Immediate postoperative CPAP in patients with OSA can act as a bridge therapy until the patient can maintain their baseline oxygen saturations without additional support.
- *See Figure 58.1 and* ⓒ ***Video 58.1*** *for additional details.*

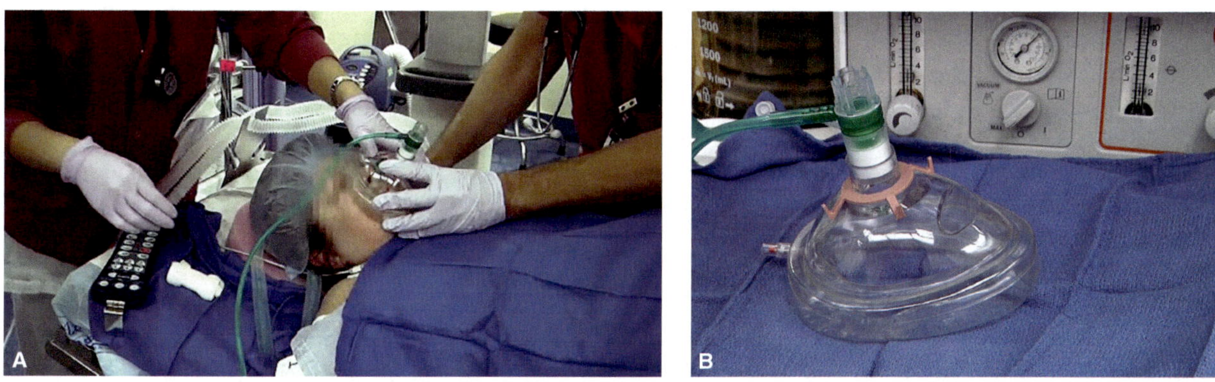

Figure 58.1. **A:** A single-use CPAP mask is applied immediately after extubation with a tight handheld seal. Mask straps will be used to secure the mask until the patient is stable without continuous positive pressure or a fitted mask can be secured. **B:** The Boussignac CPAP mask is one of several single-use devices available.

Suggested Readings

American Society of Anesthesiologists Task Force on Perioperative Management. Practice guidelines for the perioperative management of patients with obstructive sleep apnea: an updated report by the American Society of Anesthesiologists Task Force on Perioperative Management of patients with obstructive sleep apnea. *Anesthesiology*. 2014;120(2):268–286

Chung F, Nagappa M, Singh M, Mokhlesi B. CPAP in the perioperative setting: evidence of support. *Chest*. 2016;149(2):586–597.

Kumar A, Guilleminault C, Certal V, Li D, Capasso R, Camacho M. Nasopharyngeal airway stenting devices for obstructive sleep apnoea: a systematic review and meta-analysis. *J Laryngol Otol*. 2015;129(1):2–10.

Liao P, Luo Q, Elsaid H, Kang W, Shapiro C, Chung F. Perioperative auto-titrated continuous positive airway pressure treatment in surgical patients with obstructive sleep apnea. *Anesthesiology*. 2013;119:837–847.

Wong DT, Tam AD, Van Zundert TC. The usage of the Boussignac continuous positive airway pressure system in acute respiratory failure. *Minerva Anestesiol*. 2013;79(5):564–570.

59 Airway Management During Cardiopulmonary Resuscitation

Michael Ancuta

Clinical Scenario: A 72-year-old patient is in full cardiopulmonary arrest and CPR is in progress. A nurse is attempting bag-valve-mask ventilation, but there is no chest movement. No pulse nor oxygen saturation is being appreciated. On cursory examination, the external airway appears unremarkable. Per hospital protocol, you have been summoned for tracheal intubation.

1 What are the anesthetic and airway management considerations for this case?

Current management of cardiopulmonary arrest is primarily focused on providing effective chest compressions with the shortest periods of disruption. All other elements of resuscitation are determined by the patients' location, either in-hospital or out-of-hospital. This factor determines the timing of resuscitation events, expectations of personnel training, and equipment and medication availability.

This principle does not necessarily apply to in-hospital resuscitation, depending on the availability of personnel and equipment. Chest compression should be started the moment an arrest is recognized. Face mask ventilation is begun in the nonintubated patient at compression-to-breath ratio of 30:2, with compression pauses during ventilation. Advanced airway devices are applied after appropriate equipment and personnel become available. Airway decisions and attempts at tracheal intubation should not delay first shock defibrillation.

2 How would you manage the airway in this case?

Ventilation through an advanced airway device requires no interruptions in chest compressions and is therefore superior than bag-mask ventilation. Once an advanced airway is attained, the recommended rate of 8 to 10 bpm should be given concurrently with chest compressions.

The etiology of the cardiopulmonary arrest, if it can be identified, may impact the sequence of management. The Emergency Cardiac Care Committee and the National Registry of CPR Scientific Advisory Board of the American Heart Association have recommended obtaining an advanced, nonsurgical airway whenever feasible in the hospital environment. The arrest to Time-to-Invasive Airway (TTIA) is considered the "Process Gold Standard." Though the American Heart Association recommends a TTIA of 5 minutes or less, in the National Registry of Cardiopulmonary Resuscitations, the average TTIA is 5.9 minutes.

Colorimetric end-tidal CO_2 detection has been the community standard for confirmation of ETT placement during CPR. The 2020 advanced cardiovascular life support (ACLS) guidelines recommend the use of continuous capnography as opposed to a colorimetric device. Continuous capnography provides reliable information for four critical aspects of resuscitation: (1) confirmation of endotracheal tube placement, (2) quality of chest compressions (less than 10 mm Hg end-tidal CO_2 demonstrating inadequate compressions), (3) immediate detection of return of spontaneous circulation (ROSC), and (4) maintenance of tracheal tube position during patient transfer. Newer models of defibrillators have integrated end-tidal CO_2 capnographic monitors. Tracheal tube placement confirmation by an esophageal detection device or capnography had an increased rate of ROSC and survival to hospital discharge.

Three percent of CPR patients were found to have difficult airways. The ASA difficult airway algorithm should be adhered to during resuscitation and therefore necessitates that the code team have ready access to multiple modalities of airway management. The decision to use a video laryngoscope versus direct laryngoscopy will depend on the anticipated difficulty of the airway and the presence of a soiled airway.

Finally, routine administration of a hypnotic and a muscle relaxant to facilitate intubation is generally not necessary during true cardiac arrests.

3 What are the potential hazards and complications in regard to the airway?

Interruption of chest compression to allow for advanced airway management procedures compromises optimal tissue perfusion. Similarly, continuing resuscitation with face mask ventilation likewise requires brief cessations of compressions and exposes the patient to the hazards of pulmonary aspiration. The risk of aspiration of emesis and dental appliances is very high in the cardiopulmonary arrest population. The use of a face mask as the initial or definitive modality of airway management further increases the risk of emesis by 12%. The use of cricoid pressure is not recommended during face mask ventilation, as it can impede ventilation, can delay TTIA, and is not protective against aspiration.

Stone et al. found that the use of LMA, in lieu of a face mask, reduced preintubation regurgitation to 3.5%. In a randomized controlled trial of 9296 subjects, Benger et al. compared the insertion of a supraglottic airway with an endotracheal tube during CPR, finding no difference in survival (RR, 0.95 [95% CI, 0.82–1.10]) or survival with good neurologic outcome (RR, 0.92 [95% CI, 0.77–1.09]) at hospital discharge.

4 Are there special considerations for the emergence at the end of the case?

The ACLS 2020 guidelines recommend that all patients who maintain ROSC after resuscitation should be managed in a critical care unit and treated for the etiology of their arrest. Furthermore, Fio_2 concentration should be titrated to maintain an oxyhemoglobin saturation between 94% and 99%. This is to mitigate ischemia–reperfusion oxidative injury that is more likely during hyperoxemia.

Airway-related disposition planning depends on four major factors: (1) the etiology of the arrest, (2) the patient regaining respiratory function in the course of resuscitation, (3) patient requirement for cardiovascular support that necessitates positive-pressure ventilation, and (4) the ease or difficulty of obtaining the advanced airway.

If a respiratory arrest precipitated the resuscitation, then this cause should be addressed and the patient's airway managed in a therapeutically appropriate manner. Occasionally, during resuscitation, a patient will regain both respiratory and cardiovascular stability and may be extubated early after ROSC. However, patients requiring substantial post-ROSC cardiovascular support and advanced monitoring should be maintained with advanced airway support and positive-pressure ventilation.

- In-hospital cardiopulmonary arrest patients should have an advanced airway within 5 minutes.
- $EtCO_2$ monitoring is essential for assessing CPR quality and confirmation of ETT placement.
- Dental appliances and stomach content regurgitation are common hazards during CPR.
- With ROSC, the Fio_2 should be titrated to provide a 94% to 99% oxygen saturation level.
- *See Figure 59.1 and* **Video 59.1** *for additional details.*

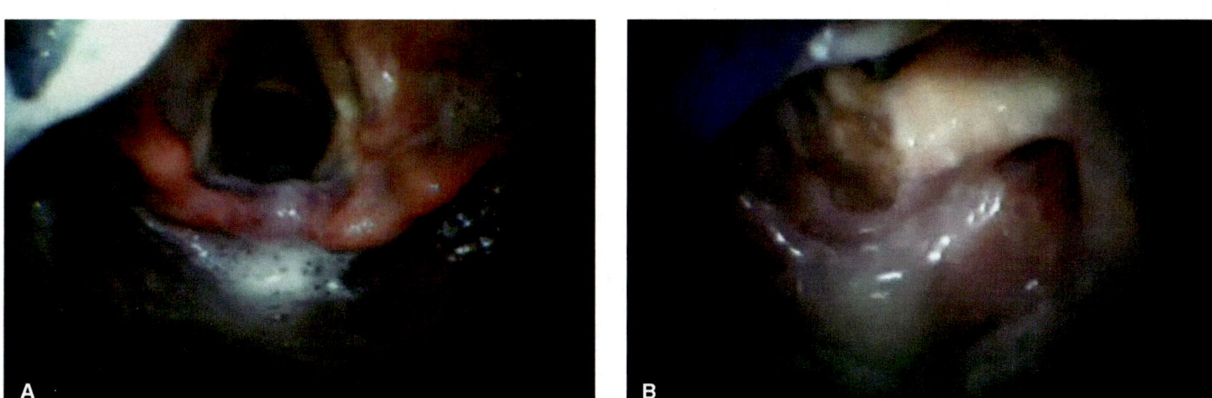

Figure 59.1. **A:** Though not appreciated in this image, rhythmic motion of the larynx should be expected to be seen in laryngoscopy during cardiopulmonary resuscitation. **B:** Regurgitated and potentially aspirated stomach contents may be seen during laryngoscopy.

Acknowledgment

We gratefully acknowledge the contributions of previous edition author, Jessica L. Feinleib, as portions of those chapters have been retained in this revision.

Suggested Readings

Benger JR, Kirby K, Black S, et al. Effect of a strategy of a supraglottic airway device vs tracheal intubation during out-of-hospital cardiac arrest on functional outcome: the AIRWAYS-2 randomized clinical trial. *JAMA*. 2018;320:779–791.

Hasegawa K, Hiraide A, Chang Y, Brown DFM. Association of prehospital advanced airway management with neurological outcomes and survival in patients with out-of-hospital cardiac arrest. *JAMA*. 2013;309(3):257–266.

Panchal AR, Bartos JA, Cabañas JG, et al. Part 3: Adult Basic and Advanced Life Support: 2020 American Heart Association Guidelines for cardiopulmonary resuscitation and emergency cardiovascular care. *Circulation*. 2020;142(16_suppl_2): S366–S468.

Phelan MP, Oranto JP, Peberdy MA, Hustey FM; American Heart Association's Get With The Guidelines-Resuscitation Investigators. Appropriate documentation of confirmation of endotracheal tube position and relationship to patient outcome from in-hospital cardiac arrest. *Resuscitation*. 2013;84(1):31–36.

Stone BJ, Chantler PJ, Baskett PJF. The incidence of regurgitation during cardiopulmonary resuscitation: a comparison between the bag valve mask and laryngeal mask airway. *Resuscitation*. 1998;38:3–6.

Sutton RM, French B, Meaney PA, et al; American Heart Association's Get With The Guidelines–Resuscitation Investigators. Physiologic monitoring of CPR quality during adult cardiac arrest: a propensity-matched cohort study. *Resuscitation*. 2016; 106:76–82.

Wong ML, Carey S, Mader TJ, Wang HE; American Heart Association National Registry of Cardiopulmonary Resuscitation Investigators. Time to invasive airway placement and resuscitation outcomes after inhospital cardiopulmonary arrest. *Resuscitation*. 2010;81(2):182–186.

The Patient with Severe Arthritic Syndrome Disease

60

Richard E. Galgon

Clinical Scenario: A 50-year-old man with severe ankylosing spondylitis (AS) presents for hip-replacement surgery under general anesthesia.

1 What are the anesthetic and airway management considerations for this case?

AS is a chronic, progressive, inflammatory disease predominately affecting the axial spine and adjacent soft tissues. The disease usually begins in the second or third decade of life, affecting more men than women at a ratio of approximately 3:1, with a prevalence ranging from 0.5% to 1.4%. It is characterized by ossification of the joints, spinal discs, and ligaments, generally beginning in the sacroiliac joints and advancing cranially to the cervical spine. Syndesmophytes form via continued endochondral ossification and ultimately bridge adjacent vertebral bodies, leading to the classic, rigid "bamboo spine" (see **Video 60.1**) and the development of spinal fixation or severe limitations in range of motion, including cervical spine immobility. With severe disease, as suggested by this patient requiring total hip arthroplasty, osteoporosis is common and leads to an increased rate of vertebral fractures and the development of hyperkyphosis, particularly in male patients. In extreme cases, "chin-on-chest" deformities have occurred, producing pressure sufficient enough to cause ulceration of the skin on both the mandible and sternum. In these severe cases, oral intubation and elective tracheostomy are often precluded due to extremely limited mouth opening and lack of access to the anterior neck, respectively. Extra-axial joint involvement, including the temporomandibular and vertebrocostal joints, may also limit mouth opening and produce restrictive lung disease, respectively. The eyes (anterior uveitis), gastrointestinal tract (inflammatory bowel disease), genitourinary tract (urethritis), kidneys (glomerulonephritis and decreased renal function), heart (conduction disturbances, valvular lesions, and cardiomyopathy), lungs (interstitial lung disease), and skin (psoriasis) may also be variably involved. However, the disease's challenging anesthetic and airway management is mostly secondary to spine deformity, fixation, and fragility. As such, all patients with AS must be approached with a high suspicion for a difficult airway.

2 How would you manage the airway in this case?

A careful history and physical examination must be performed with particular attention given to spine deformities (eg, hyperkyphosis), cervical spine fixation or range of motion limitations, mouth opening and tongue volume, dentition, beard presence, mandibular mobility, nares patency, and anterior neck soft tissue mobility and access. The medical record should be reviewed, and the patient questioned for any evidence of difficult or impossible bag-mask ventilation or intubation events. Review any available thoracic or cervical imaging for evidence of airway distortion. If significant spine deformity is present, such as hyperkyphosis, consider performing preoperative indirect mirror laryngoscopy or an endoscopic airway examination to assess the position of the epiglottis, as it oftentimes will be laying near the posterior wall of the hypopharynx and may be difficult to navigate beneath.

The main principle in managing this patient's airway is to maintain spontaneous ventilation until relative or absolute control of the airway is gained, particularly if severe spinal deformity or cervical spine fixation is present. The second principle is to always maintain support of the thoracocervical spine and to avoid the application of significant bending forces, as relatively minor forces have resulted in thoracocervical spine fractures with devastating neurologic consequences. Thus, direct laryngoscopy should be considered a relative contraindication in this patient, and awake intubation with a flexible intubating scope (either orally or nasally) should be considered the first approach. More recently, awake indirect laryngoscopy (optical or video) has proven successful, as has the use of the intubating SGA. However, intubation using these later methods must be achieved with minimal application of force, as reports of airway management-related cervical spine fractures continue to be reported even when "normal" clinical forces are applied. Awake management provides the advantage of maintaining patient feedback as an assessment of neurologic adequacy.

If this patient's disease process has not produced significant spine deformity and the airway examination is reassuring for bag-mask ventilatory adequacy, an asleep flexible scope or optical or video laryngoscopic intubation would also be reasonable. If a preoperative endoscopic airway examination revealed a marginal hypopharyngeal space or significant epiglottic obstruction, the application of CPAP during an awake, fiberoptic nasal intubation should be considered. Supplemental oxygen should be continuously administered during the intubation process. Minimally, this should be by nasal cannula or a face mask with portal openings for airway instrumentation. However, the use of high-flow nasal cannula oxygen therapy would be preferred if available. With any approach, additional advanced airway management equipment should always be immediately available.

3 What are the surgical considerations that impact anesthetic management?

Once the patient's airway is secured, attention must be turned to positioning the patient safely in a manner that provides for adequate surgical exposure, which is usually in the lateral decubitus position for the procedure above. The patient's spine, and particularly the thoracocervical spine, must be supported at all times as iatrogenic spinal fractures have been reported in these patients.

4 What are the potential hazards and complications in regard to the airway?

Patients with AS can be difficult or impossible to bag-mask ventilate and/or intubate. Therefore, they are at higher risk of oropharyngolaryngotracheal injuries, spine fracture with or without cord compromise and neurologic sequelae, the need for emergency cricothyrotomy or tracheotomy, pulmonary aspiration, hypoxic injury, and death.

5 What distinct airway device might be used in this case, and what are the special considerations?

If this patient presents with a severe spine deformity, the use of a wire-reinforced tracheal tube should be considered to prevent tracheal tube kinking.

6 Are there special considerations for the emergence or the end of the case?

The patient with AS should be extubated awake after full recovery or reversal of any neuromuscular blockade. In cases of severe spinal deformity or a particularly challenging intubation, consider extubating the patient to an airway exchange catheter. Finally, multimodal analgesia should be used to decrease opioid requirements in this patient who is at increased risk for complications if emergent reintubation is required.

- AS patients often present airway management challenges due to spine deformities and fixation.
- Relatively minor bending forces may lead to serious spine fractures.
- Awake, flexible fiberoptic intubation remains the safest airway management technique in these patients.
- Fastidious support of the thoracocervical spine during airway management and the surgical procedure is a requirement to minimize the risk of spinal injuries.
- *See Figures 60.1 and 60.2 for additional details.*

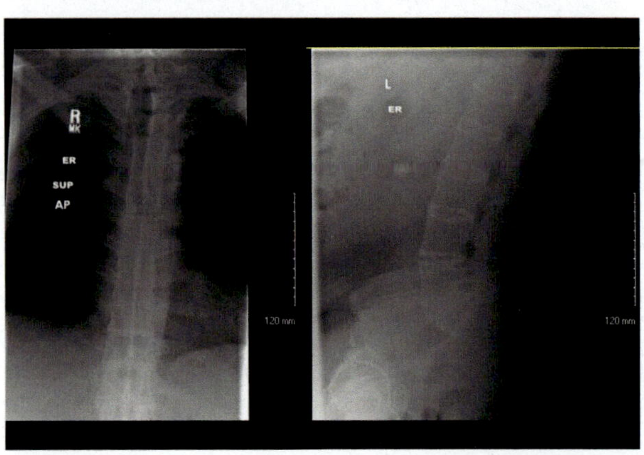

Figure 60.1. X-ray of a patient with ankylosing spondylitis shows the fusion of vertebra throughout the spine.

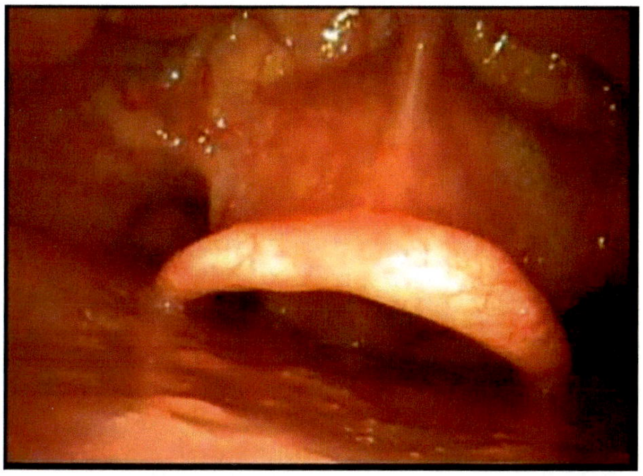

Figure 60.2. A feature of the upper airway of the patient with severe arthritic disease is the inability to move the epiglottis from a fixed position. This results in difficult exposure of the larynx, especially after the induction of anesthesia and the cessation of spontaneous respiratory efforts [**Video 60.1**].

Suggested Readings

Epaud A, Levesque E, Clariot S. Dramatic cervical spine injury secondary to videolaryngoscopy in a patient suffering from ankylosing spondylitis. *Anesthesiology*. 2021;135:495–496.

Heier JM, Schroeder KM, Galgon RE, Arndt GA. Wire-guided (Seldinger technique) intubation through a face mask in urgent, difficult and grossly distorted airways. *Saudi J Anaesth*. 2012;6:292–294.

Mort T. Continuous airway access for the difficult extubation: the efficacy of the airway exchange catheter. *Anesth Analg*. 2007; 105:1357–1362.

Rosenblatt W, Ianus AI, Sukhupragam W, Fickenscher A, Sasaki C. Preoperative endoscopic airway examination (PEAE) provides superior airway information and may reduce the use of unnecessary awake intubation. *Anesth Analg*. 2011;112:602–607.

Woodward LJ, Kam PCA. Ankylosing spondylitis: recent developments and anaesthetic implications. *Anaesthesia*. 2009;64: 540–548.

61 Angioneurotic Edema

Adriana D. Oprea • Roberto Larios

Clinical Scenario: A 62-year-old female presents to the emergency department with swelling of the tongue and face that has been worsening over a 3-hour period. She has no respiratory distress. Nasal pharyngoscopy reveals swelling of the epiglottis and the aryepiglottic fold on one side. Her past medical history includes essential hypertension that is being treated with an ACE inhibitor.

1 What are the anesthetic/airway management considerations for this case?

Angioneurotic edema (more commonly referred to as angioedema) is characterized by extravasation of intravascular fluid into the subcutaneous or submucosal space, which leads to an acute onset and often self-limited tissue swelling. Angioneurotic edema can be hereditary or acquired, the latter being most likely medication induced.

Hereditary angioneurotic edema is caused by C1 esterase inhibitor deficiency, an enzyme that normally limits the extent of complement activation. In cases of C1 esterase inhibitor deficiency, complement activation is uncontrolled, resulting in the release of bradykinin and other vasoactive substances responsible for increased vascular permeability and the development of subsequent tissue edema. In addition to laryngeal edema, which usually presents as voice hoarseness, swallowing difficulties, or throat tightness, hereditary angioedema can involve the subcutaneous tissue or the bowels, leading to diarrhea.

Nonhereditary angioedema is most commonly due to medication use, but it can also be caused by an acquired deficiency of C1 esterase inhibitor seen in lymphomas and other malignancies. Most cases of medication-induced angioedema are due to use of angiotensin-converting enzyme inhibitors (ACE inhibitors). More than 1% of patients treated with the use of ACE inhibitors develop angioedema. Angioedema has also been described with the use of angiotensin II receptor blockers, aspirin, nonsteroidal anti-inflammatories, and certain antibiotics. While most cases of angioedema develop within 4 weeks of treatment initiation, many presentations are delayed even years after the medication was started, making the diagnostic correlation more difficult. Up to 20% of these patients present with dyspnea, stridor, and dysphagia due to supraglottic tissue involvement, and subglottic swelling is uncommon. As with the hereditary form, ACE inhibitor–induced angioedema is due to bradykinin excess due to the drug's interference with its metabolism.

Both hereditary and acquired forms of angioedema are usually nonlife threatening unless the airway is involved, which can prompt concern for impending obstruction or development of an anaphylactic reaction. Treatment for angioedema includes airway protection if necessary and the administration of intravenous steroids and antihistamines. In addition, intramuscular epinephrine should be administered in cases thought to be related to anaphylaxis.

Acquired angioedema that is suspected to be caused by medications (ie, ACE inhibitors) should prompt discontinuation of the inciting therapy. Patients with hereditary angioedema may benefit from a C1 esterase inhibitor concentrate, kallikrein inhibitor, or a bradykinin receptor antagonist administration as well as administration of fresh frozen plasma.

2 How would you manage the airway in this case?

The airway management of patients presenting with angioedema varies depending on the clinical severity. A classification system was developed by Chiu that is based on the extent of airway edema on initial presentation (Table 61.1).

Patients presenting with less severe symptoms are appropriate for expectant management with serial clinical evaluations plus administration of humidified oxygen and the medical modalities described in the previous section. Patients who respond rapidly to medical treatment can also be managed without intubation. Patients presenting with significant tongue, floor of the mouth, or oropharyngeal edema are at risk of impending respiratory compromise and should be electively intubated. Patients who present with severe clinical symptoms such as stridor, hoarseness, and hypoxemia should be emergently intubated.

TABLE 61.1 Class Airway Involvement

I	Isolated facial swelling and oral cavity edema, excluding the floor of the mouth
II	Floor of mouth and/or oropharyngeal edema
III	Oropharyngeal edema with glottic and/or supraglottic involvement

Adapted from Wood A, Choromanski D, Orlewicz M. Intubation of patients with angioedema: A retrospective study of different methods over three year period. *Int J Crit Illn Inj Sci.* 2013;3(2):108–112; Chiu AG, Newkirk KA, Davidson BJ, Burningham AR, Krowiak EJ, Deeb ZE. Angiotensin-converting enzyme inhibitor-induced angioedema: a multicenter review and an algorithm for airway management. *Ann Otol Rhinol Laryngol.* 2001;110(9):834–840; and Ishoo E, Shah UK, Grillone GA, Stram JR, Fuleihan NS. Predicting airway risk in angioedema: staging system based on presentation. *Otolaryngol Head Neck Surg.* 1999;121(3):263–268.

Direct laryngoscopy (DL) can trigger worsening of the edema, potentially causing airway trauma that can convert an impending or partial airway obstruction into a complete obstruction. Awake orotracheal flexible fiberoptic intubation (FFOI) may not be feasible due to massive tongue swelling. Therefore, the awake nasotracheal approach to intubation is preferable for these patients. A retrospective analysis study by Sandefur et al. looked at 14,000 patients who presented to the emergency department with angioedema. FFOI was used in 49% of these patients (nasal route most commonly being used), video laryngoscopy was used in 41%, and DL was used in only 10%. The most successful airway technique was nasal FFOI with an 88% success rate, whereas DL was the least successful with a success rate of 50%.

When neither oral nor nasal flexible scope intubation is feasible and the patient is maintaining the appropriate oxygen saturation, retrograde wire-aided intubation has also been successfully reported. If endotracheal intubation is unsuccessful or deemed completely unfeasible, surgical tracheotomy or percutaneous tracheostomy, done under local anesthesia, can quickly reestablish airway patency.

Sedation during the airway management of these patients should be administered with extreme caution to avoid loss of upper airway muscle tone and the collapse of the pharyngeal wall, causing a complete airway obstruction. Emergency cricothyroidotomy can be used as a last resort when establishing a surgical airway is not possible due to neck edema.

3 What are the potential hazards/complications in regard to the airway?

Upper airway angioedema can progress rapidly, leading to extremely difficult conditions for airway management with any device or technique. Once recognized, emergency procedures should be activated to secure the airway as quickly as possible.

Repeated or less than gentle manipulation of the airway can lead to worsening edema, or in a patient with hereditary angioedema, precipitate an acute attack. It is important to plan airway management thoughtfully, considering experience of the intubating provider, the resources available, and the acuity of the clinical symptoms.

4 Are there special considerations for the emergence or the end of the case?

Patients who require intubation for angioedema require careful assessment of their airway patency prior to attempts at extubation. Standard extubation precautions should be exercised, and the possibility of a recurrent angioedema episode after extubation should be considered. The presence of an endotracheal tube cuff leak and resolution of any facial and oropharyngeal swelling are reassuring signs that the angioedema episode is resolving. Patients should be followed closely for the development of laryngeal edema post extubation, which can present as stridor.

- ACE inhibitors and angiotensin II receptor blockers are responsible for most cases of medication-induced angioedema.
- Intubation should be considered during an acute episode of angioedema involving the floor of the mouth and the oropharynx.
- Airway manipulation during an acute episode should be minimized due to the possibility worsening the angioedema.
- After resolution of the angioedema, careful extubation precautions should be followed.
- *See Figures 61.1 and 61.2 for additional details.*

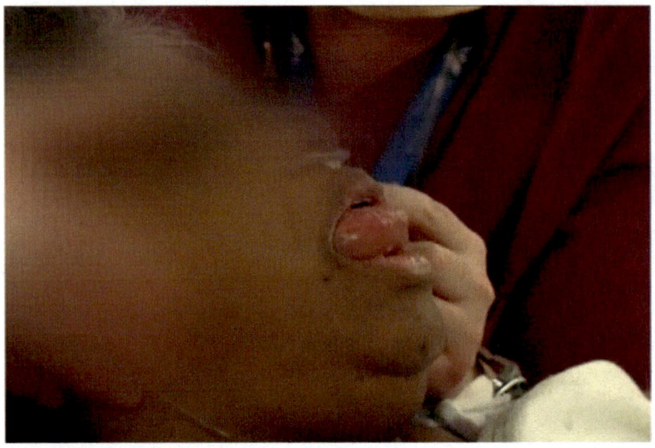

Figure 61.1. A patient who presented to the emergency department with rapidly evolving swelling of the tongue. See also **Video 61.1**.

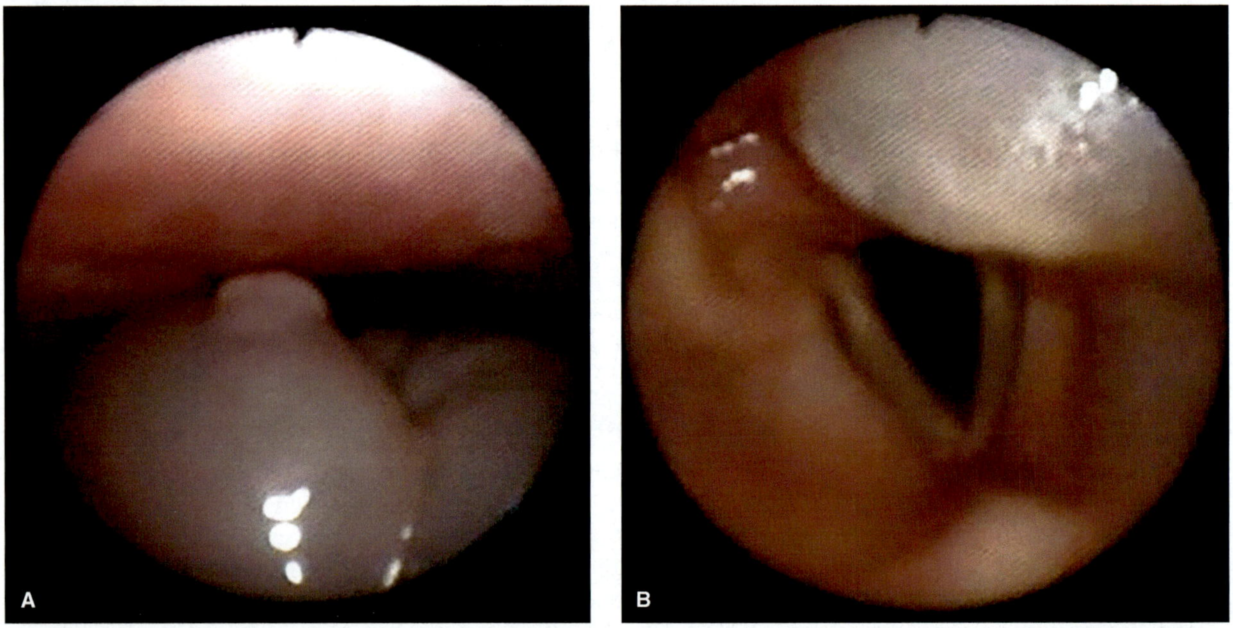

Figure 61.2. A: During flexible endoscope exam of a patient with a presumptive diagnosis of angioneurotic edema, a markedly edematous epiglottis is encountered. **B:** Unilateral aryepiglottic swelling is noted in the same patient.

Suggested Readings

Barbara DW, Ronan KP, Maddox DE, Warner MA. Perioperative angioedema: background, diagnosis, and management. *J Clin Anesth.* 2013;25(4):335–343.

Chiu AG, Newkirk KA, Davidson BJ, et al. Angiotensin-converting enzyme inhibitor-induced angioedema: a multicenter review and an algorithm for airway management. *Ann Otol Rhinol Laryngol.* 2001;110(9):834–840.

Lewis LM. Angioedema: etiology, pathophysiology, current and emerging therapies. *J Emerg Med.* 2013;45(5):789–796.

Sandefur BJ, Liu X, Kaji AH, et al. Emergency department intubations in patients with angioedema: a report from the National Emergency Airway Registry. *J Emerg Med.* 2021;61(5):481–488.

Temiño VM, Peebles RS. The spectrum and treatment of angioedema. *Am J Med.* 2008;121(4):282–286.

Neck Trauma

62

Emily Kahn • Guy Talmor • Boris Paskhover

Clinical Scenario: A 34-year-old man presents to the emergency department after sustaining a gunshot wound to the left cheek. His vital signs are stable and a computed tomography (CT) scan shows the bullet located in his neck near the larynx. There is evidence of a hematoma around the bullet, which is displacing the larynx to the right.

1 What are the anesthetic and airway management considerations for this case?

After penetrating trauma to the neck, associated injuries should be sought. Cervical spine injury should be considered prior to any neck manipulation. Vascular injury to the major vessels of the neck must be ruled out. The potential for airway obstruction with time (eg, continued bleeding or edema) or with further acute interventions (eg, anesthetic induction) is contemplated. Even if an initial assessment reveals an intact, uncompromised airway, the injury offers a host of threats via edema, hematoma, or the potential instability of fractures in the area. Patients without any signs or symptoms of airway obstruction should be admitted and closely monitored for insidious or rapid deterioration.

A normal external examination can hide an unstable airway. Careful attention should be paid to signs or symptoms of underlying airway compromise, including dyspnea, stridor, changes in voice quality, subcutaneous emphysema, odynophagia, or an inability to protect the airway. A thorough clinical evaluation can typically establish significant airway injuries. In stable patients, CT and CT angiography may delineate disruptions to the airway as well as reveal vascular injuries that merit urgent intervention. In patients who are at risk for rapid hemodynamic decompensation, early airway intervention is advised.

Once the need for securing the airway has been determined, a laryngotracheal inspection by either direct visualization or endoscopy is the next reasonable step. This approach assesses the extent of airway trauma and minimizes manipulation and secondary trauma.

If a patient with penetrating neck trauma is protecting their airway at the time of evaluation, an awake intubation using a flexible intubating scope (FIS) is the most conservative approach. This allows for both a thorough evaluation of the airway injury and safe tracheal intubation. The time required to adequately prepare the patient for awake intubation may limit the utility of this approach. In addition, optical and video devices may also be compromised by blood, tissue debris, or edema. If airway edema or a hematoma is causing critical airway stenosis, placement of the scope in itself may lead to complete obstruction of the airway. Furthermore, awake intubation is contingent upon a cooperative patient. A combative patient may preclude this approach. Sedation must be administered with caution, as agents that cause cardiorespiratory depression may lead to rapid decompensation. Dexmedetomidine is a useful alternative that does not cause clinically significant respiratory depression.

Although a rapid sequence intubation (RSI) using direct laryngoscopy for intubation is the mainstay for airway establishment in most trauma patients, this method of securing the airway should be applied cautiously in patients with penetrating neck injuries. Direct pressure to a fractured cricoid cartilage can result in dislocation, loss of view, or complete laryngotracheal separation and subsequent obstruction. The loss in soft tissue and muscle tone that occurs following an RSI can also cause complete airway obstruction in these patients. Furthermore, anatomic distortion from direct trauma or displacement from surrounding edema or hematoma may compromise the success of direct laryngoscopy. Although it is important to consider these factors, multiple review articles still support the use of RSI with direct laryngoscopy. In their retrospective review article, Shearer and Giesecke found a 98% success rate with RSI.

Any intervention should be done in conjunction with personnel experienced in emergency surgical airway access. If the initial presentation includes dyspnea, stridor, hemoptysis, or subcutaneous emphysema, a surgical airway should be considered from the outset. If impending obstruction is a concern or there is significant disturbance of laryngeal anatomy, tracheostomy should be performed under local anesthesia. Tracheostomy should also be performed if endotracheal intubation has failed or if endotracheal intubation would be unsafe due to affiliated craniofacial injuries. If tracheotomy is not feasible and the physical examination supports intact cricoid and tracheal cartilages, then cricothyroidotomy may be considered. Furthermore, if the injury provides a direct communication between the airway and the skin, then intubation through the existing communication is an option.

2 How would you manage the airway in this case?

The patient requires that his airway be emergently secured. Ideally, this would be performed in an operating room setting. Manipulation should only be attempted by a skilled provider with a surgical team available at the bedside. Many surgical providers will examine the patient and mark external airway landmarks prior to attempts at noninvasive intervention.

The initial approach to the airway will largely depend on the patient's respiratory status. As explained above, RSI can lead to obstruction if the airway is dependent upon the intact soft tissue and muscular tone of surrounding structures. In addition, in the patient who already has laryngeal displacement, direct laryngoscopy may not be possible as the normal view of the laryngeal inlet may be severely displaced. However, if the patient is already demonstrating evidence of airway obstruction (stridor, difficulty with phonation) or has significant respiratory distress, RSI may enable providers to secure the airway quickly.

3 What are the surgical considerations that impact anesthetic management?

Penetrating neck trauma and an expanding hematoma in zone II (the area between the cricoid cartilage to the angle of mandible) will require neck exploration and possible tracheotomy. If the patient is likely to have an extended period of intubation, a tracheotomy may be performed early. Due to the presence of hematoma, laryngeal structures may be displaced to the contralateral side, making a tracheotomy more difficult. The use of paralytic agents should be avoided during neck exploration in order to reduce the risk of injury to nervous structures (see Chapter 75: Soft Tissue Cancers of the Neck). Zone II also houses the major vessels to the neck, and the presence of a large, expanding hematoma may be indicative of injury to these structures. Large-bore IV access and possible arterial access should be secured.

4 What are the potential hazards and complications in regard to the airway?

Penetrating neck injuries can cause a multitude of airway injuries both via direct trauma and due to surrounding soft tissue swelling and hematoma. These patients carry a high risk for failure of tracheal intubation, so simultaneous preparation for a surgical airway should be practiced. Furthermore, obstruction of the airway from edema, hematoma, or significant bleeding into the airway can make mask ventilation impossible. Blind intubation in these patients should always be avoided.

- Following a penetrating neck trauma, rapid respiratory decompensation due to a hematoma or edema may occur.
- In the stable patient, awake intubation with a FIS is often the safest method to secure the airway.
- Most patients can be successfully managed with RSI and direct laryngoscopy.
- Personnel experienced in performing an emergency surgical airway should be present at the bedside.
- *See Figures 62.1 and 62.2 for additional details.*

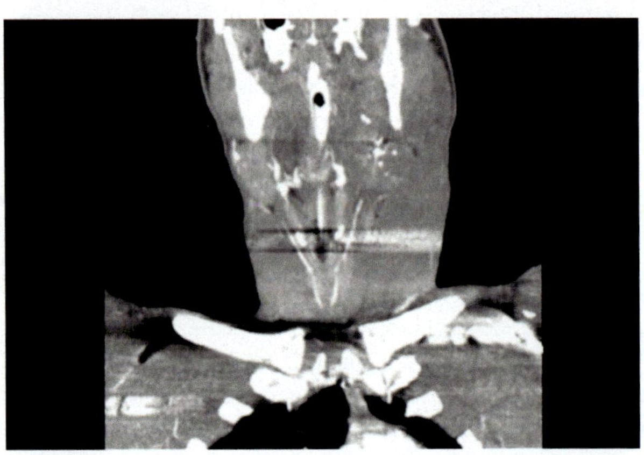

Figure 62.1. In a coronal plane section of a patient with a bullet wound to the neck, a hematoma without airway compression is noted on the left side. See also **Video 62.1**.

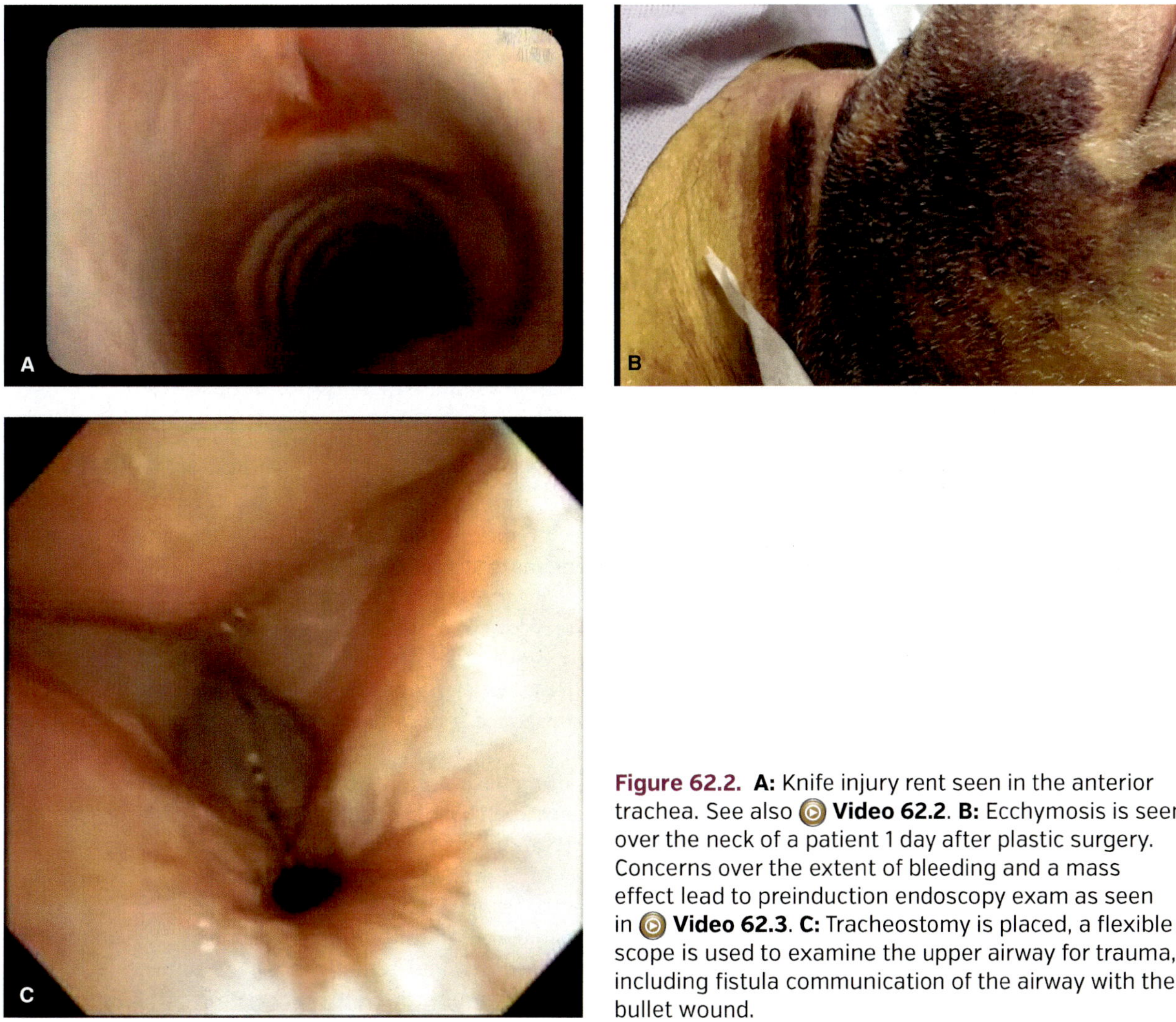

Figure 62.2. **A:** Knife injury rent seen in the anterior trachea. See also **Video 62.2**. **B:** Ecchymosis is seen over the neck of a patient 1 day after plastic surgery. Concerns over the extent of bleeding and a mass effect lead to preinduction endoscopy exam as seen in **Video 62.3**. **C:** Tracheostomy is placed, a flexible scope is used to examine the upper airway for trauma, including fistula communication of the airway with the bullet wound.

Suggested Readings

Burgess CA, Dale OT, Almeyda R, Corbridge RJ. An evidence based review of the assessment and management of penetrating neck trauma. *Clin Otolaryngol*. 2012;37(1):44–52.

Kummer C, Netto FS, Rizoli S, Yee D. A review of traumatic airway injuries: potential implications for airway assessment and management. *Injury*. 2007;38(1):27–33.

Mandavia DP, Qualls S, Rokos I. Emergency airway management in penetrating neck injury. *Ann Emerg Med*. 2000;35(3):221–225.

Schaefer SD. Management of acute blunt and penetrating external laryngeal trauma. *Laryngoscope*. 2014;124(1):233–244.

Shearer VE, Giesecke AH. Airway management for patients with penetrating neck trauma: a retrospective study. *Anesth Analg*. 1993;77(6):1135–1138.

63 Emergent Airway Management in the Unstable At-Risk Cervical Spine Patient

Lisa K. Torres • Seth Manoach

Clinical Scenario: A 56-year-old woman with a BMI of 35 status post anterior cervical discectomy and fusion (ACDF) of C3–C6 was placed in a rigid neck collar and extubated postoperatively to nasal cannula oxygen. In the post anesthesia care unit (PACU), she developed expanding neck hematoma, respiratory distress, and confusion despite an initial SpO_2 of 100%. During preparation for reintubation, she subsequently desaturated to an SpO_2 of 25% with bradycardia to 40 beats per minute (bpm).

1 What are the anesthetic/airway management considerations for this case?

Although airway maneuvers will result in some degree of neck movement, both in general and at the site of injury, their impact on secondary neurologic injury remains undefined. Despite the frequency with which airway maneuvers are performed in the at-risk patient with a cervical spine (c-spine) injury, the incidence of secondary injury associated with airway interventions is very low. In addition, limited evidence shows that failed intubation in the setting of spinal immobilization is rare. Since both failed airway management and spinal cord injury may have devastating consequences for the patient, clinicians must balance these risks when selecting an airway management approach. Previously accepted practice is that spinal movement should be limited as much as practical during airway management using manual in-line stabilization (MILS) or neck collar, however, recent challenges to this practice have emerged in the face of limited evidence of their effectiveness in preventing secondary injury. Airway management using a neck collar, especially a rigid brace, is associated with higher rates of first-pass intubation failure. The recommended approach is to detach the neck collar and use MILS to facilitate airway opening while limiting head and neck movement. However, use of MILS has been shown to worsen the view particularly during direct laryngoscopy (DL). Additional challenges accompany the care of these patients due to the potential for a substantial amount of blood, secretions, or gastric contents, high risk of vomiting and/or aspiration, deforming facial injuries, and hemodynamic instability.

Rapid sequence induction (RSI) is the most common technique utilized to quickly protect the airway while minimizing aspiration risk. We avoid bag-mask ventilation when possible, which is associated with c-spine movement, risk of gastric insufflation, and vomiting. Induction agents that have limited effects on hemodynamics, such as etomidate or ketamine, are useful medications in settings with high risk of hemodynamic compromise. After the induction agent is given, a neuromuscular blocking agent is administered, such as succinylcholine or rocuronium, prior to intubation attempt.

In addition, an expanding neck hematoma may cause airway compression, requiring the incision to be opened at bedside.

2 How would you manage the airway in this case?

Historically, airway management in the pre–video laryngoscope (VL) era of the patient with suspected or confirmed c-spine instability was managed with DL or awake versus asleep fiberoptic bronchoscopic (FOB) intubation. Unlike other airway devices, DL is not susceptible to a compromised view from a soiled airway impeding optics. On the other hand, use of FOB limits c-spine motion during intubation. There is evidence that nasal FOB intubation is associated with less posterior displacement in injured cadaveric spines than other modalities, including DL, supraglottic airways, intubating supraglottic airway (SGA), and mask ventilation. However, many trained airway managers are less experienced with the use of FOB intubation, and it is more time consuming than an RSI followed by DL.

Intubation technology has advanced in recent years to include VL, which may be supplanting DL as the default technique for endotracheal intubation. Use of VL is also associated with improved glottic view compared with DL. It is important to recognize that VL devices that pass near or through the posterior pharynx may be more susceptible to soiling than devices that are hyperangulated and remain anterior during placement. A recent systematic review and meta-analysis by Singleton et al. showed that a variety of VLs had increased probability of first-pass intubation success when compared to DL with a Macintosh blade. However, this finding was not replicated in a subgroup analysis of studies using MILS during intubation. Furthermore, no device was associated with a faster time to intubation when compared to DL with a Macintosh blade. Although intubating time may be greater with the use of VL (other studies have demonstrated time to be less than 1 minute), it is likely of little clinical relevance. Available evidence shows that overall intubation success rates with VL and DL are similar. Thus, in an unstable patient, we recommend providers use the most rapid approach with the greatest chance of first-pass success after considering patient cooperation, injuries, airway difficulty, aspiration risk, and the experience of the operator with available devices. (See Table 63.1 for a summary of interventions, considerations, and recommendations for management of patients with the unstable c-spine.)

TABLE 63.1 Interventions, Considerations, and Recommendations for Management of Patients with the At-Risk c-Spine

Intervention	Considerations	Intubating Practice or Recommendation
Neck collar	Neither soft nor semirigid collars effectively immobilize the neck for basic[a] or advanced airway[b] procedures.	Remove or disconnect anteriorly to facilitate mouth opening and application of anterior airway pressure, if needed. Can be kept on during FOB.
Manual in-line stabilization (MILS)	International standard, although efficacy questioned. May impede rapid intubation.	Used when rigid collar removed during intubation to facilitate mouth opening.
Intubating instrument		
DL	More difficulty obtaining a view with MILS. May be more rapid than VL or FOB.	Select an intubating device with which operator has most experience.
VL	Reduced spinal movement compared with DL. Higher first pass success. Anteriorly placed devices less susceptible to soiling.	
FOB	Head and neck can be left in a neutral position. Least c-spine movement to achieve intubation. Patient cooperation/airway soiling are potential issues.	Consider nasal or orotracheal intubation with FOB.
SGA (both standard and intubating)	May exert high pressures against the upper cervical vertebrae, producing posterior displacement of the upper c-spine. Associated with less c-spine movement than jaw thrust and bag mask ventilation.	Temporizing adjunct during failed airway or difficult mask ventilation. Reserve for cannot-intubate, cannot-ventilate scenarios.

DL, direct laryngoscopy; VL, video laryngoscopy; SGA, supraglottic airway; FOB, fiberoptic bronchoscopy.
[a]Basic airway procedures: chin lift, jaw thrust, head tilt, placement of oral and esophageal airways.
[b]Advanced airway procedures: placement of orotracheal tube with straight or curved laryngoscopic blade, nasotracheal tube blindly placed, or placement of an esophageal obturator airway.

3 What are the potential hazards/complications regarding the airway?

Manipulation of an unstable c-spine for successful intubation via laryngoscopy may further worsen the injury. In addition, an airway may be lost due to efforts to maintain c-spine neutrality. Efforts should be made to minimize major variations in hemodynamics during airway management and during subsequent mechanical ventilation. Hypotension (systolic blood pressure less than 90 mm Hg) must be corrected as soon as possible to prevent ischemic insult to the spinal cord and to potentially enhance neurologic outcomes. Peripheral oxygen saturations below 90% should be avoided for similar reasons, highlighting the importance of selecting the device with which the intubating provider is most comfortable to achieve a timely, first-pass success.

Rescue SGA is reserved for cannot-intubate, cannot-ventilate situations as it may cause high pressures against the upper cervical vertebrae during insertion, inflation, and while in situ. These elevated pressures may produce posterior displacement of the upper c-spine. However, the clinical relevance of these findings remains unclear, and if an SGA becomes necessary to salvage the airway, it should be used. Ultimately, an emergency surgical airway with cricothyroidotomy is warranted when available intubation and/or ventilation modalities fail.

4 What distinct airway device might be used in this case, and what are the special considerations?

In one study, the use of VL applied a reduced mean force to the c-spine of 10 Newton (N) compared with DL, which applied a mean force of 49 N. Forces causing cervical fractures or ligamentous tears have been measured in the range of 645 to 7429 N, depending on the vector. Furthermore, studies have shown that some degree of cervical spinal motion occurs during intubation regardless of the modality used. In addition, we would advocate for the use of a rigid stylet or adjunct such as a bougie to assist with intubation when a difficult airway is anticipated during use of VL or DL.

- Use of VL is becoming more common during intubation of the unstable patient with c-spine injury.
- FOB causes the least spinal movement.
- It is still standard to perform MILS, allowing some flexion or extension to facilitate rapid intubation.
- Reserve use of rescue SGA for cannot-intubate, cannot-ventilate situations as it is associated with high pressures on cervical vertebrae and posterior displacement.
- *See Figure 63.1 and* ▶ ***Video 63.1*** *for additional details.*

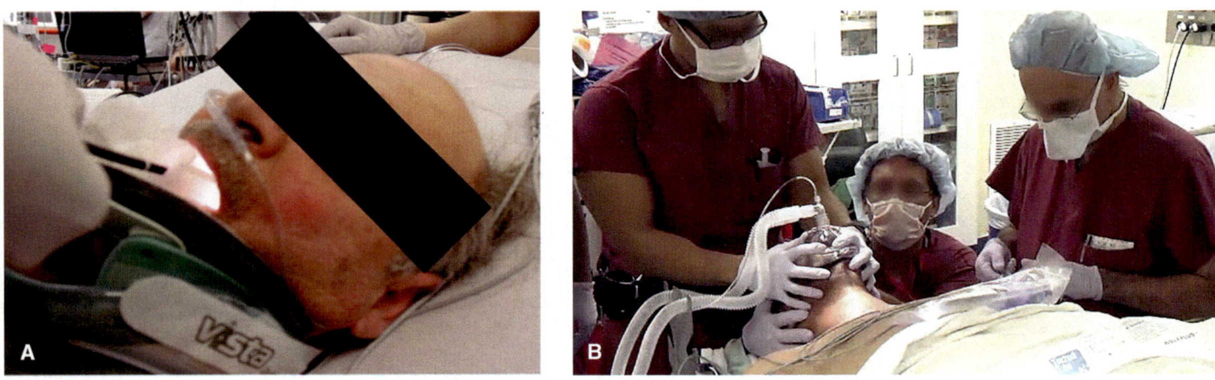

Figure 63.1. A: A patient in a cervical collar undergoes awake flexible scope intubation. **B:** A patient at risk of having an unstable cervical spine injury is placed in manual in-line axial stabilization after removal of the front section of the rigid cervical collar in preparation for anesthetic induction and tracheal intubation.

Acknowledgment

We gratefully acknowledge the contributions of previous edition author, Kapil Rajwani, as portions of those chapters have been retained in this revision.

Suggested Readings

Crosby ET. Airway management in adults after cervical spine trauma. *Anesthesiology*. 2006;104(6):1293–1318.

Estime SR, Kuza CM. Trauma airway management: induction agents, rapid versus slower sequence intubations, and special considerations. *Anesthesiol Clin*. 2019;37(1):33–50.

Holmes MG, Dagal A, Feinstein BA, Joffe AM. Airway management practice in adults with an unstable cervical spine: the Harborview Medical Center Experience. *Anesth Analg*. 2018;127(2):450–451.

Martini RP, Larson DM. Clinical evaluation and airway management for adults with cervical spine instability. *Anesthesiol Clin*. 2015;33(2):315–327.

Singleton BN, Morris FK, Yet B, Buggy DJ, Perkins ZB. Effectiveness of intubation devices in patients with cervical spine immobilisation: a systematic review and network meta-analysis. *Br J Anaesth*. 2021;126(5):1055–1066.

Wiles MD. Cervical spine injury and tracheal intubation: are we protecting patients or physicians? *South Afr J Anaesth Analg*. 2021;27(6):1260–1264.

The Stable Patient with an At-Risk Cervical Spine

64

Douglas Milano-Johnson • Seth Manoach

Clinical Scenario: A 25-year-old male presents to the emergency department after having been ejected from a motorcycle. He was conscious at the accident scene and placed in a rigid cervical spine (c-spine) collar. He sustained a laceration to his forehead and cannot recall the accident. On presentation to the emergency department, he has stable hemodynamics but requires an urgent laparotomy.

1 What are the anesthetic/airway management considerations for this case?

Until an unstable c-spine injury has been ruled out, trauma patients require cervical immobilization to prevent excessive neck movement and secondary spinal cord damage. During intubation, however, restricting cervical range of motion precludes clinicians from optimally positioning the patient's head and neck and in turn may limit glottic view. Therefore, when circumstances permit, clinical evaluation of c-spine stability, and discontinuation of c-spine precautions if indicated, should precede airway management.

Two clinical-decision tools, The National Emergency X-radiography Utilization Study (NEXUS) and the Canadian C-Spine Rule (CCR), were developed to assist clinicians in identifying low-risk trauma patients for whom cervical radiography may be unnecessary. Stiell et al. compared the sensitivity and specificity of these two tools and found the CCR to be superior in both categories. Provided an adult patient has no history of vertebral disease, is alert with a Glasgow Coma Score of 15, and has stable vital signs, the CCR excludes clinically significant cervical injury with nearly 100% sensitivity. The rule applies only to patients under age 65 without a dangerous mechanism of injury or limb paresthesias. In addition, at minimum, patients must satisfy a single low-risk criterion: they must demonstrate the ability to sit upright or ability to ambulate, have no cervical tenderness or immediate neck pain, or have been injured in a low-risk accident (such as a simple rear-end motor vehicle collision). If a patient qualifies *and* experiences no pain with 45 degrees of active bilateral head rotation, their c-spine can be cleared without radiography. Clinicians may then remove the patient's cervical collar and safely manipulate their head and neck. Unfortunately, few trauma patients requiring airway management meet these strict criteria.

When an emergent airway is required and c-spine injury cannot be excluded, clinicians should perform rapid sequence intubation (RSI) with either direct laryngoscopy (DL) or video laryngoscopy (VL) and manual in-line stabilization (MILS) to limit neck movement and establish a secure airway as quickly as possible. After removing the anterior portion of the patient's cervical collar, to perform MILS, an assistant uses both hands to hold the patient's head in a neutral position. Secondary c-spine injury attributed to airway management has become vanishingly rare since popularization of this technique in the 1980s, however, cervical stabilization can complicate airway management. Studies suggest MILS degrades laryngoscopic view and may limit mouth opening. Clinicians must therefore bear in mind that both secondary spinal cord injury and prolonged or failed intubation have potentially devastating consequences. We suggest that in difficult cases clinicians apply less rigid MILS, as momentary flexion-extension of the c-spine is unlikely to cause harm and may facilitate intubation.

Since the advent of indirect laryngoscopy, VL has become the intubation technique of choice for most clinicians in the context of suspected c-spine injury. When compared with DL, VL improves glottic view and reduces the amount of force placed on the c-spine during airway management, although it remains unclear whether these benefits make VL safer overall. While clinicians have traditionally been taught to use DL when the airway is soiled to avoid obscuring the video laryngoscope's lens, recent data indicate hyperangulated VL and DL achieve equal levels of first-pass success in this setting.

In cooperative, hemodynamically stable patients, fiberoptic bronchoscope-assisted (FOB) intubation is another important option as it causes less cervical movement than any other airway maneuver. FOB intubation can be performed on awake or sedated patients, but if injury distorts airway anatomy, or limits mouth opening, clinicians should avoid pharmacologic suppression of spontaneous respiration. An awake approach also permits postintubation neurologic assessment. FOB intubation may be performed via the nose or mouth, but a nasal approach is contraindicated in patients with facial trauma.

Ultimately, while VL has become increasingly popular and indirect laryngoscopy offers the benefit of improved glottic view, as yet, there is no conclusive evidence proving superiority of any one intubation device or method over another in the context of c-spine instability. We therefore encourage airway managers to take into consideration available expertise, resources and patient-specific factors when approaching intubation in this population.

2 How would you manage the airway in this case?

This patient's dangerous mechanism of injury precludes clearance of his c-spine without radiography, so cervical immobilization is mandatory until imaging can be performed. He requires urgent surgery but is hemodynamically stable and mentating normally, therefore his intubation qualifies as nonemergent. This would permit us to consider all available approaches to airway management.

First, we would assess the patient's airway by performing an "AMPLE" (Allergies, Medications, Past medical history, Last meal, Event) history. If the patient phonates clearly in response to questioning, this suggests his airway is not in immediate jeopardy. Next, we would perform a neurologic assessment and examine the patient's c-spine for midline tenderness and his face and mouth for predictors of difficult laryngoscopy or bag-mask ventilation.

A stable trauma patient with a dangerous mechanism of injury and loss of consciousness requires CT imaging of both the head and cervical spine. CT is more sensitive for detection of unstable c-spine fractures and dislocations than plain film radiography but cannot rule out spinal cord contusion, vascular damage or ligamentous injury. In this case, we would favor awake FOB intubation with MILS over RSI given the patient's high-risk mechanism of injury, stable hemodynamics, and nonemergent airway requirement. CT evidence suggestive of c-spine injury would reinforce our decision to pursue this technique.

Before starting, we would prepare the patient by explaining the procedure. We would then topically anesthetize the airway using atomized and viscous lidocaine and administer low-dose systemic anxiolysis. After bronchoscopically confirming successful intubation, we would perform a brief postintubation neurologic assessment prior to increased sedation or induction of anesthesia.

3 What are the potential hazards/complications in regard to the airway?

Awake FOB intubation is more time consuming than RSI, therefore its use should be reserved for stable patients. It also requires more expertise and inexperienced providers may find the technique difficult. Topical lidocaine can cause airway obstruction or toxicity. Failure to sufficiently suppress protective airway reflexes during awake intubation may precipitate vomiting, coughing or agitation, threatening both the airway and the cervical spine. In the context of acute trauma and active resuscitation, even low-dose sedatives may induce apnea, hemodynamic instability and loss of airway patency. Use of ketamine may preserve respiratory drive but can lead to hypersalivation and laryngospasm. Procedural sedation with dexmedetomidine can cause hypotension and bradycardia. Anticholinergics, including glycopyrrolate and atropine, may counteract these side effects. Initiation of positive pressure ventilation reduces preload and can cause hemodynamic collapse in hemorrhaging patients. While performing FOB intubation, the endotracheal tube may catch on the arytenoids preventing its advancement. To ease the tube's passage, while maintaining MILS, clinicians can elevate the patient's head (up to 30 degrees), provide gentle jaw thrust and rotate the tube 90 degrees counterclockwise.

4 What distinct airway device might be used in this case, and what are the special considerations?

During FOB intubation, an appropriately sized intubating oral airway can serve as a bite block and allow airway managers to maintain midline position while accessing the glottis. Clinicians should also be prepared for conversion to RSI and have DL, VL, and salvage equipment available.

- Clinical evaluation can rarely exclude an unstable c-spine injury in trauma patients requiring emergent or urgent intubation.
- Positive findings on either clinical examination or cervical CT should raise suspicion for unstable c-spine injury.
- Most trauma intubations are performed safely with RSI, MILS and VL or DL.
- Consider awake FOB intubation in cooperative, hemodynamically stable patients at high risk for unstable c-spine injury.
- *See Figure 64.1 and* **Video 64.1** *for additional details.*

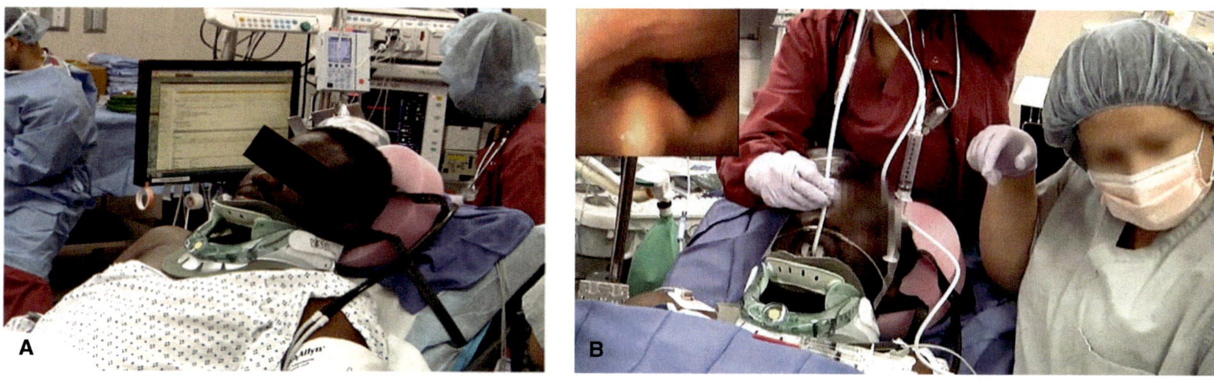

Figure 64.1. **A:** A patient in a rigid cervical collar is prepared for awake intubation. **B:** During the awake intubation the rigid collar is left in place to minimize movement that may occur.

Acknowledgment

We gratefully acknowledge the contributions of previous edition author, David Berlin, as portions of those chapters have been retained in this revision.

Suggested Readings

Brimacombe J, Keller C, Kunzel KH, et al. Cervical spine motion during airway management: a cinefluoroscopic study of the posteriorly destabilized third cervical vertebrae in human cadavers. *Anesth Analg.* 2000;91:1274–1278.

d'Arville A, Walker M, Lacey J, et al. Airway management in the adult patient with an unstable cervical spine. *Curr Opin Anesthesiol.* 2021;345:97–602.

Manoach S, Paladino L. Manual in-line stabilization for acute airway management of suspected cervical spine injury: historical review and current questions. *Ann Emerg Med.* 2007;50:236–245.

Sakles JC, Corn GJ, Hollinger P, et al. The impact of a soiled airway on intubation success in the emergency department when using the glidescope or the direct laryngoscope. *Acad Emerg Med.* 2017;24:628–636.

Stegmann G, Llewellyn R, Hofmeyr R. Global airway management of the unstable cervical spine survey (GAUSS). *South Afr J Anaesth Analg.* 2021;27(6):278–285.

Stiell IG, Clement CM, McKnight RD, et al. The Canadian c-spine rule versus the NEXUS low-risk criteria in patients with trauma. *N Engl J Med.* 2003;349:2510–2518.

65 Cervical Osteophytes and Airway Management

Ha V. Nguyen • Trevor M. Banack

Clinical Scenario: An 83-year-old man presents for resection of a large anterior cervical osteophyte (C3–C6). This osteophyte is causing symptomatic dysphagia, airway obstruction, changes in voice, weight loss, and chronic aspiration.

1 What are the anesthetic and airway management considerations for this case?

Cervical osteophytes are a subset of diffuse idiopathic skeletal hyperostosis (DISH). Forestier et al. first described DISH in 1950 as findings of spinal hyperostosis distinct from ankylosing spondylitis. These authors observed this form of hyperostosis in elderly male patients, anterior outgrowths from the vertebral bodies, primarily in the lumbar region. These findings were made on radiologic examinations (x-ray) and on postmortem gross specimens. However, anterior cervical osteophytes are best diagnosed with computed tomographic (CT) imaging and oropharyngeal swallow study. In rare cases, vocal fold paralysis can occur with compression of the recurrent laryngeal nerve, typically originating at the C6–C7 vertebrae.

The pathogenesis of DISH is not well known. Excessive bone formation leads to ossification of the anterolateral aspect of the spine. Extraspinal locations, such as in peripheral joints, have also been described. It is observed predominantly in patients older than 50 years of age with a 2:1 preponderance in males to females. While the frequency of the disease increases after the fifth decade of life, the incidence of secondary dysphagia typically presents in patients greater than 65 years of age. The most common level of bridging cervical osteophytes occurs in the lower cervical spine at C3–C5. Anterior cervical osteophytes are found in 20% to 30% of elderly patients; however, very few are symptomatic. In addition to excess bone formation, DISH has also been associated with metabolic syndrome—obesity, dyslipidemia, hypertension, and insulin resistance—and an increased risk of coronary artery disease and stroke.

The pathophysiologic changes that occur in DISH can have several effects on airway management. Rarely, patients with DISH are symptomatic. However, depending on location and size, osteophytes can pose major problems. Large anterior cervical osteophytes can cause extrinsic compression. Dysphagia is the most common symptom of cervical osteophytes, but other symptoms may include airway obstruction, dyspnea, dysphonia, and aspiration. Conservative measures of management for osteophytic changes of the airway include treatment with a gastrostomy tube, especially in the setting of aspiration pneumonia. The ossification that occurs in DISH results in stiffening of the spine, which can increase the risk of spinal fractures due to the lack of mobility in affected joints and decreased neck range of motion. Positioning can be difficult in the small subset of patients who exhibit stooped postures. It has been reported that DISH may be a cause of obstructive sleep apnea. These anatomic changes can result in difficulty with tracheal intubation.

2 How would you manage the airway in this case?

In the current presentation, a history of dysphagia, changes in voice, weight loss, and chronic aspiration demonstrates that the patient's osteophyte is causing distinct symptomology. During this patient's preoperative workup, a CT scan was obtained and a nasopharyngoscopy was performed by an otolaryngologist. The current authors would elect to proceed with an awake flexible scope intubation. The consulting otolaryngologist should be present at all times and prepared for surgical access to the airway should intubation attempts fail. A wire-reinforced tracheal tube is selected due to concerns for possible extrinsic compression by the large osteophyte. A dose of dexamethasone would be administered intraoperatively to help minimize airway edema.

3 What are the potential hazards and complications in regard to the airway?

The majority of patients with DISH are asymptomatic. The patient in this case displayed symptoms suggestive of an alteration in the airway anatomy. When large anterior cervical osteophytes are present, they can cause extrinsic compression or distortion of the airway anatomy. Also, a difficult intubation can occur as a result of cervical spine ossification, resulting in a limited neck range of motion. Severe DISH may place the patient at risk of a cervical spine fracture. Patients with DISH have been reported to be at increased risk of gastric content aspiration.

Formation of a hematoma in the operative field can cause airway compromise, requiring reexploration and evacuation. Postoperative airway edema may be present immediately following surgery or may develop several hours later. A course of steroids may be considered to help decrease edema formation. Patients with continued dyspnea in the PACU that are found to have a hematoma may require a temporary tracheostomy until swelling decreases and/or hematoma is evacuated.

4 Are there special considerations for the emergence or the end of the case?

Resection of this patient's cervical osteophyte should be curative in relieving the obstruction or compression in most instances. However, removal may be incomplete or inadequate. In addition, the airway may be edematous and the anatomy distorted following surgery, potentially making reintubation even more challenging in the event that the patient does not tolerate extubation. In dealing with a possible difficult airway, the period of emergence is as equally important as the initial induction. A plan should be formulated for the emergence and extubation. Given the higher risk of requiring reintubation, an awake extubation strategy is suggested in these patients. A cuff-leak test should be performed at the end of surgery to estimate patency of the airway. If the initial intubation was difficult, extubation over an airway exchange catheter may be considered. During the initial securing of the airway, an array of airway equipment should be immediately accessible, and a surgeon should be available to provide assistance if a surgical airway is needed. It is also important to note that while asymptomatic anterior osteophytes may not cause a problem initially, postoperative swelling can create newfound dysphagia and dyspnea after laryngeal or oropharyngeal surgery, possibly necessitating continued steroid administration or a tracheostomy.

- Diffuse idiopathic hyperostosis, specifically cervical osteophytes, can cause difficultly with intubation.
- Awake intubation is suggested, although it may still prove to be difficult.
- A surgical airway may be necessary, and skilled surgeons should be on standby and immediately available.
- The patient should be treated as a potential difficult extubation.
- The patient with severe DISH can suffer cervical spine fracture if not handled gently.
- *See Figure 65.1 and* ***Video 65.1*** *for additional details.*

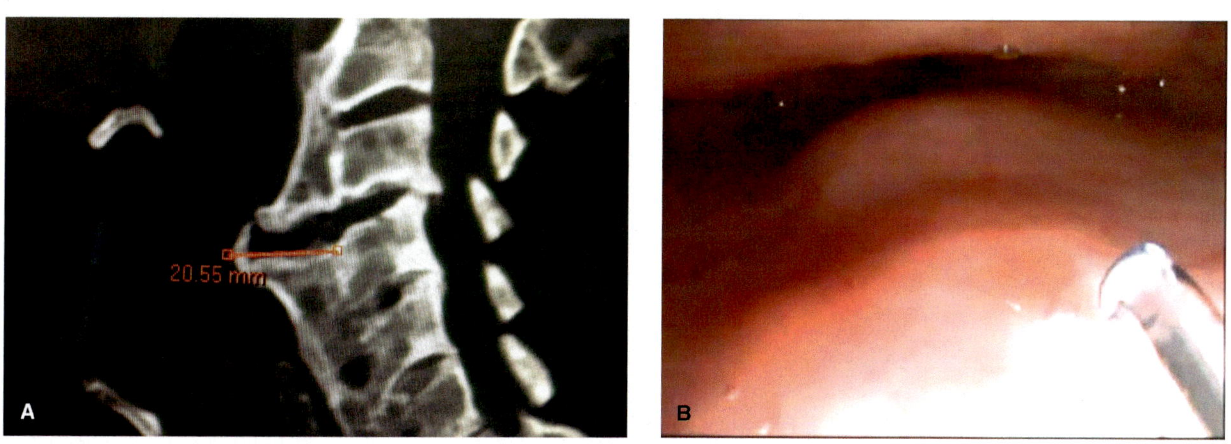

Figure 65.1. A: Cervical osteophyte is seen on lateral spine film. **B:** A cervical osteophyte causes a protuberance in the posterior pharyngeal wall.

Suggested Readings

Babores M, Finnerty JP. Aspiration pneumonia secondary to giant cervical osteophyte formation (diffuse idiopathic skeletal hyperostosis or Forrestier's disease): a case report. *Chest*. 1998;114(5):1481–1482.

Bunmaprasert T, Keeratiruangrong J, Sugandhavesa N, Riew KD, Liawrungrueang W. Surgical management of Diffuse Idiopathic Skeletal Hyperostosis (DISH) causing secondary dysphagia (Narrative review). *J Orthop Surg (Hong Kong)*. 2021;29(3):23094990211041783.

Chen YR, Sung K, Tharin S. Symptomatic anterior cervical osteophyte causing dysphagia: case report, imaging, and review of the literature. *Cureus*. 2016;8(2):e473.

Forestier J, Rotes-Querol J. Senile ankylosing hyperostosis of the spine. *Ann Rheum Dis*. 1950;9(4):321–330.

Jabarkheel R, Chen YR, Xu L, Yan CH, Patel ZM, Desai AM. Transoral endoscopic resection of high cervical osteophytes with long-term symptom resolution: case series, imaging, and literature review. *World Neurosurg*. 2018;120:240–243.

Mader R, Buskila D, Verlaan JJ, et al. Developing new classification criteria for diffuse idiopathic skeletal hyperostosis: back to square one. *Rheumatology*. 2013;52(2):326–330.

The Patient with a History of Neck Irradiation

66

Adriana D. Oprea • Haitham Ibrahim

Clinical Scenario: A 54-year-old man with a remote history of laryngeal cancer presents for direct laryngoscopy to evaluate a new soft tissue mass in the neck. He had previously been treated with a full course of chemotherapy combined with radiation to the neck. He has no new respiratory symptoms and is not suspected to have any obstruction at the level of the larynx.

1 What are the anesthetic/airway management considerations for this case?

Radiation to the head and neck has been used for decades in the treatment of thyroid and airway malignancies. Potential difficulty with bag-mask ventilation or intubation should always be considered in patients who have previously undergone radiation therapy. Radiation therapy causes both early and late consequences. Early side effects of radiation include xerostomia, loss of taste, and skin and mucosal inflammation. Late complications include stenosis or necrosis of any exposed tissues, including the oropharynx, larynx, and facial soft tissues and bones. The most significant late complication of neck irradiation is radiation fibrosis syndrome, which is estimated to affect 25% to 50% of patients exposed to neck irradiation. Patients with this complication can experience significantly limited neck range of motion and an increased Mallampati score compared to their preirradiation airway exam. Direct laryngoscopy can be difficult or impossible due to limited neck range of motion and inability to displace the tongue into the submental space. Trismus or restricted movement of the temporomandibular joint (TMJ) is another late complication due to neck irradiation. In severe cases, it can restrict the airway exam and make laryngoscopy difficult or impossible.

A proper mask seal may be difficult to obtain due to orofacial pain, swelling from mucositis, orocutaneous fistulae, or decreased tissue elasticity. Osteonecrosis of the jaw is another well-described complication of radiotherapy due to the jaw's extensive vascularization. Pathologic fractures can result from an overly aggressive grip of the mask during ventilation, especially in the presence of mandibular osteonecrosis.

Another well-described consequence of neck irradiation is hypopharyngeal stenosis, which can lead to a false recognition of the glottic opening and improper positioning of the tracheal tube during intubation. In these cases, the endotracheal tube may inadvertently be placed in the esophagus or in a position which occludes the true airway. The laryngeal inlet exists distal to the stenosis and may not be distinguishable from the esophagus in these cases. In addition, glottic and epiglottic edema secondary to radiation can also impede visualization of the glottic aperture during laryngoscopy.

Table 66.1 summarizes head and neck changes that can occur due to radiation therapy.

2 How would you manage the airway in this case?

In all cases where there are concerns related to airway management, a thorough preoperative evaluation is key. Neck range of motion, oral aperture, the relationship between the tongue and the oropharynx, Mallampati score, and thyromental distance are all important parts of the airway examination. The neck should be palpated to determine the extent of soft tissue fibrosis. Indirect laryngoscopy or a nasal–laryngeal endoscopy, if available, can provide more detail regarding anatomy of the airway. In addition, the local effect of neck masses external to the airway need to be considered before proceeding with the induction of general anesthesia. In addition to a thorough airway exam as noted above, seeking out prior imaging studies in the patient's chart can be extremely informative.

TABLE 66.1 Radiation Therapy: Head and Neck

Site of Malignancy	Pathology	Disability: Early	Disability: Late	Anesthetic Implications
Face and buccal mucosa	Necrosis Mucositis	Oral thrush Orofacial pain	Ulceration Orocutaneous fistula with purulent discharge	Difficult mask holding and ventilation Hemorrhage
TM joint	Fibrosis		Trismus	Difficult laryngoscopy and intubation
Tongue	Fibrosis Inflammation	Glossitis	Glossomegaly Decreased tongue mobility	Falsely obscures Mallampati classification Difficult laryngoscopy Hemorrhage
Dentition	Increased risk of caries	Increased mobility	Loss of teeth	Difficulty in mask holding and ventilation Dislodgement of teeth during laryngoscopy
Floor of mouth	Fibrosis		Decreased mobility of tongue	Difficult laryngoscopy
Mandible	Osteonecrosis or osteomyelitis Pathologic fracture	Asymptomatic dehiscence of mucosa	Micrognathia/ mandibular recession Extraoral/ intraoral fistulae	Reduction in mandibular space Difficult mask holding and ventilation Difficult laryngoscopy
Suprahyoid region	Fibrosis and edema		Altered consistency of neck tissue presents as firm or woody mass Skin tethering	Limitation of flexion and extension at atlanto-occipital joint
Lower airway	Epiglottic edema Glottic edema		Snoring Hoarseness of voice Irritant cough	Difficult visualization of larynx Difficult endotracheal intubation

Awake intubation is the most conservative approach to airway management in patients presenting with neck masses who have previously undergone irradiation. This approach bypasses the need for mask ventilation, supraglottic airway use, and rigid laryngoscopy, all of which can be difficult in these patients. Despite this, the literature describes cases of failed awake intubations in patients with hypopharyngeal fibrosis due to pharyngeal stenosis falsely being recognized as the as the glottic opening.

When an awake intubation is not a valid option (eg, patient refusal or inability to cooperate), an induction of anesthesia with the maintenance of spontaneous ventilation is another conservative option. In these cases, anesthesia can be induced with either an intravenous or inhalational technique. Once the ability to mask ventilate the patient is demonstrated, muscle relaxant can be given prior to intubation attempts. If the provider is unable to mask ventilate the patient, spontaneous ventilation can be maintained while the next step in airway management is determined.

Intubation following induction of general anesthesia is reasonable in patients with no evidence of jaw osteonecrosis, a preserved neck range of motion, and with a reassuring imaging and preoperative endoscopic airway exam. Many head and neck procedures involve neuromuscular testing intraoperatively, so consultation with the surgical staff should take place before a long-acting neuromuscular blocking agent is administered.

Appropriate rescue airway equipment must be immediately available during induction of anesthesia in these patients. Emergency equipment should include supraglottic airways, a video laryngoscope, a flexible intubation scope, an intubation cart, and an emergency tracheostomy kit. The surgical team should be present in the operating room during the induction of anesthesia, should the need for a surgical airway arise. When clinically appropriate, direct laryngoscopy can be attempted. Adjuncts such as an intubation bougie may prove helpful if direct laryngoscopy is used. Based on the preoperative evaluation, video laryngoscopy or a flexible intubating scope may be more appropriate choices for the first intubation attempt. The American Society of Anesthesiologists (ASA) difficult airway algorithm should be kept in mind throughout the process of securing the airway in these patients.

3 What are the potential hazards/complications in regard to the airway?

The most significant hazard when caring for these patients is underestimating the potential difficulty with airway management. As described above, radiation changes may make mask ventilation, supraglottic ventilation, and tracheal intubation difficult or impossible. Tissues may be edematous, friable, and easily traumatized, resulting in airway bleeding or the creation of false passages. Given the difficulties that can be encountered with mask ventilation, supraglottic airway devices should be available, but their use may be limited by fibrosis and stenosis of the airway tissues. Oropharyngeal stenosis can be mistaken for the true glottic opening, leading to possible erroneous intubations. Inadvertent placement of the endotracheal tube into the mediastinum has been described in these situations. Additional failed intubation attempts can create more trauma and swelling in the airway, making further attempts more difficult.

4 What distinct airway device might be used in this case, and what are the special considerations?

As described above, the difficult airway algorithm and appropriate emergency airway equipment should be readily available during airway management of a patient with prior neck irradiation.

High-flow nasal cannula during induction and intubation can be a helpful adjunct airway tool. It can improve preoxygenation in some scenarios, and it can provide continuous apneic oxygenation and prolong the apnea time during airway management.

A small, flexible intubation scope should be available in cases of severe oropharyngeal stenosis. Tracheal tubes in small sizes (eg, 5.5 and 6 outer diameter) should be available. Optical stylets or gum elastic bougies can be used in conjunction with direct or video laryngoscopy in order to facilitate the passage of a tracheal tube through a narrow tract. Unanticipated and rapid conversion to a jet-catheter ventilation technique prior to intubation due to severe oropharyngeal stenosis has also been described. Finally, an emergency cricothyroidotomy or tracheostomy kit should be available, as well as competent operators of these kits.

- Patients with a history of neck irradiation can be difficult to ventilate via mask and supraglottic airway, and intubation may also be difficult to pathologic airway changes.
- A thorough preoperative evaluation, including imaging and preoperative endoscopy, should be considered.
- Oropharyngeal stenosis can mimic the glottic opening, leading to a false intubating path.
- Flexible scope intubation is the most commonly used technique for patients with history of prior neck irradiation.
- Advanced airway tools and a tracheostomy kit with surgical operators should be present in the operating room during the induction of anesthesia in these patients.
- *See Figure 66.1 for additional details.*

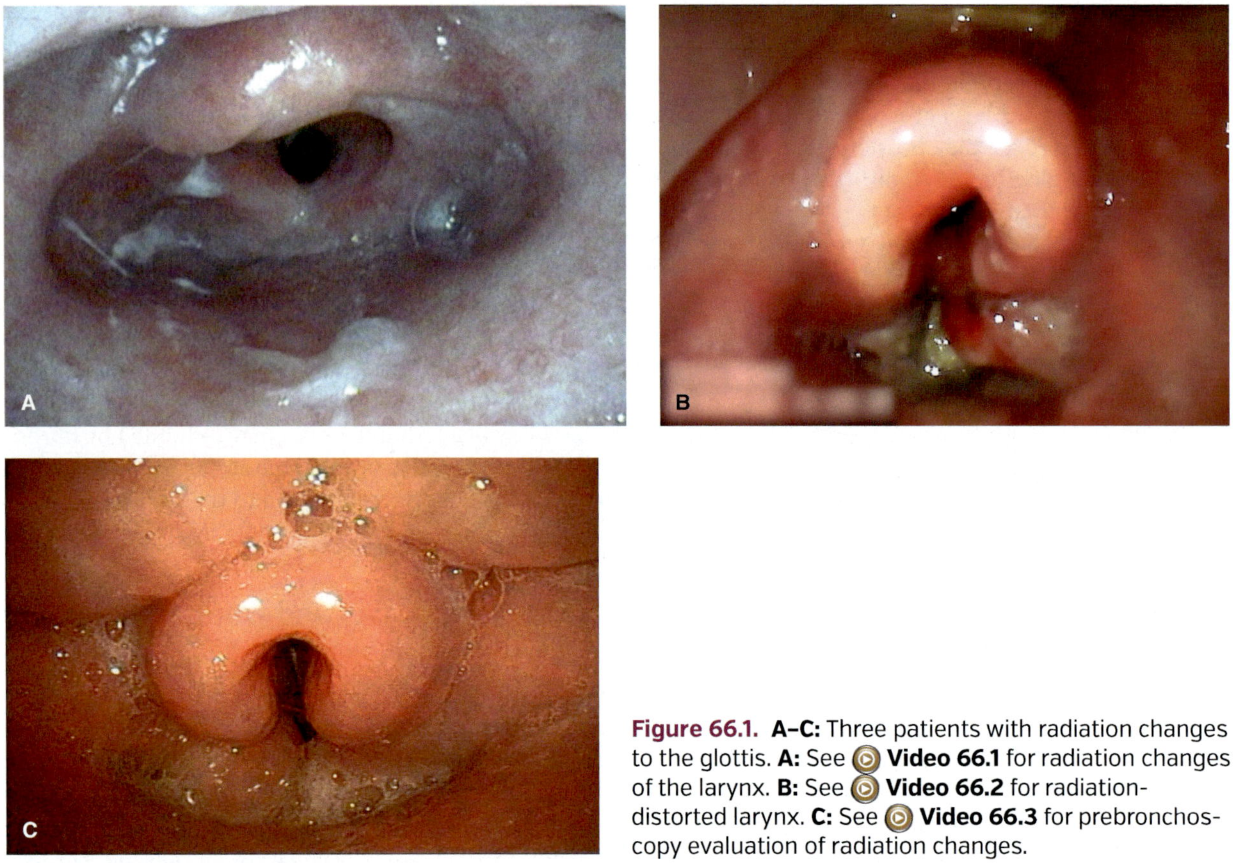

Figure 66.1. **A–C:** Three patients with radiation changes to the glottis. **A:** See **Video 66.1** for radiation changes of the larynx. **B:** See **Video 66.2** for radiation-distorted larynx. **C:** See **Video 66.3** for prebronchoscopy evaluation of radiation changes.

Suggested Readings

Balakrishnan M, Kuriakose R, Koshy RC. Radiation induced changes in the airway-anaesthetic implications. *South Afr J Anaesth Analg.* 2004;10(2):19–22.

Nageris B, Elidan J, Sichel JY. Aerodigestive tract obstruction as a late complication of radiotherapy. *J Laryngol Otol.* 1995; 109(1):68–69.

Reed AP, Frost EAM. Radiation induced hypopharyngeal stenosis masquerading as the larynx: a case report. *Middle East J Anesthesiol.* 2010;20(5):731–733.

Rosenblatt W, Ianus AI, Sukhupragarn W, Fickenscher A, Sasaki C. Preoperative endoscopic airway examination (PEAE) provides superior airway information and may reduce the use of unnecessary awake intubation. *Anesth Analg.* 2011;112(3):602–607.

Sharma I, Dong W, Vu C, Zheng G. The impact of head and neck radiation on airway management: a retrospective data review. *Can J Anaesth.* 2022;69(12):1562–1564.

Unilateral Vocal Cord Paralysis

67

Felipe Urdaneta

Clinical Scenario: A 35-year-old female presents for an urgent appendectomy. The patient has a history of unilateral vocal cord paralysis (UVCP) after a prior thyroidectomy.

1 What are the anesthetic and airway management considerations for this case?

The larynx plays a vital role in airway protection, respiration, swallowing, and phonation. Alterations in vocal cord movement are neurogenic (most commonly due to the recurrent laryngeal nerve [RLN]) or mechanical (arytenoid dislocation, joint fixation, or web formation). Abnormalities that prevent normal vocal cord function or motility interfere with the vibration of the vocal cord mucosa and manifest as voice alterations and dysphonia. Unilateral vocal cord paralysis may lead to glottic insufficiency, affecting phonation and predisposing to ineffective cough and aspiration when swallowing fluids and solids.

Vocal cord damage may result from injury to the vagus or the RLNs, and the lesion can occur at any point along the course of both nerves, from the brainstem to the larynx itself. Left vocal cord paralysis is more common than the paralysis of the right because of the longer and more complex course of the left RLN. The proximity of the RLN to the esophagus, trachea, and thyroid gland makes it vulnerable during surgical procedures involving these structures. Unilateral vocal cord palsy that occurs following surgery is not uncommon, especially during high-risk procedures such as anterior cervical spine cases, cardiac and aortic procedures, especially those involving the aortic arch. Thyroid surgery is another high-risk procedure, especially if it involves bilateral dissection or reoperation. Vocal cord paralysis (VCP) caused by a COVID-19 infection has also been recently described, even in patients who were never intubated.

The preoperative evaluation will allow the team to establish the potential impact of the lesion with regard to bag-mask ventilation, laryngoscopy, and ease of intubation. A complete clinical evaluation, including alcohol and smoking history (risk factors for malignancy), prior trauma, surgeries, prolonged intubations, upper or lower respiratory infections, history of gastroesophageal reflux, and the presence of any chronic inflammatory or neurodegenerative conditions, should be determined. Adult patients with UVCP have a greater incidence of malignant etiology, while younger patients and children with UVCP typically present with benign conditions such as vocal cord nodules and papillomas.

The anesthetic and airway management plan will be influenced by the cause of the VCP and the type of procedure planned. If general anesthesia is needed, the main consideration is to decide whether an awake intubation is needed. Proper and careful placement of the endotracheal tube (ETT) will still cause some mechanical trauma to the vocal cords. Problems associated with intubation can be worse during emergent situations or after multiple intubation attempts. Following intubation, the ETT cuff pressure should be kept at or below 30 cm H_2O. A deep plane of anesthesia and adequate muscle relaxation to prevent local irritation and coughing are recommended while the ETT is in situ. Conservative and careful airway management techniques should always be used if the proposed surgical procedure and patient conditions allow. Avoiding intubation altogether with supraglottic airway is an attractive choice, but VCP has even been described from the use of SGAs.

2 How would you manage the airway in this case?

Airway and anesthetic plans depend highly on the type of surgery being performed. For example, a quick endoscopic evaluation may not require general anesthesia or muscle relaxation. A more involved procedure on the airway may involve suspension laryngoscopy and microlaryngeal equipment. The surgery may also be completely unrelated to the airway. The most common procedures patients with VCP undergo are medialization procedures, including injection laryngoplasty and laryngeal framework surgery. The requirements for microlaryngeal surgery include an unobstructed and "motionless" surgical field, muscle relaxation, prevention of airway fires, protection from aspiration, and control of hemodynamics during periods of surgical stimulation, adequate ventilation and oxygenation, and smooth emergence and extubation.

Regardless of the procedure, further laryngeal damage should be avoided during all interventions by the anesthesiologist and surgeon. Trauma to the contralateral vocal cord may predispose to bilateral VC damage and paralysis, which can cause acute respiratory failure.

3 Are there special considerations for emergence or extubation at the end of the case?

A plan of action for extubation of a patient with a suspected or confirmed VCP must be established with surgical colleagues. A smooth extubation can help prevent further damage to the VC. Various options have been described with varying degrees of success. Administration of IV lidocaine and topicalization of the ETT cuff with lidocaine have been used with success.

- UVCP may be transient or permanent and is most commonly iatrogenic from prior surgeries or airway management.
- An awake intubation may be necessary if the patient has significant airway obstruction due to UVCP.
- No single airway management technique will work for all patients with UVCP, so the anesthesia team must be proficient in many techniques and options.
- *See Figure 67.1 and* ***Videos 67.1*** *to* ***67.3*** *for additional details.*

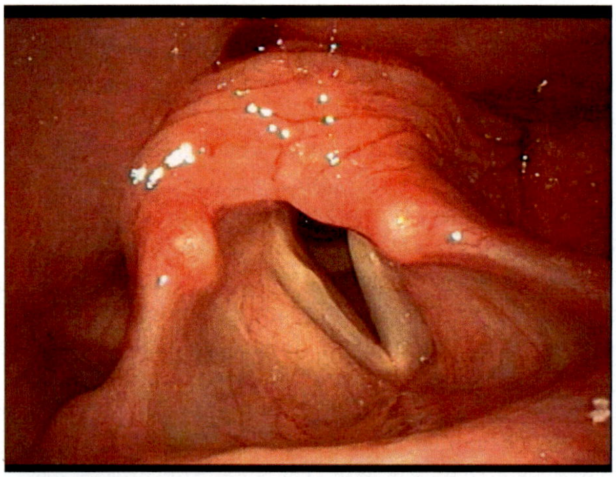

Figure 67.1. In this patient with right-sided vocal cord paralysis, the left vocal cord is abducted and the right vocal cord is medialized.

Suggested Readings

DiLisio RP, Mazzeffi MA, Bodian CA, Fischer GW. Vocal cord paralysis after aortic surgery. *J Cardiothorac Vasc Anesth.* 2013;27(3):522–527.

Mendels EJ, Brunings JW, Hamaekers AE, Stokroos RJ, Kremer B, Baijens LW. Adverse laryngeal effects following short-term general anesthesia: a systematic review. *Arch Otolaryngol Head Neck Surg.* 2012;138(3):257–264.

Vachha B, Cunnane MB, Mallur P, Moonis G. Losing your voice: etiologies and imaging features of vocal fold paralysis. *J Clin Imaging Sci.* 2013;3:15.

Zamzam SM, Hanafy RG. Impact of COVID-19 on vocal cord mobility: a case series study. *Egypt J Otolaryngol.* 2021;37(1):93.

Bilateral Vocal Cord Paralysis

68

Felipe Urdaneta

Clinical Scenario: An 85-year-old man presents to the emergency department with increasing stridor over the past week. He was examined by an otolaryngologist and found to have bilateral vocal cord paralysis. He is now coming to the OR for his airway to be secured and for a panendoscopy, a posterior cordectomy, and a search for a precipitating lesion (see Figure 68.1).

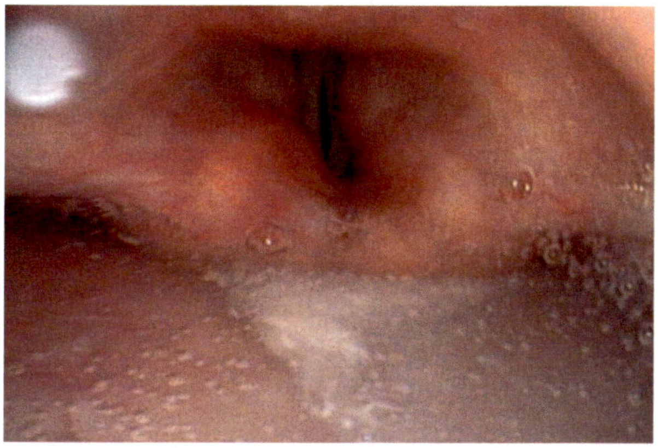

Figure 68.1. Patient with bilateral vocal cord paralysis. The vocal cords are fixed in an adducted position making the patient at risk of obstruction. See **Video 68.1**.

1 What are the anesthetic and airway management considerations for this case?

Abnormalities in vocal cord movement can be neurogenic (most commonly due to the recurrent laryngeal nerve) or mechanical (arytenoid dislocation, joint fixation, or web formation). Bilateral vocal cord paralysis (BVCP) is a potentially life-threatening condition. *Acute glottic obstruction* is a surgical emergency that requires immediate recognition and treatment and usually occurs immediately following extubation. Any procedure around the airway can cause vocal cord issues due to direct trauma to airway structures or indirectly secondary to nerve injury, hematomas, or edema. Patients with BVCP will exhibit biphasic stridor and respiratory distress. Surgical intervention is typically required to prevent acute asphyxiation.

2 What are the potential concerns in regard to the anesthetic and airway management?

Patients with BVCP present unique challenges to the anesthesia and surgical teams. No single anesthetic technique will work for all patients with BVCP. The approach to the patient with a suspected or confirmed diagnosis of VCP should include a complete clinical evaluation, including alcohol and smoking history, prior trauma, surgeries, prolonged intubations, upper or lower respiratory infections, history of gastroesophageal reflux, and the presence of chronic inflammatory or neurodegenerative conditions. Important clues to determine the cause and extent of the disease include questions about the onset, duration, and progression of symptoms. Vocal cord damage may result from injury to the vagus or the recurrent laryngeal nerves, and the inciting lesion can occur at any point along the course of either nerve. However, the great majority of cases involve nerve damage along the peripheral course of the nerve. Normal vocal cord movement and function require input from the recurrent laryngeal nerve (RLN) and superior laryngeal nerve (SLN). The RLN carries both abductor and adductor fibers to the vocal cords. The abductor fibers are more vulnerable to injury, and mild/moderate trauma can cause pure abductor paralysis. Severe trauma affects both abductor and adductor fibers.

Thus, incomplete bilateral damage to the RLN is more dangerous than complete damage. When incomplete bilateral damage to the recurrent laryngeal nerve occurs, the adductor fibers draw the cords toward each other, the glottic opening is severely compromised, and severe respiratory distress ensues. In contrast, if complete bilateral damage occurs, the vocal cord assumes a middle position between abduction and adduction, leaving enough glottic opening to prevent major respiratory distress. In addition, damage to the external branch of the SLN or the SLN trunk causes paralysis of the cricothyroid muscle, resulting in hoarseness that improves over time due to compensatory action of the opposite side. These patients are prone to aspiration because of the sensory deficit that occurs above the vocal cords.

The cause of the VCP influences the anesthetic and airway management plan. These patients may present for diagnostic and therapeutic procedures involving the airway (VC injection, thyroplasty) or for an unrelated procedure performed in another area of the body. Patients may also present emergently due to BVCP and need a surgical airway.

Endoscopic and microlaryngeal procedures are often performed with lasers because they allow better precision, hemostasis, and less postoperative edema. Procedures include posterior cordotomy, arytenoidectomy alone, or both procedures in combination. Microlaryngeal and suspension laryngoscopy provide optimal surgical exposure. Phonosurgery requires general anesthesia and muscle relaxation to keep a motionless surgical field to improve precision. Conventional endotracheal tubes may obstruct views of the glottis. Alternative "tubeless" techniques can be used, which include intermittent apnea-extubation and jet ventilation (JV). Subglottic administration of JV can be accomplished using flexible double-lumen catheters like the Hunsaker–Mon Jet Ventilation Tube (Medtronic Xomed Inc., Jacksonville, FL) or the LaserJet device (Acutronic Medical Systems, AG, Hirzel, Switzerland). In adults, intravenous induction, intubation using smaller-sized endotracheal tube (ETT), and maintenance with general anesthesia with positive-pressure ventilation remain a common anesthetic management method for these cases.

Heightened awareness must always be present during extubation and the postoperative period, as complications due to BVCP may manifest more insidiously.

3 What are the potential hazards/complications with regard to the airway?

Laryngeal procedures often require a compromise between optimal surgical exposure and control of ventilation. No single technique or method allows adequate surgical exposure, ventilation control, aspiration prevention, airway fire, and a motionless field. JV techniques allow the surgeon great exposure and an unobstructed view of laryngeal anatomy while eliminating the source of combustion (ETT) during laser surgery. In cases of complete airway obstruction, JV is contraindicated. Barotrauma from JV outflow obstruction can occur at any time due to surgical instrumentation, glottic edema, or laryngospasm. Modern JV systems incorporate safety features such as automated shutdown if pressure limits are exceeded.

4 Are there special considerations for emergence/extubation at the end of the case?

A smooth and careful extubation strategy must be planned in conjunction with the ENT surgical team. Coughing and bucking on emergence is not uncommon and may lead to further vocal cord damage, edema, and/or laryngospasm. Airway surgery causes airway edema, which can lead to acute airway obstruction postoperatively if severe enough. Airway obstruction should be suspected if a patient develops stridor (especially inspiratory) and other signs of respiratory distress. The administration of humidified oxygen, nebulized racemic epinephrine, and intravenous steroids are commonly used for initial treatment. There is a strong possibility that reintubation may be needed, so the necessary equipment and medications should be immediately available. Extubation with the aid of an airway exchange catheter (AEC) is sometimes used to maintain a conduit within the trachea.

- BVCP can lead to acute glottic obstruction, constituting an airway emergency.
- Etiology of BVCP can be neurogenic (most commonly damage to the RLN) or mechanical.
- Communication/cooperation between surgeons and the anesthetist is essential throughout the care of patients with BVCP.
- *See Figure 68.2 for additional details.*

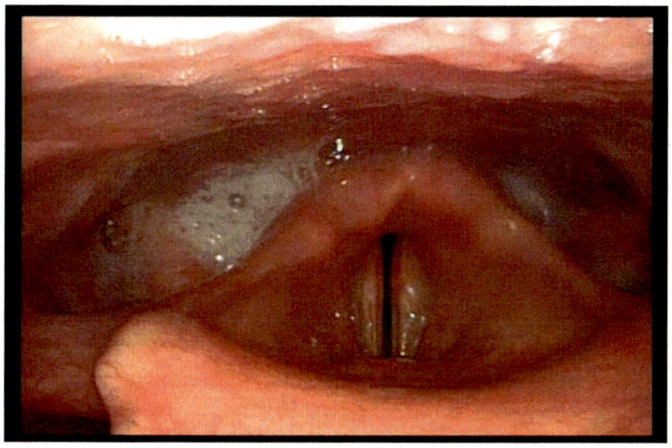

Figure 68.2. Another example of a patient with bilateral vocal cord paralysis. The vocal cords are fixed in an adducted position making the patient at risk of obstruction. See **Video 68.2**.

Suggested Readings

Brake MK, Anderson J. Bilateral vocal fold immobility: a 13 year review of etiologies, management and the utility of the Empey index. *J Otolaryngol Head Neck Surg*. 2015;44(1):27.

de Almeida RBS, Costa CC, Silva Duarte PLE, et al. Surgical treatment applied to bilateral vocal fold paralysis in adults: systematic review. *J Voice*. 2023;37(2):289.e1–289.e13.

Prasad VMN, Remacle M. Medialization thyroplasty and arytenoid adduction for management of neurological vocal fold immobility. *Adv Otorhinolaryngol*. 2020;85:85–97.

69 The Patient with a Previous Tracheostomy (Resolved)

Christopher Szabo

Clinical Scenario: A 65-year-old woman presents for urgent appendectomy. She previously had a tracheostomy, which was inserted for prolonged ventilation after a motor vehicle accident. The stoma is now closed.

1 What are the anesthetic and airway management considerations for this case?

Patients with a resolved tracheostomy often present for unrelated surgical procedures. In most cases, this historical finding may be inconsequential to airway management, however, the anesthesiologist caring for these patients should consider the enduring consequences of prior tracheostomy, including scarring, granuloma formation, airway deformation, subglottic stenosis, tracheal stenosis, tracheomalacia, or even an unrecognized tracheoesophageal fistula. Though, as in the current situation, the historical cause of the patient's tracheostomy may have been elective airway maintenance, this information may not always be available. Emergency tracheostomy or cricothyrotomy due to failed airway management may have been the trigger for invasive airway access. Clues to this critical and very relevant history should be sought from the patient, the family, and the physical examination. If this possibility cannot be excluded, appropriate airway management should be considered.

If a patient with a previous tracheostomy has signs or symptoms of airway compromise, including stridor, dyspnea, accessory muscle use, sternal retraction, tachycardia, and hypoxia, airway imaging may be revealing. CT scanning has been found helpful in diagnosing posttracheostomy or posttracheal intubation tracheal stenosis. Multidetector CT had an 89.4% sensitivity and a 95.2% specificity in detecting these injuries. Other techniques such as preoperative endoscopy or bronchoscopy may help describe distorted airway anatomy.

The patient in the current case has a history of tracheostomy. In 1921, Chevalier Jackson at Jefferson University in Philadelphia reported 158 cases of subglottic stenosis in 170 patients who had undergone cricothyroidotomies, otherwise called "high tracheostomy." This corresponded to a 93% rate of subglottic stenosis. The technique used at that time did not utilize the cricothyroid membrane, as is done currently. Brantigan and Grow challenged that rate in 1975 when they presented a series of 655 cricothyroidotomies, with no reported incidence of subglottic stenosis. More recently, the rate of subglottic stenosis has been estimated to be 0.5% to 0.7% with elective cricothyroidotomy in oral and maxillofacial surgery.

2 How would you manage the airway in this case?

The management of the airway starts with a good preoperative assessment and physical examination. It is important to determine the previous anesthetic and airway management history and fasting status. One should carefully examine for signs or symptoms of stridor, frequent aspirations and pneumonias, and dyspnea at rest or on exertion. External airway assessment can be misleading, and if the patient's history is concerning, a preoperative endoscopic airway assessment or imaging can provide useful additional information. When preparing for tracheal intubation, multiple sizes of cuffed endotracheal tubes should be readily available. If there is low level of concern regarding the ability to manage the patient's airway, routine laryngoscopy (with rapid sequence induction in the current case) can be performed. If there is concern regarding a compromised lower airway, precautions must be taken based on the nature of the evaluation. In the current case, although a significant gastric content aspiration risk exists, awake intubation with minimal sedation should be considered (see Chapter 11: Preparation for Awake Intubation). In other situations, a variety of techniques might be employed including, but not limited to, awake intubation, general anesthesia with maintenance of spontaneous ventilation, inhalation induction, and use of a flexible intubation scope (FIS) after routine induction of general anesthesia.

3 What are the potential hazards and complications in regard to the airway?

Although, in the current scenario, the patient was aware of the rationale for her prior tracheostomy (ie, prolonged mechanical ventilation), it is important to consider the scenario in which a patient is unsure of the reason for the surgical airway, such as an instance of inability to ventilate and intubate. The patient who has undergone a prior surgical airway may have undetected subglottic or tracheal stenosis that may obstruct passage of a tracheal tube. In addition, forceful or inadvertent trauma to a stenotic airway may increase tissue injury, cause bleeding, and subsequently lead to a clinically important stenosis in the future. Airway deformity, without frank stenosis from prior surgical manipulation, may also result in trauma during passage of the tracheal tube, with similar consequences.

4 Are there special considerations for the emergence or the end of the case?

As discussed previously, existing scar or lower airway deformity may result in inadvertent tissue injury, edema, and bleeding from the intubation. Extubation precautions may be in order if there is a significant suspicion that such conditions exist (see Chapter 44: Extubation of the Difficult Airway Patient). The anesthesiologist should wait for the patient to be fully emerged, neuromuscular function should be intact, and the airway cleared of secretions prior to tracheal extubation.

- When presented with a patient with a history of previous tracheostomy, determining the cause for the surgical airway is vital.
- The history of a prior tracheostomy should raise concerns regarding scar and anatomic deformity in the airway.
- A variety of tracheal tube sizes and a FIS should be immediately available during tracheal intubation.
- At emergence, the patient should be fully awake and extubation precautions should be exercised when necessary.
- *See Figure 69.1 for additional details.*

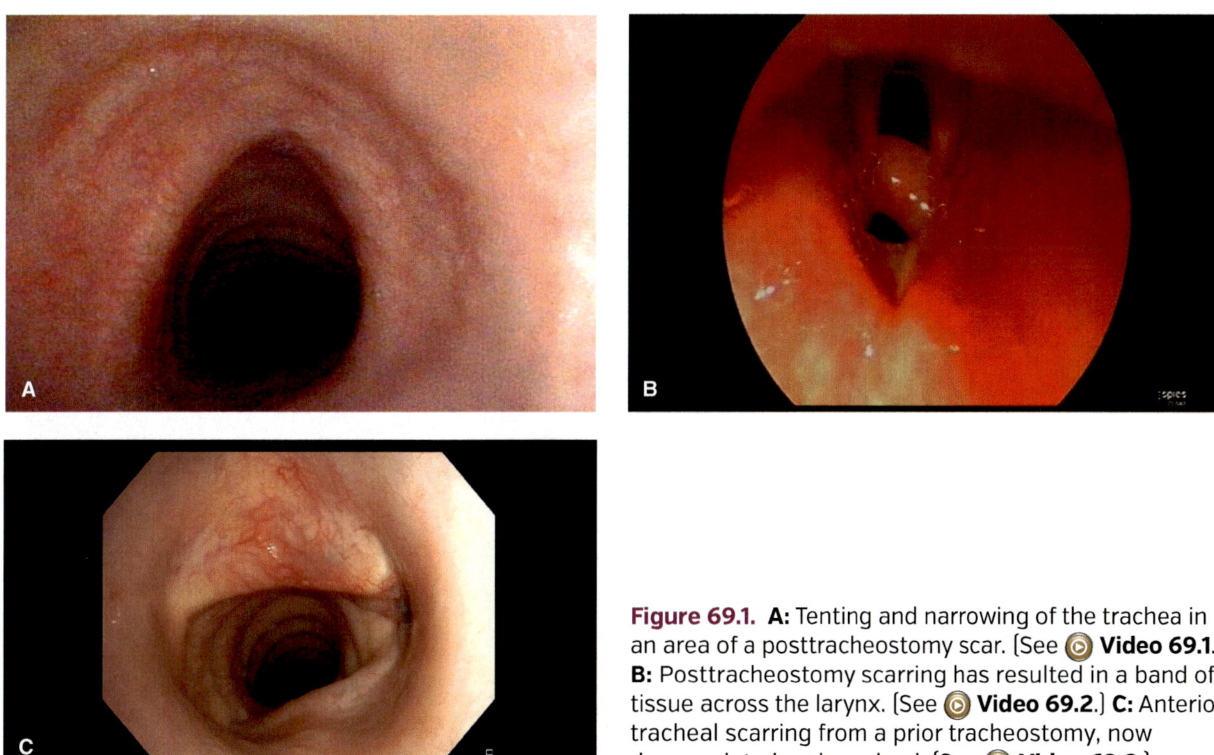

Figure 69.1. **A:** Tenting and narrowing of the trachea in an area of a posttracheostomy scar. (See **Video 69.1.**) **B:** Posttracheostomy scarring has resulted in a band of tissue across the larynx. (See **Video 69.2.**) **C:** Anterior tracheal scarring from a prior tracheostomy, now decannulated and resolved. (See **Video 69.3.**)

Suggested Readings

Brantigan CO, Grow JB Sr. Cricothyroidotomy: elective use in respiratory problems requiring tracheotomy. *J Thorac Cardiovasc Surg*. 1976;71(1):72–81.

Delaney A, Bagshaw SM, Nalos M. Percutaneous dilatational tracheostomy versus surgical tracheostomy in critically ill patients: a systematic review and meta-analysis. *Crit Care*. 2006;10(20):R55.

Epstein SK. Late complications of tracheostomy. *Respir Care*. 2005;10(4):542–549.

Higgins K, Punthakee X. Meta-analysis comparison of open versus percutaneous tracheostomy. *Laryngoscope*. 2007;117(3): 447–454.

Jackson C. High tracheotomy and other errors: the chief causes of laryngeal stenosis. *Surg Gynecol Obstet*. 1921;32:392–398.

Sun M, Ernst A, Boiselle PM. MDCT of the central airways: comparison with bronchoscopy in the evaluation of complications of endotracheal and tracheostomy tubes. *J Thorac Imaging*. 2007;22(2):136–142.

Teo N, Garrahy A. Elective surgical cricothyroidotomy in oral and maxillofacial surgery. *Br J Oral Maxillofac Surg*. 2013;51(8): 779–782.

Oropharyngeal Stenosis

70

David W. Healy

Clinical Scenario: A 55-year-old woman with a history of prior laryngeal carcinoma treated with chemotherapy and radiation now presents with dysphagia and is only tolerating liquid nutrition. The otolaryngologist is planning direct laryngoscopy with biopsy and esophagoscopy.

1 What are the anesthetic and airway management considerations for this case?

The impact of radiation therapy alone or combined with chemotherapy (chemoradiation) on airway management is often underreported and underestimated. Both therapies have been linked to challenges in laryngoscopy, face mask and supraglottic airway (SGA) ventilation, and significant oropharyngeal constriction. External beam radiation, contingent upon dosage and administration levels, can lead to dryness, scarring, and reduced mobility of airway structures. Recent studies have identified neck radiation-induced changes as an independent predictor of difficulty with bag-mask ventilation alone and in conjunction with direct laryngoscopy.

A thorough airway risk assessment is crucial prior to caring for these patients. Begin by obtaining a comprehensive patient history and a meticulous clinical examination. Additional information can be gathered from nasoendoscopy results (obtained during a surgical clinic visit) and radiologic imaging. The assessment should determine the anticipated ease of bag-mask ventilation, direct or video laryngoscopy, insertion and positioning of an SGA, and the execution of a surgical airway, such as cricothyrotomy or formal tracheostomy.

2 How would you manage the airway in this case?

According to the American Society of Anesthesiologists Guidelines on management of the difficult airway, when anticipating difficulties with airway management, it is advised to choose a technique that maintains spontaneous ventilation, if possible. In such situations, the preferred approach involves awake intubation using a flexible bronchoscope. An awake intubation allows patients to maintain their airway reflexes and breathe spontaneously during the procedure, reducing the risk of complications.

Patients with oropharyngeal stenosis following chemoradiation often present with minimal airway obstruction symptoms, which sets them apart from those with subglottic tracheal stenosis. In addition, they typically have minimal dysphagia, unlike patients with supraglottic stenosis. Although this condition may appear relatively asymptomatic, anesthesiologists must proceed with caution when managing the airways of these patients.

To ensure optimal patient care, anesthesiologists should adopt a stepwise approach that includes multiple airway management plans. This approach allows for the flexibility to switch between plans if one method proves unsuccessful or encounters complications. Furthermore, readily available equipment to support each plan is essential for efficient and safe airway management. By following these guidelines and maintaining high vigilance, anesthesiologists can provide appropriate care and minimize the risk of complications for potentially complex patients.

3 What are the surgical considerations that impact anesthetic management?

For optimal glottic exposure and access to airway instrumentation, surgeons often request small endotracheal tubes (ETTs). The author recommends either 6.5- or 6.0-mm internal diameter regular tubes or size 5.0 microlaryngeal tubes (Mallinckrodt, St. Louis, MO) designed for adult use. These microlaryngeal tubes feature narrow diameters, adequate tube length, and high-volume, low-pressure cuffs. In cases where surgical access is severely limited, jet ventilation using a Hunsaker tube (Medtronic Xomed, Jacksonville, FL) may be necessary. Jet ventilation is generally performed to improve surgical access and is considered safe only when proper gas egress (escape) is ensured and maintained.

These surgical procedures may present unique anesthetic challenges, as they often require a short duration of surgery but necessitate sufficient muscle relaxation and intense analgesia for airway instrumentation and tissue dilation. Total intravenous anesthesia (TIVA) with propofol and remifentanil infusions is practical. Both drugs can be adjusted according to the surgical stimulus and have a rapid pharmacologic washout when used for short periods. During intubation, the author prefers to combine TIVA with an initial low dose of a nondepolarizing neuromuscular blocker (eg, rocuronium). This facilitates immobility, stability, and surgical access to the airway at the beginning of the procedure. Inhalation anesthesia may not be viable if jet ventilation or an intermittent extubation technique is employed.

4 How can an anesthesia provider optimize communication with the surgical team?

The operative and anesthesia team should maintain an open dialogue regarding the patient's airway status, anticipated challenges, and potential changes in the management plan. Close collaboration helps to ensure that everyone is prepared to address any complications that may arise during airway management and the surgical procedure.

5 Are there special considerations for the emergence or the end of the case?

In cases involving patients with severe oropharyngeal stenosis who have undergone a surgical procedure, it is crucial to take appropriate precautions during extubation, especially when intubation has proven difficult or complex. The following measures should be considered to enhance patient safety and ensure a smooth extubation process:

1. Complete reversal of neuromuscular blockers: This ensures that the patient has adequate muscle strength and can protect their airway effectively. Administer a reversal agent, such as neostigmine or sugammadex, as needed.
2. Achievement of standard extubation criteria: Confirm that the patient meets the standard extubation criteria, which typically include being fully awake and responsive, having adequate spontaneous ventilation and oxygenation, and demonstrating effective coughing and swallowing reflexes. These criteria help ensure the patient can maintain their airway after removing the endotracheal tube.
3. Use of an airway exchange catheter (AEC): An AEC (Cook Medical, Bloomington, IN) is a flexible, hollow tube that can be inserted into the endotracheal tube before extubation. The endotracheal tube is removed while the AEC remains in place, providing a conduit for reintubation. This can be particularly useful when airway reestablishment is difficult, as it allows for rapid reintubation without repeating the challenging initial intubation process.

- External beam radiation in the head and neck region can cause airway stenosis at various levels.
- Oropharyngeal stenosis may be relatively asymptomatic but can still result in procedural difficulty during multiple aspects of airway management.
- The presence of radiation changes to the neck is an independent predictor of difficult bag-mask ventilation alone and in combination with direct laryngoscopy.
- *See Figure 70.1 and* ***Video 70.1*** *for additional details.*

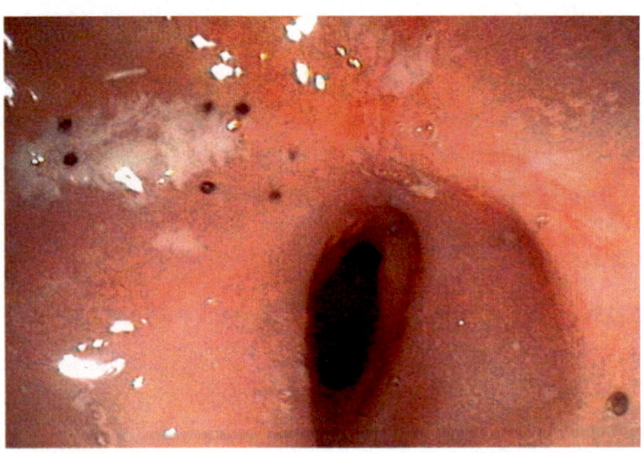

Figure 70.1. A patient with a history of chemo and radiation therapies for pharyngeal cancer is found to have oropharyngeal stenosis on preoperative endoscopic airway evaluation.

Suggested Readings

Apfelbaum JL, Hagberg CA, Connis RT, et al. 2022 American Society of Anesthesiologists Practice Guidelines for management of the difficult airway. *Anesthesiology*. 2022;136(1):31–81.

Kheterpal S, Healy D, Aziz MF, et al. Incidence, predictors, and outcome of difficult mask ventilation combined with difficult laryngoscopy: a report from the multicenter perioperative outcomes group. *Anesthesiology*. 2013;119(6):1360–1369.

Kheterpal S, Martin L, Shanks AM, Tremper KK. Prediction and outcomes of impossible mask ventilation: a review of 50,000 anesthetics. *Anesthesiology*. 2009;110(4):891–897.

Isshiki Thyroplasty

71

Yi Deng • Ashutosh Wali

Clinical Scenario: A 36-year-old female presents with unilateral vocal cord paralysis for more than 1 year following a thyroidectomy. She has undergone vocal cord augmentation in the past, but the paralysis has persisted. She now presents for an Isshiki thyroplasty.

1 What are the anesthetic and airway management considerations for this case?

Unilateral vocal cord paralysis can occur due to prior surgery (intrathoracic or head/neck), malignancy, trauma, neurologic and/or connective tissue disorders. It can be idiopathic in up to 25% of cases. A medialization thyroplasty procedure is the definitive surgical correction, often resulting in immediate and long-term improvement in phonation, breathlessness, hoarseness, and aspiration reduction. First described by Payr in 1915 and rediscovered by Isshiki in 1974, the type 1 thyroplasty is still commonly performed today. This procedure poses potential challenges to the anesthesiologist, including a shared, unprotected airway, titration of sedation, and potential postoperative complications.

Laryngeal framework surgery, like the Isshiki type 1 thyroplasty, is typically performed under local anesthesia in an awake patient to allow for intraoperative voice assessment. After adequate local anesthesia is achieved, a horizontal incision is made at the level of the vocal cords in the anterior neck, and platysma and strap muscles are divided to expose the thyroid cartilage. The lateral surface of the cartilage is then skeletonized, and a small window is incised at the level of the paralyzed true vocal fold. An implant (usually silastic, but can be Gore-Tex, titanium, or calcium hydroxyapatite) is then inserted through the window while pushing the midmembranous vocal fold medially, thus approximating the function of the paralyzed thyroarytenoid muscle. The patient is then asked to phonate, and the surgeon adjusts the size and placement of the implant until optimal vocal results are achieved. In more recent years, a nasopharyngeal flexible fiberoptic scope is often used during surgery as well for continuous monitoring of the vocal cord function. When surgical correction is complete, the strap muscles are then reapproximated and the skin incision is closed.

For a type 1 thyroplasty, monitored anesthesia care (MAC) with light sedation has been the traditional anesthetic approach. The surgery site is away from the intraoral or intrapharyngeal space in this type of procedure, so aspiration and airway compromise are of less concern. Potential drawbacks of this procedure include patient discomfort, excess laryngeal movement, and incomplete blockade of laryngeal nerves eliciting cough reflexes. A well-sedated but cooperative patient and a quiet surgical field are thus paramount for the success of this procedure.

2 How would you manage the airway in this case?

Typically, a type 1 thyroplasty is performed under MAC with infiltration of local anesthetic by the surgeon. The internal branch of the superior laryngeal nerve is blocked by infiltration at the thyrohyoid membrane, and the glossopharyngeal nerve is blocked at the inferior pole of the tonsils. Usually, a mix of lidocaine and bupivacaine with dilute epinephrine solution is used. A topical spray (ie, phenylephrine) is used to vasoconstrict vessels in the nose prior to placement of the flexible nasopharyngoscope, if indicated. Glycopyrrolate (0.1 to 0.2 mg IV) is administered upon arrival in the operating room (OR) to decrease oropharyngeal secretions. Dexamethasone (4 to 8 mg IV) is also given to decrease potential airway edema and prevent postoperative nausea and vomiting. An additional antiemetic (ie, ondansetron) may also be administered at this time. After attaching standard noninvasive monitors, patients are usually placed on nasal cannula with continuous monitoring for end-tidal carbon dioxide.

This surgery can last up to 2 to 3 hours, so sedation is important to improve both patient comfort and anxiolysis. Caution must be exercised to avoid over-sedation, which can lead to loss of airway muscular tone and compromise control of the airway. A variety of different sedative and anxiolytic regimens have been described in the literature, but the preference is to use agents that are fast onset, short acting, easily reversible, and have large therapeutic windows. To that end, a short-acting benzodiazepine such as midazolam (0.5 to 2 mg IV) is used for anxiolysis, while short-acting opioid like fentanyl (25 to 50 mcg IV) can be supplemented for analgesia. The combination of midazolam and fentanyl can synergistically inhibit respiratory drive, so careful monitoring and titration is needed to avoid oversedation. Subanesthetic doses of propofol (10 to 50 mcg/kg/min IV) are generally well tolerated and can provide adequate sedation for the duration of the procedure. In recent years, dexmedetomidine (0.3 to 1 mcg/kg/h IV) has been increasingly used for both anxiolysis and sedation with the added benefit of preserving central respiratory drive. In certain patient populations who are at an increased risk of respiratory depression (eg, severe chronic obstructive pulmonary disease, obstructive sleep apnea, etc.), dexmedetomidine can be a reasonable anesthetic choice for this procedure.

3 What are the surgical considerations that impact anesthetic management?

In general, a type 1 thyroplasty is a procedure that can be accomplished in under 3 hours. Variations in anesthetic management are more often dictated by patient factors than by differences in surgical technique. However, in certain cases of severe unilateral vocal cord paralysis, the surgeon may decide to perform arytenoid adduction in addition to the thyroplasty in order to better approximate the posterior gap of the vocal cords, which can then significantly prolong the procedure. Arytenoid adduction alone is performed under local anesthesia with MAC, but given the extended nature of the combined procedure, patient comfort and sedation can become an issue if MAC is used. A general anesthetic technique using a supraglottic airway (SGA) with subsequent intraoperative wake-up has produced positive results. In short, the patient is induced with an intravenous anesthetic of choice, and the SGA is placed for ventilation. The patient is then maintained on a volatile anesthetic (typically sevoflurane) under spontaneous ventilation. Once the thyroid window is made, the patient is woken up, the SGA is removed, and the patient can then participate in the phonation and implantation portion of the surgery. A propofol infusion may then be titrated until the termination of procedure. If an inhaled anesthetic is chosen, desflurane and nitrous oxide should be avoided due to their tendency to cause airway irritation and nausea, respectively. More recently, several case series have described the successful use of concurrent infusions of dexmedetomidine, propofol, and remifentanil for thyroplasty with arytenoid adduction. This technique allows for deeper levels of sedation than achieved under MAC during the dissection phase, with the ability of rapid titration needed during the wake-up phase.

4 What are the potential hazards/complications regarding the airway?

The three main complications of Isshiki thyroplasty are airway edema, hemorrhage, and implant dislodgement. Typically, the surgeon will account for some degree of edema to resolve postoperatively and, therefore, "overcorrect" for the degree of medialization, which can lead to stridor if the overcorrection is too zealous. Other risk factors for increased airway edema include prolonged dissection and excessive manipulation of the implant. Stridor can be treated with steroids and nebulized racemic epinephrine, or in the case of excessive overcorrection, lessening of the degree of medialization by the surgeon. Even after postoperative edema resolves, patients who have undergone a type 1 thyroplasty will have gross anatomical distortion of the glottic opening under direct laryngoscopy. However, no special precaution is necessary for future airway management. Hemorrhage leading to hematoma and airway obstruction is rare but may necessitate an immediate tracheostomy. Finally, extrusion or displacement of the implant is more commonly described with Gore-Tex or implants without outer phalanges. The implants are usually too small to cause complete obstruction of the trachea, but can become dislodged in a main stem bronchus, which requires retrieval by a rigid bronchoscope.

- Isshiki type I thyroplasty is a procedure used to correct unilateral vocal cord paralysis.
- Most laryngeal framework surgery, including an Isshiki thyroplasty, is done under local anesthesia with MAC, however, general anesthesia with SGA and intraoperative wake-up have been successfully performed, as well.
- Postoperatively, the patient should be closely monitored for laryngeal edema, hematoma, and implant dislodgement.
- *See Figure 71.1 and* **Video 71.1** *for additional details.*

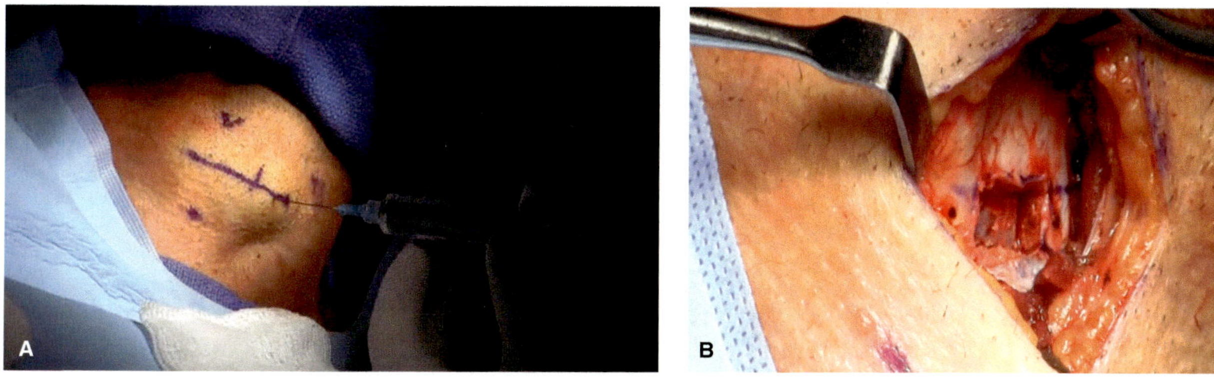

Figure 71.1. A: With the patient sedated but awake, local anesthetic is injected over the thyroid cartilage on the side ipsilateral to the nonfunctional vocal cord. **B:** A Gor-Tex wedge has been inserted into a window in the thyroid cartilage and will medialize the nonfunctional vocal cord.

Suggested Readings

Crolley VE, Gibbins N. One hundred years of external approach medialization thyroplasty. *J Laryngol Otol.* 2017;131(3):202–208.

Hamre M, Ekbom D, Handlogten KS, Weingarten TN, Seelhammer TG. Anesthetic management of medialization laryngoplasty performed under concurrent dexmedetomidine, remifentanil, and propofol infusions. *J Voice*. 2020;34(1):134–139.

Hess M, Fleischer S. Laryngeal framework surgery: current strategies. *Curr Opin Otolaryngol Head Neck Surg*. 2016;24(6):505–509.

Kanazawa T, Iino Y, Hara M, et al. Arytenoid adduction combined with medialization laryngoplasty under general anesthesia using a laryngeal mask airway. *Am J Otolaryngol*. 2012;33:303–307.

72 Esophageal Dilation

William H. Rosenblatt • Christopher Szabo

Clinical Scenario: A patient with a history of laryngeal cancer treated with radiation therapy presents with dysphagia. The surgical procedure calls for esophageal dilation.

1 What are the anesthetic and airway management considerations for this case?

Esophageal stricture is a common complication from radiation therapy in the head and neck cancer patient. Although this is the likely cause of the dysphagia in the current clinical scenario, recurrence of the primary malignancy will also be ruled out during the procedure and should be considered in planning the airway management of the patient.

In our institution, most esophageal dilations are performed with a Savary-Gilliard bougie over a guidewire dilator (Cook Medical, Bloomington, IN). Esophageal perforation can occur with bougie insertion and carries a mortality rate of up to 20%. The risk of esophageal perforation is increased with malignant disease, an inexperienced operator, and the technique and instruments used. For example, in the study by Mandelstam et al., Hurst or Maloney mercury-filled rubber bougies had the lowest complication rate (6.1/1000 cases), whereas pneumatic or mechanical dilators had the highest (18.4/1000 cases). Fortunately, the incidence of esophageal rupture during dilatation of a benign stricture is low, in the 0.1% to 0.3% range. Though also a rare complication, esophageal dilation may be complicated by bleeding in 0.2% of patients. The placement of an esophageal scope can cause cardiovascular stimulation, accompanied by wide swings in blood pressure and heart rate. In the susceptible patient, bronchospasm can also be triggered. Esophageal tear or rupture may also occur due to aggressive device insertion or patient movement.

2 How would you manage the airway in this case?

A decision must be made as to the ease or difficulty of airway management in this patient with a history of laryngeal cancer. If routine anesthetic induction is chosen, standard monitors are placed, and the patient is preoxygenated. General anesthesia with muscle relaxation is induced. In our institution, an intermediate-acting nondepolarizing neuromuscular blocking agent that may be reversed with Sugammadex is most often used. This technique provides adequate neuromuscular relaxation, which helps reduce the risk of esophageal injury with patient movement, while still being reliably reversible if needed. If a contradiction to these agents is present (eg, allergy), a succinylcholine infusion can be used. After successful tracheal intubation, airway management is passed off to the surgical team. A short-acting potent opioid, remifentanil, is administered as an infusion (0.1 to 0.5 mcg/kg/min) to mitigate the cardiovascular response to suspension laryngoscopy. Hypnosis is provided with a propofol infusion or a potent halogenated gas such as sevoflurane. The anesthesiologist should be prepared to treat sudden hypertensive episodes during the positioning of the suspension laryngoscope.

If the presenting patient has a suspected or known difficult airway, the approach to management will likely be different. The process of choosing an awake intubation versus airway management after the induction of anesthesia is discussed in a separate chapter.

Similar patients may have undergone laryngectomy previously and will present with a terminal tracheostomy. Airway management of these patients is discussed in a separate chapter.

3 What are the potential hazards and complications in regard to the airway?

A still surgical field is critical to avoiding the complications of esophageal perforation and bleeding. If the patient has unremitting moderate or severe chest pain in the postanesthesia care unit, they should be monitored closely and remain NPO in the event that the patient needs to return to the OR. If the chest pain continues 1 to 2 hours after the procedure, then further investigation into cardiac and noncardiac etiologies ought to be performed.

4 Are there special considerations for the emergence or the end of the case?

This population of patients presenting with dysphagia may be malnourished and/or hypovolemic. The clinician should adjust their induction and anesthetic maintenance accordingly and be prepared to treat hypotension. Reduced doses of induction hypnotics should be considered.

After successful esophageal dilation, the patient may be at risk for gastric contents regurgitation and aspiration. Tracheal extubation should not occur until the patient is fully awake and there is complete return of neuromuscular function. If the patient is deemed to have a difficult airway, extubation precautions should be taken accordingly.

- A still surgical field is required to avoid complications such as esophageal perforation, which carries a mortality rate of up to 20%.
- Stimulation from esophageal scope insertion may cause wide swings in blood pressure and heart rate.
- Due to the risk of aspiration, it is imperative that the patient be awake and neuromuscular function intact before extubation of the trachea.
- *See Figure 72.1 and* ***Video 72.1*** *for additional details.*

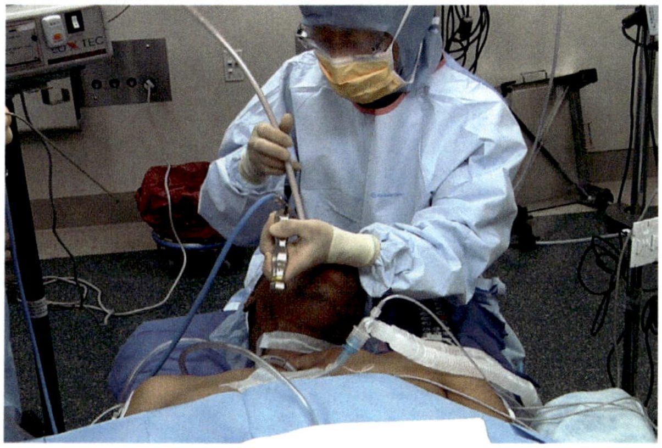

Figure 72.1. During suspension esophagoscopy, the surgeon inserts a series of esophageal dilators.

Suggested Readings

Brinster CJ, Singhal S, Lee L, et al. Evolving options in the management of esophageal perforation. *Ann Thorac Surg.* 2004;77: 1475–1483.

Lerner MZ, Bourdillon AT, Dai F, Brackett A, Kohli N. Safety considerations for esophageal dilation by anesthetic type: a systematic review. *Am J Otolaryngol.* 2021;42(5):103128.

Piotet E, Escher A, Monnier P. Esophageal and pharyngeal strictures: report on 1,862 endoscopic dilatations using the Savary-Gilliard technique. *Eur Arch Otorhinolaryngol.* 2008;265:357–364.

73 Recurrent Airway Papillomas

Karl Nazareth • Ashutosh Wali

Clinical Scenario: A 45-year-old man presents for resection of airway papillomas. He has a history of multiple prior papilloma resections since age 38. He is aphonic and has dyspnea that has been increasing since his prior resection. In the past, his airway has been managed with direct laryngoscopy (DL) without difficulty.

1 What are the anesthetic and airway management considerations for this case?

Airway papillomas are epithelial tumors of the upper respiratory tract associated with human papillomavirus (HPV). They are the most common neoplasm in humans and are almost always benign, rarely undergoing malignant transformation. Papillomas occur most commonly in children under age 10, but can extend later into life for many adults in the form of recurrent respiratory papillomatosis (RRP). Adult-onset RRP is typically less severe and more localized than the childhood variety. Papillomas usually begin on the true vocal folds and grow outward. Symptoms often start with mild hoarseness but can progress to life threatening including respiratory distress and full obstruction of the glottis. Even with the knowledge of previously uneventful anesthetics and tracheal intubations, patients presenting with RRP are at risk for an increase in the number, size, and severity of the papillomas since prior surgeries. As a result, anesthesiologists approach these cases with caution in the rare event of complete airway obstruction after the induction of general anesthesia (GA). Repeated attempts at tracheal intubation may cause bleeding in the airway and further obscure visualization of the larynx. If a patient with RRP previous tracheostomy—accelerated papillomatosis should be anticipated after such procedures.

The most effective treatment modality for RRP is resection or ablation of the lesions, which may require the use of an intraoperative laser in the airway. As a result, appropriate precautions must be taken to reduce the risk of airway fire.

2 How would you manage the airway in this case?

A thorough preoperative history and airway examination must be performed. A detailed history should include an assessment of the severity of the patient's symptoms, including the presence and degree of hoarseness, tachypnea or frank respiratory distress, and the use of accessory muscles of respiration. A thorough review of the most recent surgical airway evaluation, including commentary, pictures, and videos can be helpful. When a patient presents with actively worsening hoarseness or dyspnea, it is reasonable to perform a preoperative endoscopic airway examination (PEAE) on the day of surgery to guide the airway management plan. If the surgical evaluation or PEAE findings are concerning for a risk of obstruction or impaired visual access to the airway, an awake tracheal intubation should be performed. Recent airway surgery should heighten the anesthesia provider's suspicion. Although awake tracheal intubation can often be too difficult in the pediatric population, a planned approach can facilitate the process in adults. Although the patient in the clinical scenario was intubated via DL during his prior anesthetic, his disease may have progressed considerably as evidenced by his aphonia and increasing dyspnea. He remains at risk for airway obstruction after the induction of GA secondary to crowding and/or prolapse of the papillomatous tissue, compounded by relaxation of the laryngeal musculature due to muscle relaxants. If the patient's symptoms and presentation are similar to the previous examination, a standard induction of GA and airway management with DL is reasonable. In this case, it would still be prudent to have a flexible bronchoscope readily available in the event that visualization of the vocal cords is not readily achieved with DL.

The surgical team should be present during induction and prepared to immediately proceed with surgical airway access in case of an emergency. Unless absolutely necessary, a tracheostomy should be avoided as it has been demonstrated to provoke subglottic extension of the disease. It should also be noted that the use of an SGA, an important part of the difficult airway algorithm, may be potentially ineffective in this patient population as the obstruction occurs at the glottis itself.

3 What are the surgical considerations that impact anesthetic management?

There are various treatment modalities for RRP including surgical techniques which have progressed from cold excision to carbon dioxide/pulse dye lasers and precision microdebridement. The mainstay of treatment for RRP has been the repeated excision/ablation of the lesions with the goal of minimizing symptoms and preventing recurrence of the disease while also avoiding excessive debridement and scarring of the larynx. With the use of laser ablation, several precautions should be taken for both the patient and the anesthesiologist. Protective eye gear should be worn intraoperatively by all staff, and a laser-safe endotracheal tube should be used to reduce the risk of airway fires. Repeated manipulations of the endotracheal tube potentiate the risk for spreading disease along the airway, so it is preferred that the endotracheal tube not be removed once the procedure begins. Prior to tracheal extubation at the end of the procedure, suctioning should be carefully performed to remove as much debris and blood as possible.

4 What are the potential hazards and complications in regard to the airway?

In addition to the risks of obstruction and inability to ventilate postinduction, additional airway-related hazards may occur. As mentioned, a common treatment modality is surgical ablation with the use of a laser. Airway fires are discussed in more detail in a separate chapter.

- Despite previous uneventful intubations, patients with RRP remain at risk for difficult intubation due to the unexpected growth of airway papillomas.
- Preparation includes a detailed history of current symptoms, prior surgical history, and a review of the most recent endoscopic airway examination.
- Laser ablation requires specific airway fire precautions and an emergency plan to handle possible intraoperative airway fires.
- *See Figure 73.1 for additional details.*

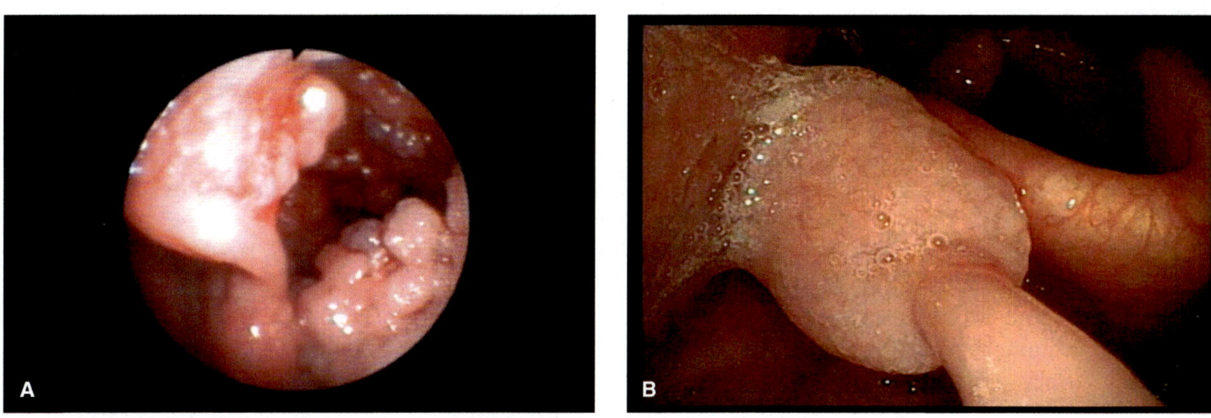

Figure 73.1. A: Papilloma-filled larynx (see **Video 73.1**). **B:** Papillomas seen on the uvula (see **Video 73.2**).

Suggested Readings

Alanazi AO, Karas AF, Husain IA. Recurrent Respiratory Papillomatosis: An Update. *Int J Head Neck Surg*. 2022;13(1):1–7.

Andrus JG, Shapshay SM. Contemporary management of laryngeal papillomas in adults and children. *Otolaryngol Clin North Am*. 2006;39:135–158.

Rosenblatt WH, Ianus A, Sukhupragarn W, Fickenscher A, Sasaki C. Preoperative endoscopic airway examination (PEAE) provides superior airway information and may reduce the use of unnecessary awake intubation. *Anesth Analg*. 2011;112:602–607.

74 Vocal Cord Polyp Surgery

Rainer Lenhardt • Matthew B. Hirsch

Clinical Scenario: A 31-year-old woman presents with progressive hoarseness and has been diagnosed with a benign vocal cord polyp for resection.

1 What are the anesthetic and airway management considerations for this case?

Vocal cord polyps and nodules are frequently seen in patients with high voice demands, predominantly women in teaching professions. This phenomenon is termed "phonotrauma." Polyps frequently interfere with vocal cord closure, and these patients typically present with progressive hoarseness. Vocal cord polyps usually consist of benign hyperplastic tissue. The decision to resect vocal cord polyps depends on the symptoms which affect voice function.

Due to the close spatial relationship of the patient's airway and the surgical region of interest, the anesthesiologist and the otolaryngologist jointly manage the airway in these procedures. Polyps can be removed by laser ablation or microsurgical resection (often termed "cool-steel" resection).

In conjunction with the surgical team, the anesthesiologist can choose an "open"- or "closed"-airway approach. An open approach provides a minimally obstructed surgical field. This can be accomplished with either intermittent intubation or jet ventilation. In a closed-airway approach, a specialized laser-resistant microlaryngeal tube will be used.

2 How would you manage the airway in this case?

If laser resection is to be used, the author's preference would be a closed-airway management system with the placement of a laser-resistant tracheal tube (TT) with a small internal diameter (6.0 to 6.5 mm). Polyp-removal surgery tends to be short in duration. Most patients can be adequately oxygenated with a small-diameter TT, though some degree of hypercapnea may need to be tolerated. A variety of laser-resistant tubes are available and may be laser type specific (eg, CO_2, potassium titanyl phosphate, or Nd-YAG laser). Fire and other laser precautions (eg, staff eye protection) must also be followed.

After intubation, the cuff of the TT is filled with saline. The TT maintains airway patency while protecting the lower airway from debris, blood, and secretions.

During the procedure, a low fraction of inspired oxygen (30% or less) concentration is used to reduce the risk of intratracheal burn injury and TT fire from the laser energy. The surgical team should be reminded that any TT can burn if exposed to enough laser energy.

Alternatively, the operative team may choose an open-airway management approach that affords the surgeon unobstructed access to the airway. The open approach is often performed via a rigid-suspension endoscope with or without high-frequency jet ventilation (HFJV). HFJV can be applied via a side-stream ventilation port of the surgical endoscope or via a subglottic jet ventilation catheter. Total intravenous anesthesia (TIVA) is mandatory during this approach.

A second open-airway approach, termed "intermittent extubation" may be employed. A standard, small-diameter TT is repeatedly inserted and removed via the endoscope. One hundred percent oxygen is used to fill the patient's functional residual capacity during periods of ventilation, extending the safe apneic time. When the patient is adequately preoxygenated, the TT is removed (typically by the surgeon) and the resection takes place. During the periods of apnea, the anesthesiologist and surgeon pay close attention to changes in the oxygen saturation. Slow desaturation is an indication for reintubation of the airway, which is performed by the surgeon, employing their suspension endoscope. The advantage of intermittent extubation is the uninhibited surgical field exposure. Because the TT never occupies the glottis simultaneously with laser use (if employed), it is safe to administer 100% oxygen during the periods of ventilation. Most clinicians prefer to use TIVA with this technique.

3 What are the surgical considerations that impact anesthetic management?

The need for excellent surgical exposure, the potential use of laser resection, and the need for nontraumatic emergence impact anesthetic management.

4 What are the potential hazards and complications with regard to airway management?

Though a rare complication of vocal cord polyps, large and polypoid masses may obstruct the view of the larynx during laryngoscopy and obstruct airflow during mask ventilation.

It is essential that the anesthesiologist and otolaryngologist communicate preoperatively regarding the nature of the polyp and the surgical plan (eg, risk of airway obstruction, the need for an open or closed approach, and the use of lasers). The otolaryngologist will have recently visualized the polyp via a mirror or nasoendoscopic examination. When this is not available, a preoperative endoscopic airway examination is an alternative.

The anesthesiologist should strive for a minimally traumatic intubation. The otolaryngologist may even request to perform the intubation themselves. Since vocal quality is the main outcome measure for this surgery, any trauma to the larynx, especially to the vocal folds themselves, can result in a degradation of vocal quality and the patient perceiving the surgery as unsuccessful or even damaging.

5 Are there special considerations for the emergence at the end of the case?

Any manipulation of the airway may cause bleeding and edema. Thus, strict hemostasis is necessary before the patient can emerge from general anesthesia. Intravenous dexamethasone may be given early in the procedure to reduce airway swelling. Techniques of intravenous anesthesia or deep extubation may be employed to reduce trauma during emergence and extubation. It is important to monitor the patient closely after extubation to detect airway edema and resecure the airway immediately if the patient has stridor.

The otolaryngologist will likely desire a smooth emergence from anesthesia. Any increase in pressure in the vocal fold microvasculature, whether from coughing, laryngospasm, Valsalva maneuver, generalized hypertension, or other etiology, can cause vocal fold hematomas or varix and result in a significant degradation of the postoperative voice quality. Laryngotracheal lidocaine may be sprayed on the vocal folds at the conclusion of the procedure to minimize coughing and spasm.

- Vocal cord polyps can be removed by laser ablation or microsurgical resection.
- An open-airway approach can be chosen with either intermittent intubation and ventilation or HFJV.
- During the closed-airway approach, a special laser-resistant microlaryngeal tube will be used.
- In the postoperative period, bleeding and edema may cause severe dyspnea.
- *See Figure 74.1 and* ***Video 74.1*** *for additional details.*

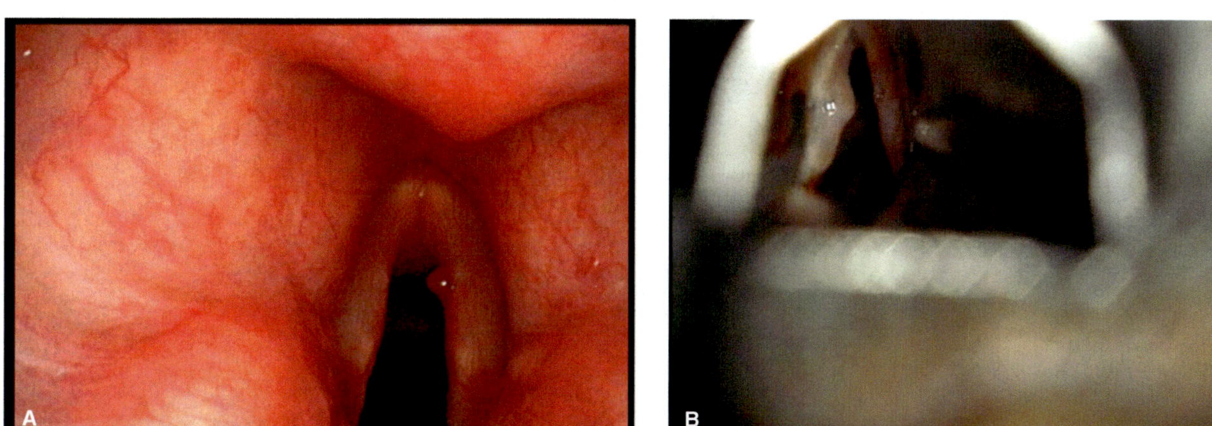

Figure 74.1. A: A single papilloma is seen on the right vocal cord. **B:** With suspension laryngoscopy in place, microlaryngeal instruments will be used to incise and remove a left-sided vocal cord polyp. The airway is being managed with a jet ventilation technique.

Suggested Readings

Barakate M, Mayer E, Wotherspoon G, Havas T. Anaesthesia for microlaryngeal and laser laryngeal surgery: impact of subglottic jet ventilation. *J Laryngol Otol.* 2010;124(6):641–645.

Benninger M. Laser surgery for nodules and other benign laryngeal lesions. *Curr Opin Otolaryngol Head Neck Surg.* 2009;17:440–444.

Kim HJ, Asai T. High-flow nasal oxygenation for anesthetic management. *Korean J Anesthesiol.* 2019;72:527–547.

Naunheim, M, Carroll. Benign vocal fold lesions: update on nomenclature, cause, diagnosis, and treatment. *Curr Opin Otolaryngol Head Neck Surg.* 2017;25:453–458.

Yoo MJ, Joffe AM, Meyer TK. Tubeless total intravenous anesthesia spontaneous ventilation for adult suspension microlaryngoscopy. *Ann Otol Rhinol Laryngol.* 2018;127:39–45.

Soft Tissue Cancers of the Neck

75

James C. DuCanto • Khalid G. Al Abdul Raheem

Clinical Scenario: A 75-year-old man presents for bilateral neck dissection. He is on anticoagulation for atrial fibrillation, which has been held preoperatively. He is maintained on adult aspirin daily.

1 What are the anesthetic and airway management considerations for this case?

The most common indication for neck dissection is squamous cell carcinoma of the head and neck. These patients often have histories of current or prior smoking, alcohol abuse, and a variety of cardiopulmonary comorbidities. Head and neck mobility, mouth opening, and pharyngeal space may be limited secondary to the patient's underlying disease process, previous therapies (eg, radiation or surgery), or other comorbidities. Masses may distort the upper airway or displace the larynx. A change in voice, worsening dyspnea, dysphagia, or exercise intolerance should increase suspicion of airway obstruction. Records of prior tracheal intubations should be reviewed to check for difficulty with airway management in the past. Preoperative findings of indirect laryngoscopy or radiographic imaging may also be useful. If there is any question of potential airway management difficulty, preoperative flexible laryngoscopy may be used for assessment.

For lesions isolated to the soft tissues of the neck, routine airway management is a reasonable approach. Suspicion of airway pathology should prompt further investigation and/or consideration of alternative approaches to airway management. Awake intubation is the typical approach when airway obstruction is suspected. Alternatively, an inhalational induction may be performed with the maintenance of spontaneous ventilation when it is expected that intubation, but not mask ventilation, will be difficult. Injuries to the 9th, 10th, and 12th cranial nerves from local tumor invasion or due to prior surgical resection can predispose the patient to aspiration or obstruction.

2 What are the surgical considerations that impact anesthetic management?

The need for surgical exploration in and around the airway will limit access to the tracheal tube. Some surgical services request that the OR table be rotated with the patient's head 180 degrees away from the anesthesia machine. Careful tracheal tube fixation is paramount to prevent migration, kinking, disconnection, and pressure on the skin, nose, and eyes. Surgical operators may inadvertently "lean" on the airway, leading to the problems mentioned above.

Neuromuscular blockade may need to be avoided during the dissection phase of the procedure to identify and test the integrity of the nerves (eg, spinal accessory, facial nerve) by direct stimulation. Strategies include tracheal intubation without neuromuscular relaxation, the use of rapidly acting depolarizing agents (ie, succinylcholine), the use of short-acting nondepolarizing agents in concert with the plan of the surgical team, or reversal of neuromuscular block with intravenous Sugammadex as needed. Many of these procedures may include surgical direct panendoscopy, which may require profound neuromuscular block and allow opportunity for block dissipation. The anesthesiologist should communicate with the surgeon regarding the current neuromuscular blockade before dissection begins.

Venous air embolism (VAE) is a rare event but can be life threatening. Suspicion should arise for VAE if end-tidal CO_2 suddenly decreases, and a precordial Doppler probe should reveal the murmur of VAE. Treatment includes increasing venous pressure with volume resuscitation, positive-pressure ventilation, jugular venous compression, discontinuation of nitrous oxide, ventilating with 100% oxygen, flooding the surgical field with saline, changing position to left lateral decubitus with Trendelenburg, and aspiration of air from a central venous catheter placed in or near the right atrium.

Internal carotid or other artery punctures may also occur during this procedure. The tissues in and around the artery may be affected by the surgical pathology, previous surgical exploration and scarring, and prior radiation therapy. Blood loss can be sudden and significant, and cross-matched blood should always be immediately available. Immediate surgical compression risks cerebral ischemia, as cerebral perfusion will depend on contralateral intracranial arterial flow. Modest hypertension should be induced during the compression and surgical repair for this reason. Invasive arterial blood pressure monitoring, which is often not otherwise required in these surgeries, should be started, and intravenous heparin administration may be requested by the surgical team. Postoperatively, the patient should be monitored for signs of cerebral ischemia.

Manipulation of the carotid sinus and stellate ganglion has been associated with wide swings in blood pressure, arrhythmias, sinus arrest, and prolonged QT intervals. Pressure on the carotid sinus can elicit a vagal reflex, resulting in bradycardia and hypotension. Ablation of the right sympathetic stellate ganglion increases the QT interval of the electrocardiography and may lower the threshold for ventricular fibrillation. Infiltration of the carotid sheath with local anesthetic will usually prevent these problems. Bilateral neck dissection may result in postoperative hypertension and loss of hypoxic drive as a result of denervation of the carotid sinuses and bodies. Patients with carotid atherosclerosis are at increased risk of stroke during neck surgery, and it has been suggested that some patients need to have prophylactic endarterectomy.

Following neck surgeries, hematomas may form postoperatively, which can compress the airway and lead to respiratory compromise. Intubation may be difficult if hematoma formation distorts the airway anatomy. Reopening of the surgical site with manual evacuation of the hematoma may help to reduce respiratory compromise and facilitate intubation.

There may be a request by the surgical team for the use of steroids to reduce postoperative edema. These should be administered early in the case to be effective.

3 Are there special considerations for the emergence or the end of the case?

Hemostasis is particularly important due to the risk of airway compromise with hematoma formation. It has been suggested that a "Valsalva maneuver" (creating a prolonged, increased intrathoracic pressure) helps to achieve hemostasis by increasing internal jugular venous pressure and by causing reflux of venous blood. In the intubated patient, the Valsalva maneuver is executed by closing the anesthesia circuit's adjustable pressure-limiting valve and administering a manual insufflation of the lungs until 30 to 35 cm H_2O of airway pressure is attained. This pressure is held for up to 20 seconds. Leakage from the thoracic duct is also investigated in this way. However, this maneuver carries its own risks, such as barotrauma, and may be accompanied by bradycardia and hypotension. Placing the patient in a steep head-down (Trendelenburg) position has proven to be more sensitive in identifying bleeding vessels not seen by a Valsalva maneuver. The Trendelenburg position poses the potential risk of increased intracranial pressure. Intracranial complications are not usually a concern when tilt time is limited to 6 minutes and tilt angle is less than 50 degrees.

A smooth emergence with avoidance of coughing and straining is important to avoid postoperative bleeding and hematoma formation. The administration of topical lidocaine at the time of tracheal extubation, the use of total intravenous anesthesia techniques, small boluses of potent opioids or dexmedetomidine, and/or deep extubation are all recommended ways to achieve a smooth emergence. If the airway was difficult to manage at the time of tracheal intubation, extubation criteria should be carefully reviewed prior to extubation.

See Figure 75.1 and ***Video 75.1*** *for additional details.*

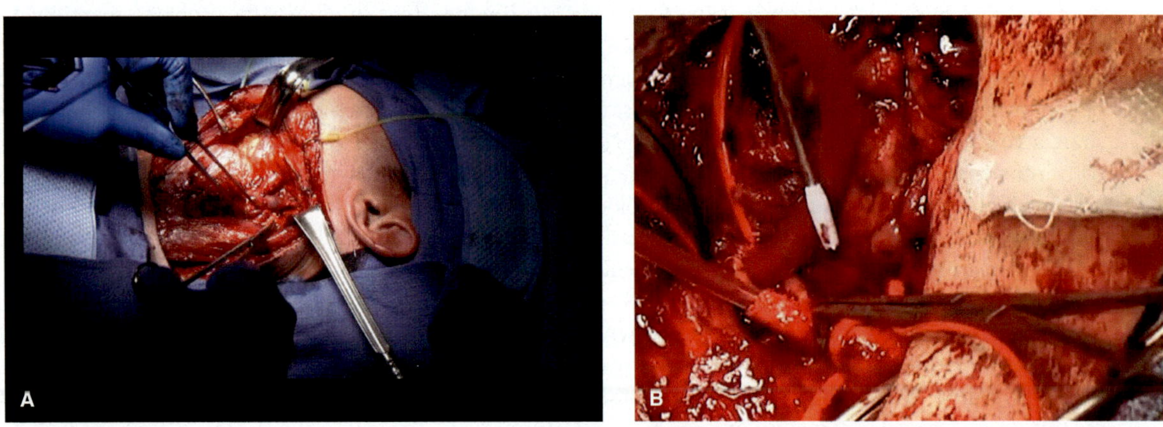

Figure 75.1. A: Left-sided neck dissection. **B:** Catastrophic carotid disruption is a risk during neck dissection. Here, a patient undergoes carotid repair.

Suggested Readings

Garg R, Darlong V, Pandey R, Punj J. Anesthesia for oncological ENT surgeries: review. *Internet J Anesthesiol.* 2008;20(1).

Moumoulidis I, Martinez Del Pero M, Brennan L, Jani P. Haemostasis in head and neck surgical procedures: Valsalva manoeuvre versus Trendelenburg tilt. *Ann R Coll Surg Engl.* 2010;92(4):292–294.

Nagarkar R, Kokane G, Wagh A, et al. Airway management techniques in head and neck cancer surgeries: a retrospective analysis. *Oral Maxillofac Surg.* 2019;23(3):311–315.

Substernal Thyroid

76

Lorraine J. Foley

Clinical Scenario: A 30-year-old woman presents for resection of a substernal thyroid goiter. She is clinically euthyroid but has significant rightward tracheal deviation as a result of the goiter. At its narrowest portion, the trachea has a diameter of 5 mm on CT scan. The patient has modest dyspnea when lying on her right side and when exercising.

1 What are the anesthetic and airway management considerations for this case?

All patients with thyroid disease should be rendered euthyroid before elective surgery. As in this case, CT or MRI should be considered the gold standard for preoperative evaluation of the airway. These modalities allow cross-sectional images that can identify tracheal deviation or compression and the degree of invasion of the mass into surrounding tissues. These issues all have significant anesthetic and surgical implications.

Substernal thyroids represent a small percentage of all goiters. The chronicity of the mass may have important implications. A substernal goiter, which has been present for a long period (eg, 15 years) and is causing tracheal deviation, may be associated with significant tracheal atrophy and erosion of the tracheal rings, resulting in loss of supporting structures (tracheomalacia). Collapse of the tracheal airway can lead to obstruction in both awake and anesthetized patients. A rapidly growing malignant goiter may indicate airway management difficulties due to tracheal invasion by tumor-associated fibrosis, resulting in a reduced elasticity of the tracheal–laryngeal tissues. Substernal thyroids may compress surrounding structures and cause superior vena cava syndrome or involve the recurrent laryngeal nerve, resulting in unilateral vocal cord dysfunction.

The span of the affected trachea should be investigated. Thyroid masses extending to the level of the carina or below should prompt consideration for preinduction institution of extracorporeal circulation (extracorporeal membrane oxygenation [ECMO] or cardiopulmonary bypass [CPB]). The potential need for extracorporeal support requires definitive preoperative decision making: ECMO or CPB "standby" (including surgeon, CPB or ECMO machine, and perfusionists). Establishing extracorporeal support may require at least several minutes for arterial-venous cannulation, so preoperative planning is imperative.

Surgically, most substernal thyroids can be removed through a cervical neck incision. This will require the surgeon to manipulate the thyroid within the narrow confines of the thoracic outlet. Compression of the trachea and great vessels may occur with this approach, potentially leading to changes in airway pressures and hemodynamics, respectively.

Though few substernal thyroidectomies will require an upper sternotomy, the anesthesiologist should always be prepared for this possibility. Major blood loss may occur with sternotomy. Due to limited access to the patient's extremities during this procedure, large-bore intravenous access and, depending on the patient's comorbidities, invasive arterial blood pressure monitoring should be established prior to surgical draping.

2 How would you manage the airway in this case?

Substernal thyroids typically do not affect the upper airway, but preoperative vocal cord examination should still be performed to evaluate for vocal cord paralysis. Laryngoscopy is generally expected to be unremarkable unless the patient has unrelated predictors of a difficult airway. The author would place this patient into an intermediate to high surgical and anesthetic risk based on signs, symptoms, and radiologic findings.

Assuming this patient's airway examination was otherwise unremarkable, the author would choose an inhalational induction with sevoflurane and 100% oxygen, maintaining spontaneous ventilation. In most circumstances, the patient is kept in an upright sitting position to avoid avert tracheal compression that might occur as the laryngotracheal musculature relaxes. Left lateral decubitus position may be helpful if respiratory compromise occurs during anesthetic induction.

Once the patient has reached an appropriate anesthetic depth, direct or video laryngoscopy can be used to examine the vocal cords prior to intubation with a small, 5.5- to 6.0-mm reinforced tracheal tube (TT). Although there may be a surgical request for a neuromonitoring TT, the narrowed tracheal lumen may preclude its use. The pathologically narrowed regions of the trachea are often pliable, but the anesthesiologist should be prepared for restrictions that might require TT downsizing.

Alternatively, intubation using a flexible bronchoscope may provide information about tracheal wall narrowing and pliability. The operator must keep in mind that the eventual placement of the TT is a blind procedure: resistance met during the TT "railroading" should not be overcome with undue force. TT downsizing may be necessary requiring FIS removal and reinsertion.

In the event of major airway or vascular compromise during the inhalational induction, the patient should be woken up to attempt restoration of native ventilation. An awake intubation technique would be the next reasonable step. If acute compromise does not immediately resolve, total body repositioning may be needed (eg, left lateral decubitus position). Further difficulty may require emergency rigid bronchoscopy with jet ventilation distal to the obstruction. Finally, emergent sternotomy to reduce tracheal compression is another option. The above rescue procedures require thoughtful preparation. Acute decompensation will leave little time for equipment assemblage.

3 What are the potential hazards and complications with regard to the airway?

The major airway issues to anticipate include tracheal obstruction, breath holding, and laryngospasm during inhalation induction or awake intubation and tracheal and TT compression and obstruction during surgical manipulation. It is also important to note that a narrowed tracheal lumen may not accept an adequately sized TT.

Vascular compression, which can occur during anesthetic induction or from surgical manipulation, may cause hemodynamic instability. The retrosternal mediastinum contains major vascular structures such as the brachiocephalic veins, the superior vena cava, the aortic arch, and the brachiocephalic, left common carotid and subclavian arteries. Major blood loss during surgery should always be considered a possibility. Other possible complications during retrosternal dissection include pneumothorax and bilateral recurrent laryngeal nerve injury, resulting in vocal cord dysfunction and potential airway obstruction at emergence and extubation.

4 Are there special considerations for the emergence or the end of the case?

A smooth emergence is important. Undue coughing, bucking, and blood pressure increases may cause bleeding, which can cause a substernal hematoma. Tracheal incompetence (from tracheomalacia or surgical repair), recurrent laryngeal nerve injury, and laryngeal edema may result in airway compromise following extubation.

For these reasons, a deep extubation technique should be considered if appropriate. The Bailey maneuver, where an SGA is substituted for the TT, might be considered prior to emergence. A video laryngoscope or FIS can be used to evaluate vocal cord function and the condition of the trachea prior to extubation. Significant findings may initiate placement of an airway exchange catheter for extubation.

- Inhalational induction and awake intubation are commonly used to secure the airway in the case of a large, substernal goiter.
- Acute airway or hemodynamic compromise during anesthetic induction may warrant awakening, body repositioning, rigid bronchoscopy, and/or emergency CPB.
- Major postoperative complications include retrosternal hematoma, vocal cord paralysis, tracheomalacia, and pneumothorax.
- *See Figures 76.1 and 76.2 for additional details.*

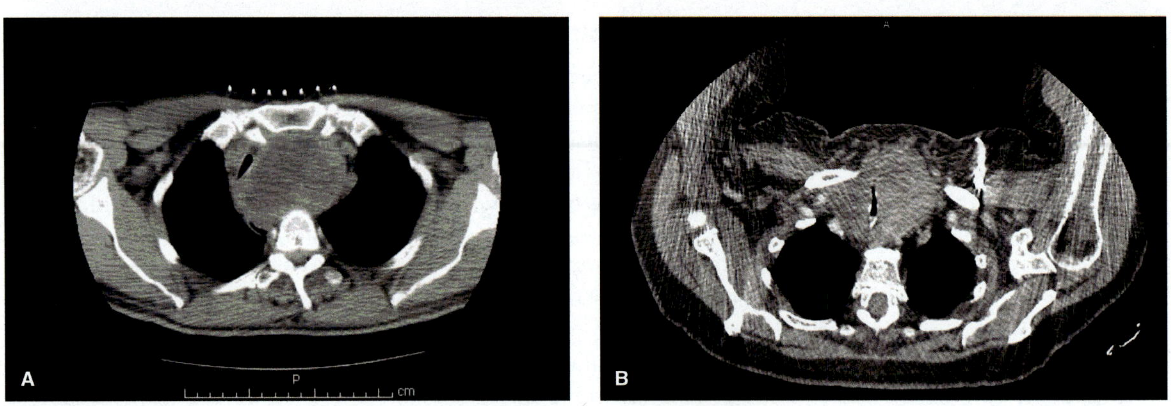

Figure 76.1. **A:** A large substernal thyroid is seen on CT scan. The trachea is seen displaced to the right side. (See **Video 76.1.**) **B:** The trachea is encased within a large, substernal thyroid.

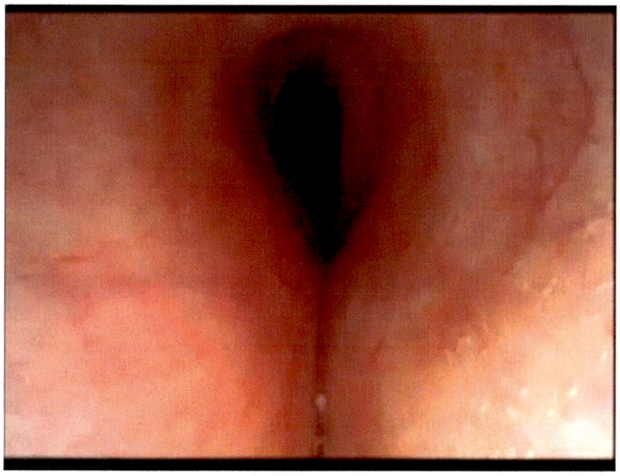

Figure 76.2. Tracheal compression is seen during intubation with a flexible intubation scope. (See **Video 76.2**.)

Suggested Readings

Blank R, de Souza D. Anesthetic management of patients with an anterior mediastinal mass: continuing professional development. *Can J Anesth*. 2011;58:853–859, 860–867.

Lee C, Cooper R, Goldstein D. Management of a patient with tracheomalacia and supraglottic obstruction after thyroid surgery. *Can J Anesthes*. 2011;58:1029–1033.

Simo R, Nixon I, Vander Poorten V, et al. Surgical management of intrathoracic goiters. *Eur Arch Otorhinolaryngol*. 2019;276:305–314.

Unlu MT, Aygun N, Kostek M, Isgor A, Uludag M. Substernal goiter from definitions to treatment. *Sisi Etfal Hastan Tip Bul*. 2022;56:167–176.

77 Neuromonitoring Tracheal Tubes

Lorraine J. Foley

Clinical Scenario: A 48-year-old woman presents for thyroidectomy for papillary carcinoma. The surgeon requests the use of a neural integrity monitor (NIM) neuromonitoring tube.

1 Describe the device in detail.

Neuromonitoring tracheal tubes (TTs), such as the NIM Standard and Contact Reinforced EMG TT (Medtronics, Minneapolis, MN), allow intraoperative nerve monitoring and are used as an adjunct in identifying the recurrent laryngeal nerve during surgery of the thyroid, parathyroids, and other paratracheal pathology. Unlike visual identification, intraoperative neuromonitoring allows the surgeon to confirm the functional integrity of the intact nerve. The NIM is a flexible silicone elastomer TT with four stainless steel wire electrodes embedded in its barrel approximately 30 mm proximal to the inflatable cuff. Sections of the steel wire immediately proximal to the cuff are exposed to make contact with the mucosa of the vocal cords. The area of electrode exposure is indicated by a contrasting color of the TT barrel in order to facilitate proper placement during laryngoscopy. The steel wires are connected to an electromyographic monitoring device via external wiring.

The NIM tube is usually placed into the larynx with video laryngoscopy, allowing both the anesthesia provider and surgeon to visualize proper positioning. Ideally, the midpoint of the contrast-colored TT barrel area is positioned juxtaposed with the vocal cords. It is recommended to reverify the placement once the head is positioned for surgery. Reexamination may be easily achieved with repeat video laryngoscopy.

Some operators advise using a TT size larger than would normally be chosen for a particular patient, in order to improve electrode–vocal cord contact. This should be balanced by the knowledge that the outer diameter of the NIM tube is 0.5 to 0.7 mm larger than that of a same internal diameter standard TT.

Neuromuscular monitoring requires that the patient not be paralyzed during the procedure. The use of short-acting or avoidance of all muscle relaxants are options for induction and intubation. Succinylcholine (1 mg/kg) has the shortest recovery time for the larynx, ranging from 5.7 to 14.5 minutes. The use of topical local anesthetics on the vocal cords or in TT lubricants should be avoided as this may prevent vocal cord movement with nerve stimulation.

The patient should be kept in a deep plane of anesthesia to prevent spontaneous respiratory efforts, which can give false-positive readings during electromyography. A bite block is recommended to prevent damage to the NIM TT.

The International Neural Monitoring Study Group has published guidelines to help standardize the application of intraoperative neuromonitoring. The study group's recommendations include standards for equipment setup, TT placement, and an algorithm for evaluating intraoperative signal loss and other problem-solving. The recommendations applicable to the anesthesiologist are discussed above. Significant equipment problems have been reported at a rate of 3.8% to 23%, mostly related to the TT. Overinflation of the cuff pressure (not to exceed 25 cm H_2O) can result in tracheal damage and cuff distortion which may lead to airway blockage. The guidelines recommend that the ground electrodes be placed on the patient's shoulders or on the sternum if the shoulder placement results in a noisy baseline. The monitor should be set at a 100 µV event threshold with a stimulation current of 1 to 2 mA and an impedance of less than 5 kΩ per electrode. It is also important that the NIM monitor is at least 10 feet away from electrocautery units.

2 Where or when is this device used in airway management?

Although the appropriate identification and preservation of the recurrent laryngeal nerve require the surgeon to have direct visualization of the nerve, postoperative vocal cord dysfunction remains a major complication of thyroid and parathyroid surgery. The rates of permanent and transient paralysis of the recurrent laryngeal nerve have been reported as 1.2% and 3.2%, respectively. Some patients with more invasive pathology, such as those with Graves disease, or recurrent surgery, are at higher risk of nerve injury (12.5% transient injury and 5% permanent injury). In these cases, NIM seems to improve outcome. For patients undergoing robotic minimally invasive video-assisted thyroidectomy, the use of intraoperative NIM is helpful due to the limited view of the structural nerve during surgical dissection.

A recent study by Eid, et al. showed that neuromuscular monitoring had an overall sensitivity of 98.4%, specificity of 62.5%, positive predictive value of 98.6%, and negative predictive value of 58.8% for predicting recurrent laryngeal nerve dysfunction.

Injury to the recurrent laryngeal nerve is of significant concern to the anesthesiologist. Although unilateral paralysis is unlikely to cause airway obstruction at the time of extubation, caution should still be exercised during bilateral dissections and when contralateral paralysis is known to exist preoperatively. When the use of neuromonitoring reveals that unilateral injury has occurred, a decision may be made to delay contralateral surgery.

3 What distinguishes this device from similar airway management methods?

Traditional laryngeal electrodes were made using conductive ink on a polyester substrate attached to the surface of a standard TT. Studies have shown no statistical difference between traditional laryngeal electrodes and the NIM tube in the ability to detect nerve injury.

Other noninvasive monitoring techniques involve visualization of the vocal cords intraoperatively. This may be done with an flexible intubating scope (FIS) in a patient being managed with an supraglottic airway device. This technique has been inadequately studied. Some authors discourage these techniques; nerve injuries, though recognized, may be difficult to treat (eg, tracheal intubation) due to poor intraoperative access to the airway. Patients intubated with a standard TT may be extubated after the return of spontaneous ventilation, but in a deep anesthetic state. The vocal cords are visualized during the extubation (by direct or video laryngoscopy). If critical paralysis is noted, the trachea can be immediately reintubated.

Invasive intraoperative monitoring may be achieved with intramuscular vocal cord needle electrodes placed through the cricothyroid membrane. The disadvantage of the needle electrodes is the risk of trauma to the vocal cords, cuff perforation, and accidental needle dislodgement during surgery.

- Confirmation of NIM TT placement after the patient is positioned for surgery should be achieved with a video laryngoscope or FIS.
- Evaluate the patient's vocal cord movement preoperatively and postoperatively.
- Avoid neuromuscular blockade and local anesthetic lubrication to optimize intraoperative neuromonitoring.
- *See Figure 77.1 and* ***Video 77.1*** *for additional details.*

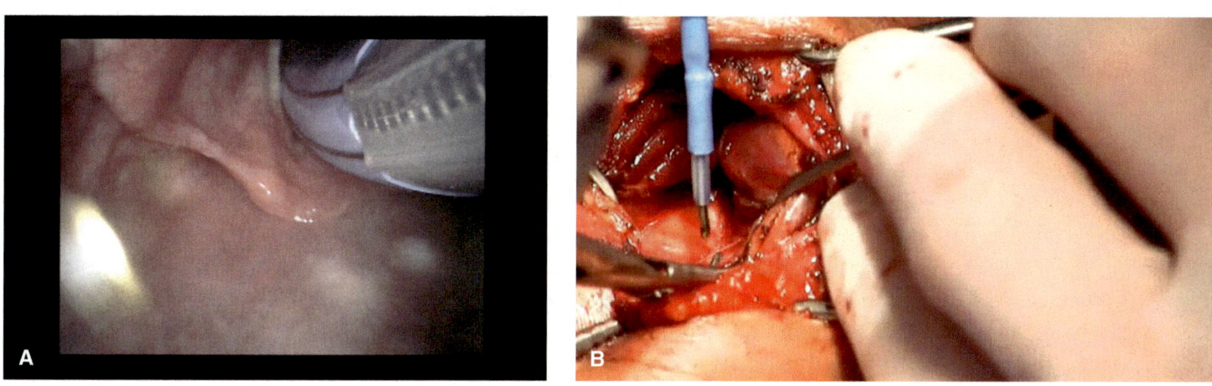

Figure 77.1. A: The wire electrodes of a neuromonitoring tracheal tube are seen against the left vocal cord. **B:** A nerve stimulator is used to isolate the recurrent laryngeal nerve. Monitoring is being performed with a neuromonitoring tracheal tube in place (not seen).

Suggested Readings

Eid I, Miller F, Rowan S, Otto RA. The role of nerve monitoring to predict postoperative recurrent laryngeal nerve monitoring during thyroid and parathyroid surgery. *Laryngoscope*. 2013;123:2583–2586.

Liang KY, Scharpf J. Avoiding complications of thyroidectomy: recurrent laryngeal nerve and superior laryngeal nerve preservation. *Otolaryngol Clin North Am*. 2024;57(1):75–82.

Medtronic Instruction Manual for NIM Standard Reinforced EMG Endotracheal Tube and NIM Contact Reinforced EMG Endotracheal Tube.

Pardal-Refoly JL, Ochoa-Sangador C. Bilateral recurrent nerve injury in total thyroidectomy with and without interoperative monitoring. Systematic review and meta-analysis. *Acta Otorrinolaringol Esp*. 2016;67:66–74.

78 Hypopharyngeal Masses

Felipe Urdaneta

Clinical Scenario: A patient with a newly diagnosed base of tongue squamous cell carcinoma presents for surgical resection (Figure 78.1).

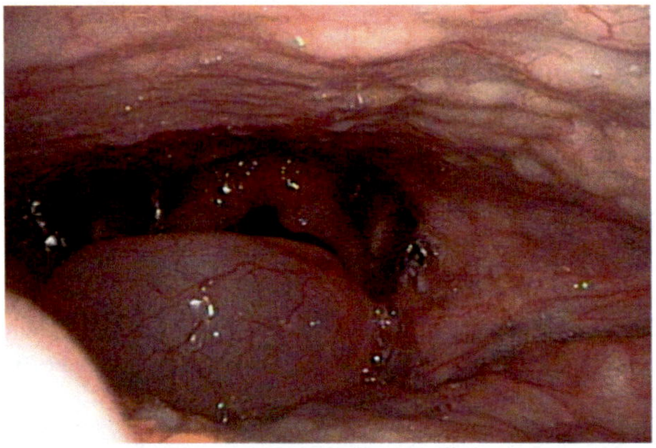

Figure 78.1. A large mass was seen in the hypopharynx during a preoperative endoscopy. [See **Video 78.1**.]

1 What are the anesthetic and airway management considerations for this case?

Preoperative evaluation of the head and neck cancer patient should always include noting the presence and extent of any airway issues that may impact the anesthesiologist's airway management. A patient presenting with a history of a hypopharyngeal mass should undergo a comprehensive preoperative airway evaluation to determine the best option for airway management (awake intubation vs induction followed by intubation). Clinical evaluation methods alone have historically lacked sensitivity and specificity. The airway architecture observed in the awake examination is not entirely translated to the anesthetized state. Assessment of the sagittal plane of the airway in an awake patient does not provide a dynamic examination of the airway structures or give any information about the subglottic region. It may lead to overestimating difficulty or, worse, creating false reassurance about how best to manage the airway. It is also associated with intense adrenergic response, which may predispose to its own complications. After induction of general anesthesia and administration of neuromuscular blocking agents, anteroposterior displacement of the larynx occurs, which can cause a change in the airway architecture compared to the awake state. Diagnostic imaging techniques, such as x-rays, CT, MRI, and ultrasound, can also be used as part of the preoperative airway exam. However, they do not provide dynamic airway information, can be costly, and at present, lack adequate evidence of their effectiveness.

2 What are the potential hazards and complications in regard to the airway?

Patients with hypopharyngeal pathology have a higher incidence of difficult airways due to anatomical and physiologic distortions in the airway. Technologic advancements in airway management, such as more routine use of video laryngoscopy, have made it reasonable to question whether the use of awake flexible intubation (AFI) is necessary in all patients with airway-related problems.

ENT providers routinely use endoscopic evaluation to assess vocal cord mobility and swallowing. It is usually performed via the nasal route, requires minimal preparation, and is well tolerated by most patients. Anesthesiologists may use documentation from prior endoscopic exams as part of their current airway exam. However, the exam performed by ENT providers focuses on evaluating the location and extent of any airway lesions rather than on variables relevant to airway management and intubation. Due to time between the endoscopic evaluation and the day of surgery, there is always the risk of disease progression, making a preoperative endoscopic exam valuable. Moorthy et al. reported their 10-year experience with 801 patients with laryngeal tumors who had endoscopic evaluation under topical anesthesia before anesthetic instrumentation. They classified laryngeal tumors into four classes depending on the type of lesion, visibility of the vocal folds, and laryngeal opening. Lower-grade lesions (I and II) could be intubated after induction of general anesthesia, but higher-grade lesions needed either awake or invasive instrumentation of the trachea. Although the study was descriptive only, they concluded this approach allowed them to avoid more airway emergencies, bleeding, and dislodgment of laryngeal tumors. Rosenblatt et al. have also evaluated whether the preoperative endoscopic exam could reduce the number of unnecessary awake intubations. In a study of 138 patients, the airway management plan was altered in 26% of patients, and awake intubation was avoided in 36%. A small percentage (5%) showed extensive airway pathology that could not be detected based on clinical examination alone.

3 Describe in detail the device or technique.

The endoscopic evaluation may be performed in the preoperative clinic, the preoperative holding area, or the operating room. The patient is usually placed in a sitting or recumbent position. The nasal approach is preferred to avoid issues with a gag reflex and the need for topicalization of the oropharynx. Sedation can usually be omitted as this exam is well tolerated by most awake patients. Topicalization can be achieved with a vasoconstrictive nasal spray in both nostrils, followed by lidocaine. The exam is usually quick and does not require any special monitoring.

Performing a preoperative endoscopic airway exam can be a time-saving strategy because the anesthesiologist can use this objective evaluation of the airway to tailor the airway management approach appropriately. This means that there will be less chance of delays due to unexpected emergencies or complications.

- The preoperative endoscopic examination gives the anesthesiologist the ability to identify significant airway pathology that may impact the plan for airway management.
- In patients presenting with hypopharyngeal masses or other pathology, the endoscopic examination may provide invaluable information that routine preoperative airway assessment may otherwise not.
- The endoscopic airway evaluation can be quickly performed with minimal preparation.
- *See Figures 78.2 and 78.3 for additional details.*

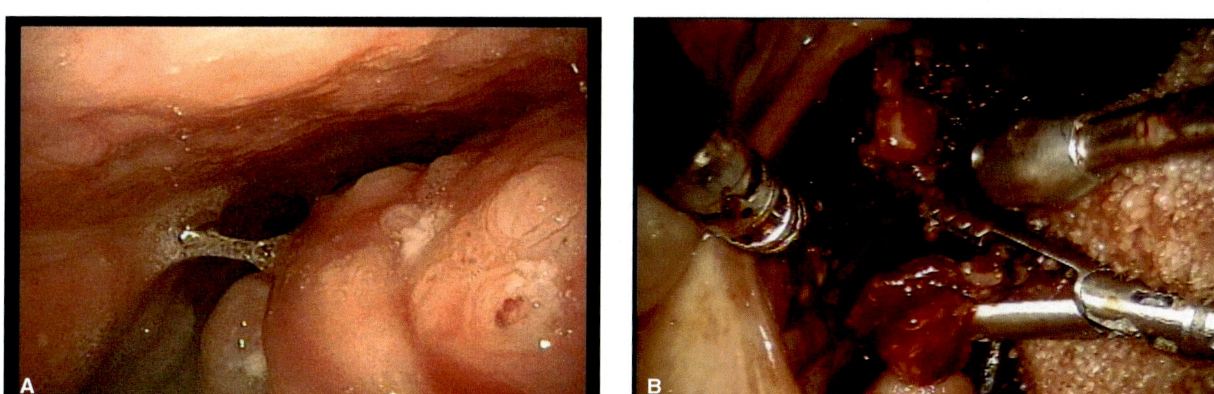

Figure 78.2. A large base of tongue mass is seen during intubation (**A**) and is being removed with a robotic surgery technique (**B**). (See **Video 78.2.**)

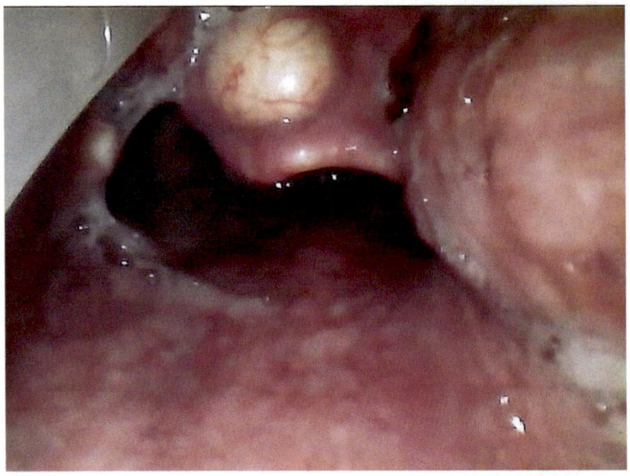

Figure 78.3. An epiglottic cyst. (See **Video 78.3.**)

Suggested Readings

Apfelbaum JL, Hagberg CA, Connis RT, et al. 2022 American Society of Anesthesiologists Practice Guidelines for management of the difficult airway. *Anesthesiology.* 2022;136(1):31–81.

Moorthy SS, Gupta S, Laurent B, Weisberger EC. Management of airway in patients with laryngeal tumors. *J Clin Anesth.* 2005; 17(8):604–609.

Rosenblatt W, Ianus AI, Sukhupragarn W, Fickenscher A, Sasaki C. Preoperative endoscopic airway examination (PEAE) provides superior airway information and may reduce the use of unnecessary awake intubation. *Anesth Analg.* 2011;112(3):602–607.

Sasu PB, Pansa JI, Stadlhofer R, et al. Nasendoscopy to predict difficult videolaryngoscopy: a multivariable model development study. *J Clin Med.* 2023;12(10):3433.

Subglottic Stenosis–Noncritical/ Supraglottic Jet Ventilation

79

James Turnbull • Anil Patel • Claudia Fernandez Robles

Clinical Scenario: A 35-year-old woman presents for laser treatment of idiopathic subglottic stenosis (SGS). The patient is otherwise healthy but experiences dyspnea with vigorous exercise, which led to her current diagnosis. She has a 5-mm airway lumen at the point of obstruction on preoperative CT scan.

1 What are the anesthetic and airway management considerations for this case?

SGS in adults is a rare but potentially life-threatening condition with an incidence of approximately 1:200,000. The most common cause is a history of prolonged endotracheal intubation, particularly in patients who have been critically ill. Other causes include benign or malignant neoplasms, granulomatous disease (such as sarcoid and tuberculosis), granulomatosis with polyangiitis, mucocutaneous disease (such as pemphigoid), thyroid or mediastinal masses, trauma, and idiopathic laryngotracheal stenosis. Severity of symptoms depends on the degree of stenosis, with most patients being asymptomatic at rest until there is more than 70% reduction in the lumen.

If minimal symptoms are present, ventilation following induction of anesthesia is generally straightforward. Induction can be achieved with either spontaneous breathing using a volatile inhalational anesthetic or through intravenous induction. While spontaneous ventilation can help maintain airway patency, failure may result in the need for emergency intubation and potentially a difficult airway due to airway collapse. Intravenous induction with muscle relaxation, in a controlled environment with close communication between the surgeon or proceduralist and the anesthesiologist, may offer better outcomes by ensuring a secure airway and improved ventilation.

Optimal management for airway surgery should prevent aspiration, afford complete control of the airway, provide an unobstructed and motionless surgical field, put no time restrictions on the surgeon, and facilitate the use of lasers. Unfortunately, the "ideal" technique does not exist, and some compromises have to be made. Anesthetic techniques can broadly be divided into two categories: "open" and "closed" systems. "Closed" systems use a cuffed tracheal tube to provide optimal protection against lower airway soiling, but with the potential for laser-related problems and limited surgical field exposure. When an endotracheal tube (ETT) is used, the surgeon may choose to use an intermittent extubation technique (the ETT is removed during laser use). Oxygenating with maximum oxygen concentrations (eg, FIO_2 of 1.0) while the ETT is in place prolongs the safe apneic period. "Open" systems employ no ETT and instead rely on spontaneous or jet ventilation techniques. This technique provides an unobstructed operating field but leaves the lower airway at risk of soiling. These systems are interchangeable, but the choice of system used depends on surgeons' and anesthesiologists' preferences and patient safety.

Jet ventilation techniques can be used for most adult vocal cord and tracheal lesions, including benign laryngeal lesions, airway stenosis, rigid bronchoscopy, airway stent insertion, tracheal resection, and airway tumors. Anesthesiologist experience with jet ventilation technique and machines is crucial for these cases. Jet ventilation can be applied at different frequencies (high, low, or superimposed) and through three distinct routes (supraglottic, subglottic, and transtracheal). High-frequency rate (100 to 50 per minute) is generally preferred as peak and mean pressures are lower, cardiovascular stability is greater, and respiratory gas exchange is more efficient. Each route has risks and benefits, and the decision of which to use is dictated by the planned surgery and individual preferences. In our practice of more than 2000 patients, a noncritical stenosis would be managed with supraglottic high-frequency jet ventilation (SGHFJV).

2 How would you manage the airway in this case?

Airway management begins with a thorough preoperative assessment, including a history of current symptoms, exercise tolerance, previous surgeries, and an airway examination. Reviewing flow-volume loops and CT imaging provides further information regarding the site and severity of the obstruction. Flexible nasoendoscopy can be part of the airway exam and should be reviewed when available. A complete discussion of the airway plan with the surgical team is also essential to keep the patient safe.

Intravenous induction, including muscle relaxation, is performed, and maintenance through intravenous anesthesia is preferred to decrease operating room air contamination and to achieve a more reliable level of anesthesia. In this case, after establishing the airway with mask ventilation, laryngoscopy is performed and local anesthetic is applied to the vocal cords (tracheal intubation is not performed). Continued ventilation is achieved by a face mask or supraglottic airway. The surgeon performs suspension laryngoscopy. An injector needle is connected to the laryngoscope, and once aligned, high-frequency jet ventilation (HFJV) is started via an automated jet ventilator. Typical initial settings would be a driving pressure of 1 to 2 bar, frequency of 100 to 120 per minute, and FIO_2 of 1.0. Chest excursion and recoil should be monitored, and the settings should be adjusted accordingly. At the end of the procedure, the suspension laryngoscope is removed, the ease of ventilation is confirmed, the anesthetic is discontinued, and the muscle relaxant is reversed. The patient should be allowed to slowly reestablish spontaneous respiration without stimulation.

3 What are the Surgical Considerations that Impact Anesthetic Management?

In supraglottic techniques, the responsibility of maintaining a patent airway is handed over to the surgeon. If airway anatomy is abnormal, positioning of the scope may be difficult, and face mask ventilation and oxygenation may be required. Any malalignment or displacement of the scope can result in inadequate ventilation and gastric insufflation. While surgical access and effective ventilation are interrelated, the operative field remains the surgical priority, so the anesthetic team must remain vigilant to detect ineffective ventilation. The teams should maintain constant communication to ensure patient safety.

The use of SGHFJV provides the surgeon with an excellent view of the larynx and surrounding structures. Compared with other techniques, it also decreases the incidence of hypoxemia, especially in high-risk patients. There is some movement of the vocal cords during ventilation, but in most cases, this does not impact the surgical field. During dilation of the stenosis, ventilation is stopped, thus introducing a time limit before oxygen desaturation occurs and jet ventilation needs to be resumed. Although airway fire is less of a concern, standard laser precautions should be used to decrease the risk of ignition of surrounding materials.

4 What are the potential hazards and complications in regard to the airway?

SGHFJV can maintain oxygenation even in patients with significant stridor and severe airway stenosis. Common complications include inability to ventilate, prolonged hypoxemic events, laryngospasm, and, less commonly, pneumothorax. Occasionally, in patients with significant obesity who require a neutral or head-down position, desaturation can occur despite maximal driving pressures, oxygen concentrations, and rate optimization. In such patients, conversion to a cuffed tracheal tube may be required. Alternatively, a manual jet ventilator used at low frequency with a shorter length of tubing provides increased distal pressure and oxygen flow and may succeed where HFJV has failed. Another theoretical hazard is the blowing of blood and debris into the lungs, although a recent case series suggests this is of little clinical relevance. The effect of dry gases must also be considered. Tracheobronchitis and destruction of the mucociliary transport system can occur with prolonged SGHFJV.

- Routine induction of anesthesia is typically safe in patients with noncritical stenosis.
- SGHFJV provides excellent operating conditions and gas exchange with minimal risk of airway fires.
- *See Figure 79.1 and* ***Video 79.1*** *for additional details.*

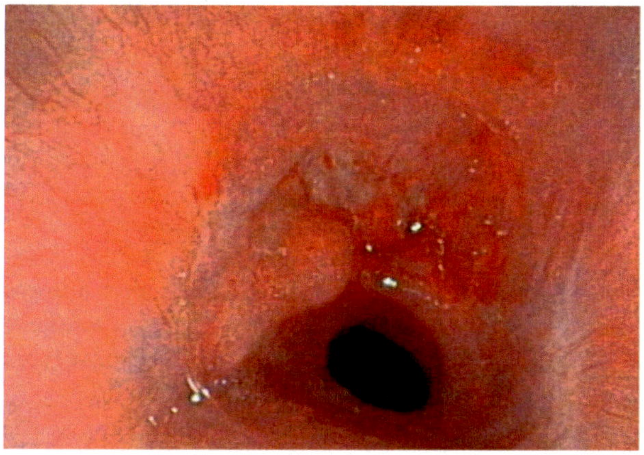

Figure 79.1. A patient with subglottic stenosis–6 weeks earlier, the patient had undergone tracheal intubation after a traumatic event.

Suggested Readings

Daumerie G, Su S, Ochroch EA. Anesthesia for the patient with tracheal stenosis. *Anesthesiol Clin*. 2010;28(1):157–174.

Nouraei SAR, Giussani DA, Howard DJ, Sandhu GS, Ferguson C, Patel A. Physiological comparison of spontaneous and positive-pressure ventilation in laryngotracheal stenosis. *Br J Anaesth*. 2008;101(3):419–423.

Rezaie-Majd A, Bigenzahn W, Denk DM, et al. Superimposed high-frequency jet ventilation for endoscopic laryngotracheal surgery in more than 1500 patients. *Br J Anaesth*. 2006;96(5):650–659.

Rodney JP, Shinn JR, Amin SN, et al. Multi-Institutional analysis of outcomes in supraglottic jet ventilation with a team-based approach. *Laryngoscope*. 2021;131(10):2292–2297.

Xu R, Li Z, Jiang X, et al. Effect of supraglottic jet oxygenation and ventilation on hypoxemia in patients undergoing endoscopic surgery with sedation: A meta-analysis of randomized controlled trials. *J Clin Anesth*. 2024;97:111559.

80 Subglottic Jet Ventilation

James Turnbull • Anil Patel • Claudia Fernandez Robles

Clinical Scenario: A 50-year-old woman presents with subglottic stenosis 6 months after a previous prolonged intubation. She has significant respiratory stridor and has undergone an elective awake intubation. The surgeon has established a view of the larynx with suspension laryngoscopy and now requests the use of subglottic jet ventilation via a microcatheter to provide access to the stenotic area.

1 What are the anesthetic and airway management considerations for this case?

The use of subglottic jet ventilation for suspension laryngoscopy was first described by Benjamin in 1979. Modifications to the original catheter by Hunsaker in 1994 led to further acceptance of this technique, particularly for the treatment of vocal cord pathologies. The use of subglottic catheters in patients with subglottic stenosis is more controversial as the severity of the stenosis increases. Insertion of subglottic catheters can be difficult, and further reductions in tracheal lumen diameter may completely occlude the expiratory pathway.

The Hunsaker Mon-Jet catheter (Xomed, FL) is made from Teflon, making it highly resistant to laser strike. It measures 35.5 cm long with an external diameter of 3 to 4.3 mm. A metal stylet provides rigidity. It incorporates a self-centering basket at the distal portion, reducing the risk of trauma to the tracheal mucosa and preventing movement at the tip. It has two connection ports: one for the ventilator and the other to monitor pressure and $ETCO_2$. An alternative, the LaserJet microcatheter (Acutronic, Switzerland), has similar properties with a rounded-off tip instead of a basket and an adjustable red band to help estimate insertion depth. It is stiffer than the Hunsaker and therefore less prone to kinking, but movement at its tip can be a problem.

Compared to supraglottic jet ventilation, subglottic techniques are more efficient because gases are delivered directly into the trachea. Driving pressures are reduced and exact alignment of the laryngoscope is not required for effective ventilation. Moreover, there is minimal movement of the vocal cords and less drying effects. Protection against airway contamination is better as the jet tends to blow blood and debris upwards and outwards through the larynx. Unlike supraglottic techniques, instrumentation through the glottis is still required, so trauma to the vocal cords or surrounding lesions can occur. From a surgical perspective, subglottic catheter techniques allow excellent, uninterrupted visualization of the larynx and surrounding structures with reduced tissue movement.

Laser safety is an important consideration when using subglottic catheters. As mentioned, both microcatheters are made from nonflammable Teflon. These catheters have been extensively tested against maximum power strikes from potassium titanyl phosphate and neodymium-doped yttrium aluminum garnet lasers in 100% oxygen. If struck by a CO_2 laser, a self-sustaining flame will not develop but catheters may still burn and perforate at a power of 2 to 10 W. If jet ventilation is then continued, a fragment can be forced into the distal airways.

2 How would you manage the airway in this case?

Effective airway management in patients with subglottic stenosis requires careful planning and technique based on the degree of stenosis. Options include awake or asleep fiberoptic endotracheal intubation, placement of a supraglottic airway, and transtracheal jet ventilation in severe cases.

When an endotracheal tube (ETT) is used, selecting a downsized or microlaryngoscopy tube is recommended to reduce trauma and minimize the risks of swelling or bleeding that could complicate airway management further. The smaller size helps prevent damage to the narrow subglottic space, facilitating a safer and more controlled intubation.

The supraglottic airway (SGA) is another choice, offering advantages such as minimal tracheal manipulation, which reduces the potential for trauma. It maintains a patent airway and enables fiberoptic evaluation, which is especially valuable in assessing and managing subglottic stenosis.

In this specific case, after carefully removing the existing ETT, a jet ventilation microcatheter is introduced, positioning the distal end in the mid-trachea to minimize the risk of dissection through the mucosa which can lead to pneumomediastinum or pneumothorax. The catheter should be secured to the left side of the mouth to avoid displacement. Attention must be given to prevent kinking by ensuring the ventilator tubing is well supported.

When the surgeon is ready for suspension laryngoscopy, the microcatheter can be adjusted to ensure a snug fit that optimizes ventilation while allowing the procedure to safely occur. Following placement of the microcatheter, high-frequency jet ventilation (HFJV) with an automated ventilator can then begin. Initial settings depend on the size of the patient and the anticipated lung compliance. Usually, initial settings include a driving pressures of 1 to 2 bar (15 to 30 psi), frequency of 100 to 120 per minute, inspiratory pressure of 40%, pause pressure of 20 cm H2O, pressure dial of 20 psi, and FIO_2 of 1.0. End-tidal CO_2 can be checked through the monitoring port to confirm ventilation. If laser is used, the FIO_2 should be reduced if tolerated by the patient's oxygen saturation. Maintenance of anesthesia is accomplished using total intravenous anesthesia. Muscle paralysis should be maintained throughout the procedure to prevent the possibility of laryngospasm and subsequent barotrauma. At the end of the procedure, jet ventilation is stopped and the microcatheter is removed. The SGA (or Guedel airway) is reinserted, mask ventilation initiated, and neuromuscular blockade reversed. The patient should then be allowed to slowly regain spontaneous respiration with the SGA in situ or assisted with mask ventilation.

3 What are the potential hazards and complications in regard to the airway?

The most serious risk from subglottic jet ventilation is barotrauma. This is because inflow of air is unimpeded as the catheter bypasses the lesion, whereas outflow may be restricted, in particular in stenotic pathology. Even in benign vocal cord surgery, the onset of laryngospasm can quickly lead to barotrauma if undetected. Ensuring an adequate depth of anesthesia, sufficient analgesia, and muscle relaxation is extremely important. Despite this, published complication rates are low, with one case series suggesting a 0.2% risk of barotrauma. The most common complications in this series are reversible hypoxia (3.6%) and hypercarbia (2%).

The risk of barotrauma can be minimized with the use of an automated jet ventilator. These machines include an automatic cut-off facility should either peak inspiratory or end expiratory pressure (or pause pressure in some machines) exceed a set limit. The alternative is to use a manual device such as the Manujet III (VBM Medizintechnik GmbH, Germany) which has an adjustable pressure regulator starting at 3.5 bar. These devices are common in centers that perform only occasional laryngeal surgery, and perhaps unsurprisingly, are associated with an increased risk of barotrauma.

Technical considerations when using a microcatheter include difficulty with insertion and kinking of the catheter. Inadvertent esophageal intubation and gastric perforation have been described. The Hunsaker catheter has a port for monitoring $ETCO_2$ and pressure, which opens 3.2 cm proximal to its tip. While this is satisfactory to confirm catheter placement and ventilation, it should not be relied upon as a true reflection of $Paco_2$ or to measure true intraluminal pressure. Pressure monitoring from this will not affect the shutdown facility of the automated ventilator.

- Subglottic HFJV provides excellent operating conditions with minimal vocal cord movement.
- Subglottic catheters are relatively safe when used for laser surgery, but fracture and transection of the distal portion can rarely occur.
- There is a risk of barotrauma when using jet ventilation, and vigilant avoidance of laryngospasm is important.
- *See Figure 80.1 and* **Video 80.1** *for additional details.*

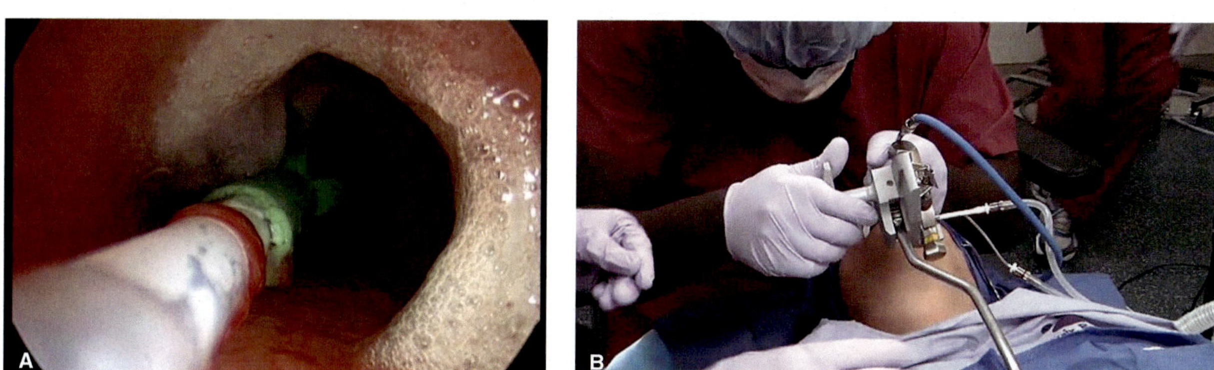

Figure 80.1. **A:** Hunsaker jet ventilation tube is seen mid-trachea. **B:** The Hunsaker jet ventilation tube can be seen emanating from the mouth to the patient's left of the suspension laryngoscope.

Suggested Readings

Benjamin B, Gronow D. A new tube for microlaryngeal surgery. *Anaesth Int Care*. 1979;7(3):258–263.

Cook TM, Alexander R. Major complications during anaesthesia for elective laryngeal surgery in the UK: a national survey of the use of high-pressure source ventilation. *Br J Anaesth*. 2008;101:266–272.

Hu A, Weissbrod PA, Maronian NC, et al. Hunsaker Mon-jet tube ventilation: a 15 year experience. *Laryngoscope*. 2012;122(10): 2234–2239.

Mangahas AM, Talugula S, Husain IA. Anesthesia considerations during management of airway stenosis: a systematic review. *Am J Otolaryngol*. 2023;44(2):103767.

Patel A, Rubin JS. The difficult airway: the use of subglottic jet ventilation for laryngeal surgery. *Logoped Phonniatr Vocol*. 2008; 33(1):22–24.

Elective Transtracheal (Transcricothyroid Membrane) Jet Ventilation

81

Ramneek Maan

Clinical Scenario: A 45-year-old man with a glottic tumor presents for laser debulking. He is a lifelong smoker and has morbid obesity with a body mass index of 45 kg/m^2. He has stridor at rest and is unable to lie flat for long periods. The lesion is thought to be highly vascular and extends into the subglottic region.

1 What are the anesthetic and airway management considerations for this case?

Patients with critical airway stenosis pose some of the most complex and demanding challenges in airway management for the anesthesiologist. A variety of approaches, including awake tracheostomy and awake intubation, have been advocated. Inserting a transcricothyroid membrane transtracheal catheter (TTC) prior to anesthesia induction serves two critical functions: (1) as a contingency route for oxygenation or ventilation in case of airway difficulties, and (2) as a primary technique to facilitate surgical intervention. This approach provides both a safeguard and a functional option for airway management, enhancing patient safety in challenging cases.

TTCs are relatively easy to insert, eliminate the need for direct laryngoscopy and intubation, and significantly reduce the risk of airway trauma, particularly to existing lesions. This method provides a safer and more efficient alternative for airway management in certain clinical scenarios, ensuring both simplicity and reduced risks. They can be inserted preemptively with the patient awake when a difficult airway is anticipated and may improve the view at subsequent direct laryngoscopy. Following surgery, they can be left in situ for up to 24 hours in case of airway deterioration. From a surgical perspective, transtracheal jet ventilation (TTJV) allows an uninterrupted view of the larynx with minimal movement at the surgical site. In contrast to supraglottic techniques, it tends to force blood and debris out of the lungs.

2 How would you manage the airway in this case?

The airway plan must be discussed with the surgical team preoperatively. A clear idea of the level of obstruction is vital so that the site of TTC insertion can be planned. The cricothyroid membrane is the preferred site as it is relatively superficial and provides rigidity. The upper trachea can be used if the pathology involves the glottis or subglottis.

TTC insertion should be performed with the patient awake and in a 45-degree head-up position. With the neck in maximal extension, local anesthetic can be infiltrated over the cricothyroid membrane, which may be identified by palpation or ultrasonography. Using a fluid-filled syringe, a dedicated TTC is inserted with constant aspiration. A 13G VBM (Medizintechnik, Germany) catheter is typically used for this procedure. Once air is freely aspirated, the needle should be inserted 2 to 3 mm further in a slight caudal direction. Air aspiration is then reconfirmed, and the cannula is threaded over the needle. Once the needle has been removed, the position of the TTC is again confirmed by air aspiration and capnography. Some authors recommend performing nasoendoscopy to verify the cannula's position in the larynx before initiating jet ventilation, although this procedure may be poorly tolerated.

Following preoxygenation by face mask, the patient is induced and an intermediate-duration muscle relaxant administered. Succinylcholine may be considered. The ability to perform face mask ventilation should be checked, followed by careful laryngoscopy. At this stage, it may be possible to pass a laser-resistant tracheal tube. If this is not possible, jet ventilation should commence, ensuring there is some upper airway patency by a jaw thrust type maneuver to allow gas egress. Following suspension laryngoscopy by the surgeon, TTJV at high frequency can be started using an automated ventilator. Initial settings would depend on the size of the patient and the anticipated lung compliance. Typical initial settings would be as follows: driving pressure (DP) 1 to 2 bar (15 to 30 psi), frequency 100 cycles per minute, inspiratory to expiratory (I:E) ratio of 1:2.5, pause pressure of 10 mbar, and an F_{IO_2} of 1.0. These settings can be adjusted depending on chest excursion and recoil. A reduction in the frequency is often required in these patients to allow sufficient time for expiration. The cut-out facility of the automated ventilator does not limit the first tidal volume given, and thus it is better to use low DPs initially and titrate up if required. Maintenance of anesthesia is with total intravenous anesthesia (TIVA).

3 What are the potential hazards and complications in regard to the airway?

The major concern with TTJV is barotrauma, with one study showing an 8.4% risk of surgical emphysema, 1% risk of pneumothorax, and 2.5% risk of pneumomediastinum. Additionally, the technique may result in suboptimal ventilation or aspiration, particularly if not properly executed. This risk appears to be greater for transtracheal compared with transglottal routes. This is because ingress of gases through the catheter is unimpeded, but egress may be limited by a combination of pathology, airway collapse, laryngospasm, and instrumentation. Misplaced or migrated cannulas and multiple puncture attempts increase the risk of developing barotrauma. Risk can be minimized by using an automated ventilator with cut-out facility (ie, when increased luminal pressure is detected) and ensuring adequate depth of anesthesia and analgesia, continuous muscle relaxation, and an open upper airway. Excellent communication between the surgeon and the anesthesia provider is needed to ensure that the removal of the suspension laryngoscope is anticipated and jet ventilation is stopped. If the suspension laryngoscope is removed for a significant length of time, an oral airway or supraglottic airway can be placed and jet ventilation resumed.

Other hazards include direct injury to the larynx and trachea, particularly with repeated punctures over the cricothyroid membrane. While failure of insertion is rare, complications such as bleeding, kinking, occlusion, and catheter displacement are more common. These issues are particularly prevalent in patients with abnormal anatomy, obesity, or when a nondedicated catheter, like an angiocatheter, is used. Proper technique and catheter selection are essential to minimize the risk. Most dedicated, commercial TTCs are made from fluoroplastic Teflon and therefore have low flammability. However, damage to the catheter with life-threatening consequences has been described following perforation and continued attempts at jet ventilation.

Oxygen desaturation and hypercapnia are other concerns. Risk factors for these complications include longer duration of surgery, use of laser (and therefore a low FIO_2), obesity, and preexisting chronic pulmonary disease.

4 Are there special considerations for the emergence or the end of the case?

Much depends on the success of the surgical procedure and if an immediate improvement in obstructive symptoms is anticipated. If minimal surgery has been possible or significant swelling anticipated, the need for postoperative tracheostomy should be discussed. If tracheostomy is deemed unnecessary but airway swelling still remains a concern, leaving the TTC in situ for 24 hours is advisable. In most cases, a significant improvement in the patency of the airway is attained, and ventilation via a face mask or SGA is straightforward. The TIVA infusion(s) is discontinued, the neuromuscular relaxation reversed, and the patient is allowed to recover spontaneous respirations.

- TTJV is an alternative means of oxygenation and ventilation.
- TTJV provides an unobstructed surgical view of the vocal cords and laryngeal structures.
- The transtracheal route carries a greater risk of barotrauma than other approaches to jet ventilation.
- TTJV should only be used in conjunction with an automated ventilator.
- *See Figures 81.1 and 81.2 for additional details.*

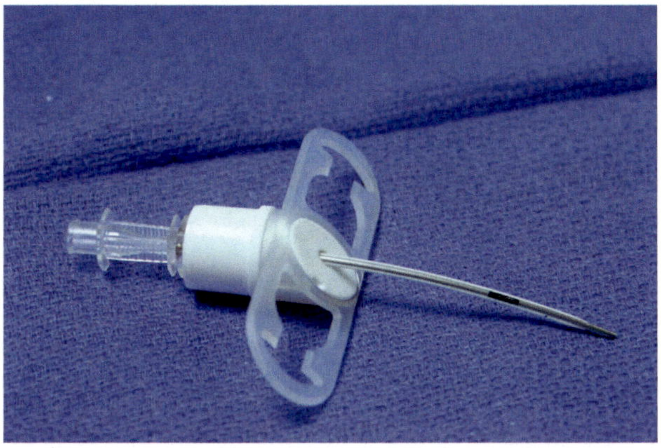

Figure 81.1. A Ravussin catheter is constructed with a precurved shaft. (See **Video 81.1.**)

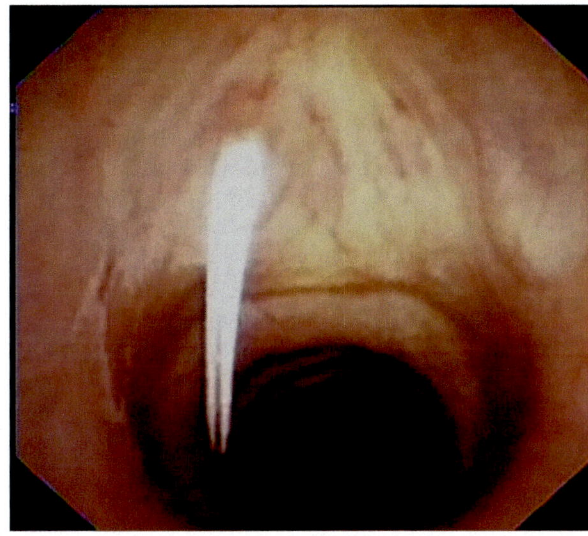

Figure 81.2. A translaryngeal catheter is seen coming through the cricothyroid membrane (**Video 81.2**). (Video courtesy of Dr. Jaime Hyman.)

Suggested Readings

Bourgain JL, Desruennes E, Fischler M, Ravussin P. Transtracheal high frequency jet ventilation for endoscopic airway surgery: a multicentre study. *Br J Anaesth*. 2001;87:870–875.

Cook TM, Alexander R. Major complications during anaesthesia for elective laryngeal surgery in the UK: a national survey of the use of high-pressure source ventilation. *Br J Anaesth*. 2008;101:266–272.

Evans E, Biro P, Bedforth N. Jet ventilation. Continuing education in anaesthesia. *Crit Care Pain*. 2007;7(1):2–5.

Ross-Anderson DJ, Ferguson C, Patel A. Transtracheal jet ventilation in 50 patients with severe airway compromise and stridor. *Br J Anaesth*. 2011;106(1):140–144.

82 Laser Airway Surgery

Felipe Urdaneta

Clinical Scenario: A 62-year-old male patient is scheduled to undergo microlaryngoscopy and removal of a vocal cord polyp with the use of CO_2 laser.

Introduction

Upper airway surgical techniques continue to evolve. Advances such as high-magnification operating microscopes, microlaryngoscopy equipment, robotic procedures, and lasers have created new challenges for anesthesia providers. The word laser is an acronym for light amplification by stimulated emission of radiation. Laser electromagnetic particles are high in density and monochromatic, coherent, and collimated, allowing large amounts of energy to be transferred to specific targets. Lasers allow more precision and better hemostasis with minimal postoperative edema and pain. Laser airway surgery requires close attention to airway management principles, the pathology being addressed, and any special equipment needed. Laser surgery is performed on a broad spectrum of patients. Some patients may present for surgery due to critical airway obstruction, while others present for treatment of phonation-related pathology.

1 What are the anesthetic and airway management considerations for this case?

The use of general anesthesia requires the implementation of advanced airway and ventilation strategies. The trachea may be intubated, or a "tubeless" technique is used. During the procedure, the patient may breathe spontaneously or ventilation is controlled with the use of neuromuscular blockers, which is more commonly used in the adult population if the airway lesion allows. In pediatrics, inhalational induction and maintenance of spontaneous ventilation are commonly used. In adults, intravenous induction and intubation using small-diameter endotracheal tubes and balanced general anesthesia with positive-pressure ventilation remains the most common anesthetic management. If jet ventilation is used instead of an endotracheal tube, total intravenous anesthesia is the appropriate anesthetic choice since inhaled agents cannot be administered via jet ventilators.

Airway fires should be a concern anytime a laser is used in the airway. An endotracheal tube is a potential "fuel source" for an airway fire. There are several methods used to lower the risk of airway fires during laser airway surgery:

1. Using FDA-approved laser-resistant endotracheal tubes (ETT). Laser-resistance grade implies that the ETT provides some degree of protection to airway fires but still remains vulnerable. Laser-resistance refers to the shaft of the ETT but not the cuff, which remains unprotected.
2. Intermittent apnea/extubation–reintubation. Patients are intubated with small-diameter ETTs and a technique of extubation–apnea–reintubation and ventilation is repeated until the laser portion of the surgery is completed.
3. Jet ventilation (supraglottic, subglottic, and transtracheal)

2 Potential hazards/complications with regard to the airway?

There are significant risks with the use of lasers for airway surgery. Laser system hazards by the laser beam can cause direct tissue injury (laryngeal and tracheal perforation, pneumothorax, pneumomediastinum, venous gas embolism, eye injury) or indirectly, including toxic waste from tissue vaporization and effects from the plume (odor, biohazard, and radiation). Plume content biohazard relates to the presence of fine particles, which can be toxic (mutagenic and teratogenic) and can contain genetic material of viral origin. Although there is no documented human transmission of papilloma from laser plum, proper evacuation of the plume is essential at the surgical site, and medical providers must wear special surgical masks throughout the procedure. As mentioned above, a major concern when using airway lasers is the possibility of airway fires. The exact incidence of ENT laser airway fires is unknown. Some airway fires are localized, causing minor thermal effects on the tissue surrounding the ETT. Airway fires can also involve the inside of ETTs. If the gas mixture inside the ETT is rich with an oxidizer such as O_2, the fire causes a "blowtorch effect" creating local and distal parenchymal damage, causing permanent disability and even death.

3 Are there special considerations for the emergence at the end of the case?

A smooth and safe extubation strategy must be planned ahead of time and in coordination with the surgical team. Airway surgery causes some degree of airway edema, which can lead to acute airway obstruction postoperatively if the edema is severe in an already vulnerable airway. Airway obstruction should be suspected if a patient develops stridor, especially inspiratory, and respiratory distress. Administration of IV dexamethasone and racemic epinephrine can be used in these situations. Other methods include (a) the exchange of the ETT for a supraglottic airway (Bailey maneuver), (b) The use of a short-acting opioid such as remifentanil by continuous infusion to prevent coughing during emergence from anesthesia, (c) the use of airway exchange catheters (AECs) in case there are concerns for reintubation. Delayed glottic and subglottic edema are potential side effects of laser surgery, so patients need to be monitored closely postoperatively. Respiratory distress may also be sign of other more rarer complications such as pneumothorax or pneumomediastinum.

- Lasers increase precision in targeting airway lesions, decrease bleeding and edema, and preserve surrounding structures. However, their use requires additional special equipment and more advanced airway management techniques.
- Airway fires are a main concern when using lasers for airway surgery.
- Airways fires are potentially fatal. Their prevention requires surgical and anesthetic planning, communication, vigilance, and an airway fire protocol if a fire inadvertently occurs in the OR.
- *See Figures 82.1 and 82.2 for additional details.*

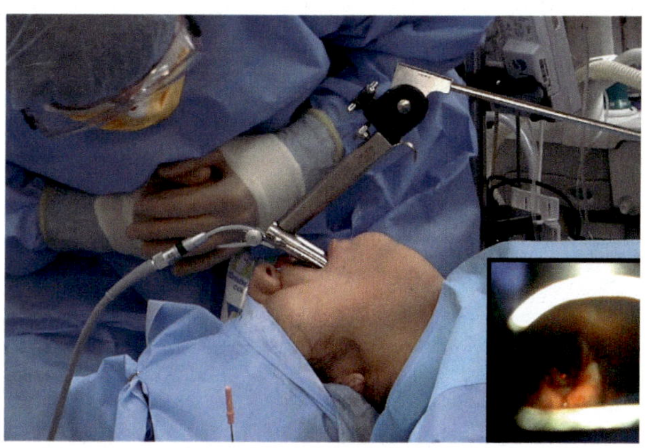

Figure 82.1. A patient in suspension laryngoscopy. (See also **Video 82.1.**)

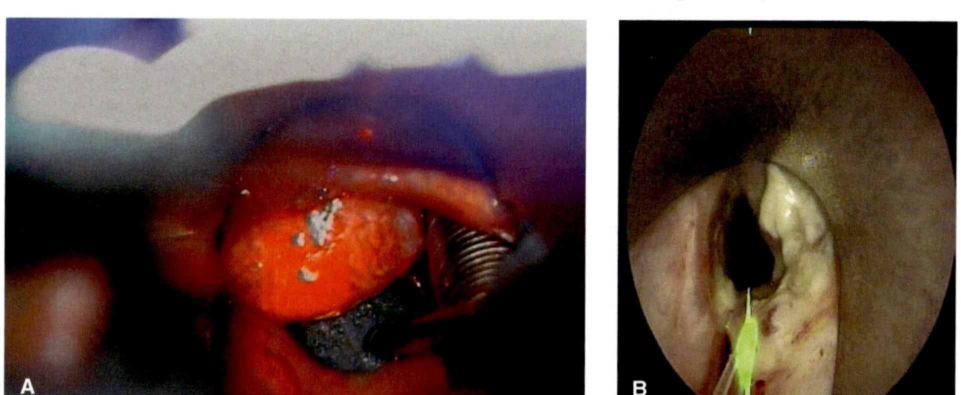

Figure 82.2. A: As seen through a suspension laryngoscope, a spatula is placed behind a mass in preparation for laser excision (**Video 82.2**). **B:** The light from a potassium titanyl phosphate (KPT) laser is seen (**Video 82.3**).

Suggested Readings

Burns JA, Adlard SD, Kobler JB, Tynan MA, Petrillo RH, Tracy LF. A comparison of laser-protected endotracheal tubes. *Otolaryngol Head Neck Surg*. 2018;159(5):871–878.

Roy S, Smith LP. Preventing and managing operating room fires in otolaryngology-head and neck surgery. *Otolaryngol Clin North Am*. 2019;52(1):163–171.

Swerdlow BN. Surgical smoke and the anesthesia provider. *J Anesth*. 2020;34(4):575–584.

Managing an Airway Fire

83

Ann Marie Melookaran Iliff

Clinical Scenario: A patient with a supraglottic mass is undergoing neodymium-doped yttrium aluminum garnet (Nd:YAG) laser-assisted resection of the mass. The surgeon suddenly yells "FIRE!"

1 What are the anesthetic and airway management considerations for this case?

Airway surgery involving lasers requires consideration of the risk of an airway fire. Airway fires are reported 550 to 650 times a year in the United States, but the actual number is most likely far higher. When the three elements necessary to start and propagate the fire (ignition/heat source, oxidizer, and fuel) are likely to interact in the airway, planning and preparation for prevention are essential. Once the fire occurs, actions aimed at limiting injury to the patient, as well as the OR staff, must be immediate. Once the fire is detected, one or more components of the "fire triad" (heat source, fuel, and an oxidizer) must immediately be removed from the airway. Postfire tracheal injuries with abnormal scarring or healing may lead to stenosis and airway obstruction.

If the source of the fire is the ETT, it should immediately be disconnected from the oxidizer source and simultaneously removed from the patient. In addition, water or saline should be poured in the mouth. If the fire is on the patient, it should be extinguished with saline. Singed paper drapes should be removed and thrown to the floor. Materials that continue to burn once removed from the patient (eg, paper drapes, the tracheal tube) should be dowsed with saline or treated with a carbon dioxide fire extinguisher. The availability of saline and the location of the fire extinguisher should be discussed during the preoperative "time-out."

2 How would you manage the airway in this case?

During the laser procedure, the lowest tolerable oxygen concentration should be used. This can be accomplished by blending oxygen with air, nitrogen, or helium via the anesthesia machine. Nitrous oxide should be avoided. Although the use of a low concentration of oxygen is good practice to reduce the risk of fires, it also reduces the safe apneic period when the tracheal tube is removed. After the burnt tracheal tube is removed, the airway should be inspected to ensure that no other burning material has been retained. The patient should be mask ventilated while the OR staff ensures that burning materials are removed from the vicinity of the patient and all fires are extinguished. If mask ventilation is not adequate, the airway should be rescued with an SGA. The patient will then need to be reintubated, and the airway should then be inspected with a flexible bronchoscope to assess any injuries to the trachea or to remove any foreign materials that may have been aspirated.

3 What are the surgical considerations that impact anesthetic management?

When airway laser surgery is planned, the surgical, anesthesia, and operating room staff should all be aware of the risk of airway fire and their individual roles in patient management should an airway fire occur. In the event of an airway fire, the removal of the burning tracheal tube and/or extinguishing of burning materials and the reestablishment of oxygenation and ventilation are priorities. Due to the nature of the surgery planned, there is a high possibility that the patient has a known difficult airway. This may now be complicated by burn injury, surgical debris, blood, and an incomplete surgical procedure (eg, retained mass), so the OR team must be prepared for a surgical airway. Help should be called for immediately in anticipation of difficulty with either upper airway management or invasive airway access.

4 What distinct airway device might be used in this case, and what are the special considerations?

Rubber endotracheal tubes wrapped or covered by foil, such as the Rusch LaserTubus, can be used with the Nd:YAG laser. The sponge jacket on the LaserTubus should be kept moist with saline. Saline, rather than air, should be used to fill the cuff. The cuff should be inflated adequately to prevent oxygen leakage into the area of laser or cautery use. If a tracheostomy is to occur, the anesthesia provider should advance the tracheal tube so the cuff is beyond the site of surgical interest.

5 Are there special considerations for the emergence at the end of the case?

Patients who experience an airway fire should remain intubated and will likely need to be admitted to the ICU postoperatively. If there is extensive airway damage, it may be beneficial to utilize a fiberoptic bronchoscope to inspect and assess the injury prior to extubation.

Author Caveats

If, from the outset, the site of surgical interest is the airway, special consideration should be given to the prevention of fire. Surgery of the airway often involves the use of heat sources such as electrocautery and lasers. Appropriate heat-resistant tracheal tubes should be used, but the surgeon should still be made aware that these materials can still burn with enough energy. Lasers should be placed on standby mode when not in use. Electrosurgery electrodes should not have rubber sleeves, should not be activated until the working tip is within the surgeon's view, and should be placed in a location away from the patient when not in use. Bipolar cautery should be used in lieu of monopolar settings. Facial and head hair can be prepared with surgical lubricant. The eyes, teeth, and skin should be protected from accidental laser discharge.

The OR team should know the location of an ABC fire extinguisher, and saline should be available on the surgical technician's table. A surgical airway kit should be in the room. If possible, the anesthesia provider should monitor the surgical use of the heat source (eg, observing tracheal tube location and proximity to the heat source via secondary microscope monitors).

- Airway fire prevention and the emergency plan in case a fire does occur should be discussed at the surgical time-out.
- At the first recognition of a fire, immediately remove components of the fire triad (ignition source, fuel, oxidizer) from the airway.
- Extinguishing any burning materials and reestablishing the patient's airway are the main priorities in airway fire management.
- Once the fire is extinguished and the patient is stabilized, the airway should be examined for any remaining debris and to determine the extent of injury.
- *See Figure 83.1 and* ***Video 83.1*** *for additional details.*

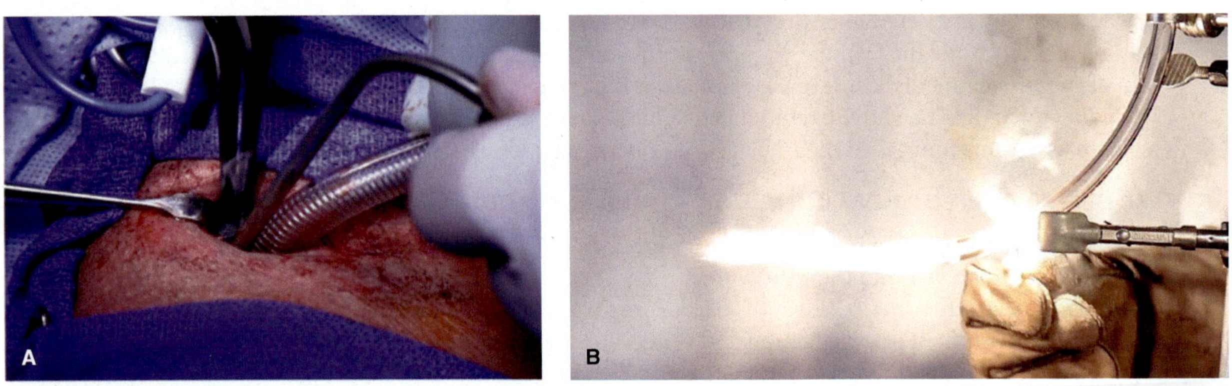

Figure 83.1. A: LaserFlex LASER-resistant tracheal tube is seen passing through a laryngeal stoma. **B:** Demonstration of a PVC tracheal tube fire when 100% oxygen is used and heat is applied to a puncture site.

Suggested Readings

Akhtar N, Ansar F, Baig MS, Abbas A. Airway fires during surgery: management and prevention. *J Anaesthesiol Clin Pharmacol.* 2016;32(1):109–111.

Apfelbaum JL, Caplan RA, Barker SJ, et al. Practice advisory for the prevention and management of operating room fires: an updated report by the American Society of Anesthesiologists Task Force on Operating Room Fires. *Anesthesiology.* 2013; 118(2):271–290.

Pozin IE, Zabida A, Friedman Z, et al. Simulation training results in performance retention for the management of airway fires: a prospective observational study. *Anaesth Intensive Care.* 2023;51(2):114–119.

Aintree Catheter Use for Supraglottic Airway to Endotracheal Tube Conversion

84

Lauren C. Berkow

Clinical Scenario: You are asked to assist in the tracheal intubation of a patient in the emergency room. After several attempts at direct laryngoscopy by both paramedics and the emergency medicine staff, a first-generation supraglottic airway (SGA) was placed and the patient is being ventilated.

1 What are the anesthetic and airway management considerations for this case?

In the emergency department setting, patients who require airway management nearly always require tracheal intubation. Though many other clinical situations can be managed with supraglottic ventilation, these patients are typically at high risk for gastric content aspiration. The decision to remove the SGA and attempt intubation by other means (eg, video laryngoscopy) in the current case should not be taken lightly. The tissues of the upper airway have likely suffered trauma from multiple intubation attempts. In this case, even an "easy" airway may be difficult to secure by direct or indirect laryngoscopy. In addition, the patient is being oxygenated and ventilated successfully with the SGA, which stabilizes the situation. If the decision is made to intubate, a technique that allows gas exchange through the SGA during the procedure should be considered. Finally, should tracheal intubation fail, providing a means for facilitating SGA return or providing oxygenation during performance of a surgical airway (if needed) is desirable.

2 How would you manage the airway in this case?

There are several approaches to exchange an SGA for a tracheal tube. Not all have the desired features noted above.

A well-described technique uses the SGA as a conduit for intubation with the aid of an Aintree Intubation Catheter (AIC) (Cook Medical, Bloomington, IN). The AIC is a hollow-bore, stiff plastic catheter with an inner diameter of 4.8 mm. The AIC can be fitted over a FIS of not more than 4.2 mm outer diameter (OD). The FIS is then inserted into the trachea using the SGA as a conduit. Once the midtrachea is visualized, the AIC is positioned likewise and the FIS is removed. Though oxygenation and ventilation are often halted to allow FIS-AIS placement, the assemblage can also be inserted via a bronchoscope circuit adaptor, thereby allowing uninterrupted gas exchange. The SGA is then removed leaving the AIC in situ. A tracheal tube sized 6.5 OD or larger can then be passed over the AIC and into the trachea. Oxygen can also be insufflated through the AIC lumen via either a 15-mm airway adaptor or a Luer-lock adaptor packaged with the AIC. This might be necessary if some obstruction to tracheal tube placement is encountered.

As an alternative to instrumentation via the SGA, the anesthesia provider might consider removal of the SGA and attempting direct, video, or FIS-aided intubation. As discussed previously, the operator may encounter an intrinsically difficult airway with edema or airway trauma from previous intubation attempts, and this approach does not allow for continuous or backup gas exchange.

Blind or FIS-aided intubation via the indwelling SGA may also be attempted. In this approach, it may be difficult or even impossible to remove the SGA after successful intubation or to adequately secure the tracheal tube due to the overall length of the SGA.

Retrograde wire intubation techniques have also been described in this situation. After preparation of the skin, a hollow bore needle is percutaneously inserted into the larynx via the cricothyroid membrane. A wire, at least twice the length of the tracheal tube to be used, is inserted via the needle, which is aimed in a rostral direction. The wire will often emerge from the barrel of the SGA. If the SGA is poorly positioned, it may emerge laterally to the device or not at all due to obstruction. Once the wire is retrieved from the mouth, the SGA is removed and a small tracheal tube inserted over the wire. The wire is then removed via the upper airway.

If the appropriate equipment is not available or significant airway trauma has occurred, a surgical airway may be the appropriate next step. If the indwelling SGA is functioning to maintain oxyhemoglobin saturation and ventilation, a surgical airway can be performed under controlled conditions. If, on the other hand, gas exchange is inadequate, an emergency cricothyrotomy should be considered.

3 What are the potential hazards and complications in regard to the airway?

In the current case, the airway has most likely been traumatized by previous attempts at intubation, and there may be tissue edema, blood, and traumatic debris in the airway. These factors may contribute to difficulty or even failure with SGA-to-tracheal tube exchange. Likewise, in a full-stomach patient, there is a persistent risk of gastric contents aspiration (if it has not already occurred). Hang-up may occur when either the AIC mounted on the FIS or the tracheal tube mounted on the AIC is passed into the airway. Rotating the tracheal tube 90 degrees counterclockwise and/or performing a jaw thrust can often facilitate advancement of the AIC or tracheal tube. At any point in the procedure, gas exchange may be lost due to displacement of the SGA or failure to place the tracheal tube.

4 Are there special considerations for the emergence or the end of the case?

As discussed previously, the airway of this patient must be considered traumatized. When it is clinically appropriate to extubate, strict extubation precautions should be exercised.

- An airway rescued after multiple previous intubation attempts should be considered traumatized.
- Although not an ideal airway in this case, the indwelling SGA does provide oxygenation and ventilation and should not be removed without much consideration.
- The Aintree Intubating Catheter in conjunction with a FIS provides a safe method for converting an SGA to an endotracheal tube conversion (ETT).
- Strict extubation precautions must be exercised.
- *See Figures 84.1 and 84.2 for additional details.*

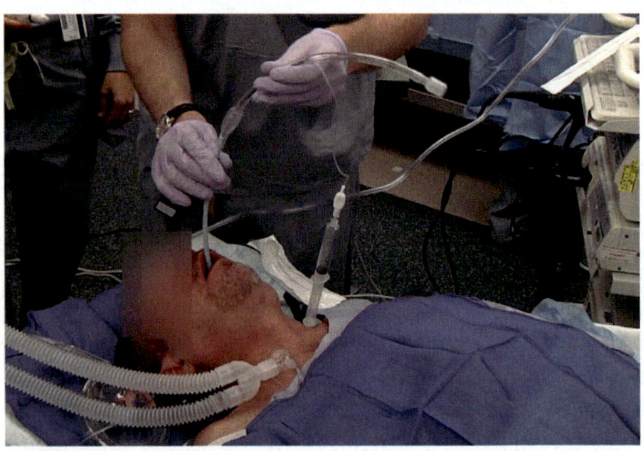

Figure 84.1. After placing an Aintree catheter with the aid of a flexible intubation scope, a tracheal tube is advanced into the airway. (See **Video 84.1.**)

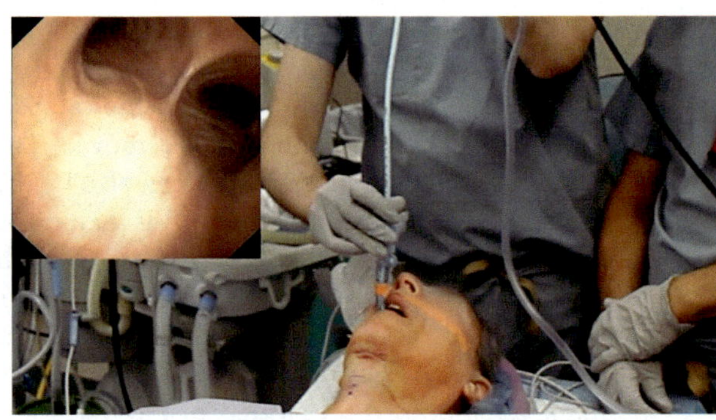

Figure 84.2. A flexible intubation scope is used to advance an Aintree catheter into position about the carina (**Video 84.2**).

Suggested Readings

Berkow LC, Schwartz JM, Kan K, Corridore M, Heitmiller ES. Use of the laryngeal mask airway-Aintree Intubating Catheter-fiberoptic bronchoscope technique for difficult intubation. *J Clin Anesth*. 2011;23:534–539.

Cook TM, Seller C, Gupta K, Thornton M, O'Sullivan E. Non-conventional uses of the Aintree Intubating Catheter in management of the difficult airway. *Anaesthesia*. 2007;62:169–174.

James GI, Williams D. Challenges with tracheal tube exchange using a flexible bronchoscope and an Aintree Intubation Catheter. *Anaesth Rep*. 2021;9(1):120–121.

Wong DT, Yang JJ, Mak HY, Jagannathan N. Use of intubation introducers through a supraglottic airway to facilitate tracheal intubation: a brief review. *Can J Anesth*. 2012;59:704–715.

Management of the Previously Surgically Manipulated Larynx

85

Boris Paskhover • Guy Talmor

Clinical Scenario: A 64-year-old former smoker who has undergone hemilaryngectomy for vocal cord cancer, now presents with a bowel obstruction and is scheduled for an urgent laparotomy.

1 What are the anesthetic and airway management considerations for this case?

Conservation laryngeal surgery is used to preserve the function of the larynx in patients presenting with early-stage squamous cell carcinoma. The patient may have undergone a variety of procedures that could alter the structure of the upper aerodigestive tract and impede routine airway management. With the patient presenting for urgent surgery, the anesthesia provider should assume that significant changes in the upper airway exist.

First, an attempt should be made to clarify the details of the prior surgery. Likewise, prior anesthetic records may reveal information regarding the ease or difficulty of past management, including endotracheal intubation. Though obstructive lesions may have been removed during prior surgery, changes in architecture, edema of the remaining structures, and changes related to radiation therapy may complicate management. The laryngeal structures may be difficult to recognize or delineate from other anatomy. Landmarks frequently used in standard orotracheal intubation may be absent. Restrictions in the laryngeal inlet may also prevent the passage of a normally sized tracheal tube. Changes to tissues remote from the larynx (eg, submentum, tongue) may impede tongue displacement for direct or indirect laryngoscopy.

Endoscopic transoral laryngeal-preserving procedures are often performed with either laser or transoral robotic resection of laryngeal structures. Classically, this group of procedures includes partial endoscopic cordectomies, which involve the removal of mucosa and possibly the underlying musculature of the vocal cords. A "supraglottic laryngectomy" may include procedures on the false cords, aryepiglottic folds, and/or epiglottis.

Open procedures on the upper airway include vertical partial laryngectomy, often termed "hemilaryngectomy"—the larynx is approached anteriorly with a vertical en bloc excision of the tumor, most often sacrificing one vocal cord with or without inclusion of the arytenoid cartilage.

Last, there are variations on horizontal laryngeal conserving surgeries. The supracricoid laryngectomy with cricohyoidoepiglottopexy often involves removal of both vocal cords with preservation of one arytenoid unit and surgical removal of structures up to the hyoid. An open supraglottic laryngectomy involves removal of the supraglottic structures with preservation of the vocal cords.

2 How would you manage the airway in this case?

For the anesthesia provider caring for these patients, an understanding of the patient's prior surgical procedures (via past medical records or a discussion with the head and neck surgeon) may be helpful but inadequate. A detailed physical examination can provide useful details. An intraoral examination with manual palpation of the oral cavity and tongue base may detect the presence of a tumor. Fibrosis of the skin of the neck is a sign of prior radiation therapy, which frequently results in changes to the upper aerodigestive tract. Given that the majority of partial laryngectomy procedures are performed due to oncologic indications, it is imperative that the patient's full oncologic history is reviewed. Recent imaging including computed tomography (CT) and positron emission tomography (PET) should be closely examined. Patients lost to follow-up with no recent imaging are at risk of tumor recurrence, and the possibility of an obstructive lesion in larynx should be ruled out prior to proceeding. Asking the otolaryngologist to document a preoperative fiberoptic laryngoscopy is reasonable but may not be practical in an urgent presentation for non-airway surgery. The anesthesia provider should consider performing their own upper airway endoscopy if possible. Regardless of who performs the preoperative endoscopy, the following information should be documented: (1) Are there obstructions to a single, anatomic plane of access to the larynx? (2) Are there lesions or architectural changes which might prevent the placement or seating of an SGA (in case one should be needed for emergency ventilation)? (3) Are there lesions or architectural changes which might be traumatized during airway manipulation? A positive answer to any of these three questions should lead the anesthesia provider to consider the following: (1) Should specialized equipment be available at the bedside prior to the induction of anesthesia? (2) Should awake intubation be pursued? (3) Should awake surgical airway be pursued, or should a qualified surgical team be made immediately available for an emergency surgical airway, should efforts at upper airway cannulation fail?

Last, any suspicious findings or bleeding during upper endoscopy or airway manipulation may represent malignant recurrence and should be brought to the attention of the patient's otolaryngologist.

3 What are the potential hazards and complications in regard to the airway?

Apart from failure to secure the airway in a timely manner, other hazards exist when managing these patients. Alterations in the complex functions of the normal larynx, upper esophagus, and hypopharynx may result in the regurgitation and aspiration of gastric contents after minimal sedation during awake intubation or awake tracheostomy. Trauma to an occult recurrence of the prior airway malignancy may result in significant bleeding, obscuring attempts to visualize and secure the airway.

4 What distinct airway device might be used in this case, and what are the special considerations?

As discussed above, if the anesthesia provider's evaluation results in a suspicion that airway management may be difficult, advanced equipment should be prepared at the bedside. The provider may also seek the consultation of personnel experienced in the case of such patients. It is not unreasonable to delay the surgical procedure (if possible) until a qualified surgeon is available at the bedside to perform an elective tracheostomy or to stand by in case of failure to secure the upper airway. In the latter situation, skin marking of the surface landmarks of the larynx, the injection of local anesthetic and vasoconstrictor drugs into the skin over the trachea, and setup of surgical cautery and suction are often undertaken prior to the induction of anesthesia or efforts at awake intubation.

5 Are there special considerations for the emergence or the end of the case?

If airway management proved to be at all difficult during the induction of anesthesia or if significant changes in the airway architecture were found during airway visualization, strict extubation precautions should be exercised. Even if tracheal intubation is straightforward, these patients may be at risk of extubation failure and postextubation aspiration of gastric contents due to functional changes in the upper aerodigestive tract.

- Prior oncologic surgery and radiation may result in significant changes to the airway, which may hinder both routine and advanced management efforts.
- An effort must be made to delineate airway changes through the examination of past records or direct communication with the patient's otolaryngologist.
- Preoperative endoscopy may be performed by an otolaryngologist or the anesthesia provider to define the current airway architecture.
- Securing a surgical airway prior to the induction of anesthesia or having a qualified surgeon on "standby" during attempts at upper airway cannulation are both reasonable approaches.
- Suspicious findings in the airway, including bleeding during manipulation, should be reported to the patient's oncologic surgeon.
- *See Figures 85.1 and 85.2 for additional details.*

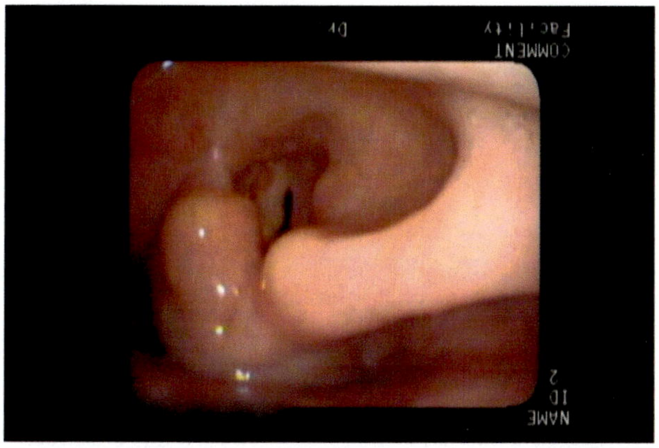

Figure 85.1. In this patient who underwent a hemilaryngectomy, the left-sided aryepiglottic fold is missing [**Video 85.1**].

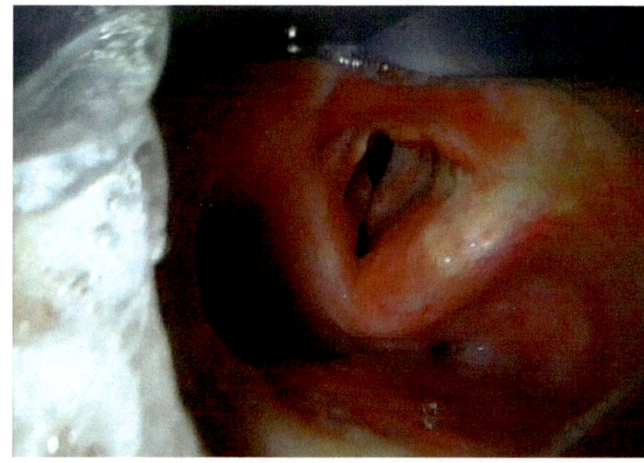

Figure 85.2. In this patient with a history of epiglottic cancer, the epiglottis has been removed and the results of radiation therapy can be appreciated [**Video 85.2**].

Suggested Readings

Apfelbaum JL, Hagberg CA, Connis RT, et al. 2022 American Society of Anesthesiologists Practice Guidelines for management of the difficult airway. *Anesthesiology*. 2022;136(1):31–81.

Rosenblatt WH, Ianus AI, Sukhupragarn W, Fickenscher A, Sasaki C. Preoperative endoscopic airway examination (PEAE) provides superior airway information and may reduce the use of unnecessary awake intubation. *Anesth Analg*. 2011;112:602–607.

Weinstein GS, Laccourreye O, Rassekh CH, et al. Conservation laryngeal surgery. In: Flint PW, Haughey BH, Lund VJ, et al., eds. *Cummings Otolaryngology: Head and Neck Surgery*. 5th ed. Mosby Elsevier; 2010:1539–1562.

86 Free Tissue Transfer Surgery

David W. Healy

Clinical Scenario: A 65-year-old male presents with a 4-cm left mandibular mass. He is scheduled for tracheostomy, mandibular resection, and free tissue transfer from the fibula. Pain restricts his mouth opening to 2 cm, and he has been unable to eat solid food recently, leading to significant weight loss. He is 5′11″ tall, weighs 136 lb, and has a BMI of 19. He has been smoking for 50 years but quit 2 weeks ago after his diagnosis. His medical history includes well-controlled hypertension and atrial fibrillation treated with radio-ablation 2 years ago.

1 What are the anesthetic and airway management considerations for this case?

A perioperative nutritional assessment and interventions such as dietitian referrals and consideration of supplemental feeding can improve patient outcomes in malnourished patients such as this one. Preoperative cessation of tobacco is recommended, with consideration for the use of a nicotine patch through recovery. Evaluating and managing alcohol withdrawal syndrome may mitigate adverse outcomes, including withdrawal phenomena during recovery. Head and neck pathology and neck radiation changes can impair the ability to perform mask ventilation and tracheal intubation. In each case, a thorough airway risk assessment informed by available preprocedural nasoendoscopy and radiologic imaging must be performed. Communication between the anesthesia and surgical teams regarding optimal airway management strategies is essential. Limited mouth opening due to the tumor location or temporomandibular joint involvement may complicate airway management. Poor tissue mobility and friability from prior neck radiation pose additional risks for procedural failure.

2 How would you manage the airway in this case?

The decision to manage the patient's airway before or after inducing anesthesia is made after careful evaluation and communication between anesthesia and surgical teams. In the patient in the scenario, the author would recommend an awake endoscopic intubation using a low-dose remifentanil infusion (0.02 µg/kg/min) for sedation after adequate topicalization has been performed. After induction of anesthesia and successful intubation, a temporary tracheostomy is commonly created in the context of extensive facial and/or airway surgery. To avoid airway fires, constant communication between the surgical team and anesthesia provider is essential during tracheostomy creation. An armored tracheal tube can be placed through the fresh stoma until the procedure's conclusion, when it is then replaced with a regular tracheostomy device.

3 What are the surgical considerations that impact anesthetic management?

The anesthetic plan must take into consideration all portions of the surgery, including tumor resection, tissue and functional reconstruction, and closure. Given the high prevalence of pathology-related factors impacting the ability to ventilate and/or intubate in this patient population, awake airway management techniques that maintain spontaneous ventilation should always be carefully considered. These techniques include awake endoscopic intubation, awake video laryngoscopy, or awake tracheostomy. Effective communication between the surgical and anesthesia teams is crucial in comprehending the surgical plan and regulating the patient's physiologic parameters throughout the procedure. The surgical team must clearly state the specific areas and laterality for tissue transfer which is vital information when placing intravenous and arterial lines. This communication not only enhances patient safety but also prevents the unnecessary placement of lines and facilitates an uninterrupted workflow. An arterial line allows close monitoring and optimization of the patient's blood pressure, hematocrit, and volume status.

During extended periods of surgical preparation, dissection, or reconstruction with limited surgical stimulation but a need for immobility and cardiovascular stability, vasopressors are often necessary to maintain adequate tissue perfusion. However, their use is still debated due to potential vasoconstriction in transposed tissue, which has not been supported by studies. Thus, current recommendations advise using vasopressors judiciously after identifying and addressing factors contributing to hypotension, such as hypovolemia, deep anesthesia, anemia, and electrolyte imbalances. To reduce the risk of free flap failure caused by venous engorgement and tissue edema, it is advised to avoid fluid overload. Maintaining hematocrit levels between 24 and 28 and a transfusion trigger of 24 is also recommended in the absence of myocardial disease.

During parotid or thyroid resections or neck dissections, it may be necessary to monitor nerve function. Before beginning the procedure, the surgical team must be informed if muscle relaxants were used for tracheal intubation and tracheostomy creation. For extended surgeries, some anesthesiologists administer a potent opioid infusion (such as sufentanil at 0.3 μg/kg/h or remifentanil at 0.05 to 0.3 μg/kg/min) to maintain immobility and tracheal tube tolerance. Please note; if relying on sufentanil, sufficient time must be allowed for the drug to approach a steady plasma state before relying on its ability to prevent response to surgical stimulation.

4 Are there special considerations for the emergence or the end of the case?

Following head and neck procedures that involve extensive tissue resection and reconstruction, a smooth emergence from anesthesia is important to minimize coughing or bucking on the endotracheal tube. In addition, blood pressure should be closely monitored as uncontrolled hypertension can result in hematoma formation at the tissue transfer site, potentially compromising tissue perfusion and airway patency. To ensure patient comfort and stable hemodynamics during emergence, multimodal analgesia including opioids plus adjunct medications such as a dexmedetomidine infusion (0.2 to 0.7 μg/kg/h) can be utilized.

If a surgical airway has been performed, the armored tube is replaced with a regular tracheostomy tube or stoma obturator at the end of the procedure. This airway device exchange is a stimulating procedure that demands a careful balance between allowing the return of spontaneous ventilation and preventing coughing and bucking, especially if the chosen airway lacks a cuff (stoma obturator or uncuffed tract). Anesthetic agents should be titrated appropriately to prevent overstimulation during this procedure.

The anesthesia, surgical, and postoperative teams must communicate clearly and effectively when planning for extubation with the potential for reintubation. Standardized notes in the electronic health record, clear patient handoffs, and bedside equipment availability and signage should be used to enhance this communication. At the end of the case, patients should be breathing spontaneously with adequately maintained minute ventilation. Postoperative care requires specialized attention and monitoring, which can be provided in an ICU or floor setting with appropriate surveillance and skilled nursing.

- A comprehensive preoperative assessment should include evaluating nutritional status, tobacco use, and potential alcohol withdrawal syndrome with necessary interventions.
- It is recommended that a thorough airway risk assessment be conducted before any procedure, taking into account information available from endoscopic evaluation and radiologic imaging.
- Over administration of IV fluids should be avoided, and hematocrit levels should be monitored and maintained between 24% and 28%.
- To minimize coughing and hemodynamic instability during emergence, the use of long-acting opioids or supplemental infusions such as dexmedetomidine may be beneficial.
- The surgical and anesthesia care teams should discuss plans for extubation and reintubation (if needed) before emergence.
- *See Figure 86.1 and* **Video 86.1** *for additional details.*

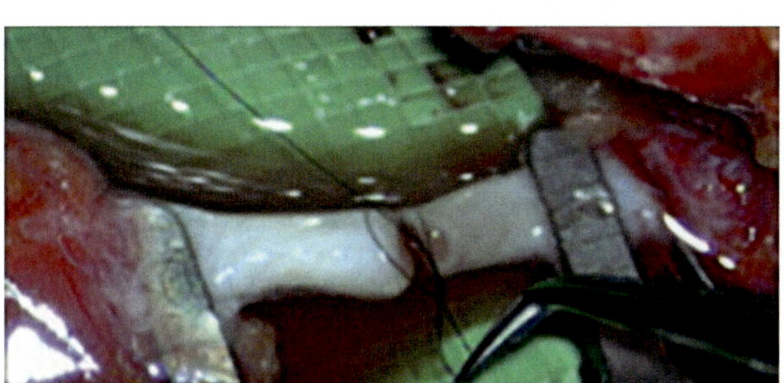

Figure 86.1. Arterial vascular anastomosis in progress during a free tissue transfer implant.

Suggested Readings

Healy DW, Cloyd BH, Straker T, et al. Expert consensus statement on the perioperative management of adult patients undergoing head and neck surgery and free tissue reconstruction from the society for head and neck anesthesia. *Anesth Analg*. 2021;133:274–283.

Kheterpal S, Healy D, Aziz MF, et al; Multicenter Perioperative Outcomes Group (MPOG) Perioperative Clinical Research Committee. Incidence, predictors, and outcome of difficult mask ventilation combined with difficult laryngoscopy: a report from the multicenter perioperative outcomes group. *Anesthesiology*. 2013;119:1360–1369.

Dental Restoration

87

Andrew Herlich • Paul J. Schwartz

Clinical Scenario: A 24-year-old man with severe cognitive delay requires dental restoration. Apart from very poor dentition and a difficult exam (refuses to open his mouth), he appears to have an otherwise normal airway. He is obese with a BMI of 30, and he snores loudly but has never been evaluated for sleep apnea because of his cognitive deficiencies.

1 What are the anesthetic/airway management considerations for this case?

Prior to making any anesthetic plans, the anesthesiologist and the dentist must confer as to the dental care plan. An accurate medical history and a physical examination within the limits of patient cooperation should be obtained. If available, previous anesthetic records are helpful in formulating an anesthetic plan. Preoperative sedation for this patient population may pose a number of obstacles. In the cognitively challenged patient, the ability to perform preoperative intravenous insertion is unpredictable. In an obese patient who likely has obstructive sleep apnea, soft tissue obstruction from standard sedatives such as intravenous midazolam or opioids is potentially troublesome. Moderate or deep sedation in this uncooperative patient population is typically inadequate to provide anesthesia to perform necessary procedures. Fortunately, these patients usually are accompanied by a caretaker who is familiar with the patient's medical history and activities of daily living. These caregivers, who often provide a calming influence on these patients, can be helpful in the administration of preoperative sedation. It is frequently difficult for this patient population to cooperate with awake IV placement. Intramuscular ketamine administered possibly combined with midazolam, glycopyrrolate, or atropine is a preoperative sedative option. Another suitable alternative is oral or intranasal midazolam. These sedatives will likely be administered in the holding area/waiting room or occasionally outside of the hospital with constant supervision. If an IV is placed preoperatively, titrated doses of dexmedetomidine is another reasonable sedation technique that is associated with less respiratory obstruction. The anesthesiologist should be prepared to monitor the patient and manage the airway at any time after the sedation is administered until the patient is safely transported to the operating room or dental operatory.

If an inhalation induction of anesthesia is the only choice, additional personnel help will likely be needed to provide gentle but firm restraint if cooperation from the patient is not likely. Alternatives to traditional mask inhalation induction include a "game" approach using either the elbow or Y-piece of the breathing circle (without the mask) and having the patient breathe the anesthetic gases as if they were snorkeling. This technique is very effective with mask-phobic patients who are also needle phobic.

Once induction and initial airway management have been completed, the use of additional long-acting neuromuscular blocking agents is unwarranted. Additional fixed agents, such as opioids or sedatives, may make emergence less predictable. In addition to any local anesthetic agents administered by the dentist, adjuvant agents such as intravenous acetaminophen or ketorolac as supplements are ideal. Bilateral inferior alveolar nerve blocks, in addition to local infiltration of the maxilla, may create some dysphoria for the patient if they are unable to sense the structures in the mouth. The patient may not be able to sense that they are biting their tongue.

After emergence from general anesthesia, the patient is likely to have a rapid transition from recovery to discharge if additional opioids and sedatives such as midazolam are avoided.

Finally, postoperative nausea and vomiting are rarely problematic in these cases. However, administration of ondansetron and dexamethasone are helpful to further prevent postoperative nausea and vomiting.

2 How would you manage the airway in this case?

Nasotracheal intubation is traditionally the preferred route of tracheal intubation for dental cases. Oxymetazoline spray requires a minimum of 10 to 15 minutes to exert its maximal affect. In the uncooperative, awake patient, application of nasal sprays may sometimes be difficult or impossible. Epistaxis is most often caused by the tracheal tube bevel traumatizing the mucosal surfaces of the nose. This trauma can be reduced with the use of a nasogastric (NG) sump malleable guide. The NG sump is inserted into the tracheal tube so that it extends beyond the bevel by 9 to 12 inches. After induction of anesthesia, both nares should be lubricated with surgical gel. When the patient is ready for tracheal intubation, the NG sump is inserted into the nostril and advanced gently until it is in the pharynx. The nasotracheal tube is advanced over the NG tube into the pharynx and the NG sump is removed. Finally, laryngoscopy is performed and the nasotracheal tube is advanced into the glottis under direct vision.

If nasotracheal intubation is not possible, orotracheal intubation or use of a flexible laryngeal mask are alternatives. The disadvantage of oral intubation is the requisite moving of the tube in the mouth during the procedure and testing of the occlusion after restoration. Folding the barrel of the flexible supraglottic airway into the mouth during occlusion testing has been described.

3 What are the surgical considerations that impact anesthetic management?

It is important to remember that most dental care is not emergent. The anesthesia provider should be empowered to delay a case if medical history, oral intake status, or other physical findings initiate any concerns.

Finally, economic considerations will likely dictate the location of such care in the future. Hospital costs have become relatively prohibitive for dental care and will force such care into ambulatory care centers, dental schools, and the office-based setting. As a result, the most challenging of this patient population may not get care due to the anesthetic challenges in the office-based or ambulatory care setting.

4 What distinct airway device (eg, specialized tracheal tube, rigid bronchoscope, bronchial blocker) might be used in this case, and what are the special considerations?

Preformed nasotracheal tubes, preformed orotracheal tubes, standard endotracheal tubes or flexible laryngeal masks are the airway devices of choice and necessity. Although the nasal route is preferred, the oral route and its appropriate tubes are also satisfactory alternatives.

5 Are there special considerations for the emergence or the end of the case?

Administration of intravenous opioids prior to emergence from anesthesia is often not necessary if local anesthetics have been administered by the dentist. As previously stated, these opioids and benzodiazepines may delay emergence and discharge.

- Preanesthetic discussion with the operating dentist is important to gaining the best understanding of the unique requirements for each patient.
- Nasotracheal intubation is almost always preferred in dental cases.
- Minimize opioid and benzodiazepines as much as possible. Adjuncts such as local anesthetics, dexmedetomidine, acetaminophen, and intravenous nonsteroidal medications will improve analgesia and shorten time to discharge from the PACU.
- *See Figure 87.1 and* ***Video 87.1*** *for additional details.*

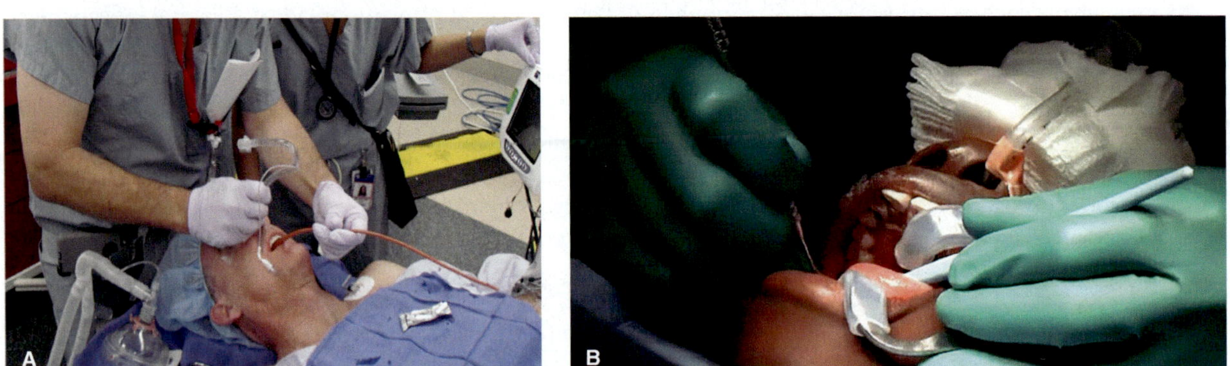

Figure 87.1. A: Nasotracheal intubation being performed for a dental restoration case (**Video 87.1**). **B:** Dental restoration in a child.

Suggested Readings

Brimacombe J, Binn B. Malocclusion testing with the flexible laryngeal mask airway. *Anaesthesia*. 2002;57:410.

Herlich A, Cladis FP, Studen-Pavlovich D, et al. Anesthesia for pediatric dentistry. In: Davis PJ, Cladis FP, eds. *Smith's Anesthesia for Infants and Children*. 10th ed. Elsevier Mosby; 2022:1132–1147.

Rashewsky S, Parameswaran A, Sloane C, Ferguson F, Epstein R. Time and cost analysis: pediatric dental rehabilitation with general anesthesia in the office and the hospital settings. *Anesth Prog*. 2012;59:147–153.

Wong A. Treatment planning considerations for adult oral rehabilitation cases in the operating room. *Dent Clin N Am*. 2009;53:255–267.

88 Cleft Palate Surgery

Andrew Herlich • Paul J. Schwartz

Clinical Scenario: On an international plastic surgery mission trip, you are caring for a 4-year-old child with a cleft palate. His cleft lip was repaired the previous year.

1 What are the anesthetic/airway management considerations for this case?

When evaluating a child with cleft disorders, the anesthesiologist must consider associated comorbidities. Prior to planning the anesthetic, the anesthesiologist and surgeon should have a discussion regarding the surgical needs and approach.

Patients who present with both a cleft lip and cleft palate often have a syndrome disorder such as fetal alcohol, Crouzon, CHARGE Sequence, or holoprosencephaly. These syndromes can also affect the brain, face, cervical spine, and heart. Syndromal patterns such as Pierre–Robin sequence, Treacher–Collins syndrome, or Klippel–Feil sequence are associated with cleft palate alone. Facial asymmetry, micrognathia, and macroglossia may make inhalational induction and mask ventilation extremely challenging. Many practitioners will choose to maintain spontaneous ventilation via an inhalation technique until intravenous access and the airway are secured. Gentle but continuous positive airway pressure during mask induction will be helpful in maintaining airway patency and reducing early oxygen desaturation.

The anesthesiologist should also anticipate the possibility of difficult laryngoscopy. Anatomic findings such as microstomia, exposure of the nasal passages, clefting of the soft palate and uvula, as well as relative glossomegaly or glossoptosis can contribute to difficult laryngoscopy. The premaxillary segment may be rotated and malformed. The laryngoscope can also slip into the cleft and cause soft tissue damage. A moistened gauze square placed into the cleft may reduce such trauma. In patients with bilateral clefts, the premaxillary segment may be mobile prior to any airway maneuvers and subject to fracture or avulsion if care is not taken. A hard gum or acrylic shield may aid intubation and reduce laryngeal trauma.

Associated limb anomalies may make intravenous access challenging as well. The anesthesiologist must be creative to obtain intravenous access if the patient has arthrogrypotic limbs.

During the maintenance phase of anesthesia, opioids should be used judiciously. Mechanical ventilation to eliminate volatile agents at the end of the procedure may be quite helpful since residual volatile agent is the most frequent cause of hypoventilation in the postanesthesia recovery unit. Analgesics such as intravenous acetaminophen or acetaminophen suppositories are helpful additions to the analgesic plan. In addition, maxillary nerve blocks that include the anterior alveolar nerve, palatal blocks, sphenopalatine blocks, and local tissue infiltration with longer-acting local anesthetics such as bupivacaine may reduce the need for postoperative opioids.

2 How would you manage the airway in this case?

The airway requires an orotracheal approach to facilitate the surgery. Direct laryngoscopy with a Wis–Hippel design laryngoscope may be less traumatic than other pediatric blades. Thanks to technological advancements in airway management, video laryngoscopy (VL) using a pediatric blade or flexible intubation scope are reasonable approaches that help reduce trauma during laryngoscopy.

Alternatively, a supraglottic airway (SGA) may be initially inserted. Subsequent tracheal intubation through the SGA using a flexible intubation scope may be used. Once the orotracheal tube is secured in the trachea, the laryngeal mask can be carefully removed. A preformed orotracheal tube (RAE) is often used in the management of cleft lip and palate surgery. Alternatively, a flexible, armored orotracheal tube can be used but may have a propensity for becoming dislodged at the level of the glottis. The dislodging of the armored tube may be reduced by the use of a throat pack.

The flexible SGA has also been described for cleft surgery. However, this technique must be used with great care since careless SGA removal may cause avulsion of a pharyngeal flap or disruption of the palatal suture line. The placement of nasopharyngeal airways secured with sutures prior to emergence from anesthesia should be strongly considered to maintain airway patency prior to extubation of the trachea. The surgeon should cut and place the airways so that they do not create airway irritation in the hypopharynx and do not interfere with the lips and nasal passages anteriorly. Oropharyngeal airways are contraindicated after a palatal repair due to pressure on the repaired surface. A traction suture placed into the anterior portion of the tongue may be a suitable alternative to the placement of an oropharyngeal airway. Tracheostomy may be required as a last resort in patients with extremely difficult airways.

3 What are the surgical considerations that impact anesthetic management?

The age and type of palatal repair vary and depend upon the extent of the cleft and age of the patient. If the patient is obviously malnourished from his or her inability to chew and swallow adequately, it is unwise to proceed with surgery until the patient has a positive caloric balance.

There are a number of other surgical considerations that directly impact the anesthetic management. The surgeon will be working in a small space that will make it difficult for the anesthesiologist to have immediate access to the airway during surgical repair. The operating table is usually turned 90 degrees with the patient's head to the anesthesiologist's right. A specialized mouth gag will be placed so that the mouth gag blade may be attached to a Mayo stand, which is placed above the patient's chest. This arrangement permits the greatest surgical access to the entire oropharynx once the head is extended. Unfortunately, the design of a common mouth gag, the Dingman style gag, is such that it may partially or completely obstruct the tracheal tube at three points. The visible point of obstruction is the compression of the tracheal tube in the region of the mandibular incisors from the blade of the mouth gag. Most gags have obviated that compression point by including a "cut-out" where the tracheal tube, the teeth, and the blade meet. The second point of obstruction is on the dorsum of the tongue, although tongue compression is more likely. The third point of obstruction is in the hypopharynx, at the level of the tongue base. The latter points of obstruction may cause significant soft tissue compression, edema, and venous engorgement. The surgeon and anesthesiologist must have continuous communication with respect to the effects of the mouth gag during the procedure and be prepared to adjust the gag's position and compression along the tongue.

4 What are the potential hazards/complications in regard to the airway?

Emergence should only occur after excellent hemostasis has been achieved. Blood is removed with a soft suction catheter, directed by the surgeon to prevent injury to any of the repair sites. As previously mentioned, one or both nares should have nasopharyngeal airways cut to appropriate length and sutured into position to maintain airway patency. A smooth emergence and extubation is preferable. Emergence agitation in this patient population may compromise the cleft repair. Consider adding a dexmedetomidine continuous infusion 0.8 μg/kg beginning after induction as an adjunct. It may also be advisable to avoid sevoflurane in favor of total intravenous anesthesia (TIVA) to decrease incidence of emergence delirium and agitation.

- The anesthesiologist and surgeon should communicate regarding surgical and anesthetic plans prior to speaking with the patient's parents.
- Anticipate a difficult airway and intubation.
- Limit opioids and benzodiazepine sedatives when possible; use adjuvants including local anesthesia.
- Addition of a dexmedetomidine infusion can significantly decrease emergence agitation, protecting the cleft repair during emergence.
- Consider avoiding potent inhalation agents in favor of TIVA to reduce emergence delirium.
- Place individually prepared nasopharyngeal airways prior to extubation of the trachea.
- *See Figure 88.1 for additional details.*

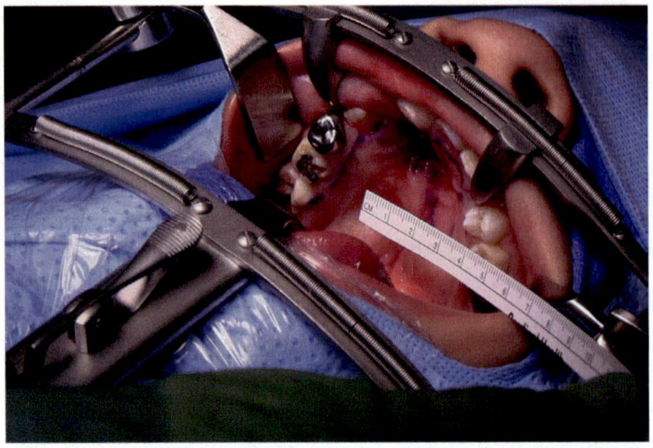

Figure 88.1. A palate defect is being measured in preparation for surgical repair.

Acknowledgments

We gratefully acknowledge the contributions of previous edition author, Brian C. Paterson, as portions of those chapters have been retained in this revision.

Suggested Readings

de Beer D, Bingham R. The child with facial abnormalities. *Curr Opin Anaesthesiol.* 2011;24:282–288.

Liu D, Pan L, Gao Y, et al. Efficaciousness of dexmedetomidine in children undergoing cleft lip and palate repair: a systematic review and meta-analysis. *BMJ Open.* 2021;11(8):e046798.

Mahmoud AAA, Fouad AZ, Mansour MA, Kamal AM. A novel intubation technique in bilateral cleft palate pediatric patients: hard gum shield-aided intubation. *Pediatr Anesth.* 2012;23:349–354.

Le Fort 1 Facial Advancement

89

Andrew Herlich • Paul J. Schwartz

Clinical Scenario: An 18-year-old male with dysmorphic facial features including a depressed midface presents for facial advancement. The maxillofacial surgeon is planning to perform a Le Fort 1 osteotomy.

1 What are the anesthetic/airway management considerations for this case?

Maxillary hypoplasia may commonly present as an isolated finding but may also be associated with Crouzon, Apert, and other congenital syndromes. Comorbidities, such as obstructive sleep apnea, must be considered in the preoperative evaluation. Occasionally, patients with these syndromes have had previous cleft lip and palate repairs or pharyngeal flaps for speech improvement. In these cases, the management of the airway is likely to require a flexible intubation scope to guide the nasotracheal tube through the previously repaired palate or nasal aperture.

An effective anesthetic helps to safely reduce the patient's arterial blood pressure during the maxillary down fracture (wherein the surgeon separates the lower portion of the maxilla containing the teeth from the upper portion, which contains the sinuses). This same surgical access may be used to correct a nasal septal deviation or to perform inferior turbinectomies. This single access approach typically avoids the need to exchange a nasotracheal tube for an orotracheal tube during surgery. Maxillomandibular interfixation is not common postoperatively since the bone components are usually repaired with a rigid plate and screw fixation.

Brisk bleeding can occur from numerous branches of the maxillary artery and venous plexuses in the surgical field. The surgeon's ability to identify specific bleeding vessels in the confined surgical space can be a challenge. Deliberate hypotension with a mean arterial pressure of 60 to 70 mm Hg is ideal to assist with limiting blood loss. This can be achieved with various techniques, including deepening the anesthetic or the administration of additional doses of intravenous opioids or beta blockers. A single large-bore intravenous cannula is typically sufficient for vascular access. Careful use of intravenous fluids helps to reduce edema in the surgical field. Early administration of either intravenous (IV) dexamethasone or methylprednisolone will help to reduce surgical edema and can also help prevent postoperative nausea and vomiting.

Effective pain management is an important consideration in these surgeries. During the procedure, the soft tissues are retracted superiorly causing temporary neuropraxia, which minimizes postoperative pain. The greater palatine nerves are necessarily transected and sacrificed during the procedure, depending upon the degree of maxillary movement. Palatal hypesthesia is a consequence of the dissection, as well. Most surgeons will use local anesthetics with epinephrine to minimize blood loss as well as reduce pain. It is most helpful to administer the majority of the opioid analgesics early in the procedure to assist in maintaining the lower mean arterial pressure. Administration of long-acting opioid analgesics such as morphine or hydromorphone should be discouraged since they are rarely needed and will increase the likelihood of post-anesthesia care unit (PACU) respiratory problems. Intravenous acetaminophen is an excellent nonopioid analgesic that should not impact surgical hemostasis.

2 How would you manage the airway in this case?

Nasotracheal intubation is the most common approach to airway management in Le Fort I osteotomy. Some surgeons may request staged nasal and oral tracheal intubations, which will require an intraoperative tube exchange.

The smallest caliber, clinically acceptable nasotracheal tube should be used, but the tracheal tube length should also be considered. A practical guide for sizing the nasotracheal tube includes the use of a 6.0- to 6.5-mm tubes for adolescent and older females and a 6.5- to 7.0-mm tubes for adolescent and older males. The nasotracheal tube may more easily kink if it is placed in warm water prior to intubation. After application of vasoconstrictors and generous lubrication of both nasal passages, nasotracheal intubation can be performed using the anesthesia provider's method of choice. Following intubation, multiple points of tube fixation should be utilized. Careful attention to prevent nasal traction must also occur.

Submental intubation, where the tracheal tube is surgically passed through the floor of the mouth, is a technique that is used mainly in Great Britain and Europe. It is rarely used in the United States. It has the purported advantage of having the entire nasal canal free of a nasotracheal tube without distortion of external structures. It is considered preferential to tracheotomy in certain circumstances.

3 What are the potential hazards/complications in regard to the airway?

Difficult intubation should be anticipated in patients with mid-face syndromes. Failure to use a flexible intubation scope may increase intubation difficulty.

Surgical disruption of the nasotracheal tube with saws or osteotomes has been reported. The anesthesiologist must have a formulated plan if such an event occurs.

Bradycardia or asystole can occur with maxillary down-fracture or mobilization due to the trigeminocardiac reflex. This reflex can be elicited during procedures that involve manipulation of the central or peripheral branches of the trigeminal nerve. To ameliorate the reflex, it should be treated in the same fashion as the more familiar oculocardiac reflex. The surgeon should cease the inciting surgical activity, and the anesthesiologist should administer a vagolytic agent such as glycopyrrolate 0.2 mg IV or atropine 0.5 mg IV. Once the reflex ceases and the heart rate improves, the surgeon may proceed.

At the end of surgery, the removal of all throat packs must be confirmed. The presence of a retained throat pack should be the first consideration if airway obstruction occurs during extubation or in the postoperative setting.

4 What distinct airway device might be used in this case, and what are the special considerations?

Preformed nasotracheal tubes are ideal for the surgical procedure. Flexible intubation scopes and rigid video laryngoscopes with Magill forceps are important devices to have available during the induction of anesthesia and airway management. An airway exchange catheter can add increased security during tracheal tube exchange.

5 Are there special considerations for the emergence or the end of the case?

Gastric decompression with an orogastric tube is indicated at the end of the case. The surgeon will be in the best position to guide the orogastric tube prior to emergence. Additional administration of oxymetazoline spray to both nostrils prior to extubation will reduce the risk and severity of postoperative epistaxis. If maxillomandibular fixation is performed, wire or band cutters must be immediately available at all times.

Prior to extubation, it is helpful to slowly deflate the pilot balloon of the endotracheal tube to prevent sudden coughing from tracheal recoil.

If emergence delirium is likely, administration of intravenous dexmedetomidine boluses 0.1 to 0.2 mcg/kg may be helpful in preventing or lessening delirium.

- Preoperative discussion between the surgeon and anesthesiologist should address optimal anesthetic and airway management.
- Deliberate hypotension and restriction of intravenous fluids help to reduce surgical hemorrhage and edema.
- Use of a flexible scope for intubation can help to reduce nasal trauma.
- Avoid long-acting opioids to help prevent postoperative respiratory distress in the PACU.
- *See Figure 89.1 and* ▶ ***Video 89.1*** *for additional details.*

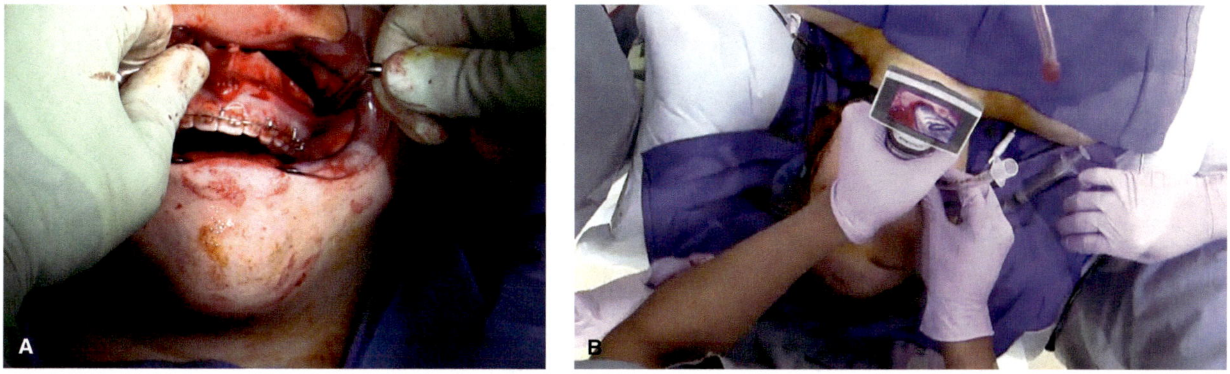

Figure 89.1. **A:** The maxillary down fracture is performed. **B:** Where nasal procedures will be performed after completion of the advancement, conversion to orotracheal intubation takes place.

Acknowledgments

We gratefully acknowledge the contributions of previous edition author, David W. Parker, as portions of those chapters have been retained in this revision.

Suggested Readings

Busaidy KF, Seabold C, Khalil S. Kinked endotracheal tube: possible complication of softening in warm water. *J Oral Maxillofac Surg*. 2011;69:3129–1330.

Lim D, Ma BC, Parumo R, Shanmuhasuntharam P. Thirty years of submental intubation: a review. *Int J Oral Maxillofac Surg*. 2018;47(9):1161–1165.

Lin S, McKenna SJ, Yao CF, Chen YR, Chen C. Effects of hypotensive anesthesia on reducing intraoperative blood loss, duration of operation, and quality of surgical field during orthognathic surgery: a systematic review and meta-analysis of randomized controlled trials. *J Oral Maxillofac Surg*. 2017;75(1):73–86.

Somers M, Tsakiris P, Isert P, Kim S. Management of total transection of nasoendotracheal tube during LeFort I osteotomy. *Case Rep Anesthesiol*. 2020;2020:2097240.

90 Mandibular and Temporomandibular Joint Surgery

Andrew Herlich • Paul J. Schwartz

Clinical Scenario: A 35-year-old female with severe temporomandibular joint (TMJ) internal derangement presents for total joint replacement surgery.

1 What are the anesthetic/airway management considerations for this case?

The TMJ may require an arthroplasty reconstruction due to numerous conditions. These include a spectrum of arthritic conditions, idiopathic resorption, avascular necrosis, neoplastic disorders, trauma, and previous surgical attempts at correction.

Proper mandibular function involves both a gliding and hinge motion. In pathologic TMJ motion, the disc will have anterior displacement that does not relocate properly. Patients may have limited function due to disc malposition or ankylosis. In some instances, the TMJ locks in an open or closed position. Females are more likely to have TMJ problems than males.

Prior to deciding on an anesthetic plan, the anesthesiologist and surgeon should discuss the surgical plan, airway access during the procedure, and the need for mandibular fixation at completion of the procedure. Awake intubation is often chosen if the surgical evaluation reveals significant restriction of mouth opening, such as in bony ankylosis. Isolated trismus may be managed by a skilled operator using techniques such as inhalation induction in the absence of other contraindications.

Total intravenous anesthesia and administration of several antiemetics are strongly recommended to prevent postoperative nausea and vomiting (PONV). Vomiting after TMJ surgery should be prevented to minimize the risk of aspiration and risk of compromising the surgical repair.

2 How would you manage the airway in this case?

Nasotracheal intubation will likely be required. The decision to perform the airway management before or after induction of general anesthesia is aided by the surgeon's understanding of the patient's mandibular function with respect to pain versus anatomical limitations and the involvement of other systems.

The author would secure the airway of the current patient with an awake intubation. If the assessment reveals that the trismus is mechanical and isolated without other evidence of airway obstruction or significant risk of aspiration, an inhalation induction technique followed by nasal intubation is another reasonable approach.

3 What are the surgical considerations that impact anesthetic management?

Nasal intubation is preferred so the surgeon can test the mobility and function of the joint continuously during the procedure. Some surgeons prefer a submental intubation technique. To perform this technique after oral or nasal intubation, a surgical incision is made in the floor of the mouth, and the in-situ tracheal tube is passed via the submental space.

The classic surgical approaches to the TMJ may be classified as preauricular, endaural, and postauricular. The choice of approach is usually a matter of operator preference, clinical experience, and prior training. Cosmetic considerations may also have a significant influence on the choice of surgical approach. The facial nerve lies in close proximity to the area of incision. Some surgeons will use nerve stimulators to assess the function and proximity to the nerve. Consequently, the use of nondepolarizing neuromuscular blockade must be discussed with the surgeon prior to its use. In some instances, the use of nondepolarizing neuromuscular blockade will aid in the surgeon's ability to move the mandible.

4 What are the potential hazards/complications in regard to the airway?

A complex surgical dissection may create edema medial to the muscles of mastication, creating airway edema. Excessive jaw motion during the procedure is not likely to create nasotracheal tube movement since the nasotracheal tube is securely "housed" in the nares and appropriately taped in position.

5 What distinct airway device might be used in this case, and what are the special considerations?

Flexible fiberoptic laryngoscopy and rigid video laryngoscopy are the most successful approaches in managing the airways of patients with temporomandibular joint disorders. Although a standard endotracheal tube may be inserted nasally, preformed nasotracheal tubes Ring, Adair, and Elwyn are the most commonly used tubes for TMJ surgery.

6 Are there special considerations for the emergence or the end of the case?

A stormy emergence and extubation may disrupt the TMJ surgical repair. The anesthesiologist should administer multimodal PONV medication at the onset of surgery to reduce the likelihood and severity of PONV. Decompression of the stomach prior to emergence will also reduce the severity of PONV. Slow deflation of the endotracheal tube cuff will reduce coughing and bucking. If the patient has the propensity for a stormy emergence, judicious titration of dexmedetomidine intravenously can help reduce emergence delirium. Infiltration of local anesthesia to reduce postoperative pain around the auricle is also helpful. The greater auricular nerve is easily blocked by superficial infiltration of local anesthetics along the anterior and posterior aspects of the auricle.

- The anesthesiologist and surgeon must discuss the surgical plans and severity of TMJ disease prior to creating an airway management plan.
- Administration of nondepolarizing neuromuscular blockade should be discussed with the surgeon.
- Awake intubation should be strongly considered in these patients who typically have limited mouth opening.
- A smooth emergence without retching will reduce trauma to the repaired TMJ.
- *See Figures 90.1 and 90.2 for additional details.*

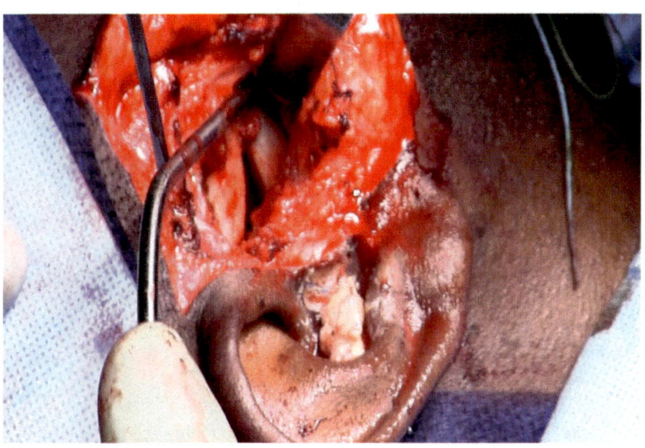

Figure 90.1. Exposure of the tempromandibular joint. (See also **Video 90.1.**)

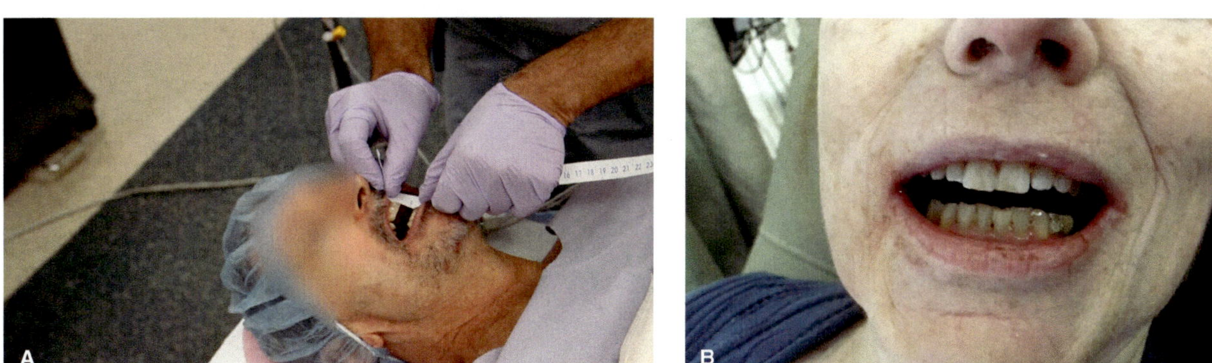

Figure 90.2. **A, B:** Patients presenting for temporomandibular joint surgery may have severe trismus. (See also **Video 90.2.**)

Acknowledgments

We gratefully acknowledge the contributions of previous edition author, Jev A. Clark, as portions of those chapters have been retained in this revision.

Suggested Readings

Chung CJ, Choi YJ, Kim IS, Huh JK, Kim HG, Kim KH. Total alloplastic temporomandibular joint reconstruction combined with orthodontic treatment in a patient with idiopathic condylar resorption. *Am J Orthod Dentofacial Orthop*. 2011;140:404–417.

Henein P, Ziccardi VB. Temporomandibular disorders: surgical implications and management. *Dent Clin North Am*. 2023;67(2):349–365.

Kumar S, Khanna V, Singh BP, Mehrotra D, Patil RK. Impact of technology in temporomandibular joint reconstruction surgeries: a systematic review. *J Plast Reconstr Aesthet Surg*. 2021;74(6):1331–1345.

Ram SPSA, Bhatia N, Jain K, Gupta T, Hazarika A. A prospective, randomized comparison of the classical Altemir's method with the newer Seldinger's technique of submental intubation. *Anesth Analg*. 2023;137(3):638–647.

Robotic Surgery in the Airway

91

Lauren C. Berkow

Clinical Scenario: An otherwise healthy adult patient is having resection of a base of tongue mass with a robotic surgical system. The surgery will be proceeded by panendoscopy.

1 What are the anesthetic and airway management considerations for this case?

Transoral robotic surgery (TORS) is increasing in popularity as it provides better exposure of the oral cavity and a decreased risk of blood loss. The robotic approach is now commonly used for the resections of oral cavity cancer and lingual tonsillectomies.

Any patient with a known mass in the upper airway should be assessed for the risk of difficulty with ventilation and intubation. Preoperative airway assessment should include an airway exam, review of any available radiologic studies, and a discussion with the surgeon to determine the location and extent of any mass. These patients frequently undergo preoperative endoscopy or panendoscopy, so the surgeon has likely recently assessed the extent of the pathology.

Depending on the configuration of the robotic system in the OR, the head of the patient may need to be turned 180 degrees away from the anesthesia provider for the surgery. Even if the patient is not turned 180 degrees, access to the airway will be limited during the procedure due to the robotic system. Multiple robotic arms are placed into the surgical field that the operating surgeon controls from a remote console. An assistant helps with "swapping out" instruments and controlling the arms, similar to a laparoscopic procedure. The endotracheal tube (ETT) should be well secured and possibly sutured in place. In addition, the OR lights will be low or off during the procedure, further limiting visualization of the patient. Finally, the use of muscle relaxants should be discussed with the surgeon. Muscle paralysis can help the patient to better tolerate suspension laryngoscopy and is preferred during the robotic procedure, but it will prohibit nerve monitoring during a neck dissection if planned. Staging of the procedure portions (eg, performance of a neck dissection prior to the robotic-assisted resection) will guide the anesthetic technique during the entirety of the procedure.

2 How would you manage the airway in this case?

Depending on the surgeon's preference and the location of the tumor, the anesthesia provider should determine whether an oral or nasal ETT is required. In addition, a reinforced tube, preshaped Ring, Adair, and Elwyn tube, or a fire-resistant tube may be needed. Jet ventilation is also an option for airway management. Airway management should be planned in collaboration with the surgical team.

If the airway pathology obstructs the glottis, difficulty with ventilation and intubation should be anticipated, and an awake intubation technique may be preferred. Backup plans for ventilation and intubation should be outlined and discussed with the surgical team prior to induction of anesthesia. Advanced airway equipment should also be available in the room prior to induction.

Perioperative tracheostomy may also be considered for patients with significant disease or to improve visualization during the procedure.

3 What are the potential hazards and complications in regard to the airway?

The risk of ETT tube obstruction is significant in these cases because the robotic arms move in close proximity to the airway. Increases in airway pressure should be immediately reported to the surgical team and may prompt repositioning of the ETT or robotic arm. Depending on the experience of the surgeon, these cases may be several hours in length, which can cause significant laryngeal edema. The use of cautery or lasers in the crowded confines of the upper airway presents a significant airway fire risk. The lowest oxygen concentration the patient will tolerate should be used, and all members of the OR team should discuss the risk, prevention, and management of an airway fire during the surgical time-out.

Emergency undocking of the robot in the event of an airway fire or other untoward event (eg, ETT disconnect or obstruction) should also be discussed during the surgical time-out. The role of each team member should be defined, recognizing that the closest personnel to the airway may not be an anesthesia provider.

4 Are there special considerations for the emergence or the end of the case?

As previously mentioned, there may be significant airway edema at the conclusion of the case, so the timing of extubation should be carefully considered. Perioperative steroids can be given to prevent airway edema. In some cases, extubation may be delayed for 24 hours to allow for the reduction of airway edema. Prior to extubation, the airway should be examined for retained mouth gags and tooth guards. Where indicated, the patient should be treated as a difficult extubation. Perioperative tracheostomy may be considered in patients at high risk of postoperative airway compromise. Post robotic airway surgery patients are also at risk of postoperative bleeding and airway obstruction, so they should be monitored closely in the postoperative period.

- Patients presenting for TORS should be carefully assessed for the risk of difficult ventilation and intubation, and the airway management plan should be discussed in collaboration with the surgical team.
- Access to the patient and the ETT are significantly restricted during TORS.
- Movement of the robotic arms can cause compression or dislodgement of the ETT.
- Postoperative airway edema and bleeding are significant postoperative complications and should influence the timing of extubation as well as consideration for perioperative tracheostomy.
- *See Figures 91.1 and 91.2 for additional details.*

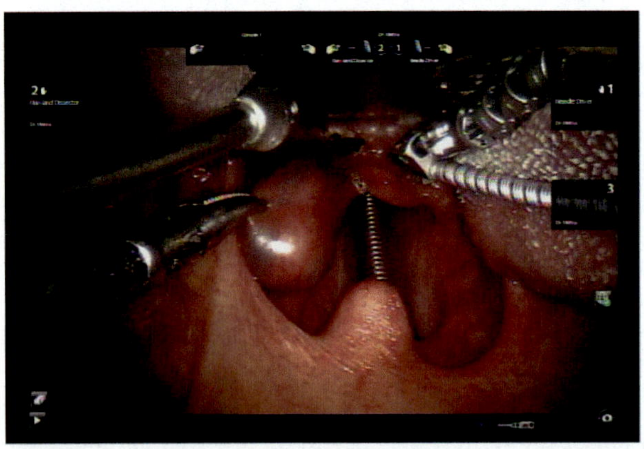

Figure 91.1. Multiple robotically operated tools as well as a suction cannula, and a laser resistant nasotracheal tube. [See also **Video 91.1.**]

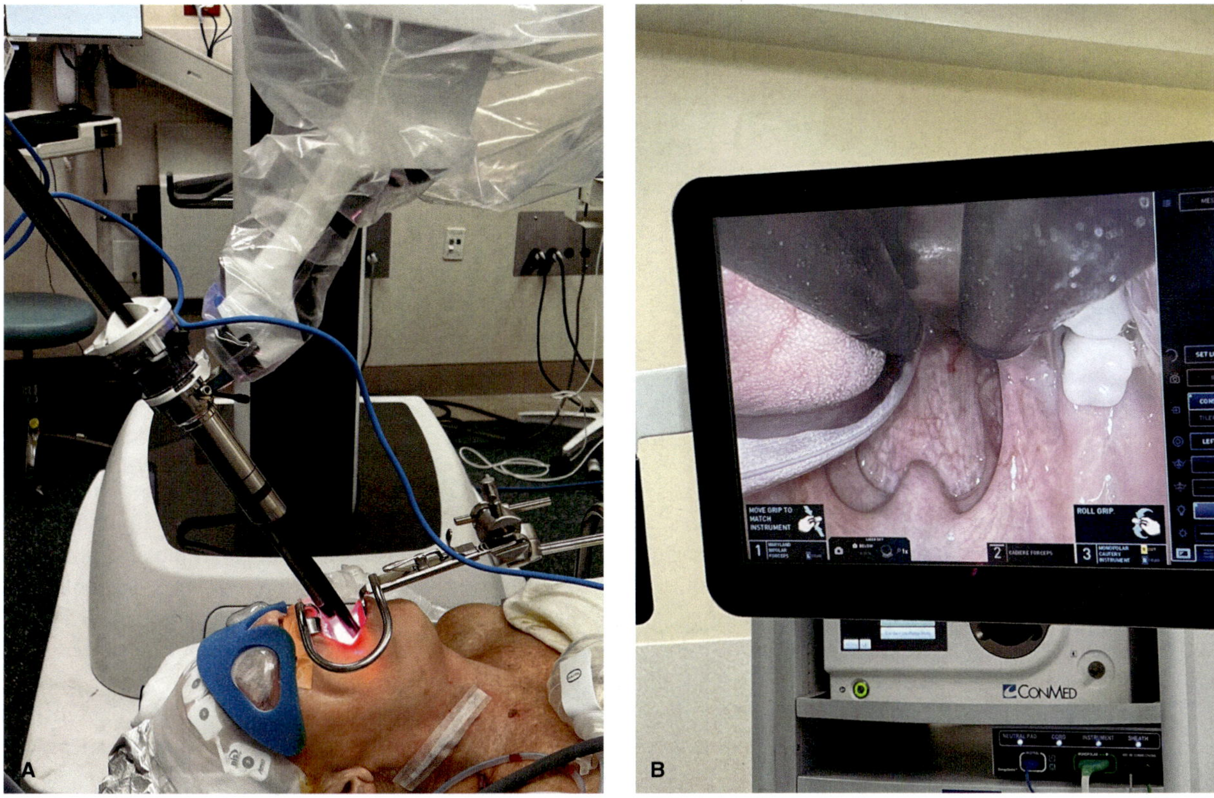

Figure 91.2. **A:** Use of a single-port robot. **B:** Note the parallel arms of the single-port robot.

Suggested Readings

Chi JJ, Mandel JE, Weinstein GS, O'Malley BW Jr. Anesthetic considerations for transoral robotic surgery. *Anesthesiol Clin.* 2010;28(3):411–422.

Krespi Y, Kizhner V, Koorn R, Giordano A. Anesthesia and ventilation options for flex robotic assisted laryngopharyngeal surgery. *Am J Otolaryngol.* 2019;40(6):102185.

Oliveira CM, Nguyen HT, Ferraz AR, Watters K, Rosman B, Rahbar R. Robotic surgery in otolaryngology and head and neck surgery: a review. *Minim Invasive Surg.* 2012;2012:286563.

Stubbs VC, Rajasekaran K, Gigliotti AR, et al. Management of the airway for transoral robotic supraglottic partial laryngectomy. *Front Oncol.* 2018;8:312.

Turner MT, Stokes WA, Stokes CM, Hassid S, Holsinger FC, Lawson G. Airway and bleeding complications of transoral robotic supraglottic laryngectomy (TORS-SGL): a systematic review and meta-analysis. *Oral Oncol.* 2021;118:105301.

92 Tracheostomy in the Intubated Patient

Andres R. Brenes Bastos

Clinical Scenario: A 35-year-old man who sustained a cervical spine injury is now ventilator dependent. He has previously undergone a neck fusion, and now presents for a permanent tracheostomy.

1 What are the anesthetic and airway management considerations for this case?

Tracheostomy is the most common surgical procedure performed on critically ill patients. Each patient presents specific anesthetic and airway challenges, and their admitting diagnosis will determine their management. Establishment of an early tracheostomy in chronically ventilated patients frees the mouth for nutrition, verbal communication, and is associated with decreased morbidity and mortality. Frequently, patients with chronic respiratory failure requiring prolonged mechanical ventilation have severe cardiopulmonary disease, metabolic, neurologic derangements, and/or have sustained major trauma. Thorough preoperative evaluation is crucial in the management of the patient scheduled for a tracheostomy to develop an anesthetic and surgical plan and to determine the feasibility of the planned procedure. The anesthesiologist should perform a thorough assessment of the airway anatomy, ventilatory parameters (FIO_2, PEEP, etc.), state of consciousness, and sedation and vasopressor requirements.

Surgical tracheostomy can be achieved in awake or lightly sedated patients, but general anesthesia with deep muscle relaxation is often preferred for patient comfort and to assure ideal surgical conditions. In the unstable patient, the transition from awake with a preserved or low support respiratory function to unconscious with positive-pressure ventilation may unmask underlying cardiovascular volatility.

During the tracheostomy procedure, the patient will be in the supine position with head extension supported with sand bags or gel pillows to achieve a stable surgical field. Ensuring proper eye and nose protection is important due to their proximity to the surgical field. Proper draping should be monitored to prevent the inadvertent creation of pockets that could lead to oxygen entrapment, increasing the risk of an airway fire. The surgical team will make a midline incision in the trachea, most frequently between the second and third tracheal rings, typically directly above an in situ translaryngeal tracheal tube (TT). A low FIO_2 should be used to reduce the risk of ignition of the TT as airway fires are a constant danger while electrocautery is in use. The recommended FIO_2 is less than 30%. This is achieved by mixing air with oxygen, and lowering the FIO_2 from 100% to the desired level of expired O_2 often requires several minutes. The anesthesia provider may be asked to deflate the TT cuff and either advance or withdraw the TT to avoid damage of the cuff by probing needles, tracheostomy hooks, scalpels, or electrocautery.

Placement of the tracheostomy might prove difficult or even fail, so there must be a backup plan to return to ventilating with an FIO_2 of 100% should hypoxia ensue. Communication with the surgeon should occur throughout this process to avoid unexpected use of electrocautery when the FIO_2 is not below 30%.

Once the trachea has been incised and before the tracheostomy device is inserted, the anesthesia provider will likely be requested to withdraw the TT and suspend positive-pressure ventilation. Deep suctioning of the airway is recommended as it will reduce the risk of the secretions going into the airway. After suctioning, special attention to not completely remove the TT should be emphasized in case tracheostomy placement fails, requiring use of the TT to resume mechanical ventilation. Once the tracheostomy is in place, the anesthesia circuit is then disconnected from the TT, connected to the tracheostomy device, and ventilation is attempted. If malposition of the tracheostomy device is suspected (ie, no or minimal end-tidal CO_2 detection, high airway resistance, lack of bilateral breath sounds), readvancement of the laryngeal positioned TT should be attempted. In patients who have known or suspected difficult airways, the readvancement of the TT may require the use of an airway exchange catheter (AEC) or a FIS to guide placement. These adjunct devices should ideally be placed prior to the initial withdrawal of the TT.

2 How would you manage the airway in this case?

The preferred anesthetic for a tracheostomy is total intravenous anesthesia due to the open airway exposure. If the patient's cardiopulmonary status does not allow for a significant reduction in FIO_2, the surgical team should be made aware of the increased fire risk and modifications to minimize or stop electrocautery use should take place. As the surgical dissection approaches the anterior tracheal surface, the surgical staff should be queried as to the continued need for electrocautery. Closed-loop communication with the surgical team is critical, especially during tracheal incision, withdrawal of the TT, confirmation of tracheostomy device placement, and removal of the TT. Constant vigilance for airway fires and/or loss of the airway should be maintained.

TT cuff puncture is a known risk during tracheal incision, leading to spillage of oxygen into the surgical field and the inability to ventilate. To minimize this risk, deep placement of the TT with a deliberate mainstem intubation and gradual withdrawal from the bronchus until the TT is positioned just above the carina (this can be achieved via auscultation or fiberoptic visualization) or complete withdrawal of the TT are techniques implemented to reduce the risk of cuff puncture.

Alternatively, in the special setting where the TT will hinder the possibility to perform the tracheostomy, airway patency can be maintained by placement of an supraglottic airway (SGA). The placement of an SGA eliminates the risk of surgical damage to the TT and leaves the trachea unoccupied. This technique is not suitable for all patients (eg, risk of gastric contents aspiration, upper airway mass or other distortion, high positive-pressure requirement), so risks versus benefits should be discussed prior to using this method.

3 What are the potential hazards and complications in regard to the airway?

As has been discussed above, the conversion from translaryngeal tracheal intubation to a tracheostomy poses a number of concerns as previously discussed. Many chronically intubated patients will have significant cardiopulmonary disease and may not tolerate a reduction in the FIO_2 or even brief periods of apnea. Prolonged interruptions of ventilation in the event of a surgical complication will not be tolerated by many of these patients.

Critically ill patients often possess significant risk factors for tracheal–mucosal separation (eg, anasarca, prolonged intubation, mucosal friability, chronic steroid use, infection, prior midline surgical procedures, or prior radiation therapy to the neck). These patients have a higher incidence of iatrogenic false passage with inadvertent insertion of the tracheostomy device. The creation of a false airway passage constitutes an airway emergency. Early signs of a false passage include loss of end-tidal CO_2, an increase in peak inspiratory pressures, and absent or distant breath sounds. Aside from loss of the airway, additional false passage complications include pneumothorax, pneumomediastinum, and aspiration of blood/secretions. Treatment should include establishment of a secure airway by either removal and replacement of the tracheostomy device, the insertion of other adjuncts (see below), or readvancement of the TT.

4 What distinct airway device might be used in this case, and what are the special considerations?

Creation of a tracheostomy in the intubated patient presents several hazards as described above. Due to the significant risk of airway fires, the surgical field should always include sterile water and a preloaded irrigation syringe. The entire OR team should be aware of an emergency plan and appropriate steps to follow in the event of a fire. Equipment for reintubation of the trachea should be readily available in the event that emergent extubation is necessary due to an airway fire or a failed tracheostomy device insertion. When a difficult intubation is known or suspected, appropriate equipment, including a rigid bronchoscope, should be made immediately available. Sterile small diameter standard TTs (eg, 6.0 internal diameter) should be available for the surgical team to place if tracheostomy device placement proves difficult. Placement of an AEC prior to withdrawal of the TT may aid in visualization of the airway for the surgical team and also guide readvancement of the TT if tracheostomy placement fails.

In light of the recent COVID-19 pandemic, there is a noted risk of infection transmission among healthcare workers performing aerosolizing procedures such as tracheostomy and intubation. Safety measures including appropriate personal protective equipment should be followed to minimize risk of transmission.

- Chronically intubated patients presenting for tracheostomy are likely to have systemic comorbidities which may present challenges with regard to positive-pressure ventilation and Fio_2 requirements.
- Creation of a false airway passage is an emergency, and the anesthesiologist should be prepared to resecure the airway in this scenario.
- Closed loop communication and timeouts during critical portions of the tracheostomy should be followed.
- *See Figure 92.1 and* ***Video 92.1*** *for additional details.*

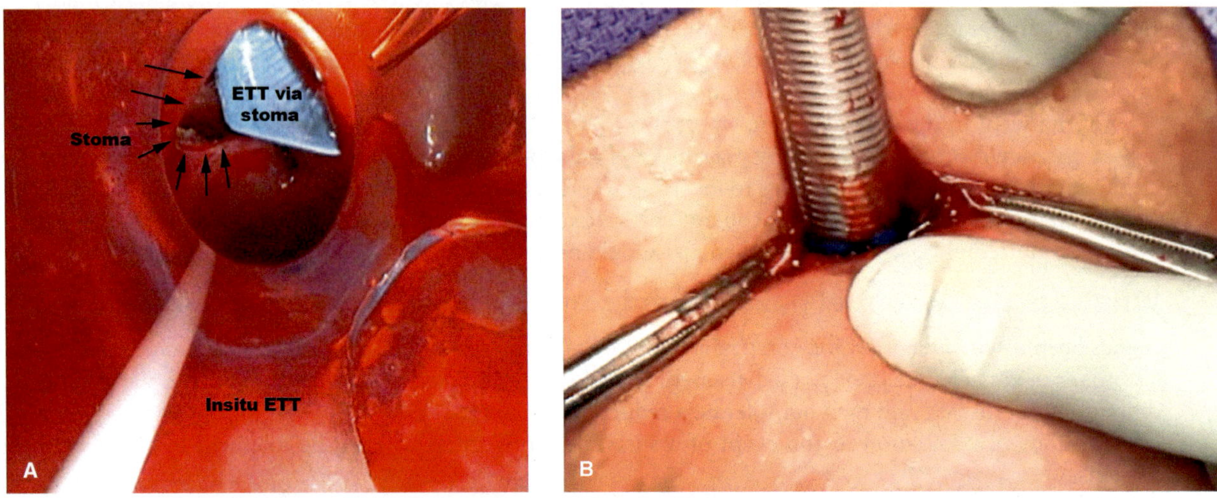

Figure 92.1. **A:** With the help of a flexible intubation scope, the insertion of a tracheal tube into a newly created tracheostomy is verified. Placement will be confirmed with the stable measurement of end tidal CO_2. **B:** A tracheal tube has been inserted into a newly created tracheostomy. Appreciating the proximal cuff (*blue*) suggests, but does not ensure, that the distal tracheal tube is above the carina.

Acknowledgments

We gratefully acknowledge the contributions of previous edition author, Lara Zador, as portions of those chapters have been retained in this revision.

Suggested Readings

Chan Y, Goddard JC, eds. *K.J. Lee's Essential Otolaryngology: Head and Neck Surgery*. 12th ed. McGraw Hill; 2019.

Gosling AF, Bose S, Gomez E, et al. Perioperative Considerations for Tracheostomies in the Era of COVID-19. *Anesth Analg*. 2020;131(2):378–386.

Jaffe RA, Schmiesing CA, Golianu B. *Anesthesiologist's Manual of Surgical Procedures*. 6th ed. Wolters Kluwer; 2020.

Laryngectomy

93

Paula Trigo

Clinical Scenario: A 58-year-old patient with a history of laryngeal cancer presents for laryngectomy. The patient has a remote history of neck radiation therapy and chemotherapy for his cancer. He recently underwent laryngeal biopsy—at that time, the anesthesia team providing anesthetic care for him noted a friable, bleeding mass on the epiglottis and recommended awake intubation when the patient presents again for definitive therapy.

1 What are the anesthetic/airway management considerations for this case?

Preoperative assessment of patients presenting for laryngectomy should include evaluations of current substance use, concomitant cardiac and respiratory disease, and occurrence of second primary cancers. A thorough history should also be taken regarding any prior surgeries or treatments to the airway which could potentially distort airway anatomy or cause tissue induration, swelling, or friability. External examination of the airway alone can be misleading because pathology that may impact airway management may not be seen on routine examinations. Consultation and review of recent anesthesia records is of paramount importance (eg, in the current case, prior anesthesiologists had demonstrated a difficult direct laryngoscopy). The preoperative evaluation of the laryngectomy patient should start with the assumption of difficulty with intubation, and awake intubation should be considered. Imaging studies and a preoperative endoscopic airway evaluation may also be helpful in this regard.

Surgical preference will dictate one of two approaches to tracheostomy creation in a laryngectomy case. In the more conservative approach, the tracheostomy is created prior to dissection and removal of the patient's larynx. Tracheostomy may be accomplished with the patient awake or immediately after anesthetic induction and intubation. The alternative is to create the tracheostomy following neck dissection. Once the larynx is isolated in the neck, the second, third, or fourth intratracheal ligament is incised, and the distal tracheal tube is removed. A wire-reinforced tracheal tube is then inserted into the tracheal stump by the surgical team. The Montandon tracheal tube is manufactured with an acute distal curve that facilitates its placement away from the surgical field. Once the anesthesiologist confirms bilateral breath sounds by auscultation, the tracheal tube is fixed to the chest wall. The larynx is then removed, and the stoma formalized. In both approaches, the risk of airway fire is constantly present and should be considered.

While some surgeons believe routine bilateral neck dissection may not be necessary in the surgical treatment of all supraglottic cancers, some studies have shown a reduction in cervical recurrence and overall higher survival with additional neck dissection. The surgical decision to perform neck dissection or not impacts the duration of the procedure and the magnitude of postoperative tissue swelling.

2 How would you manage the airway in this case?

After a thorough evaluation of the airway, the anesthesia team secures the airway with the most appropriate technique (eg, awake vs postinduction, intravenous vs inhalation induction, routine vs video laryngoscopy vs flexible intubating scope). In rare complex cases, awake tracheostomy may be elected. In circumstances where there is minimal or no obstructive disease and tracheostomy placement is planned at the outset of the case, an supraglottic airway can be placed initially for tracheostomy placement.

Regardless of the airway management technique chosen, the anesthesiologist should always have an alternative plan to secure the airway. The surgical team should be present in the OR while the airway is secured.

The FiO_2 should be reduced to 30% or less during the tracheostomy creation, and the OR team should stay aware of the increased fire risk. Although muscle relaxants can be helpful during the preneck dissection and tracheostomy creation, they are generally avoided during the neck dissection to facilitate surgical neuromonitoring.

3 What are the surgical considerations that impact anesthetic management?

The location, size, and extension of the tumor will affect airway management. Surgical dissection in the neck will be directed by neuromonitoring and will prohibit the use of neuromuscular blocking agents. Specific reconstructive tissue transfers may require muscle relaxants later in the procedure (eg, pectoralis pedicle flap), and this should be discussed with the surgical team ahead of time. In patients with significant cardiopulmonary or hepatorenal disease that necessitates central venous pressure monitoring, cannulation of the large veins of the neck may be either impossible (ie, with planned bilateral dissections) or relatively contraindicated (in unilateral disease) in a desire to preserve venous drainage from the head and neck. In these cases, alternative cannulation sites should be considered. Once the tracheostomy is created, the airway becomes part of the surgical field, so the anesthesiologist should closely monitor for tracheal tube kinking, obstruction, dislocation, circuit disconnection, or mainstem bronchus intubation.

To minimize surgical blood loss during neck dissection, a modest induced hypotension may be desired by the surgeon. Inhaled agents or infusion of a potent opioid or dexmedetomidine are often used. The close proximity of the carotid sinus to the surgical field can cause profound hypotension, bradycardia, and, rarely, asystole. The surgical team should be immediately notified of any profound hemodynamic disturbances. Stopping surgical manipulation may result in immediate recovery. Chronotropic therapy or the injection of local anesthetic into the carotid sinus may be necessary as a next step.

During neck dissection, there is a concern for possible venous air embolism (VAE). The diagnosis of VAE should be strongly considered with an acute drop in end-tidal CO_2 and blood pressure, and the surgical team should be notified immediately of this possibility. The surgical team can investigate for evidence of venous leaks and flood the surgical field with saline. Hemodynamic support with sympathomimetic agents may be the first line of therapy. Carotid injury and acute arterial bleeding are other potential complications, especially in patients who have had prior neck surgeries or radiation. A modest hypertension may be required during the vascular repair if the injured vessel needs to be temporarily occluded because ipsilateral brain perfusion will be dependent on collateral flow.

4 Are there special considerations for the emergence or the end of the case?

At the end of surgery, the tracheal tube is exchanged for a flanged tracheostomy device. This device may or may not allow connection to the anesthesia circuit, and an uncuffed device is typically preferred. The anesthesiologist should be aware of the type of device that is placed because this may help in planning the emergence of the patient. If the device will not allow positive-pressure airway control, the patient should return to spontaneous ventilation prior to airway exchange. Once an appropriate tidal volume and respiratory rate are established, the airway exchange may occur. Careful suctioning of blood and secretions from the tracheostomy should be performed to prevent plugging. Postoperatively, the head of the bed should be maintained at 15 degrees to 20 degrees angle to reduce edema.

- A patient with a history of laryngeal cancer should increase the anesthesiologist's suspicion of difficult airway management.
- Preoperative upper airway endoscopy should be considered, and recent imaging studies of the head and neck should be reviewed, if available.
- Airway fire precautions should be exercised during tracheostomy creation.
- Administration of muscle relaxants should be discussed with the surgical team.
- *See Figure 93.1 and* ***Video 93.1*** *for additional details.*

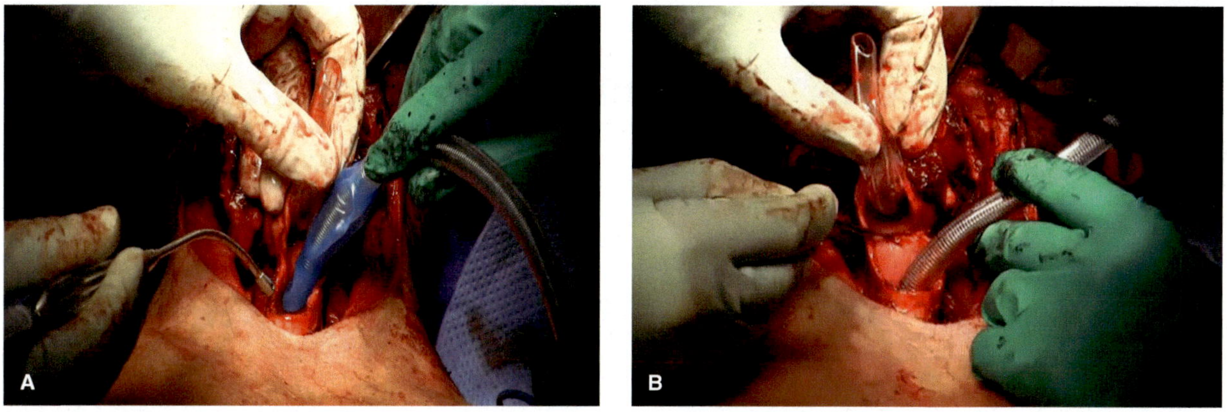

Figure 93.1. **A:** The trans-field tracheal tube is being inserted into the distal trachea after the oral tracheal tube has been retracted along with the partially separated larynx. **B:** During the final stages of larynx removal, both the proximal (oral tracheal) and distal (trans-field) tracheal tubes are seen. At this moment, the surgical and anesthesiology teams must monitor for and correct the high risk of bronchial intubation.

Suggested Readings

Baird BJ, Sung CK, Beadle BM, Divi V. Treatment of early-stage laryngeal cancer: a comparison of treatment options. *Oral Oncol.* 2018;87:8–16.

O'Carroll J, Endlich Y, Ahmad I. Advanced airway assessment techniques. *BJA Educ.* 2021;21(9):336–342.

Rosenblatt WH, Yanez ND. A decision tree approach to airway management pathways in the 2022 difficult airway algorithm of the American Society of Anesthesiologists. *Anesth Analg.* 2022;134(5):910–915.

Roth D, Pace NL, Lee A, et al. Bedside tests for predicting difficult airways: an abridged Cochrane diagnostic test accuracy systematic review. *Anaesthesia.* 2019;74(7):915–928.

94 Tube Exchange in a New Tracheostomy

Laura J. Alexander

Clinical Scenario: An 80-year-old man has just undergone a resection of a supraglottic mass and free tissue reconstruction. At the end of the case, the surgical team wishes to exchange the tracheal tube in his tracheostomy for an 8.0 ID Shiley tracheostomy tube.

1 What are the anesthetic and airway management considerations for this case?

Manipulation of a tracheostomy less than 5 to 7 days after its creation must be done with caution. The tissue surrounding a fresh, incompletely healed stoma may be fragile. Removal of an in situ tracheal tube for replacement with another device can be complicated by loss of control of the airway. This is especially true when a large and opaque device such as a Shiley tracheostomy tube is to be inserted—the flanges of the tube can obscure visual guidance of the stoma as it is being recannulated. As the in situ tube is withdrawn, the borders of the tracheostomy tract can be disrupted, risking hemorrhage and/or separation of tissue planes. In addition to blood, surgical debris can be introduced into the lower airway. False passage insertion of the airway device can also occur, resulting in damage and crepitus to adjacent soft tissues or the mediastinum. Not only does this result in the inability to oxygenate and ventilate, but may also result in pneumomediastinum, pneumothorax, subcutaneous emphysema, or air embolus. Patient characteristics, such as an elevated body mass index (BMI), large neck circumference, and previous surgery or radiation, confer a higher risk of false passage. Loss of control of the stoma can result in hypoxia, cardiovascular collapse, and death. Postoperative complications (eg, hematoma) can also cause airway obstruction and collapse of the airway during the exchange.

2 How would you manage the airway in this case?

Airway management of a newly created stoma involves taking prophylactic measures that minimize the risk of loss of control of the airway. Patient-specific characteristics should be taken into account prior to the exchange (eg, BMI, respiratory drive, hemodynamic stability). The patient should be preoxygenated with 100% FIO_2 for 3 to 5 minutes prior to the device exchange. Any residual debris, secretions, or blood in or around the airway could be aspirated during the exchange procedure and should be removed. The airway above the tracheal tube should be suctioned via the mouth, and the in situ tube should be suctioned, as well. In most cases, the patient should remain under general anesthesia, and some clinicians prefer the patient to be muscle relaxed to ensure optimal control of the airway. Pulse oximetry, capnography, and airway pressures should be continuously monitored. Where there exists a significant concern for loss of airway control (eg, in the morbidly obese patient), an intubation bougie, wire, or airway exchange catheter (AEC) can be placed into the tracheal tube, and the exchange can be performed using a modified Seldinger technique. If the stomal opening is small or obscured by adipose tissue, has poor anatomic landmarks, or if the tissue integrity is in question, one or two tracheal hooks can be used to secure the inside surface of the trachea around the tracheal tube to maintain stability and patency of the opening. Once the tracheal tube is removed, the tracheostomy tube should be immediately inserted and the cuff inflated. Tracheostomy tubes of various sizes, including smaller and larger, should be immediately available. If the device's cuff is unable to completely seal the airway, it should be immediately exchanged. The anesthesia circuit is reattached, and the anesthesiologist measures the end-tidal CO_2. If the end-tidal CO_2 is absent while the circuit and machine are otherwise properly functioning, it is likely that the tracheostomy device has been placed into a false passage, is otherwise malpositioned, or its cuff is obstructing the airway. High airway pressures (elevated from the patient's previous baseline) can also indicate tracheostomy malpositioning. Surgeon denial of false passage placement is common as the apparent ease of tracheostomy device placement can be deceiving. In the situation where multiple false placements occur, the insertion of a small, standard, cuffed tracheal tube under direct visualization of the tracheal wall can stabilize the patient and should subsequently be replaced.

3 What are the potential hazards and complications in regard to the airway?

Mortality rates from tracheostomies in the current surgery era are typically less than 1%, with the majority of deaths resulting from loss of airway control. Lack of maturation and structural integrity of the tracheostomy stoma can lead to tissue damage, damage to the surgical site, bleeding, or false passage of the new tracheostomy tube. False passage into the soft tissues of the mediastinum can further distort the anatomy and requires immediate correction. Even passage of the bougie, wire, or AEC can cause dangerous trauma to the trachea and bronchi. Improper placement of a tracheostomy device or kinking can obstruct the airway, leading to high airway pressures and loss of end-tidal CO_2 detection. Typically, this occurs during inflation of the device cuff with the open end obliquely occluded against the wall of the trachea. Mechanisms to maintain patency and identification of the stoma through manual force can further disrupt the surgical site, especially in a freshly opened trachea or fragile tissues (eg, due to chronic steroid use or prior surgery and/or radiation).

4 What distinct airway device might be used in this case, and what are the special considerations?

Although the majority of new tracheostomy exchanges will proceed without adverse incidents, difficulty in managing these airways can result in devastating consequences in a rapid manner. The availability of an AEC and small, standard, cuffed tracheal tubes (eg, 6.0 ID and 6.5 ID in an adult population) should be confirmed. The intraoperative team may decide to insert an AEC prior to the in situ tracheal tube's removal. The AEC should be of the largest size that can be inserted within both the in situ tube and the to-be-inserted tracheostomy tube. If an AEC is to be used, the equipment to deliver oxygen via its lumen should be confirmed (eg, manual jet ventilation device with Luer lock connector). Multiple tracheostomy devices in a variety of sizes, including a duplicate (in the event of a defect), should also be available.

- Tissue along the tract of a fresh tracheostomy is fragile and can be easily disrupted.
- Continuous pulse oximetry, capnography, and airway pressure monitoring should be present throughout the airway device exchange.
- Elevated peak inspiratory pressure immediately after tracheostomy changes and/or absence of end-tidal CO_2 readings usually indicate a malpositioned tube or obstruction in the trachea.
- A cuff leak around the newly introduced tracheostomy tube may require an additional tube exchange.
- Adjunctive equipment should include an AEC or bougie, duplicate and smaller tracheostomy devices, small-cuffed tracheal tubes, and tracheal hooks.
- *See Figure 94.1 and* ***Video 94.1*** *for additional details.*

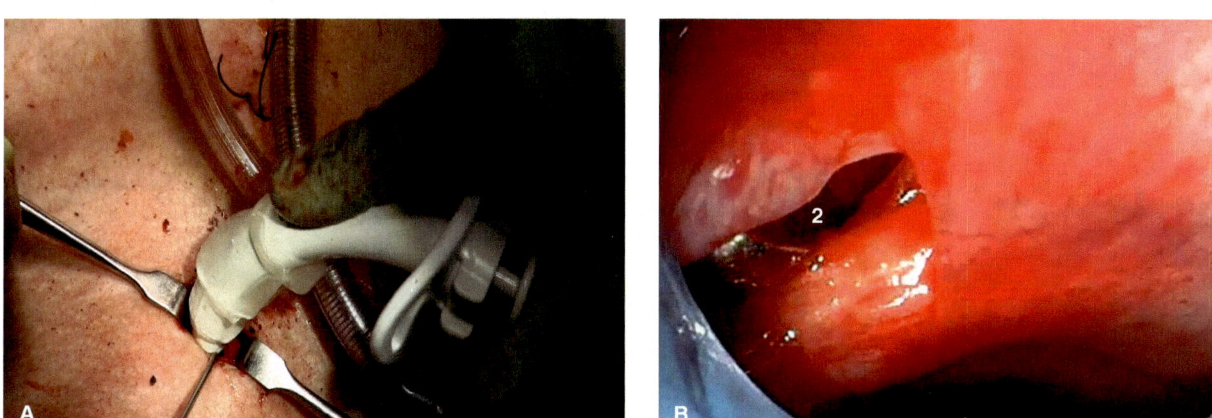

Figure 94.1. A: With the careful suspension of the edges of a recently created tracheal stoma (two surgical retractors and a tracheostomy hook in place), a Shiley Catheter is placed into a tracheal stoma that had been previously intubated with a wire-reinforced tracheal tube. **B:** During the intubation of a newly created tracheostomy, an inserted wire-reinforced trachea tube has traveled into a false lumen: (1) True tracheal lumen and (2) false lumen.

Suggested Readings

Budde AM, Kadar RB, Jabaley CS. Airway misadventures in adult critical care: a concise narrative review of managing lost or compromised artificial airways. *Curr Opin Anaesthesiol.* 2022;35(2):130–136.

Nunn C, Uffman J, Bhananker SM. Bilateral tension pneumothoraces following jet ventilation via an airway exchange catheter. *J Anesth.* 2007;21(1):76–79.

Rosero EB, Corbett J, Mau T, Joshi GP. Intraoperative airway management considerations for adult patients presenting with tracheostomy: a narrative review. *Anesth Analg.* 2021;132(4):1003–1011.

Switching from Established Shiley Catheter to Tracheal Tube

95

Christopher Szabo

Clinical Scenario: An 82-year-old man has previously undergone a supraglottic mass resection and free tissue transfer reconstruction. He has a tracheostomy with a cuffed 8.0 ID Shiley catheter in place. He now presents for emergency exploratory laparotomy due to a bowel obstruction.

1 What are the anesthetic and airway management considerations for this case?

Patients with a preexisting indwelling tracheostomy device (eg, Shiley catheter) presenting for surgery will typically require some manipulation of the device, including replacement with a tracheal tube. Often the tracheostomy device will not include a distal, inflatable cuff, or may be fenestrated (to allow speech), and replacement of the device will be mandatory if positive-pressure ventilation is planned. If the device is cuffed, or if spontaneous ventilation is to be maintained, the device may be adequate provided there is no aspiration risk.

Determining the maturity of a tracheostomy stoma is the first step in designing an airway plan. A tracheostomy is considered mature when there is sufficient epithelialization of surface-skin-to-tracheal-mucosa to prevent separation of tissue planes with minor trauma. When sufficient epithelialization has not occurred, manipulation may separate tissue planes and cause an airway emergency. Complications from creation of a false lumen include subcutaneous emphysema, mediastinitis, airway loss, and death. In a survey of 59 otolaryngology chief residents, 42% were aware of a loss of airway during a tracheostomy device exchange. Fifteen percent of respondents were aware of a death at the first tracheostomy tube exchange. Generally, the first tracheostomy tube exchange occurs between 3 and 7 days after stoma creation. In children, an earlier exchange may be safe. The maturation of the tracheostomy tract is generally complete by postoperative day 7.

The presence of a tracheostomy tube disrupts swallowing and predisposes to aspiration and pulmonary complications. Therefore, the ASA guidelines for preoperative fasting apply equally to a patient with a tracheostomy. Some liberalization of fasting guidelines may be appropriate in tracheostomy patients who have undergone laryngectomy. Patients with a full stomach presenting for emergency surgery or those with an increased aspiration risk for other reasons (e.g., bowel obstruction) require an awake tracheostomy to tracheal tube change or a rapid sequence induction technique.

2 How would you manage the airway in this case?

As with any airway manipulation, planning and the preparation of primary contingency plans should take place. The following devices must be available: (1) a replacement tracheostomy, (2) the inner cannula and obturator for the patient's in situ device, (3) small, standard tracheal tubes, and (4) FIS, airway exchange catheter (AEC), and/or Aintree catheter. The patient can be preoxygenated via the in situ tracheostomy device. Preoxygenation by anesthesia face mask is likely inefficient even in situations where the device is occluded (due to peridevice leak). In the postlaryngectomy patient, face mask preoxygenation is futile. In patients with upper airway continuity, inflation of the tracheal tube cuff ensures full tidal volume preoxygenation. If a cuffless device is in situ, patients can often control the extent of ventilation via the upper airway and should be asked to "breathe through the stoma." Secretions should be removed with gentle suctioning.

Though the tracheostomy device can be removed and a tracheal tube inserted without the use of a hypnotic, this is often unpleasant for the patient, and induction of anesthesia should be considered in most cases.

An intravenous hypnotic is administered and may be followed by muscle relaxation. In the case of a mature tracheostoma, the tracheostomy tube cuff is deflated and the device is removed. When the stoma is not mature, or there has been poor wound healing or dehiscence, further precautions should be considered. It is not unreasonable to request the presence of an otolaryngologist at the bedside. After the induction of anesthesia, a tracheal hook is advanced under the inferior edge of the device and the trachea is controlled prior to device removal. Alternatively, an AEC can be placed into the device and used for exchange to a tracheal tube.

After removal of the tracheostomy device, secretions hitherto unappreciated may be suctioned away. The tracheal tube is inserted into the tracheostoma and advanced only to a depth that will allow secure cuff sealing. In patients with significant pretracheal adipose, this will require cautious advancement—the cuff must be within the trachea, but care must be taken to assure a supracarinal position of the tracheal tube bevel. In the majority of cases, visualizing some portion of the proximal cuff will assure adequate positioning (see Chapter 61: Angioneurotic Edema). The tracheal tube cuff is subsequently inflated and ventilation is confirmed. Auscultation of the lungs confirms bilateral and equal breath sounds. A FIS can be used to verify position. After determining the proper placement of the tracheal tube, it is secured via tape or chest wall suture to avoid displacement.

3 What are the potential hazards and complications in regard to the airway?

Complications include false-lumen creation, bleeding, and difficulty with reinsertion of the tracheal tube. False-lumen creation can result in subcutaneous emphysema, mediastinitis, respiratory arrest, and death. False-lumen intubation is often difficult to recognize. High airway ventilation pressures and no or reduced end-tidal CO_2 detection should raise suspicion. Operator denial is common. False-lumen intubation constitutes an emergency, and subsequent attempts at stomal intubation may become progressively more difficult. Repeated intubation or persistent ventilation of the false lumen can worsen the situation. Insertion of a tracheal hook and preintubation with a small tracheal tube, AEC, FIS, or jet ventilation catheter should be undertaken without hesitation. Difficulty reinserting a tracheostomy tube can result from stenosis at the site of the stoma as well as granulation tissue within the trachea. Narrow device intubation, as discussed earlier, should be undertaken, and an otolaryngologist or thoracic surgeon should be consulted.

Bronchial mainstem intubation is a common complication of tracheal stoma intubation and is discussed in Chapter 96: Intubating an Existing Tracheostomy.

- Stomas less than 1-week old may be prone to false lumen creation and other complications during device manipulation.
- The presence of a tracheostomy tube disrupts swallowing and predisposes a patient to aspiration.
- The anesthesia provider should have a small tracheal tube or other bougie-like device available when exchanging the in situ device.
- *See Figure 95.1 and* **Video 95.1** *for additional details.*

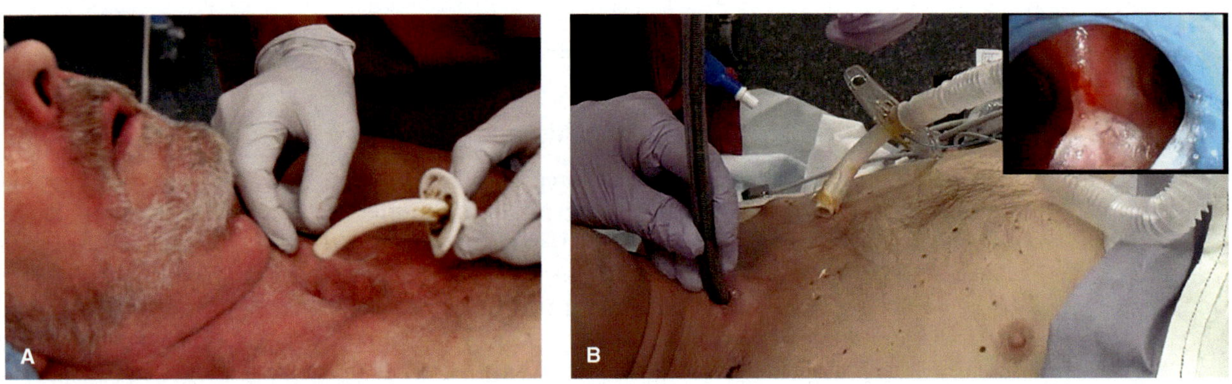

Figure 95.1. A: An uncuffed Shiley tracheal tube is removed from an established tracheostomy. **B:** In order to assure precranial positioning of a tracheal tube inserted into a preexisting stoma, a flexible intubated scope is being used.

Suggested Readings

Mitchell RB, Hussey HM, Setzen G, et al. Clinical consensus statement: tracheostomy care. *Otolaryngol Head Neck Surg*. 2013; 148(1):6–20.

Rosero EB, Corbett J, Mau T, Joshi GP. Intraoperative airway management considerations for adult patients presenting with tracheostomy: a narrative review. *Anesth Analg*. 2021;132(4):1003–1011.

Tabaee A, Lando T, Rickert S, Kuhel WI. Practice patterns, safety, and rationale for tracheostomy tube changes: a survey of otolaryngology training programs. *Laryngoscope*. 2007;117(4):573–576.

White AC, Kher S, O'Connor HH. When to change a tracheostomy tube. *Respir Care*. 2010;55(8):1069–1075.

Intubating an Existing Tracheostomy

96

Larissa I. Galante

1 Describe in detail the device or technique.

Patients may present to the OR with a variety of tracheal stomas and tracheostomy devices which require unique considerations.

A tracheostomy consists of a stomal length, which is the distance from the skin to the anterior tracheal wall (average length 2.6 cm ± 0.7 cm with ranges of 1.8 to 5.5 cm in men and 1.5 to 4.2 cm in women), and the intratracheal length, measured from the inferior edge of the tracheal opening to the carina (mean 4.3 cm, range of 2.2 to 6.6 cm). Stomal length varies depending on its location in the neck, patient body habitus, and angle of the stoma in relation to the trachea. Stomal length is increased with lower tracheal entrance sites, obesity, generalized edema, and nonperpendicular angles of insertion. Most tracheostomies are inserted at the second or third tracheal cartilage rings, and the size of the tube is determined by the internal cannula diameter.

The tracheostomy can be a midaccess point in the patient's airway as in the case of a patient with upper airway pathology or may constitute the terminal end of the airway (ie, after laryngectomy where no contiguous upper airway exists). For the purposes of this discussion, tracheostomy will refer to the former, and terminal stoma will refer to the latter. A laryngectomy tube can appear very similar to a tracheostomy, but it is important to remember that mask ventilation is not possible due to the surgical excision of the upper airway.

A number of prosthetic devices or coverings may be present on tracheostomy or terminal-stoma patients, ranging from simple metallic or plastic tubes with/without air-inflated cuffs or plastic cuffed or uncuffed tubes with fenestrations to allow speech. Well-epithelialized tracheostomies often do not require any tubular device, and the patient may be using a speech valve glued to the skin.

Stoma devices will vary in the manufactured lengths of the stomal (skin-to-airway track) and intratracheal arms, as well as in internal diameter. There are varieties with which the lengths can be actively adjusted (eg, Bivona, Smiths Medial, Dublin, OH). Almost all tubular devices will have an inner cannula that can be cleaned or replaced, and a solid obturator that occludes the lumen during reinsertion.

The proximal flange may be flush with the patient's neck, which does not allow external circuit connection as is the case with metallic tracheostomy tubes. It may have a standard 15-mm adaptor that allows connection to an anesthesia circuit or breathing bag (eg, Shiley catheter). If fitted with a cuff and nonfenestrated, these devices may be used for general anesthesia with positive-pressure ventilation. This is not recommended for long procedures, and it is crucial for the anesthesia provider or otolaryngologist to have uninterrupted access to the device if necessary. Fenestrated and uncuffed tubes will rarely provide a seal adequate for positive-pressure ventilation and should never be used with anesthetic gases due to leaks, environmental pollution, and staff exposure. It is best to exchange the tracheostomy device for a standard endotracheal tube or to intubate the uninstrumented stoma, unless a cuffed, nonfenestrated tracheostomy tube is in place. In addition, devices that meet the criteria to provide positive-pressure ventilation may need to be replaced due to interference with the surgical field, risk of dislodgement, or for longer procedures (Table 96.1).

TABLE 96.1 Preanesthetic Checklist for Tracheostomized Patients

1. Identify the indication for tracheostomy including total laryngectomy
2. Determine whether the trachea could be intubated orally
3. Determine the timing of tracheostomy: greater or less than 7 d
4. Determine the size and type of tracheostomy device
5. Confirm patient position during procedure: prone, supine, or lateral
6. Determine the need for neuromuscular blockade and positive pressure ventilation
7. Assess other relevant medical aspects of the patient: coagulation status, respiratory status, morbid obesity, thick and short neck, etc.
8. Determine the need to consult an ear, nose, and throat surgeon

Reprinted with permission from Rosero EB, Corbett J, Mau T, Joshi GP. Intraoperative airway management considerations for adult patients presenting with tracheostomy: a narrative review. *Anesth Analg*. 2021;132(4):1003–1011. Table 2. Copyright © 2020 International Anesthesia Research Society.

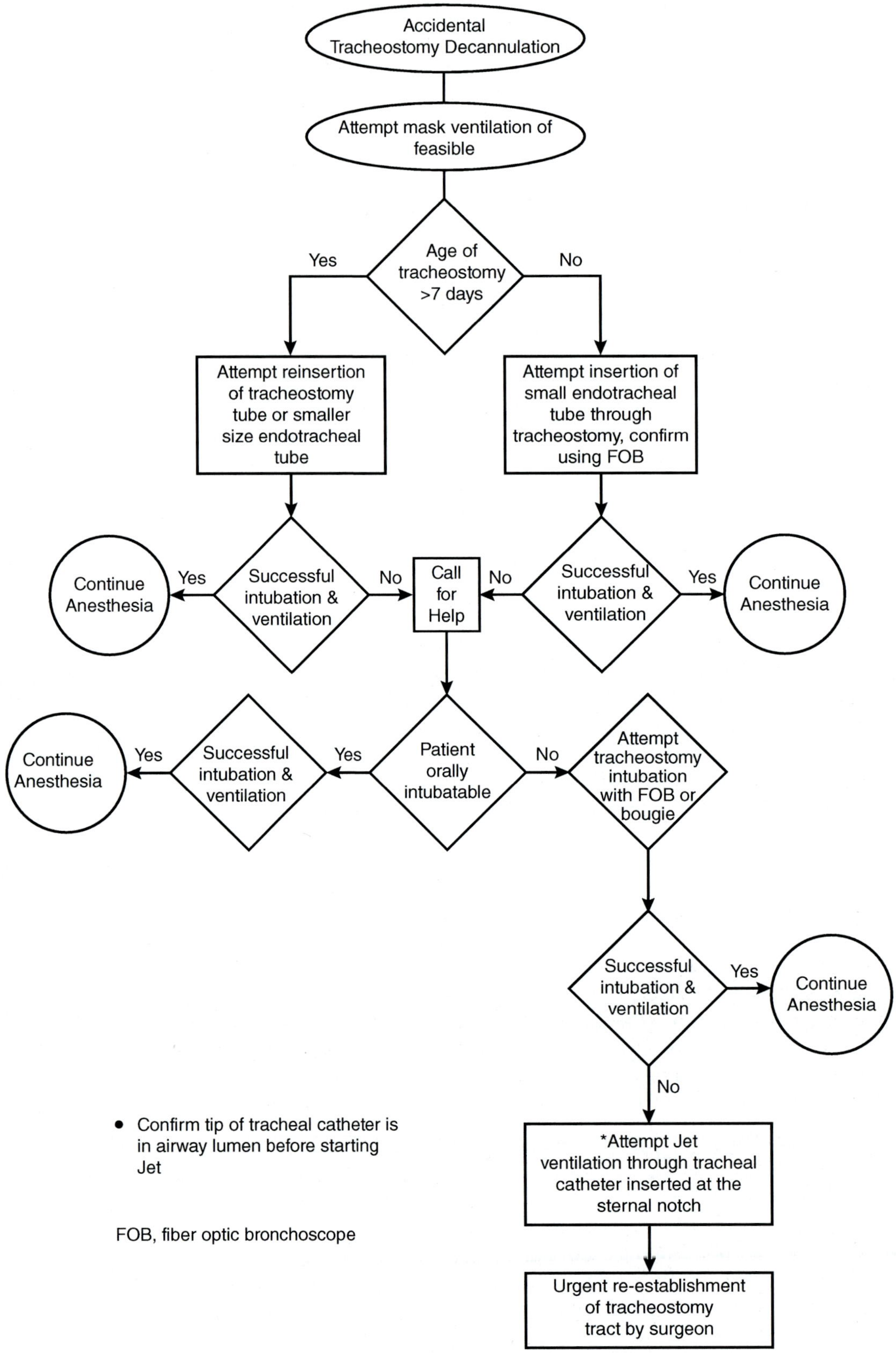

Figure 96.1. Algorithm for management of accidental tracheostomy decannulation during anesthesia. (Reprinted with permission from Rosero EB, Corbett J, Mau T, Joshi GP. Intraoperative airway management considerations for adult patients presenting with tracheostomy: a narrative review. *Anesth Analg*. 2021;132(4):1003–1011. Figure 4. Copyright © 2020 International Anesthesia Research Society.)

If there are preoperative concerns about the integrity of the tracheostomy or terminal stoma, removal of the tracheostomy device and/or reintubation can be done prior to the induction of anesthesia, maintaining spontaneous ventilation. Preparing the patient with 50 to 100 mg atomized lidocaine will reduce discomfort. If there is little concern, general anesthesia can be induced prior to manipulation of the airway. Induction may be performed either intravenously or via inhalation.

Prior to exchanging an indwelling device or otherwise manipulating a terminal stoma or tracheostomy, the patient should be preoxygenated. If the upper airway is patent, it may be necessary to occlude it or the tracheostomy to achieve effective preoxygenation.

The degree of caution that should be exercised in manipulating the stoma will depend on the type of stoma, its age, and the tissue integrity. During the creation of a terminal stoma, the tracheal mucosa is secured to the skin. Early manipulation of these stomas is generally safe. Indwelling devices can be removed and tracheal tubes inserted, with the chief caution being avoiding mainstem bronchus intubation. In most cases, visualizing the proximal tracheal tube cuff at the upper edge of the terminal stoma is sufficient. The tracheal tube should be secured to the patient's chest with wide tape or sutures (Figure 96.1).

In the surgical creation of a nonterminal tracheostomy, the skin-to-airway track is allowed to epithelialize, which may require 5 or more days. Prior to complete epithelialization, false lumens may be created during manipulation. Extreme care should be taken when removing any indwelling tracheostomy tube and placing another device. In patients with fenestrated tubes, granulation tissue may form in the posterior tracheal wall, which will make it more difficult to remove.

Often one or two tracheostomy hooks are used to secure the interior of the trachea prior to removing the indwelling device. Alternatively, an airway exchange catheter (AEC) may be inserted into the indwelling device, which is then removed. The AEC is held with a hand resting on the patient's chest for stabilization. A tracheal tube is now introduced over the catheter. Care should be taken to avoid forcible insertion of the AEC or tracheal tube, and the depth of insertion of either device should be carefully monitored. A FIS may also be used to insert the tracheal tube. A FIS, fitted with a tracheal tube, is inserted into the tracheostomy after removal of any indwelling device. The FIS is used to identify the carina. The tracheal tube is then inserted and assessed visually to remain in the trachea. When using an AEC or FIS for insertion, hang-up may occur. Tracheal tube rotation, change to a smaller tube or larger AEC or FIS, or a change to another tracheal tube design should be considered. Repeated forceful attempts at stoma intubation should be avoided. As with terminal stomas, visualizing the proximal tracheal tube cuff within the track generally assures a safe depth of insertion.

Once the tracheal tube is placed, the cuff is inflated to the minimal pressure needed to prevent air leak. Bilateral breath sounds and end-tidal CO_2 must be assessed. If bilateral ventilation cannot be verified, the location of the proximal tracheal tube cuff is again assessed in the stoma, and/or the position can be evaluated with a FIS.

In the event of difficulty with intubation of a terminal stoma or tracheostomy, insertion of a small standard tracheal tube, a jet ventilation microcatheter, or an AEC capable of oxygen-insufflation may be used successfully as a temporizing airway. Intubation via the upper airway can also be considered.

Depending on the planned surgical procedure and the position of the patient (eg, prone), a wire-reinforced, kink-resistant tracheal tube may be indicated. Problems that may occur during maintenance of anesthesia include kinking of the tube, subcutaneous emphysema if high airway pressures are used, complete dislodgement or migration into a mainstem bronchus with laparoscopic pneumoperitoneum, Trendelenburg positioning, or movement of the head and neck.

- Preoperatively assess the type of stoma, its age, and tissue integrity.
- Indwelling devices should be assessed for compatibility with controlled ventilation.
- Chief risks include false lumen creation and endobronchial intubation.
- Appropriate depth of the tracheal tube is most often verified by seeing the proximal cuff edge in the stoma.
- *See Figure 96.2 for additional details.*

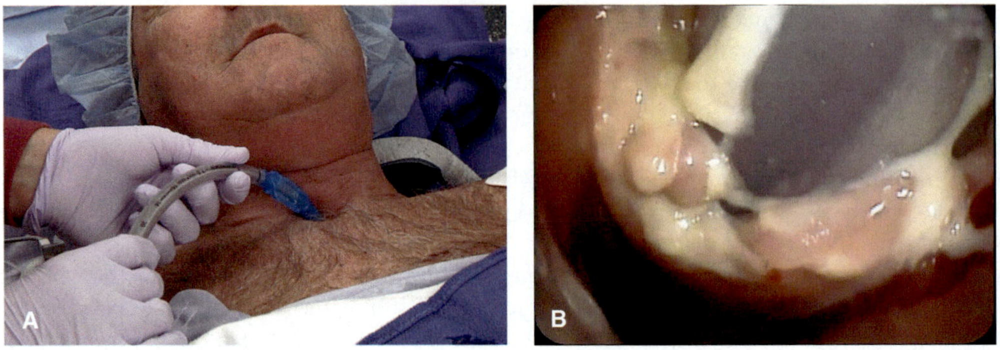

Figure 96.2. **A:** A patient with a well-established tracheal stoma is being intubated with a wire-reinforced tracheal tube. (See **Video 96.1**.) **B:** In a patient with a tracheal-esophageal fistula (iatrogenic), an esophageal stent is seen with a flexible scope in the trachea. (See **Video 96.2**.)

Suggested Readings

Chong DY, Greenland KB, Tan ST, Irwin MG, Hung CT. The clinical implication of the vocal cords-carina distance in anaesthetized Chinese adults during orotracheal intubation. *Br J Anaesth.* 2006;97(4):489–495.

Mallick A, Bodenham A, Elliot S, Oram J. An investigation into the length of standard tracheostomy tubes in critical care patients. *Anaesthesia.* 2008;63(3):302–306.

Pang G, Edwards MJ, Greenland KB. Vocal cords-carina distance in anaesthetised Caucasian adults and its clinical implications for tracheal intubation. *Anaesth Intensive Care.* 2010;38(6):1029–1033.

Rosero G, Corbett J, Mau T, Joshi P. Intraoperative airway management considerations for adult patients presenting with tracheostomy: a narrative Review. *Anesth Analg.* 2020;132(4):1002–1011.

97 One-Lung Ventilation in a Patient with Tracheostomy

Terrence Feldheim

Clinical Scenario: A 67-year-old man with a left lower lobe 2-cm mass presents to the OR for a video-assisted thoracoscopic left lower lobectomy. The patient has a history of laryngeal cancer 10 years ago for which he underwent a laryngectomy with tracheostomy. He currently has an uncuffed 8.0 Shiley catheter in place.

1 What are the anesthetic and airway management considerations for this case?

Video-assisted thoracoscopic surgery (VATS) requires one-Lung ventilation (OLV) to facilitate surgical exposure.

The most commonly used methods for OLV include either placement of a double-lumen endotracheal tube (DLT) or a bronchial blocker (BB). DLTs are still the most common devices used for lung separation. However, the design of BBs makes them especially worthy of consideration for cases requiring lung isolation in patients with preexisting tracheostomies. The presence of a tracheostomy requires adaptations of conventional lung-isolation techniques.

2 How would you manage the airway in this case?

Following preoxygenation and intravenous induction of anesthesia, the tracheostomy tube (TT) is removed and replaced by an 8.0 mm wire-reinforced endotracheal tube (ETT). The position of the ETT above the carina is confirmed using the flexible bronchoscope (FB), and the tube is sutured in place.

For the purpose of lung isolation, a BB is used.

The Uniblocker (Fuji System Corporations, Tokyo, Japan) kit consists of a BB with a fixed bent tip and an airway adaptor. The airway adaptor contains ports for the anesthesia circuit, the FB, the BB, as well as for the ETT. This adaptor is connected to the anesthesia circuit and to the wire-reinforced ETT, respectively.

The FB is inserted through the designated port, and the blocker is advanced into the left main stem bronchus under bronchoscopic visualization. The cuff of the BB is inflated and confirmed not to herniate over the carina. The port for the BB is tightened down to hold the BB in place. Once adequate occlusion of the left main stem bronchus is confirmed, the scope is removed. Alternatively, any BB can be used. For indications and instructions on how to use the Cohen BB, see the designated chapter. Following lateral decubitus positioning, the position of BB is checked again using the same technique.

At the completion of the surgical procedure, the BB is removed. The wire-reinforced ETT is carefully suctioned and removed. The TT tube is subsequently reinserted in the stoma.

3 What are the potential hazards and complications in regard to the airway?

Malposition and dislodgement of the DLT, ETT, or the BB can occur, particularly during positioning in lateral decubitus or during surgical manipulation. In general, DLTs have fewer instances of dislodgement. However, conventional DLTs placed into a tracheostoma are too long for a shortened airway and therefore, the potential for dislodgement is augmented. DLTs are bulkier and may be more likely to lead to airway trauma when inserted through the tracheostoma.

Preoperative FB examination of the stoma is essential in determining what type and what size tube can be used. Measurement of the distance from the stoma to the carina identifies if a DLT can be used. If the tracheostomy is performed very low in the airway, most likely the bronchial cuff of the DLT will herniate above the carina while the tracheal cuff will herniate above the stoma.

4 What Distinct airway device (eg, specialized tracheal tube, rigid bronchoscope, BB) might be used in this case, and what are the special considerations?

A variety of methods to achieve lung isolation in patients with preexisting tracheostomies have been described, and there are advantages and disadvantages to each technique.

Short DLTs intended for tracheostomies are not available on the US market. Conventional DLTs have been used, particularly in procedures precluding the use of BB (ie, sleeve resection or disease of the main stem bronchus). In these cases, DLT insertion can be achieved directly through the tracheostoma. Alternatively, DLTs can be inserted from above, via direct laryngoscopy, with removal of the TT as soon as the distal end of the DLT passes through the vocal cords.

BBs are more commonly employed in tracheostomized patients requiring lung isolation. With a cuffed TT in situ, the BB adaptor can be directly connected. The BB is then passed through the TT, and it is positioned under FB guidance. The adaptor is connected to the circuit, and ventilation is achieved via the cuffed TT.

Alternatively, the TT is removed and replaced by an in-stoma ETT. BBs can then be inserted either through an ETT or alongside the ETT. Very small tracheal stomas can only accommodate a small-sized ETT. Therefore, the simultaneous insertion of the BB and FB may be impossible. In this case, the FB and the BB are inserted through the stoma and the BB is positioned under direct visual guidance. The FB is removed and a small-sized ETT is passed through the stoma, alongside the BB.

OLV in the presence of a recent tracheostomy imposes further management challenges. Removal of a fresh tracheostomy is hazardous as the bleeding risk from an immature tracheostoma is high. In addition, there is an increased potential for losing the airway after TT removal and for creating a false track if reinsertion attempts are pursued. Therefore, the lung isolation will have to be achieved without removal or significant manipulation of the TT. BBs constitute the preferred option for lung isolation in patients with fresh tracheostomies. The in situ cuffed TT will be used to ventilate the noncollapsed lung, as described above for patients with a mature tracheostomy.

However, with a small-sized TT, the BB will have to be placed alongside the in situ TT. In these cases, the BB will be inserted from above via direct laryngoscopy. When the BB passes the laryngeal inlet, the TT cuff is briefly deflated to allow the BB to be positioned alongside the TT. Once the BB is positioned distal to the TT, the FB is inserted through the TT and the BB is advanced in the desired main stem bronchus. The potential for BB dislodgement as well as the potential for airway injury is higher in these cases.

If the direct laryngoscopy is known to be difficult, an supraglottic airway (SGA) could be used as a conduit for both BB and FB until the laryngeal inlet is visualized. Thereafter, the BB is allowed to pass alongside the TT (after brief cuff deflation) and the FB is reinserted through the TT to allow further BB positioning distal to the TT, in the main stem bronchus. In these cases, the SGA can also serve as an anchoring device for the BB (Figure 97.1).

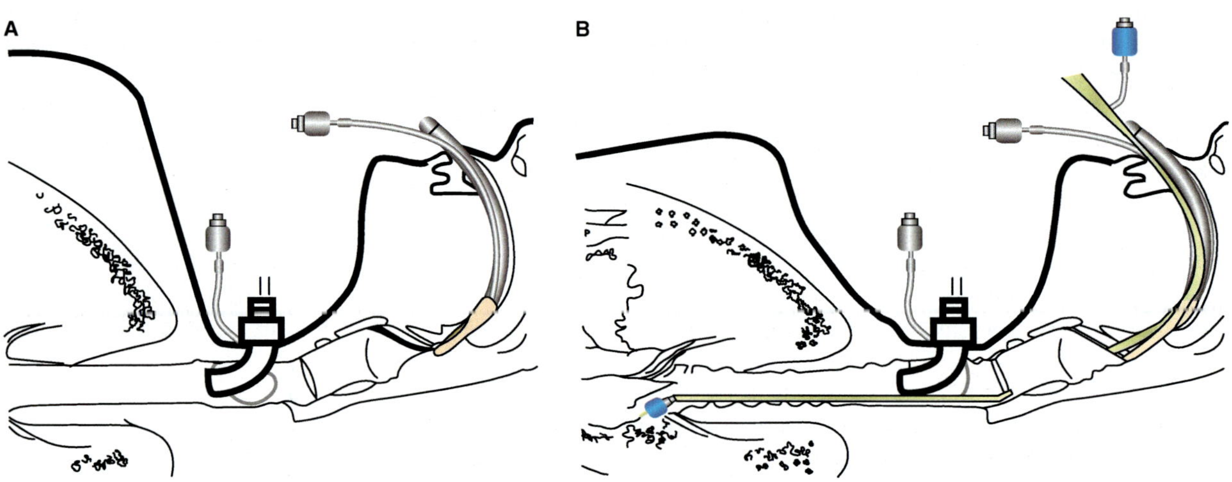

Figure 97.1. A: Schematic of tracheostomy patient with an SGA in the oropharynx. **B:** Schematic of proper position of BB in a tracheostomized patient with an SGA. (Figure used with permission of A.R. Robinson III and K. Kuck, Department of Anesthesiology, University of Florida College of Medicine. From Robinson AR III, Gravenstein N, Alomar-Melero E, Peng YG. Lung-isolation using a laryngeal mask airway and a bronchial blocker in a patient with a recent tracheostomy. *J Cardiothorac Vasc Anesth.* 2008;22(6):883–886.)

- The presence of a tracheostomy requires adaptations of conventional lung-isolation techniques.
- The preoperative FB evaluation is essential in airway management planning and in selection of the appropriate lung-isolation device.
- The choice of a specific airway technique depends on the patient's particular anatomy and clinician's experience with each device.
- *See Figure 97.2 and* ***Video 97.1*** *for additional details.*

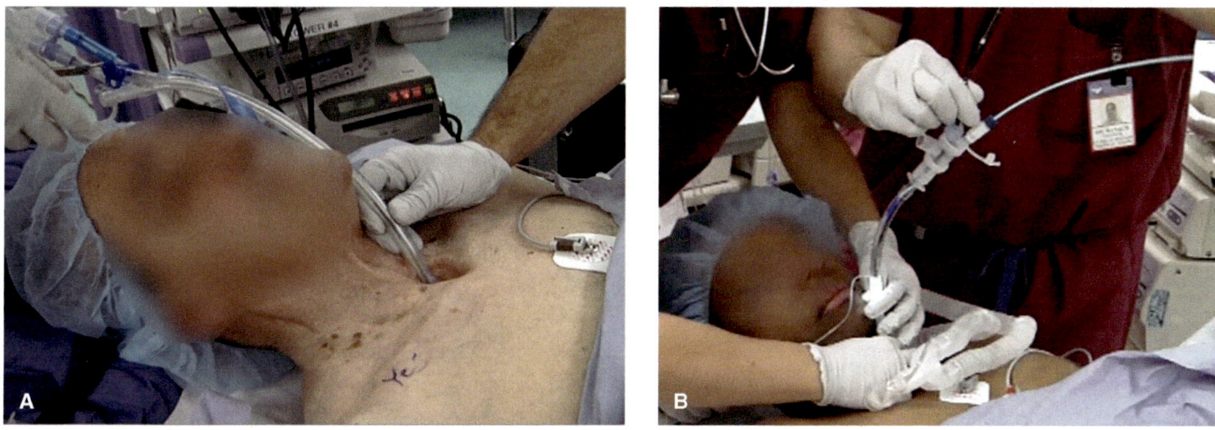

Figure 97.2. **A:** Double-lumen tracheal tube is being used to achieve lung isolation in a patient with a preexisting tracheal stoma. **B:** An 8.0 ID tracheal tube and a bronchial blocker are being used to achieve lung isolation in a patient with a preexisting tracheal stoma.

Suggested Readings

Brodsky JB. Lung separation and the difficult airway. *Br J Anaesth.* 2009;103:i66–i75.
Campos JH. An update on bronchial blockers during lung separation techniques in adults. *Anesth Analg.* 2003;97:1266–1274.
Campos JH. Lung isolation techniques for patients with difficult airway. *Curr Opin Anesthesiol.* 2009;22:1–6.
Collins SR. Lung isolation in the patient with a difficult airway. *Anesth Analg.* 2018;126(6):1968–1978.
Neustein SM. The use of bronchial blockers for providing one-lung ventilation. *J Cardiothorac Vasc Anesth.* 2009;23(6):860–868.

98 Tracheoesophageal Puncture for Voice Prosthesis Placement

Andres R. Brenes Bastos

Clinical Scenario: A 72-year-old man underwent laryngectomy 3 weeks ago. He now presents for the creation of a tracheoesophageal fistula in preparation for placement of a voice prosthesis.

1 What are the anesthetic and airway management considerations for this case?

Tracheoesophageal puncture (TEP) with voice prosthesis placement is the gold standard for vocal rehabilitation of patients who have undergone total laryngectomy. The voice prosthesis may be placed at the time of the procedure (primary) or at a later date (secondary). There is currently no consensus on superiority between primary and secondary placement, and selection is made on a patient-by-patient basis. The prosthesis is a one-way valve that allows airflow from the trachea into the pharynx. TEP involves surgical manipulation at the level of the tracheal stoma. The posterior tracheal wall and anterior esophageal wall are punctured and stented with a silicone catheter. The silicone catheter is sutured to the lateral peristomal skin, and the distal end is directed down the esophagus. When performed in the operating room, the entirety of the procedure is performed under general anesthesia and under visualization through a rigid esophagoscope by a trained endoscopist. Currently, there is evidence of the procedure being safely and comfortably performed in the office setting under flexible nasal endoscopy and local anesthesia. At the author's institution, however, preference is still to perform TEP in the operating room. Office-based TEP will not be discussed in this chapter.

Immediate complications with TEP are rare but can include aberrant perforation of the posterior esophageal wall with subsequent mediastinitis or abscess formation. Antibiotics may be given for prophylaxis against peristomal infection or cellulitis around the site of the catheter. Intraoperative aspiration of esophageal contents is possible but unlikely because the small TEP is the only communication between the esophagus and the airway. Postoperative complications include pharyngocutaneous fistula, wound infection, bleeding, and stomal stenosis.

TEP is performed under general endotracheal anesthesia. Intubation is achieved through the tracheostoma with a wire-reinforced TT. The duration of surgery is usually short (10 to 30 minutes) with a very little interval between procedure termination and need for anesthetic termination.

Total intravenous anesthesia (TIVA) is generally preferred for endoscopy. In the event of intentional or accidental intraoperative extubation, TIVA maintains an adequate depth of anesthesia. Conversely, delivery of inhalational agents relies on a continuous airway, so the removal of the TT during the procedure may cause a fluctuation of the anesthetic depth. In addition, pollution of the operating room environment is avoided with the use of TIVA.

2 How would you manage the airway in this case?

It is important to emphasize that TEP patients present posttotal laryngectomy, so there is no continuity between the upper and lower airway. Preoxygenation ($FIO_2 = 1.0$) is achieved via the tracheostoma. Patients present with any variety of tracheostomy devices or none at all. Some devices may allow attachment to the anesthesia circuit for preoxygenation. After adequate preoxygenation, general anesthesia is induced, and TIVA is initiated. Tracheal intubation is accomplished through the existing tracheostoma. Wire-reinforced ETTs are preferred as they allow more flexibility around the stoma, resist compression, and offer greater surgical exposure, but standard tracheal tubes can also be utilized.

The ETT should be advanced into the stoma until the cuff can adequately seal the airway when inflated. The distance between the tracheostoma and carina is variable. Special caution should be taken to avoid endobronchial intubation as the tracheostoma may be just a few centimeters superior to the carina. Endotracheal intubation should be confirmed with auscultation of bilateral breath sounds, symmetric chest rise, capnography and/or appropriate oxygenation and ventilation, and if needed, FIS aided inspection. The patient's head is usually positioned 90 degrees to 180 degrees away from the anesthesia machine, so special consideration should be taken to adequately secure the TT. Frequently, this will be performed by the surgical team as they will also manipulate the TT during the procedure. Stoma extubation is not uncommon given the close proximity of the surgical site. Elective, intermittent extubation may be needed to access the tracheal puncture site. This may be done by the anesthesiologist or surgeon—in either case, close communication is vital. Electrocautery is typically not required. If it must be used, the FIO_2 should be reduced to approximately 30% as the patient tolerates to reduce the risk of airway fires. A laser tracheal tube can be substituted if deemed appropriate.

TEP is a highly stimulating procedure mostly due to the rigid esophagoscopy, but has minimal postoperative pain. Short-acting opioids are preferred in this scenario. This could include remifentanil (loading dose 0.5 to 1.0 µg/kg IV, infusion 0.1 to 0.25 µg/kg/min), alfentanil (loading dose 20 to 40 µg/kg IV, infusion 0.25 to 1.0 µg/kg/min IV), or small doses of fentanyl. Of note, when compared to alfentanil, use of remifentanil for TIVA is associated with faster return of spontaneous ventilation, reduction of propofol use, and increased hemodynamic stability.

Both spontaneous and mechanical ventilation are viable options, depending on the anesthetic regimen used. Relaxation may be required for insertion of the esophagoscope as patient movement can result in esophageal trauma. If nondepolarizing agents are used, an adequate, spontaneous tidal volume should be observed before stomal extubation. Alternatively, titrated boluses of short-acting opioids may be sufficient for the endoscopy.

3 What are the surgical considerations that impact anesthetic management?

TEP patients have undergone prior total laryngectomies. Many of these patients are elderly and have a history of alcohol and/or tobacco abuse. Other common comorbidities must be considered, such as malignancy, chronic obstructive pulmonary disease, and cardiovascular disease.

Although TEP is a short procedure, esophagoscopy is highly stimulating. The anesthesia provider must ensure hemodynamic stability. TEP is associated with up to a 4% incidence of myocardial ischemia mostly due to the adrenergic response to endoscopy. Patient movement when the esophagoscope is in place can result in esophageal trauma, and so a still surgical field is imperative. Often muscle relaxation is given for endoscope placement, and opioids and other hypnotics are used to prevent further movement. Surgical puncture of the posterior tracheal wall may require intermittent extubation of the stoma.

4 What distinct airway device might be used in this case, and what are the special considerations?

During TEP, a rigid esophagoscope is used to provide visualization of the esophageal lumen and prevent puncture of the posterior esophageal wall. A flexible, wire-reinforced tracheal tube withstands compression and allows for increased surgical exposure during surgical manipulation. Adult tracheostomas will usually accept adult-sized tracheal tubes (eg, 7.0 to 8.0). Consultation with the surgeon is appropriate if there is a question for preference regarding size of the TT. A laser-resistant tracheal tube should be available if cautery must be used for a long duration.

- Deep anesthesia and neuromuscular relaxation should be used whenever the esophagoscope is in place.
- TIVA is usually preferred for TEP when performed in the operating room.
- A wire-reinforced, flexible ETT allows for maneuverability around the tracheostoma while maintaining adequate ventilation.
- *See Figure 98.1 and* ***Video 98.1***.

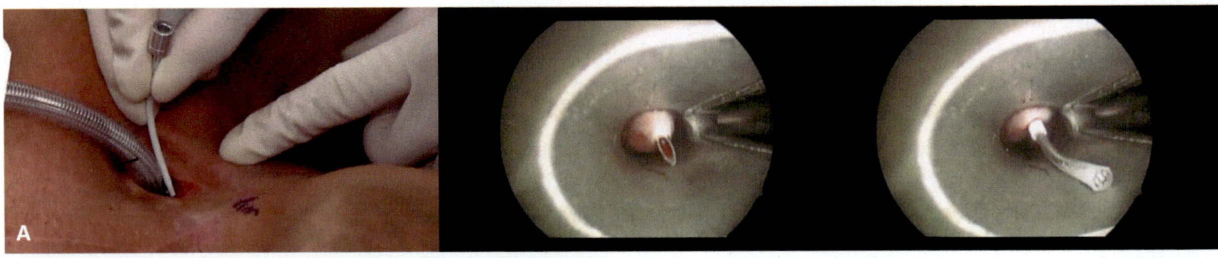

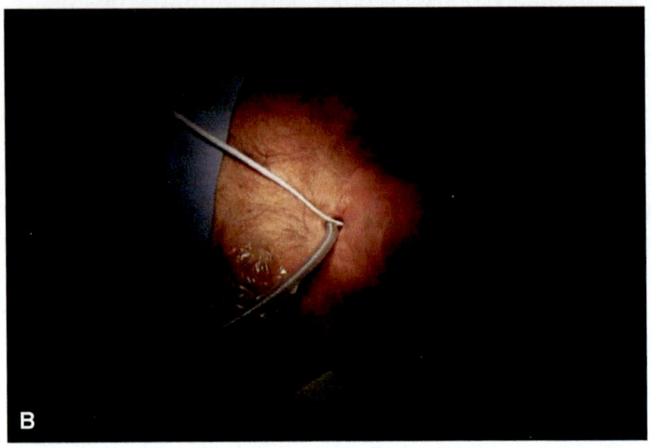

Figure 98.1. **A:** In the process of creating a tracheal–esophageal fistula and the placement of a voice prosthesis, (**left to right**) a puncture is made in the posterior tracheal wall as it is observed using a suspension esophagoscope (that also serves to protect from wayward needle advancement). A wire is passed that will be used to place the final stenting catheter. In alternative techniques, the voice prosthesis can also be placed at this time. **B:** A stenting catheter has been placed. This catheter will later be substituted by the voice prosthesis.

Acknowledgment

We gratefully acknowledge the contributions of previous edition author, Lara Zador, as portions of those chapters have been retained in this revision.

Suggested Readings

Bergeron JL, Jamal N, Erman A, Chhetri DK. Office-based tracheoesophageal puncture: updates in techniques and outcomes. *Am J Otolaryngol.* 2014;35(5):549–553.

Desyatnikova S, Caro JJ, Andersen PE, Cohen JI, Wax MK. Tracheoesophageal puncture in the office setting with local anesthesia. *Ann Otol Rhinol Laryngol.* 2001;110:613–616.

Myers J, Hanna EY, Myers EN. Chapter 15: Voice rehabilitation after total laryngectomy. In: *Cancer of the Head and Neck*. Wolter Kluwers; 2017.

Tracheostomy Revision

99

Ann Marie Melookaran Iliff

Clinical Scenario: A patient who has undergone previous laryngectomy presents with breakdown of the skin around his tracheostomy site. He is scheduled for stoma revision.

1 What are the anesthetic and airway management considerations for this case?

Tracheostomy revision post laryngectomy requires sharing of the airway by surgeon and anesthesiologist. While oxygenation and ventilation take precedence, the surgical intervention may require multiple removals and reinsertions of a tracheal tube for surgical access. Unless contraindicated (or if only brief and few removals of the tracheal tube are planned), total intravenous anesthesia is often used for tracheostomy revisions. The patient who has previously undergone a total laryngectomy will have an end-tracheostomy. Patients may present with a bare stoma, or with a metal, plastic, or silastic stomal tube in situ. Factors such as the age of the stoma, recent or ongoing therapies (eg, radiation), and surgeon and patient preference will dictate how the tracheostomy is maintained outside the OR. For the purposes of providing anesthetic care, an indwelling device is typically replaced with a cuffed tracheal tube to allow for positive-pressure ventilation if needed. The surgical team revises the tracheal stoma by either working around the tracheal tube or intermittently removing and replacing it. In patients who have a preserved larynx, upper airway intubation may be possible, averting the need for intermittent extubation. This may not be possible in all patients (eg, severe tracheal/laryngeal stenosis) and/or may require special care (eg, awake intubation). The risk of airway fires is increased in patients presenting for airway surgery. Although apneic periods may be needed for surgical access, a lower concentration of oxygen should be used whenever possible to reduce airway fire risk.

2 How would you manage the airway in this case?

In this laryngectomy patient, preoxygenation should occur via the stoma. If the patient presents with an indwelling device, it may have a fitting which allows a connection with the anesthesia circuit. Devices that do not connect to the anesthesia circuit may be replaced, and the removed device should be returned to the patient postoperatively. The anesthesia circuit with high oxygen flow may be held to the stoma or in-site device. After induction of anesthesia, a tracheal tube can be inserted into the stoma of the end-tracheostomy patient with or without the use of muscle relaxation. Though any standard tracheal tube can be used, a wire-reinforced flexible tube may have the advantages of being repositioned away from the surgical area and less likely to bend or kink. Preapplication of a topical local anesthetic to the trachea may be considered.

The depth of tracheal tube insertion through the stoma should be noted. There is always a risk of endobronchial intubation. The proximal end of the tracheal tube cuff should be visible at the skin–mucosa junction of tracheostomy. Bilateral auscultation should be performed, and flexible scope inspection can be used to verify supracarinal position of the tracheal tube bevel. The tracheal tube may be taped or sutured to the skin. Either controlled or spontaneous ventilation can be used during the procedure. Similar stomal management can be practiced in the patient with a preserved larynx, but tracheal intubation via the upper airway is another reasonable technique in these patients. A preoperative discussion with the surgical team will decide the best approach based on patient anatomy. In severely compromised airways (eg, severe breakdown of tracheal mucosa–skin junction; existence of tracheal–cutaneous, tracheal–esophageal, or other fistulas, tracheal stenosis, or tracheal mucosal tears), an airway exchange catheter (AEC) or similar device may be passed through the in situ tracheostomy device prior to removal and used as a guide for replacement with the tracheal tube. These catheters may be shortened in length to provide improved handling. If a catheter is shortened, it must still maintain twice the length of a typical tracheal tube to function as an AEC. Repositioning of the tracheal tube or complete removal from the stoma may be requested during the surgery. The duration of extubation events should be tempered by changes in the oxygen saturation and/or end-tidal CO_2. Use of 100% FiO_2 during periods of ventilation will help prolong the safe apneic period (if fire risk is low), but return of the maximal oxygen saturation may be seen before full reoxygenation occurs. Reextubation should be resisted until the anesthesiologist is satisfied with reoxygenation, which will also provide for a longer apneic and surgical access period. Each reinsertion of the tracheal tube should prompt a check of the bevel depth based on cuff position and auscultation as necessary. In the severely compromised airway, leaving in situ AEC may be helpful when reintubation is undertaken. A similar technique may be necessary for the patient with a preserved larynx who has been intubated via the upper airway. In some cases, surgical access may still require transient removal of the tracheal tube. This is an advanced technique and should be thoroughly understood before being undertaken.

3 What are the surgical considerations that impact anesthetic management?

Surgical considerations include requirements for exposure, use of electrocautery around the airway, and extent of revision. This will require diligence to the position of the tracheal tube intraoperatively. Surgery can take place while the tracheal tube is in place and also when it is intermittently removed. This requires continuous communication between the surgical and anesthesia teams. Use of a low concentration of oxygen and possibly a fire-resistant tracheal tube may be necessary to reduce the risk of airway fires.

4 Are there special considerations for the emergence or the end of the case?

Prior to removing the tracheal tube and replacing it with the patient's tracheostomy device, adequate spontaneous ventilation should be assured. If controlled ventilation will need to be maintained postoperatively, a cuffed tracheostomy device should be used (eg, cuffed tracheal tube or Shiley tracheostomy tube).

- Total intravenous anesthesia is preferred for maintenance of anesthesia during tracheostomy revision due to the nature of the shared airway and possibility of intermittent apnea.
- Wire-reinforced tubes are less likely to bend and may be easier to reposition to help facilitate surgical exposure.
- Airway fire risk should be discussed and prevented by all members of the operating room team.
- In a patient with a preserved larynx, intubation of the upper airway may be beneficial but should be discussed with the surgical team prior to proceeding as airway management will depend on the individual patient's anatomy.
- *See Figure 99.1 and* **Video 99.1** *for additional details.*

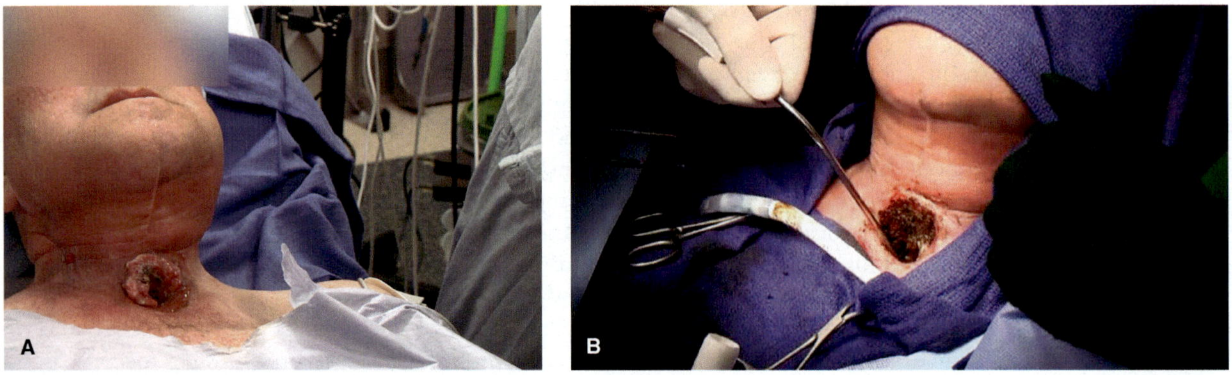

Figure 99.1. **A:** Hyperplastic (and potentially cancer recurrent) tissue around a prior tracheal stoma. The patient presents for tissue biopsy and stoma revision. **B:** During tracheal stoma revision, the patient is managed with total intravenous anesthesia. It may be necessary to remove the tracheal tube from the stoma to provide improved surgical access. Note that a heat-resistant tracheal tube is in use.

Suggested Readings

Bathula SS, Srikantha L, Patrick T, Stern NA. Immediate postoperative complications in adult tracheostomy. *Cureus.* 2020;12(12):e12228.

Freeman BD. Tracheostomy update: when and how. *Crit Care Clin.* 2017;33(2):311–322.

Jaffe R, Schmiesing C, Golianu B. *Anesthesiologist's Manual of Surgical Procedures.* 5th ed. Lippincott Williams & Wilkins; 2014:192–193.

Rosero EB, Corbett J, Mau T, Joshi GP. Intraoperative airway management considerations for adult patients presenting with tracheostomy: a narrative review. *Anesth Analg.* 2021;132(4):1003–1011.

Decannulation of the Patient with the Long-Standing Tracheostomy

100

Laura J. Alexander

Clinical Scenario: A 45-year-old obese patient had previously been treated with a tracheostomy for subglottic stenosis following a prolonged intubation. After several laser resections, she now presents for a trial of decannulation under visualization by direct laryngoscopy.

1 What are the anesthetic and airway management considerations for this case?

To be considered for decannulation, patients must be able to cough and swallow effectively, be independent of ventilatory support, alert without altered mentation, and able to tolerate deflation of the tracheostomy cuff and a capping trial. Capping trials create a scenario of "functional decannulation." These trials assess the patient's ability to move air through the upper airway and elucidate whether any clandestine stenotic lesions formed during the period of tracheostomy dependence. Before terminal decannulation, the airway will often be examined by direct laryngoscopy under general anesthesia to rule out any obstructive lesions. Terminal decannulation procedures offer a unique set of challenges for the anesthesia provider. Unlike freshly created stomas, the tract of a long-standing tracheostomy has "matured" and disruption of the tissue is less likely, except in those patients with recognized risk factors such as prior radiation or poor nutrition. Furthermore, anterior wall tracheal collapse can be masked by the tracheostomy tube's stenting of the airway. Surgeons often utilize flexible and rigid endoscopy to visualize lesions or areas of stenosis. In the case of rigid endoscopy, neuromuscular paralysis is critical for patient safety. These procedures are stimulating but have minimal postoperative pain, therefore, short-acting opioid analgesics provide sufficient intraoperative hemodynamic control without the prolonged postoperative respiratory depressant effects of long-acting opioids.

2 How would you manage the airway in this case?

Prior to induction of anesthesia, preoxygenation can be achieved via the in situ tracheostomy device or through the mouth and nose. Effective preoxygenation may require occlusion of the airway not in use as tolerated by the patient. Induction of anesthesia is most often carried out with intravenous agents and maintained with total intravenous anesthesia (TIVA). Inhalation agents are generally avoided due to the inevitable leak from the tracheostomy site or upper airway. After induction of anesthesia, the tracheostomy device is removed and replaced with a cuffed tracheal tube. A wire-reinforced, flexible tracheal tube may confer an advantage. The surgical team may request a fire- or laser-resistant tracheal tube depending on the expected treatments. In most circumstances, the proximal tracheal tube cuff should be visible in the stoma to ensure it has not been placed too deeply. The presence of bilateral breath sounds and flexible endoscopy can both be used to ensure a supracarinal placement of the tracheal tube bevel. The tracheal tube may be secured to the chest wall for the procedure. Once successful oxygenation and ventilation are confirmed, the upper airway is inspected with rigid or flexible endoscopy. Granulation tissue or stenosis compromising more than 30% of the airway is surgically addressed. Laser resection or stent placement may take place. Before emergence, a downsized and/or cuffed tracheostomy device may be placed depending on surgeon preference. The patient should emerge sufficiently from anesthesia such that he or she is breathing spontaneously with adequate tidal volumes. The surgical team may elect to decannulate the tracheostomy at this time. If there is any concern as to whether the patient will be able to maintain his or her airway, decannulation may be performed over a wire or exchange catheter. The stoma is covered with an occlusive gauze, and air is allowed to pass through the upper airway. The patient should be monitored for stridor and adequate oxygenation. Converting a patient from a tracheostomy to upper airway breathing increases physiologic dead space by 50% and work of breathing by 30%. If respiratory failure occurs during this trial, reintubation via the upper airway or through the stoma should be performed.

3 What are the potential hazards and complications in regard to the airway?

Numerous hazards exist in patients who have long-standing tracheostomies. Occult stenosis from anatomical issues or granulomas is the most common complication. This should be identified and/or addressed before or during decannulation. Unrecognized stenosis or granulation tissue causing airway compromise can quickly lead to respiratory collapse after decannulation. Tracheomalacia may be camouflaged due to splinting by the tracheostomy device. This can result in tracheal collapse and stridor after decannulation. Bleeding is common in the setting of granuloma resection, especially in the setting of anticoagulant usage. When lasers are utilized in a setting of high FiO_2, airway fires can occur. FiO_2 should be reduced to 30% during laser usage, and it is important to note that standard polyvinyl chloride endotracheal tubes are highly flammable. Laser smoke, in particular, can pose a risk to operating room staff as it can contain active viral DNA. Staff should wear N95 masks and protective eyewear during airway laser procedures.

4 What distinct airway device (eg, specialized tracheal tube, rigid bronchoscope, BB) might be used in this case, and what are the special considerations?

During decannulation, equipment for evaluation of the airway including flexible endoscopy, infant laryngoscopy, and rigid bronchoscopy should be available in the operating room. In the case of failed decannulation, a bougie wire, smaller tracheostomy tube, and tracheostomy hook should be available. Subglottic stenosis requires the presence of equipment for airway stenting.

5 Are there special considerations for the emergence or the end of the case?

Upon emergence, the patient must be monitored for adequate oxygenation, tidal volumes, airway pressures, and stridor. Stridor may be the earliest sign of airway compromise upon occlusion of the stoma, and emergency access to the stoma and replacement of the tracheostomy tube may be necessary. The patient should remain in the recovery unit for several hours to ensure adequate ventilation before discharge. A cuffed tracheostomy tube should be present at the bedside should the patient develop airway obstruction from swelling related to surgical interventions.

- Candidates for decannulation must be alert, able to clear secretions, and able to maintain ventilation without assistance.
- Granulation tissue, anatomic changes, or tracheomalacia may result in airway obstruction after decannulation.
- TIVA is the preferred maintenance anesthesia technique.
- *See Figure 100.1 and* ⊙ ***Video 100.1*** *for additional details.*

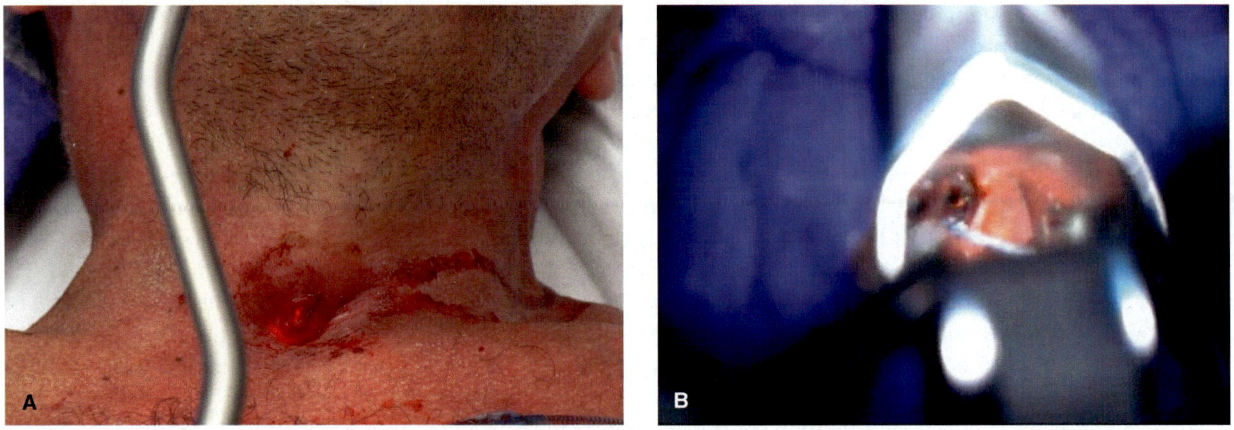

Figure 100.1. **A:** A patient with a chronic tracheostomy requires surgical opening of the upper airway before attempts at decannulation. **B:** Suspension laryngoscopy and LASER tissue resection being used to reestablish the upper airway in an attempt at decannulation of a patient with a chronic tracheostomy.

Suggested Readings

Chadda K, Louis B, Benaïssa L, et al. Physiological effects of decannulation in tracheostomized patients. *Intensive Care Med.* 2002;28(12):1761–1767.

Christopher KL. Tracheostomy decannulation. *Respir Care.* 2005;50:538–541.

Epstein SK. Late complications of tracheostomy. *Respir Care.* 2005;50:542–549.

Laser treatment for laryngeal lesions. In: Hemmings H, ed. *Yao & Artusio's Anesthesiology Problem-Oriented Patient Management.* 10th ed. Wolters Kluwer; 2026:724–735.

Pathak V, Welsby I, Mahmood K, Wahidi M, MacIntyre N, Shofer S. Ventilation and anesthetic approaches for rigid bronchoscopy. *Ann Am Thorac Soc.* 2014;4:628–634.

101 Emergency Care of Tracheostomy Tube Dislodgement

Elizabeth C. Behringer

Clinical Scenario: A 48-year-old man has ventilator-dependent respiratory failure due to adult respiratory distress syndrome. He had a bedside tracheostomy placed percutaneously this morning in the intensive care unit (ICU). You are called emergently by the nurse because the new tracheostomy tube has been accidentally dislodged while the patient was being positioned for a chest x-ray. The patient is exhibiting signs of respiratory distress and his oxygen saturation is now in the 80s.

Performance of a tracheostomy and the presence of a tracheostomy device (TD) are common findings in critically ill patients. Seven percent to 19% of ICU patients will be managed with a TD, which can be performed via an open surgical technique in the operating room or, most commonly, at the bedside via a percutaneous dilatational Seldinger technique. Indications for tracheostomy vary greatly, and may include but are not limited to upper airway obstruction and need for emergency airway access, laryngeal cancer with laryngectomy, or reprieve from prolonged tracheal intubation. Tracheostomy procedures are often considered after 7 to 10 days of mechanical ventilatory support without successful weaning. There is evidence to support early tracheostomy, as some studies cite improved outcomes and a reduction in ventilator days. An emergent surgical tracheostomy may also be necessary in a variety of clinical scenarios when acute upper airway obstruction mandates surgical access to the airway.

The decision to perform a tracheostomy is complex and requires its own chapter to discuss completely. This chapter will focus specifically on emergent tracheostomy dislodgement and aims to address the evaluation and management of this complication in the acute setting. In addition, as patients with TDs or laryngectomies are found throughout the prehospital and hospital settings, knowledge of the resources and goals of care for this patient population are important for all clinicians.

Several studies have reported that up to 30% of acutely hospitalized patients with TDs are at risk for significant morbid events or death associated with their tracheostomy. The NAP4 study reported 14 dislodged tracheostomies in ICU patients. Eleven of these led to death or hypoxic injury. Common issues cited included lack of competency, lack of capnography, inadequate staff training, lack of equipment and support, as well as lack of preformulated emergency pathways and inadequate follow-up of critical events. The National Tracheostomy Safety Project (NTSP) and the National Confidential Enquiry into Patient Outcome and Death (NCEPOD) have underscored the importance of improving care for this patient population.

Incidental TD dislodgement is a sentinel event that can lead to serious morbidity and can become rapidly fatal. TD dislodgement may present in a variety of forms:

1. A "cuff leak" in a newly tracheostomized patient indicating partial dislodgement
2. Malposition of the TD resulting in impaired or impossible gas exchange
3. Complete decannulation (removal of the TD)

It should be recognized that the TD may migrate into a false lumen of the tissues of the anterior neck, or the distal end of the TD may be obstructed with blood, mucus, or tissues of the tracheal wall.

When faced with the emergent management of a dislodged TD, understanding the indication and timing of insertion are essential for success. In short, understanding the "why," "when," and "how" the TD was placed will guide management. Attempting oropharyngeal tracheal intubation in a patient with a history of total laryngectomy would be both ineffective and traumatic, for example. The "why" can vary, and it affects decision making in emergency management of TD dislodgement. "When" your patient's tracheostomy was performed (eg, the date of the procedure) helps to narrow the differential diagnosis in the setting of a postprocedural complication and determines how to manage oxygenation and ventilation when encountering TD dislodgement. Maturation of the tracheal stoma requires approximately 5 to 7 days when placed percutaneously and a minimum of 3 days when done via an open surgical technique with stoma maturation sutures. If sutures are present, identify what kind of sutures are present, their function, and placement. Ideally, if the surgeon has placed "stay sutures" on either side of the anterior tracheal wall during tracheostomy, these can be gently pulled away from the midline on either side to open the stoma. Attempting to recannulate an immature tract after TD dislodgement without a clear and open stoma may result in the creation of a false tract into the soft tissue and/or mediastinum. If the tracheostomy is less than 7 days postplacement, as in the case described above, assume the tract is not mature. In short, three questions should immediately be asked when approaching an emergency TD dislodgement: (1) Why was the tracheostomy performed?, (2) When was the tracheostomy performed?, and (3) How was the tracheostomy performed? Due to the importance of this information in emergency situations, all patient handoffs should include the same why, when, and how. In addition, it is crucial to know the size, manufacturer, and type of TD placed at the time of insertion. It is important to note any special features of the TD, such as extra length, presence of an inner cannula, or a specialty cuff. It is recommended to have a duplicate replacement TD, including additional inner cannulas (if applicable), immediately available at the patient's bedside. Finally, it is important to assess whether the TD's cuff pressure is appropriate, as excessive cuff pressure often indicates malposition of a TD and increases its risk of accidental decannulation.

Once the outlined information has been clarified, the provider can then make an informed plan for airway management and how to safely oxygenate and ventilate the patient. The multidisciplinary NTSP has established multiple easy-to-follow algorithms for airway management of emergent tracheostomy complication or dislodgement. The starting point and choice of algorithm is based on the aforementioned "Why," "When," and "How" (http://www.tracheostomy.org.uk) (see also Figure 101.1).

All emergent TD dislodgements with respiratory compromise are airway emergencies and should begin with the same primary principles: call for help, provide supplemental oxygen via the mouth, nose, and tracheostomy stoma, have the necessary equipment immediately available at the patient's bedside (a difficult airway cart), and notify the airway team at your facility or an airway expert. After making the call for help, a primary survey of the patient, including airway, breathing, and circulation, must quickly be performed. The primary survey includes a look, listen, and feel at both the mouth and the tracheostomy/laryngectomy stoma. The use of waveform capnography is highly sensitive for airway patency with air movement and ventilation. All the NTSP decision-making trees for emergent TD displacement management start with these basic steps. If the patient is pulseless, proceed with cardiopulmonary resuscitation (CPR) and initiate chest compressions followed by basic life support or advanced cardiopulmonary life support based on the resources available.

Two main algorithms have been devised by the NTSP: Emergency management of dislodged TD in the setting of a patent upper airway and emergency management of a dislodged TD post laryngectomy. Patients who are converted to tracheostomy after emergency cricothyrotomy for difficult and failed intubation have a "patent" upper airway but are proven to have difficult upper airway management, and therefore, fall into the postlaryngectomy decision tree.

The clinical scenario at the beginning of this chapter described a patient who is postoperative day 0 from a percutaneous tracheostomy and has an incidental total TD dislodgement with respiratory distress. In most cases, these patients will have a patent upper airway and a stoma that is not mature. Assuming the patient is not experiencing cardiopulmonary arrest, high-flow oxygen should be applied to both the face and the stoma. Bag-mask ventilation with waveform capnography should be attempted while occluding the stoma, to confirm airway patency while additional help is summoned. If the patient's respiratory distress stabilizes and capnography confirms ventilation, preparations should be made for oral intubation with difficult airway equipment, including immediate availability of a fiberoptic bronchoscope. After successful intubation and stabilization of the patient, a fiberoptic scope should be used to confirm placement of the endotracheal tube below the level of the stoma and facilitate suctioning of blood and secretions.

If bag-mask ventilation is unsuccessful, an oral airway or supraglottic airway should be considered to improve oxygenation and ventilation before attempting laryngoscopy. High-flow oxygen should be administered through the stoma site. Blind attempts to pass a TD through an immature stoma are not recommended.

The Global Tracheostomy Collaborative is a superb international organization and resource for multidisciplinary teamwork, standardization, education, and patient partnership in tracheostomy care (www.globaltrach.org). Interested clinicians should be aware of this important resource.

- All inadvertent TD dislodgements are considered airway emergencies.
- Knowing the "why," "when," and "how" the TD was placed will guide further management.
- *See Figure 101.2 and* **Video 101.1** *for additional details.*

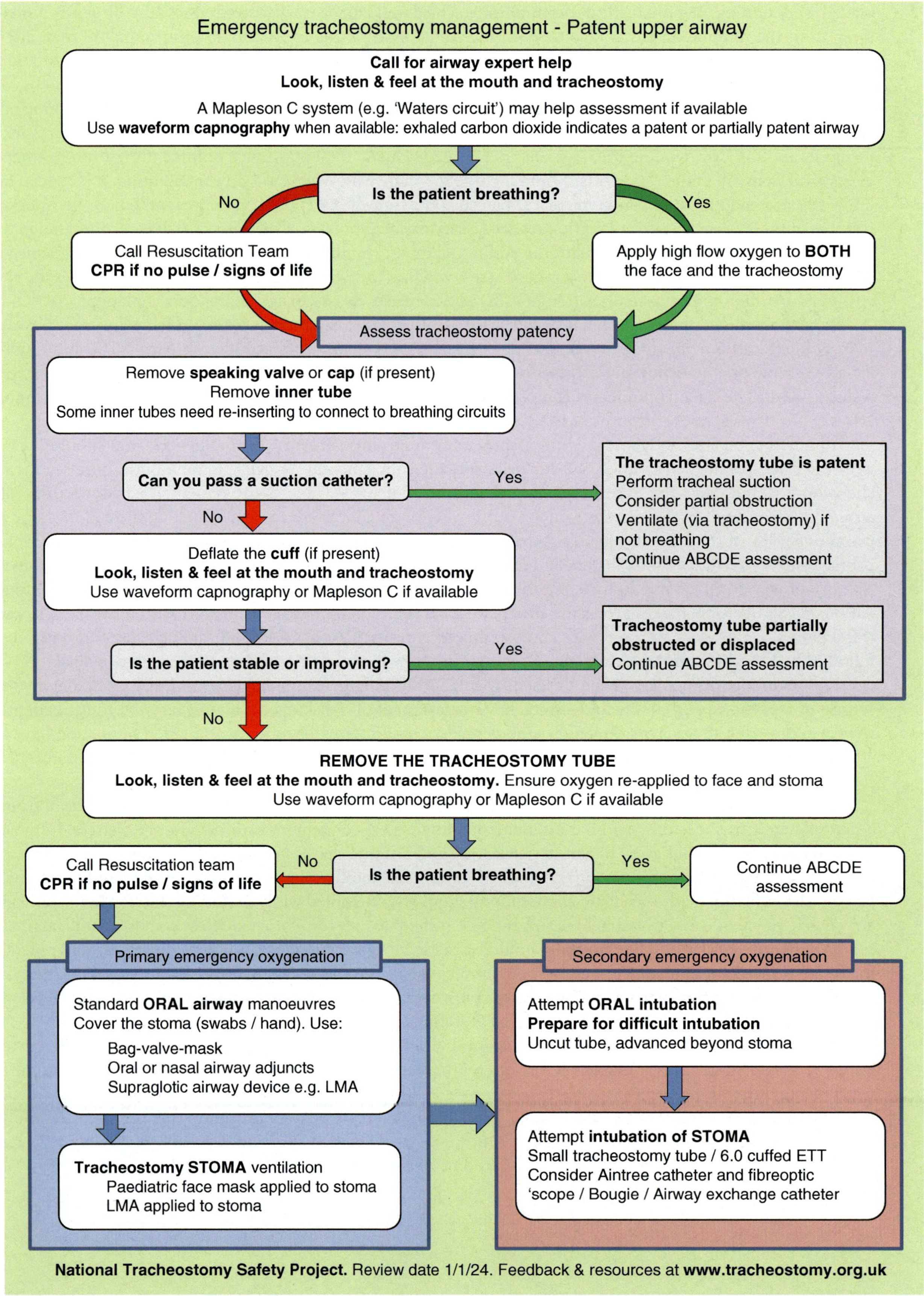

Figure 101.1. Emergency tracheostomy management: upper airway. (Courtesy of the National Tracheostomy Safety Project. Review Date 1/1/24. Feedback & resources at www.tracheostomy.org.uk.)

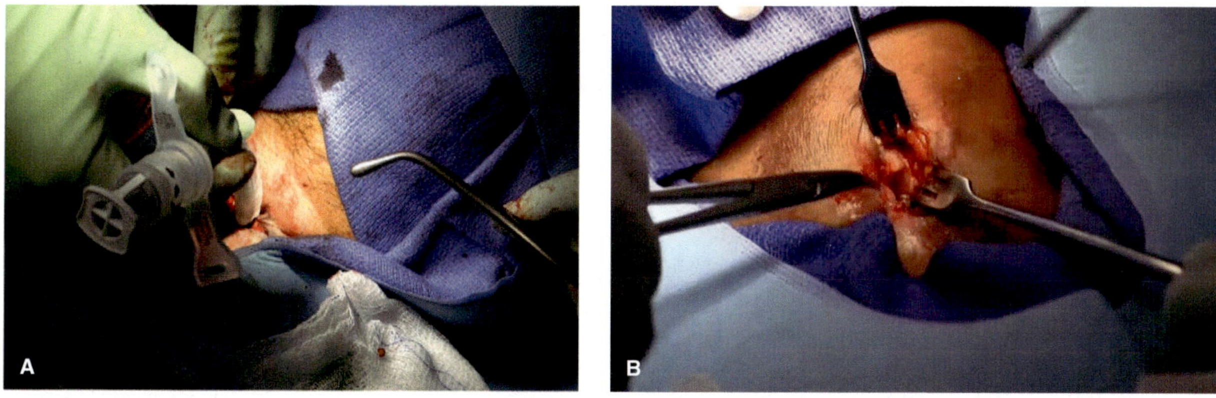

Figure 101.2. **A:** A Shiley tracheostomy catheter is replaced into a decannulated and partially closed tracheostomy. **B:** A long-standing tracheostomy that was accidentally decannulated for 48 hours requires emergency surgical exploration and reopening.

Acknowledgments

We gratefully acknowledge the contributions of previous edition authors, Wayne Lai and Taizoon Yusufali, as portions of those chapters have been retained in this revision.

Suggested Readings

Cook TM, Woodall N, Harper J, et al. Fourth National Audit Project. Major complications of airway management in the UK: results of the Fourth National Audit Project of the Royal College of Anaesthetists and the Difficult Airway Society. Part 2. Intensive care and emergency departments. *Br J Anaesth*. 2011;(5):632–642.

Lewith H, Athanassoglou V. Update on management of tracheostomy. *BJA Educ*. 2019;19(11):370–376.

McGrath BA, Wilkinson K. The NCEPOD study: on the right track: lessons for the anaesthetist. *Br J Anaesth*. 2015;115:155–158.

Mitchell RB, Hussey HM, Setzen G, et al. Clinical consensus statement: tracheostomy care. *Otolarnyngol Head Neck Surg*. 2013; 148(1):6–20.

Wallace S, McGrath BA. Laryngeal complications after tracheal intubation and tracheostomy. *BJA Educ*. 2021;21(7):25–257.

102 The Patient with a Persistent Tracheostomy Fistula

Laura J. Alexander

Clinical Scenario: A 55-year-old man who had undergone elective tracheostomy for prolonged ventilation after a motor vehicle accident now returns with a persistent air leak from his stoma. He is otherwise healthy, does not snore, and does not have gastroesophageal reflux. He has a normal BMI. The surgeon wishes to surgically close his persistent stoma.

1 What are the anesthetic and airway management considerations for this case?

A patient presenting with a persistent air leak from an incompletely closed tracheal stoma poses a unique challenge for the anesthesiologist. Air leak from the stoma may render supraglottic airway (SGA) ventilation, including face mask, inefficient or even impossible. Positive-pressure ventilation proximal to the defect will cause increased leak, loss of gas, OR pollution, and ineffective oxygenation and ventilation.

Inhalational induction may be limited by room air dilution entrained via the stoma and can result in OR pollution. In the event that the tracheal intubation is difficult, the use of face mask or SGA rescue, as suggested by the difficult airway algorithm of the American Society of Anesthesiologists, may not be feasible.

Thyroid or laryngeal malignancy and a history of airway obstruction are independent risk factors for persistent tracheocutaneous fistula. As such, this patient population is often inherently high risk. Prior to formulating an airway plan, the anesthesiologist must understand the immediate anatomy of the tracheal defect, including the existence of strictures or scarring. Typically, the surgeon will have performed a preprocedure endoscopy or imaging studies to characterize the airway above and below the defect. Significant findings might dictate alternative courses such as surgical resection of the stenosis or stenting prior to the stomal revision surgery.

If difficulty with tracheal intubation is expected, awake intubation should be pursued to secure the airway. If airway control after the induction of anesthesia is the chosen pathway, an intravenous technique and use of a nonmask or SGA for ventilation should be used.

Regardless of the method of tracheal intubation employed, the goal is to position the tracheal tube cuff distal to both the stomal defect and any tissue that will be mobilized during the surgical repair. This tube position will isolate the surgical field from positive ventilating pressures which could undermine an incomplete repair. With low-lying stomas, the possibility of bronchial intubation must be eliminated, which might require flexible intubating scope (FIS) verification. Once positioned, the tracheal tube should be adequately secured against movement.

The monitoring of the location and pressure within the tracheal tube cuff is integral to the surgical procedure. If the surgical closure involves a tracheal mucosal flap, a nearby, overinflated cuff can endanger tissue perfusion. Likewise, an inadequate tracheal tube cuff seal may allow air leakage, potentially undermining tissue used in the closure.

At the end of the procedure, the surgical team may ask for a leak test of the stoma closure. The tracheal tube cuff is deflated and pressure within the trachea is allowed to rise. The surgical team may flood the local plane with sterile saline and monitor for bubbles indicating a leak.

2 How would you manage the airway in this case?

There are a few options for management to ensure proper and adequate ventilation and control throughout the surgery. If the patient has a history of difficult laryngoscopy, the author's preference would be to use an awake FIS technique for securing airway. If there is no indication that intubation will be delayed or difficult, a nonmask/SGA induction technique combined with FIS for tracheal tube placement is a reasonable approach. During preoxygenation, the stoma can be occluded or covered. The FIS is used to assure passage of the tracheal tube beyond the stomal defect while still remaining above the tracheal carina. While advancing the FIS into the trachea, a blunt needle, wire, or a gloved finger can be placed into the stoma to identify its location from an intratracheal view, which helps with tracheal cuff positioning.

Tracheal tube cuff pressure should be monitored during the procedure.

3 What are the potential hazards and complications in regard to the airway?

In the patient with a persistent tracheal stoma, preoxygenation, mask ventilation, and inhalational induction may be difficult or futile. During tracheal intubation, it may be difficult to pass a FIS or tracheal tube beyond scarring or strictures in the airway. The risk of failure to ventilate or intubate can occur in this scenario, so the surgeon should be present in the OR during attempts to secure the airway.

Throughout the procedure, the proximity of the tracheal tube to the surgical repair must be constantly monitored. There is an ongoing risk of airway fire, and the integrity of the tracheal tube and tracheal tube cuff may become compromised which increases fire risk. Depending on the extent of the surgery and the dissection required to mobilize tissue coverage of the tract, there can be significant contamination of the airway with blood or other surgical debris. A competent tracheal tube cuff and an FiO_2 of equal or less than 30% must be maintained for this reason.

4 Are there special considerations for the emergence at the end of the case?

Strategies for emergence and extubation should be individualized and must consider the preoperative anatomy, complexity of the airway, and the extent of the surgery. In extensive reconstructions, the airway should be irrigated and suctioned proximally to remove any contaminating debris or blood products from the surgical field. The tracheal tube cuff should be deflated to test for an air leak. Of note, this is an imperfect assessment of the immediate swelling around the surgical site. The otolaryngologist may want to inspect the tract closure from the interior of the trachea with a FIS to assure the suture line and ensure the closure remains intact. This will also allow inspection of the vocal cords for swelling and, if strictures and scarring were present during intubation, identification of any airway trauma. Unless contraindication exists, extubation while the patient is spontaneously breathing at a deep plane of anesthesia may be requested. The goal of this technique is to avoid both iatrogenic positive pressure in the airway and coughing and straining. Once the patient is extubated, he or she should be monitored for stridor. To avoid disrupting the surgical closure, care should be taken to avoid positive-pressure ventilation via a face mask or SGA.

- Preoxygenation is most effective when the stomal leak is occluded.
- Mask and SGA ventilation will likely not be possible due to the stomal leak.
- Use of an FIS helps assure adequate placement of the tracheal tube past the stoma.
- Communication with the surgical team to ensure integrity of the tracheal tube and cuff during the procedure is essential.
- Whenever possible, the patient is extubated in a manner that will avoid mask ventilation, coughing, and straining.
- *See Figures 102.1 and 102.2 for additional details.*

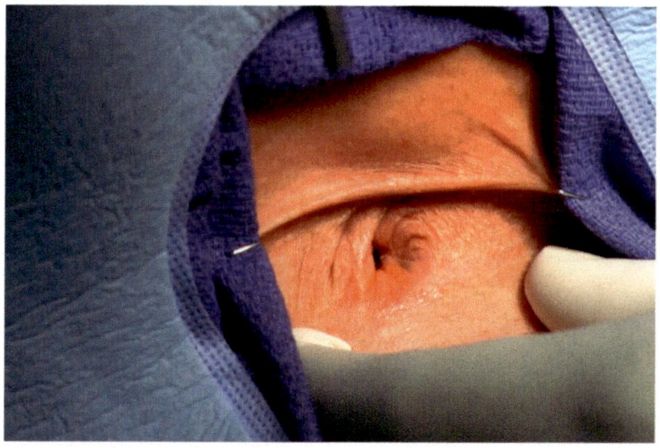

Figure 102.1. A patient decannulated from tracheostomy has a nonclosing, persistent tracheal-cutaneous fistula. See **Video 102.1.**

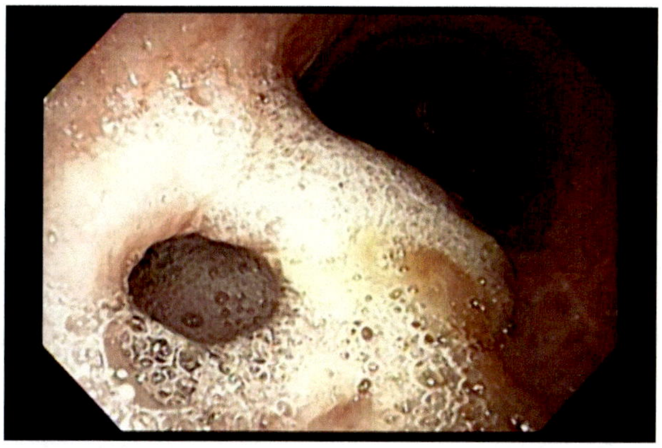

Figure 102.2. A patient with persistent tracheoesophageal fistula. See **Video 102.2.**

Suggested Readings

Apfelbaum JL, Hagberg CA, Connis RT, et al. 2022 American Society of Anesthesiologists Practice Guidelines for management of the difficult airway. *Anesthesiology*. 2022;136(1):31–81.

Gallagher TQ, Hartnick CJ. Tracheocutaneous fistula closure. *Adv Otorhinolaryngol*. 2012;73:76–79.

Mohan VK, Kashyap L, Verma S. Life threatening subcutaneous emphysema following surgical repair of tracheocutaneous fistula. *Paediatr Anaesth*. 2003;13(4):339–341.

Short JA. Temporary occlusion of a persistent tracheocutaneous fistula during anaesthesia. *Anaesthesia*. 2000;55(4):392–393.

The Adult with a Foreign Body in the Airway (Acute)

103

Melissa S. Shears • Jessica L. Feinleib

Clinical Scenario: A college-age man is brought urgently into the emergency department (ED) by ambulance. He was eating dinner and began to cough violently. He has loud stridor and is in obvious distress. Trauma surgery and anesthesia were both called urgently to the ED.

1 What are the anesthetic and airway management considerations for this case?

Most adult foreign body aspiration victims are in the seventh decade of life or older and have risk factors, which include neurologic deficits with dysphagia, altered mental status, neuromuscular disease, or intoxication. Cough is the most common presenting symptom of foreign body aspiration, but patients can also have wheezing, dyspnea, stridor, hoarseness, and hemoptysis.

Acute foreign body aspiration is an airway emergency in a potentially unfasted, high aspiration-risk patient. The obstruction may be in the upper or lower airway, and there is risk of progression to complete airway obstruction. Patients with upper airway obstruction are more likely to present with respiratory distress. Further consideration should be made for location of the foreign body retrieval (ED vs OR), multidisciplinary team members, type of anesthesia and monitoring, postprocedure disposition, and potential complications.

2 How would you manage the airway in this case?

Preprocedure planning is critical to successfully retrieve the foreign body. The perioperative plan should be designed by a multidisciplinary team, which includes anesthesiologists, otolaryngologists, and technicians. Team discussion should include characteristics of the foreign body, location in the airway, anticipated airway plan to maintain ventilation and oxygenation, as well as stepwise plan for removal of the foreign body. A designated airway equipment cart should be present in the OR/ED prior to the commencement of the procedure. Standard monitors and supplemental oxygen should be applied. The use of continuous waveform end-tidal capnography is essential to assess airway patency in real time. Auscultation is often the most readily available and rapid method for delineating the location of the obstruction: pharynx, larynx, trachea, or bronchial tree. Imaging confirmation could be considered, but can consume precious time in unstable patients when direct visualization of the airway can be diagnostic and therapeutic. In addition, caution should be taken when sending a patient to a poorly monitored and difficult-to-access setting to obtain imaging.

Expedited patient preparation, including topical local anesthetics and sedation, will facilitate the removal process. Nebulized 4% lidocaine provides airway topical anesthesia while not interrupting supplemental oxygen. Choice of anesthetic agent(s) should be done with consideration for the desire to maintain spontaneous ventilation while providing adequate depth for a highly stimulating airway procedure. Positive-pressure ventilation may increase the risk of dislodging the object further into the airway, as well as causing hyperinflation and barotrauma secondary to the ball-valve effect. Although maintenance of spontaneous ventilation is critical, steps should be taken to minimize aspiration risk given this is an emergency procedure with unknown fasting time. Utilizing a volatile anesthetic for this purpose could be considered, but often, total intravenous anesthesia is preferred. Additional adjuncts that can be considered include administration of a corticosteroid to minimize inflammation and edema, and glycopyrrolate to dry secretions.

If the foreign body is in the pharynx, then a laryngoscope or a flexible bronchoscope with a pair of Magill forceps are highly suitable tools for its brisk removal. However, if the object is lodged in the hypopharynx or more distally, then the conscious patient will require some preparation prior to retrieval of the foreign body. If at any point the patient loses consciousness, then the need for patient comfort is obviously moot, and immediate action should be taken to remove the object and ventilate the patient.

Laryngeal foreign bodies are best approached with a flexible bronchoscope equipped with a snare, forceps, basket, magnet, Fogarty balloon, suction catheter, or Magill's or any device that the user is facile with. Additional factors in the selection of a bronchoscope working channel tool are the friability of the object and its geometry.

For objects located in the central airway, carrying a higher risk of complete airway loss, a rigid bronchoscope can support the airway and facilitate removal of the foreign body. If, during the removal procedure, complete airway obstruction occurs, the bronchoscope or a tool from the working channel can be used to force the object distally past the carina. This is a temporizing maneuver to allow for patient ventilation while reevaluating possible strategies to extract the foreign body.

Patients with foreign bodies located in the distal airway or bronchopulmonary tree may require full control of the airway and intubation. If the object is smaller than the internal diameter of the ETT, then they can be retrieved with a flexible bronchoscope snare or grasper. In contrast, when the object is greater in size than the internal diameter of the endotracheal tube (ETT), the operation becomes more involved. It is tempting to break up the object and then pull fragments through the ETT; however, this can cause multiple and more distal obstructions. Alternatively, capturing the foreign body with the flexible bronchoscope and removing it in coordination with the removal of the ETT is a fine technique. To facilitate this maneuver, a laryngoscope and a pair of forceps in the pharynx can visualize and remove the object from the pharynx once it is delivered above the vocal cords.

3 What are the potential hazards and complications in regard to the airway?

In cases of critically ill patients with inextricable supralaryngeal obstructions, it is important to ensure multiple airway plans, including emergency surgical front of neck access (FONA).

With respiratory distress, an assessment of medical stability is the first priority and abnormalities in presenting vital signs are a marker for poor outcomes. The greatest complication of an acute foreign body airway obstruction is the obvious; loss of the airway. With the loss of an airway, hypoxia-induced cardiac arrest is soon to follow, and therefore, cardiac resuscitation equipment should be available in addition to airway equipment.

The removal of rigid and piercing foreign bodies located in the distal bronchial tree can present a risk of pneumothorax. Therefore, the availability of a chest tube is prudent.

There is a risk of local edema, incurred by the trauma of foreign body removal. One study found mucosal inflammation and granulation tissue in 40% of a series of 32 patients with foreign bodies. This risk can be attenuated by administration of a prophylactic dose of corticosteroids.

4 Are there special considerations for the emergence at the end of the case?

Potential postoperative airway complications to remain vigilant for include bronchospasm, laryngospasm, pneumothorax, pulmonary hemorrhage, postobstructive pneumonia, and negative pressure pulmonary edema. Postoperative negative pressure pulmonary edema can occur up to 24 hours following the removal of a foreign body. Decision regarding extubation should be made on an individual case basis. At a minimum, it would be prudent to consider ensuring these patients remain in a monitored setting postoperatively.

- Clinical signs and symptoms of airway obstruction should trump the lack of foreign body imaging confirmation.
- Regardless of the location of the foreign body, a rigid bronchoscope and resuscitation equipment should be immediately available in case of central airway obstruction.
- The use of steroids should be considered.
- Observe patient for postobstructive pulmonary edema for 24 hours after foreign body removal.
- *See Figures 103.1 and 103.2 as well as* ***Videos 103.1*** *and* ***103.2*** *for additional details.*

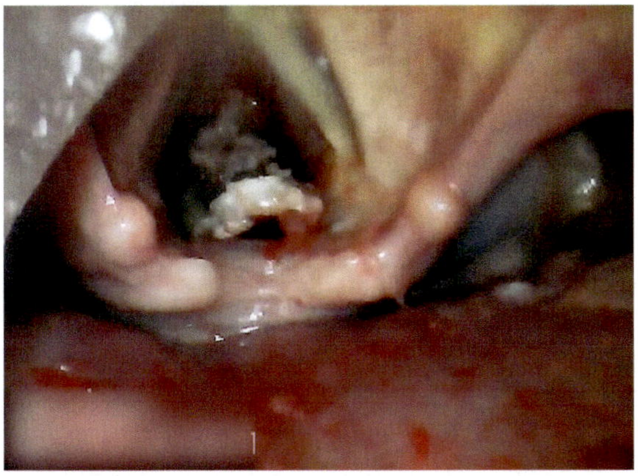

Figure 103.1. A tracheal foreign body is seen through a rigid bronchoscope.

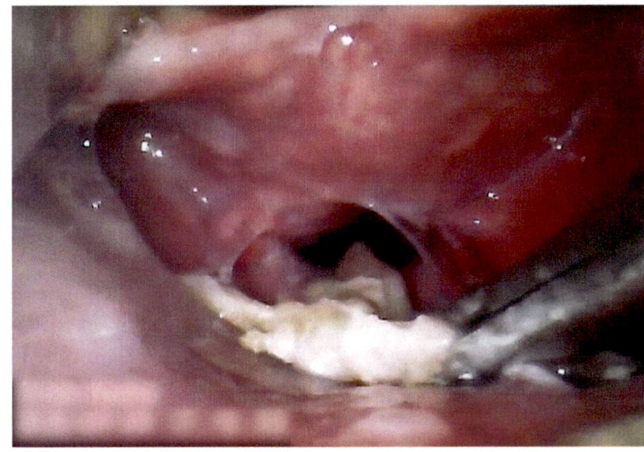

Figure 103.2. A foreign body is removed from the upper esophagus in a patient intubated using a rapid sequence technique.

Suggested Readings

Couper K, Hassan AA, Ohri V, et al; International Liaison Committee on Resuscitation Basic and Paediatric Life Support Task Force Collaborators. Removal of foreign body airway obstruction: a systematic review of interventions. *Resuscitation.* 2020;156:174–181.

Hewlett JC, Rickman OB, Lentz RJ, Prakash UB, Maldonado F. Foreign body aspiration in adult airways: therapeutic approach. *J Thorac Dis.* 2017;9(9):3398–3409.

Ramos MB, Fernandez-Villar A, Rivo JE, et al. Extraction of airway foreign bodies in adults: experience from 1987–2008. *Interact Cardiovasc Thorac Surg.* 2009;9(3):402–405.

Udeshi A, Cantie SM, Pierre E. Postobstructive pulmonary edema. *J Crit Care.* 2010;25(3):538.e1–538.e5.

White JJ, Cambron JD, Gottlieb M, Long B. Evaluation and management of airway foreign bodies in the emergency department setting. *J Emerg Med.* 2023;64(2):145–155.

104 The Adult with a Long-Standing Foreign Body in the Airway

Lena N. Glowka

Clinical Scenario: A 64-year-old man with polysubstance abuse has a 3-year history of multiple episodes of aspiration pneumonia and a discoid object in right upper bronchus. The cardiothoracic surgical team has scheduled a bronchoscopic retrieval of the foreign body.

1 What are the anesthetic and airway management considerations for this case?

Chronic airway foreign bodies often have cryptic and insidious presentations. In adults presenting with de novo occurrences of asthma, dyspnea, and recurrent pneumonias of unknown etiology, chronic foreign body obstruction should be included in the differential diagnosis. Suspicions should be further increased when the patient has a concurrent history of substance abuse, decreased mental status, or pharyngeal dysfunction.

Common foreign bodies include food, tablets, dentition, dental appliances, and coins. A careful history taken from both the patient and the family can be particularly useful in determining the foreign body's composition and can greatly affect the modes of evaluation and the subsequent removal plan.

Preoperative identification of the location, size, and nature of the object can be sought through a variety of imaging methods. Plain-film chest radiographs are often followed by thoracic CT. Ultrasonography may be useful for foreign bodies located in extremely distal branches of the bronchial tree. MRI cannot be used until the possibility of ferromagnetic properties of the foreign body has been ruled out.

2 How would you manage the airway in this case?

The optimal airway management plan for the patient will be formulated through preoperative discussion with the surgical team, establishing a series of strategies for the foreign body removal as well as contingency plans for failed attempts and untoward outcomes. The surgical team may elect to use a FIS via a large-diameter tracheal tube, a ventilating rigid bronchoscope, or a nonventilating bronchoscope that will require intermittent episodes of ventilation and oxygenation.

Corticosteroids should be considered with caution. The reduction of tissue edema can disrupt the stability of the foreign body and result in movement to a more deleterious position. Alternatively, if most of the airway obstruction is believed to be produced by reactive edema, then corticosteroids on their own may produce a cure.

The location, size, and material of the foreign body will determine removal techniques and optimal ventilation modes. In general terms, proximal foreign bodies may be removed with a rigid bronchoscope or flexible bronchoscope (FB), whereas extremely distal items may require a thoracotomy. These two surgical options have obvious airway management and anesthetic implications. A surgical approach to the foreign body should be managed as any thoracotomy case and will not be discussed here. When removing objects located below the vocal cords, but above the carina, maintenance of spontaneous ventilation may prevent the foreign body from shifting position and worsening the obstruction. The use of an supraglottic airway may be considered in order to avoid uncontrolled dislodgement of a foreign body in the larynx or trachea. If at any time the foreign body completely occludes upper airway and cannot be removed expeditiously, it should be driven distal to the carina, lessening its impact on ventilation.

Objects smaller than the internal diameter of a tracheal tube can often be extracted via the tube, with care taken not to cause tracheal tube obstruction. However, larger objects may be removed via a rigid bronchoscope or in coordination with extubation (eg, a grasped object is withdrawn and removed along with the tracheal tube, which is then reinserted). The choice of wire loop snares, wire baskets, biopsy forceps, or Fogarty balloon catheters with which to dislodge the foreign body will depend chiefly on operator comfort and the friability of the foreign body. In addition, the resection of obstructing reactive granulation tissue should be considered while the foreign body is being removed.

In the stem case above, a discoid object, a dime, lodged in the right bronchus was removed with a FB and biopsy forceps. Once the dime was brought to the distal tracheal tube, the tube cuff was deflated and the patient was extubated in conjunction with video laryngoscopy. The dime was then transferred past the vocal cords in an anterior–posterior axis, delivered to the posterior pharynx, and extracted with a McGill forceps.

3 What are the potential hazards and complications in regard to the airway?

An essential component of preoperative planning will include a treatment plan for untoward outcomes. The pre-eminent hazard is worsening of the airway obstruction caused either by loss of control of the foreign body during removal or by shifting the object from a longitudinal to a transverse position within the airway. As discussed in the preceding section, acute proximal airway obstructions that are not immediately amenable to rapid object removal may be overcome by driving the object distally past the carina. A common complication of airway manipulation is bronchospasm. Pretreatment of disposed patients with antihistamines, leukotriene inhibitors, as well as steroidal inhalers and direct bronchodilators should be considered.

There are many other less frequent, but equally deleterious, consequences associated with foreign body extraction. Type II postobstructive pulmonary edema is possible after relief from a long-standing upper airway obstruction. Sepsis can be triggered by the exposure of an endotoxin reservoir. A pneumothorax, pneumomediastinum, or hemorrhage may occur if the foreign body removal causes a significant rent in the pulmonary or tracheal tissue. Mindfulness of all of these possible sequelae, prior to embarking on foreign body extraction, will hasten diagnosis and ensure access to the necessary therapy.

4 Are there special considerations for the emergence or the end of the case?

The greatest determinants of the patient's postoperative course are the completeness of foreign body removal, surgical modalities employed, and collateral damage incurred during the retrieval of the foreign body. Prophylactic administration of corticosteroids, after removal of the foreign body, should be considered. The need for patient postoperative observation beyond the recovery room will be determined by the occurrence of interoperative complications and will necessitate patient-specific care plans. Patients suffering from obstructive pneumonia may be at risk for significant hemodynamic instability and even sepsis in the postoperative period. In addition, postobstructive pulmonary edema may occur up to 24 hours after removal of an airway obstruction. Therefore, patients should be observed for this period after the extraction of significant foreign bodies. Furthermore, postoperative imaging may be necessary to confirm complete removal of foreign body and to rule out subclinical pneumothorax or pneumomediastinum.

- Preoperative workup is used to determine the location, size, and composition of the foreign body.
- Prior to extraction attempts, a detailed discussion with surgical service must include the plans for removal of the foreign body and for untoward events such as object dropping and airway obstruction.
- Postoperative monitoring and imaging of the patient is directed at confirming complete object removal and to rule out airway damage.
- *See Figure 104.1 for additional details.*

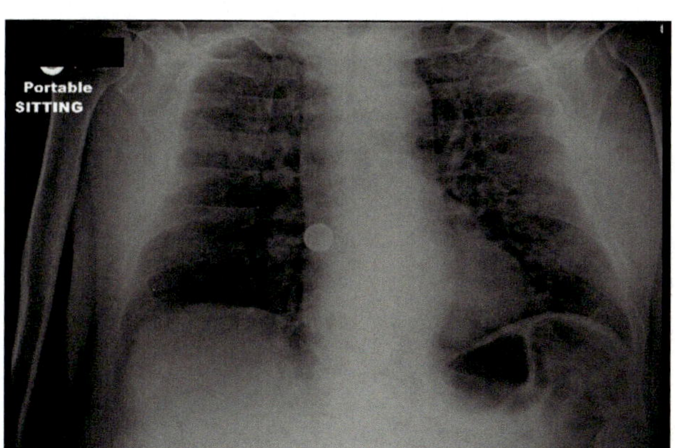

Figure 104.1. Chest x-ray of a patient with a foreign body in the right bronchus.

Suggested Readings

Fidkowski CW, Zheng H, Firth PG. The anesthetic consideration of tracheobronchial foreign bodies in children: a literature review of 12,979 cases. *Anesth Analg.* 2010;111(4):1016–1025.

Ramos MB, Fernandez-Villar A, Rivo JE, et al. Extraction of airway foreign bodies in adults: experience from 1987–2008. *Interact Cardiovasc Thorac Surg.* 2009;9(3):402–405.

Swanson KL. Airway foreign bodies: what's new? *Semin Respir Crit Care Med.* 2004;26(4):405–411.

Udeshi A, Cantie SM, Pierre E. Postobstructive pulmonary edema. *J Crit Care.* 2010;25(3):508.e1–e5.

Esophageal Foreign Bodies

105

Lorraine J. Foley

Clinical Scenario: A 2-year-old boy presents to the emergency department with hematemesis. Though the bleeding has now stopped, on chest x-ray, he is noted to have a large, irregularly shaped object in the lower esophagus. The patient's mother recalls a broken mirror at home and is concerned that her child has swallowed a fragment.

1 What are the anesthetic and airway management considerations for this case?

Over 100,000 presentations of esophageal foreign bodies (EFBs) occur in the United States each year, 1500 of which result in a patient death. Treatment and the implications for the anesthetic management of these patients depend on the type of object, the location of the object, and the child's symptoms. The objects' characteristics are important in determining the damage that might have and might still occur in the esophagus. Sharp objects carry a higher risk of complications such as an esophageal perforation and formation of an aortoesophageal fistula. In the current case, the child has presumably swallowed a large piece of a broken mirror, now lodged in the lower esophagus, and has been symptomatic with hematemesis. Vomiting in this case can be dangerous—vigorous pressure in the thin-walled esophagus could result in rupture. This sharp EFB needs to be removed urgently. The anesthetic and airway concerns include risk of pulmonary aspiration, trauma to the esophagus and trachea by perforation, and/or compression of the airway. Even though the EFB appears to be located in the lower esophagus, there is a possibility of EFB migration or position change during the chest x-ray procedure itself, as the patient may be placed in different positions to obtain images. Therefore, there should be concern about applying cricoid pressure at the time of induction. Although rare, an aortoesophageal fistula may occur. This must be differentiated from an acute esophageal mucosal lesion. Both may present with vomiting of blood, but the acute esophageal mucosal lesion will usually result in smaller quantities and appears earlier than an aortoesophageal fistula. One or two large intravenous catheters would be warranted to assist in fluid replacement if a large amount of blood loss occurs before, during, or after removal of the EFB.

2 How would you manage the airway in this case?

First, communication among the OR team is critical. The patient's airway will be shared by both the anesthesia provider and the surgeon, so a detailed plan should be developed ahead of time. This patient is a 2-year-old who most likely will not be cooperative with induction. Though parental presence is often helpful, some pediatric anesthesiologists suggest that it can be counterproductive in critical situations. Due to the patient's hematemesis, the author would intubate this patient with a rapid sequence intravenous induction, without cricoid pressure, and with the patient in a 45-degree or more sitting position. Sitting will reduce the risk of aspiration if the patient vomits during induction. No cricoid pressure should be applied to avoid the possible laceration or perforation of the esophageal mucosa by the sharp EFB. A tracheal tube can be placed with direct or video laryngoscopy. During laryngoscopy, the oropharyngeal and hypopharyngeal cavities should be evaluated for laceration or undetected foreign bodies. The tracheal tube should be passed through the vocal cords carefully, appreciating that resistance to forward advancement could indicate laryngotracheal compression or perforation by the EFB. Forcing the tracheal tube placement may cause further trauma to the airway and/or esophagus.

3 What are the surgical considerations that impact anesthetic management?

Four surgical techniques may be used to remove an EFB, depending on the type of object and its location: regurgitation, McGill forceps, rigid endoscopy, and balloon catheter. As in this case, a sharp object located anywhere in the esophagus requires rigid esophagoscopy. During rigid esophagoscopy, tracheal compression may occur. Sudden difficulties in ventilation must be immediately communicated to the surgeon, who may either adjust or abandon rigid esophagoscopy. Neuromuscular relaxation is required throughout the procedure in order to prevent movement, coughing, and bucking which could result in additional trauma from the EFB or rigid esophagoscope.

Once the object is removed, the surgeon will reevaluate the esophagus for a second EFB and lacerations or perforations. If there is any concern that an esophageal-tracheal perforation has occurred, the surgeon will continue the evaluation with flexible bronchoscopy. Depending on the location of the lesion, the tracheal tube may need to be retracted to allow for a complete laryngotracheal evaluation.

4 What are the potential hazards and complications in regard to the airway?

There are many complications associated with EFB—ulceration, necrosis, arterioesophageal fistula, tracheo-esophageal fistula, esophageal rupture, hemorrhage, mediastinitis, and stricture. The acute injury may lead to edema or compression that can compromise the airway postoperatively and make reintubation difficult. If any of these complications are present after EFB removal, the author recommends that the patient remain intubated and observed in an intensive care setting.

- Sharp EFBs require removal under general anesthesia as soon as possible.
- Communication between anesthesia provider and surgeon before, during, and after the procedure is critical, as both will be sharing the airway.
- Cricoid pressure during intubation should be avoided with sharp objects.
- *See Figure 105.1 and* ***Video 105.1*** *for additional details.*

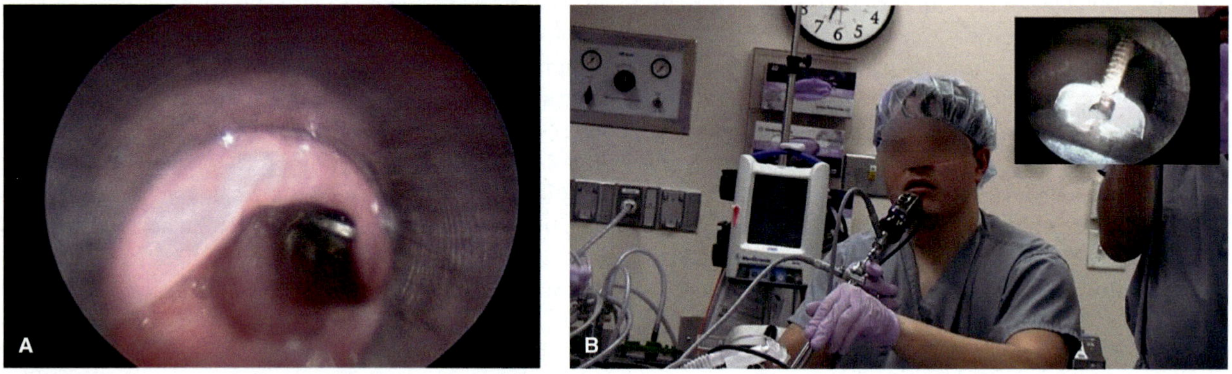

Figure 105.1. **A:** Right esophagoscope view of an object (coin) in the esophagus. **B:** The coin has been grasped through the esophagoscope and will be removed from the airway.

Suggested Readings

Dipasquale V, Romano C, Iannelli M, et al. Managing pediatric foreign body ingestions: a 10-year experience. *Pediatr Emerg Care.* 2022;38(1):e268–e271.

Rybojad B, Niedzielska G, Niedzielski A, Rudnicka-Drozak E, Rybojad P. Esophageal foreign bodies in pediatric patients: a thirteen-year retrospective study. *ScientificWorldJournal.* 2012;2012:102642.

Wright C, Closson F. Updates in gastrointestinal foreign bodies. *Pediatr Clin North Am.* 2013;60:1221–1239.

Zhang X, Liu J, Li J, et al. Diagnosis and treatment of 32 cases with aortoesophageal fistula due to esophageal foreign body. *Laryngoscope.* 2011;121:267–272.

Pediatric Postoperative Bleeding Tonsil

106

Ramneek Maan

Clinical Scenario: A 5-year-old boy with a history of obstructive sleep apnea (OSA) is in the postanesthetic care unit after having undergone a tonsillectomy 1 hour prior. His initial airway management was uncomplicated, but he is now experiencing significant bleeding from the tonsil bed. The surgeon has decided to return to the OR for further intervention.

1 What are the anesthetic and airway management considerations for this case?

A variety of surgical techniques are employed in tonsil surgery. The method used and other clinical circumstances determine the likelihood of perioperative tonsillar hemorrhage. Steel or cold-knife dissection with complete removal of the palatine tonsils is still the most common method practiced worldwide, followed by electrocautery. Additional methods include harmonic scalpel, radiofrequency ablation, laser ablation, microdebrider, and coblation (bipolar radiofrequency ablation). Intracapsular tonsillectomy, also known as tonsillotomy, for sleep-disordered breathing is also increasing in popularity.

Tonsillar surgery carries inherent risks, particularly for patients with OSA or sleep-disordered breathing. The leading causes of death or permanent brain injury are most often linked to anoxia resulting from airway obstruction or postoperative bleeding. Key considerations include airway protection, obstruction prevention, and effective blood loss management. Postoperative vigilance is essential to detect airway compromise due to swelling or bleeding. Hemorrhage occurs in the immediate postoperative period (24 hours or less) or is delayed up to several days after surgery, in 1% and 5% of all cases, respectively. Risk factors in children include a preexisting coagulopathy, allergies, male sex, longer duration of the anesthetic, and the method of surgery. The practice of obtaining coagulation tests in the absence of a history of coagulopathy lacks predicative value in identifying patients at risk for posttonsil surgical hemorrhage.

2 How would you manage the airway in this case?

By virtue of the clinical situation, the patient's airway will be shared by the anesthesiologist and surgeon, and ideally, an early discussion regarding airway management should occur. Prior to anesthetic induction, a clear airway plan should be articulated. Emergency surgical airway equipment should be present in the OR. The electrocautery dispersive pad should be applied to the patient before the induction of anesthesia, and surgical suction should be in operative order. In older, cooperative children, conscious sedation may allow "awake" video laryngoscopy and intubation. Intravenous dexmedetomidine is an excellent choice for sedation. A consciousness monitor has anecdotally proven to be helpful, especially if other intravenous induction agents are used. Overall, maintenance of the intrinsic protective airway reflexes during induction and intubation is preferred.

Anesthetic care and airway management in younger children with posttonsillar surgical bleeding has been reviewed, and most anesthetic inductions for these cases are completed with a rapid sequence technique using succinylcholine. Inhalational induction may be considered for children without intravenous access and is usually done with the child in the sitting position. An upright position is often voluntarily assumed by the child in airway distress and should be supported. Positive-pressure ventilation prior to tracheal intubation is to be avoided as this may lead to regurgitation and aspiration of gastric contents, which may include voluminous amounts of blood.

Parental attendance during inhalation induction in elective surgery is common. Conversely, during the management of a critical airway, the strain on personnel often outweighs the calming effect of parental presence. In addition, a parent's own apprehension in witnessing a child in extremis can compound the difficulty of the situation. The perspective on the benefits of parental presence may differ between the anesthesiologist and the surgeon, who likely shares a closer, ongoing relationship with the family. However, the anesthesiologist's judgment should take precedence in such decisions.

The approach to the airway during posttonsil surgery bleeding is highly dependent on the skills and experience of the anesthesiologist. This includes his or her familiarity with the available devices. The most experienced laryngoscopist present should attempt direct laryngoscopy, as there is evidence that repeated laryngoscopies increase the incidence of complications. The employment of unfamiliar devices is ill-advised. Blood and secretions impede the performance of most indirect vision devices (eg, video laryngoscopes), so their use may be limited or contraindicated in a time-critical situation. In the case of the bleeding tonsil, an supraglottic airway can be useful as a conduit to isolate the glottic inlet and allow passage of an endotracheal tube (ETT) or a flexible intubating scope preloaded with an ETT.

Attention should be given to the choice of ETT and it may be discussed with the surgical staff. Cuffed endotracheal tubes offer the benefit of reducing lower airway contamination by providing a better seal, thus minimizing the risk of aspiration.

Massive acute or chronic, subtle bleeding can lead to clotted blood partially obstructing the glottic inlet, resulting in complete airway obstruction. This can occur during nasal endoscopy, even by an experienced otolaryngologist, particularly in the event of a rapid, life-threatening airway hemorrhage, and emergency tracheostomy may be required.

3 What are the surgical considerations that impact anesthetic management?

The treatment of posttonsillar surgery hemorrhage is primarily surgical. Once the airway is secured, exploration of the wound site and attempts at stopping hemorrhage are undertaken. In the case of associated coagulopathy, indicated therapy is instituted. If hemostasis is not successful, the otolaryngologist may elect to treat the bleeding site with hemostatic and packing material and postpone exploration until the bleeding has ceased. Alternatively, interventional radiologists may be recruited to eliminate the blood supply to the site of hemorrhage via cannulation of the external carotid artery and its branches.

4 Are there special considerations for the emergence or the end of the case?

Once hemostasis is achieved, the patient should be extubated fully awake. Consideration should be given to administering antiemetics and performing orogastric suction at the end of the procedure to prevent postoperative nausea and vomiting, which could trigger rebleeding. In addition, ensuring adequate pain control is essential for a smooth extubation. If difficult extubation and reintubation are anticipated, a plan to rescue the airway should also be in place and discussed with critical care staff. As life-threatening posttonsillar hemorrhage can recur, the patient should be observed in an intensive care setting until stable.

- Posttonsillar surgical bleeding may occur immediately after surgery or several days postprocedure.
- Children are more likely to suffer anoxic injury or death because of posttonsillar surgical hemorrhage.
- Adults and cooperative older children may be managed with sedated intubation. Younger children are generally managed with rapid sequence induction and intubation.
- Patients that are at risk of rebleeding and should be admitted to an intensive care or other unit where continuous observation is available.
- *See Figure 106.1 for additional details.*

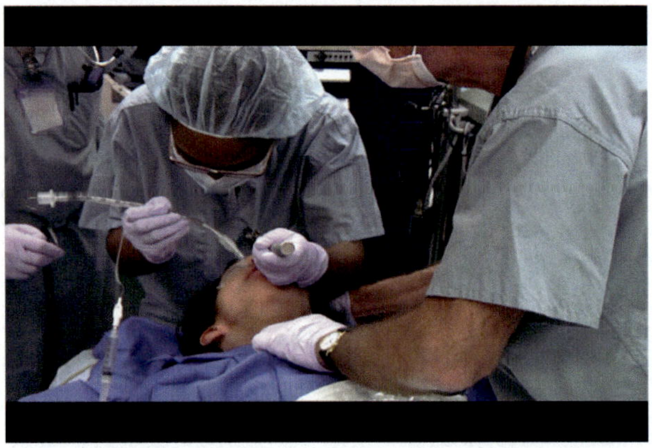

Figure 106.1. Rapid sequence intubation of a child with postoperative tonsillectomy airway bleeding.

Acknowledgment

We gratefully acknowledge the contributions of previous edition author, Valerie E. Armstead, as portions of those chapters have been retained in this revision.

Suggested Readings

Coté CJ, Posner KL, Domino KB. Death or neurologic injury after tonsillectomy in children with a focus on obstructive sleep apnea: Houston, we have a problem! *Anesth Analg*. 2014;118:1276–1283.

Fields RG, Gencorelli FJ, Litman RS. Anesthetic management of the pediatric bleeding tonsil. *Paediatr Anaesth*. 2010;20:982–986.

Goldman JL, Baugh RF, Davies L, et al. Mortality and major morbidity after tonsillectomy: etiologic factors and strategies for prevention. *Laryngoscope*. 2013;123:2544–2553.

Hessen Soderman AC, Ericsson E, Hemlin C, et al. Reduced risk of primary postoperative hemorrhage after tonsil surgery in Sweden: results from the National Tonsil Surgery Register in Sweden covering more than 10 years and 54,696 operations. *Laryngoscope*. 2011;121:2322–2326.

Suvarna D, Fernandes S. Anesthesia management of adenotonsillectomy. *Int J Otorhinolaryngol Clin*. 2015;7(1):17–21.

107 An Uncooperative Child with a Difficult Airway

Valerie E. Armstead • Ramneek Maan

Clinical Scenario: A 7-year-old presents for intra-abdominal surgery. The child has Pierre Robin syndrome and is uncooperative in the preoperative area.

1 What are the anesthetic and airway management considerations for this case?

Health care workers frequently encounter uncooperative pediatric patients in both elective and emergency surgical settings. For elective surgical cases, communication between parents, staff, and the surgical team allows for better planning. In emergencies, limited preparation time can complicate the management of children with difficult airways.

Types of Difficult Pediatric Airways

Pediatric difficult airways can be categorized as those related to trauma (bleeding) or malalignment, immobility, foreign body aspiration, infection, congenital dysmorphism, storage diseases, tumors, and morbid obesity. The patient's age (infant, toddler, older child) will also differentiate the anesthesia provider's approach to airway management.

Infant

Infants presenting in the emergency setting are usually rather robust. All but the youngest may stridently resist separation from the parent. Emergency care for those with difficult airways may require IV access, blood sampling, lumbar puncture, or imaging. These infants often present with congenital syndromes like Pierre Robin sequence, where a cleft palate and large tongue obstruct airflow when supine but improve with proper positioning. Titrated sedation that avoids respiratory compromise allows for effective evaluation and treatment. In cases without IV access, alternative routes—such as nasal, oral, intramuscular, rectal, or inhalation (eg, sevoflurane)—can be used. Rectal administration of methohexital or midazolam, for example, can provide sufficient sedation for peripheral IV placement without significant respiratory risk. Methohexital is preferred due to its predictability (10-minute onset, 45-minute duration) and suitability for short procedures. Close monitoring of vital signs, including capnography, is essential in all cases.

A common challenge arises when repeated failed intubations transform a normal airway into a severely compromised one. A pediatric-sized GlideScope Cobalt AVL video laryngoscope can help secure the airway, but both video laryngoscopes and fiberoptic scopes (FIS) may be obstructed by excessive bleeding in a traumatized airway. If video laryngoscopy fails, a supraglottic airway (SGA) can maintain patency, and it can serve as a conduit for intubation using a pediatric FIS or a Shikani intubating stylet, which can reliably deliver a 2.5-ID tracheal tube. These devices may allow oxygen delivery during intubation via accessory ports. If intubation or ventilation via face mask or SGA is inadequate, immediate surgical consultation is necessary for rigid bronchoscopy or a surgical airway. However, surgical airways in infants may have long-term consequences, such as laryngotracheal incompetence.

When an infant with a known difficult airway presents for an elective procedure, the preanesthesia induction safety checklist should alert the OR team to the airway concerns. The time-out verifies that the necessary equipment and personnel are ready while confirming the airway management plan and any backup strategies. Premedication may be administered, but airway-compromising agents should be avoided. If IV access is challenging, a specialized team may be required. In some cases, it may be prudent to intubate in the OR prior to transferring the child to a non-OR procedure site, ensuring access to familiar resources and support.

Toddlers

Emergencies involving uncooperative toddlers with difficult airways are more likely to involve trauma. An uncooperative child might also be decompensating from shock. Intravenous access may be a challenge if the child is uncooperative. Depending on the clinical situation, central or intraosseous access may be warranted if peripheral venous access is difficult to obtain.

Pediatric emergency and trauma physicians prioritize securing the airway and immobilizing the cervical spine early, as these children are prone to emesis, necessitating lower airway protection. In cases of suspected cervical trauma or spinal cord injury without radiologic abnormalities, a Pediatric GlideScope is typically employed. If intubation proves challenging with the glidescope alone, it can be combined with a FIS to facilitate oral or nasal intubation.

Elective procedures for toddlers with difficult airways are handled in a similar fashion to the infant, except that the toddler is more likely to accept oral midazolam administered by a parent. If they are still in diapers, 25 mg/kg of rectal methohexital reliably induces airway protective sedation in about 10 minutes.

Early Childhood

Uncooperative **early childhood patients** (ages 3 to 6 years) with difficult airways are handled in a similar fashion as with the toddlers, except that rectal medications are seldom used.

Middle Childhood

Middle childhood patients (ages 6 to 12 years) who are uncooperative and have difficult airways may be challenging, especially if the patient is large, strong, and obese. Emergency management of difficult airways is tailored to the patient's age, development, and clinical context. For patients who have reached menarche, it's crucial to assess the possibility of pregnancy before sedation. For larger patients, up to 20 mg of oral midazolam can be administered to initiate sedation. In emergency or elective scenarios, intramuscular ketamine and glycopyrrolate may be injected in a dart-like manner while distracting an uncooperative patient, ideally on a stretcher. This approach requires personnel to ensure the patient remains secure until they lose consciousness, which can be particularly challenging with morbidly obese individuals. All airway equipment must be prepared, as obstruction can occur suddenly. These patients often require examination under anesthesia, making supraglottic airways particularly valuable, as they can remain in place for spontaneously breathing patients until a satisfactory level of consciousness is restored.

Adolescent

Adolescent patients (12 to 18 years) are managed similarly to middle childhood patients if there is any developmental delay that causes them to be uncooperative.

2 How would you manage the airway in this case?

The overall strategy in dealing with a difficult pediatric airway is to avoid the cannot-ventilate situation.

In the current case, oral premedication of the maximal dose of midazolam syrup would be the first strategy unless the child is suffering from a bowel obstruction. If oral medication cannot be used or the child is still uncooperative, up to 5 mg/kg intramuscular ketamine can be given rapidly during a distraction maneuver. Personnel should be assembled to help transfer the patient to a waiting stretcher with oxygen, ventilation bag, mask, oral airways, and nasal airways at the ready. Typically, sedation with these agents will allow for peripheral intravenous catheter insertion. If the patient is still uncooperative, inhalation induction with sevoflurane is often possible.

The Pediatric GlideScope Cobalt AVL used as a primary or assisted intubation device (eg, with a FIS) is preferred for several reasons. There are a wide variety of single-use blade sizes that can be rapidly exchanged. It also creates an adequate space for passage of a tracheal tube with a stiff stylet for approaching the very anterior larynx.

The GlideScope can assist in guiding a pediatric FIS preloaded with a tracheal tube (preferably a Parker-type tube). Another "stiff stylet" option is the use of the pediatric Shikani optical stylet either alone or with a GlideScope.

If the patient's oxygen saturation drops below 95% during intubation attempts, the patient is ventilated with a face mask or SGA until the oxygen saturation returns to an acceptable baseline.

In conclusion, uncooperative pediatric patients with difficult airways present unique challenges based on age and clinical context. Approaching each case with caution and thorough preparation of equipment and personnel can greatly improve the chances of success.

3 What distinct airway device might be used in this case, and what are the special considerations?

Specialized equipment that should be considered for this case are the GlideScope Cobalt AVL system, Pediatric Shikani optical stylet, Clarus tube stop for holding a preloaded tracheal tube, stylets of adequate stiffness, and pediatric Parker tracheal tubes. All of the aforementioned devices have battery-power capabilities, so they are portable. It is possible to attach lightweight systems to eyepieces of optical scopes to allow sharing the view for assistance and input.

4 Are there special considerations for the emergence or the end of the case?

If the patient received ketamine in addition to midazolam, an oral gastric tube can be used to suction out any residual midazolam to prevent delayed emergence.

Extubation should be done with the patient fully awake with consideration of a nasal airway that can be removed if needed.

- The uncooperative child presents challenges that vary based on age, type of airway difficulty, and clinical scenario.
- An appropriate armamentarium of difficult airway equipment should be ready before sedating the child.
- The staff of the entire OR should be aware of the airway concerns and should know their role if a failed airway situation arises.
- *See Figure 107.1 for additional details.*

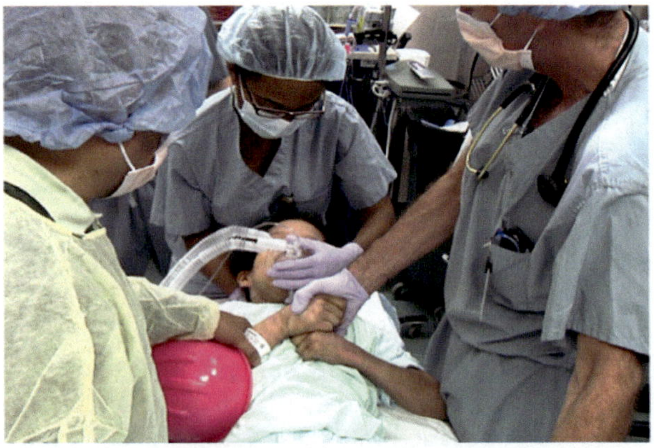

Figure 107.1. An inhalation induction takes place in a child with an at-risk, difficult airway.

Suggested Readings

Cladis F, Kumar A, Grunwaldt L, Otteson T, Ford M, Losee JE. Pierre Robin sequence: a perioperative review. *Anesth Analg.* 2014;119:400–412.

Fonte M, Oulego-Erroz I, Nadkarni L, Sánchez-Santos L, Iglesias-Vásquez A, Rodríguez-Núñez A. A randomized comparison of the GlideScope videolaryngoscope to the standard laryngoscopy for intubation by pediatric residents in simulated easy and difficult infant airway scenarios. *Pediatr Emerg Care.* 2011;27:398–402.

Gan TJ. Pharmacokinetic and pharmacodynamic characteristics of medications used for moderate sedation. *Clin Pharmacokinet.* 2006;45:855–869.

Jamora C, Iravani M. Unique clinical situations in pediatric patients where ketamine may be the anesthetic agent of choice. *Am J Ther.* 2010;17:511–515.

Kwok PC, Chan HK. Delivery of inhalation drugs to children for asthma and other respiratory diseases. *Adv Drug Deliv Rev.* 2014;73:83–88.

Pediatric Airway Foreign Body

108

Ramneek Maan

Clinical Scenario: A mother of a 2-year-old boy reports that he was playing with marbles and placing them in his mouth when he suddenly began coughing. She immediately brought him to the emergency department. Notably, there was no loss of consciousness.

1 What are the anesthetic and airway management considerations for this case?

Airway foreign body aspiration most commonly occurs in young children and is associated with high rate of airway distress, morbidity, and mortality. Presenting symptoms of foreign body aspiration can range from mild to severe airway obstruction and are often nonspecific or seemingly innocuous. In the absence of a witnessed choking or aspiration event, the diagnosis may be delayed for weeks or months and contribute to worsening disease. The common offending object is typically a seed such as a nut or a grain depending on the geographic region. Numerous studies have highlighted data indicating that infants and toddlers who lack the teeth (ie, molars) to crush these food items before being delivered to the posterior pharynx are at a higher risk of choking. Chest x-rays and high-resolution CT scans may eventually contribute to the diagnosis. Signs of obstructive emphysema may become evident when the lobe or side with the foreign body appears more transparent on imaging, while the healthy lung tissue is compressed. There may be deviation of the trachea away from the side obstructed by the foreign body. This is a result of what is referred to as a "ball valve" or air-trapping effect. In the stem scenario, the location of the foreign body may be quickly identified with anterior–posterior and lateral x-rays. Bronchoscopy is used to confirm the diagnosis and retrieve the object. Rigid bronchoscopy is useful because of the ability of the anesthesiologist to provide ventilation through the channel of the bronchoscope continuously. Resistance to ventilation increases dramatically with the telescope in place.

Flexible bronchoscopy (FB) is another important procedure for the evaluation of the pediatric airway. FB allows for a dynamic view of the trachea and the lower bronchi. It offers greater maneuverability than the rigid bronchoscope and may be used in conjunction with other procedures, such as bronchoalveolar lavage, transbronchial biopsy, endobronchial ultrasound, and electrocautery or laser treatments. Pediatric bronchoscopes are small enough in diameter to be used through tracheal tubes with internal diameters of 3.0 mm. Simultaneous ventilation through a tracheal tube obstructed by the bronchoscope is not possible. Therefore, close monitoring of oxygen saturation and end-tidal CO_2 is crucial to prevent patient deterioration while addressing the foreign body. Careful attention is needed to balance the urgency of the procedure with maintaining stable respiratory function. Although bronchospasm, transient fever, infection, and pneumothorax are rare complications of flexible bronchoscopy, these risks are minimized with careful technique and ongoing communication between the anesthesiologist and bronchoscopist.

Localized inflammation and the reaction to the foreign object, along with the trauma caused by bronchoscopy can result in damage to oral structures, tracheitis, bronchitis, atelectasis, airway reactivity, and pneumonia.

2 How would you manage the airway in this case?

The safest way to remove the foreign object is under general anesthesia. However, the type of anesthesia used will ultimately depend on the symptoms of the patient, the nature and position of the foreign body, and the planned removal strategy. Initially, induction of anesthesia is achieved with an inhalational agent such as sevoflurane to facilitate establishment of vascular access and good depth of anesthesia.

Depending on the stability of the patient and the degree of obstruction, the airway can be secured with a deep plane of anesthesia or with the use of a muscle relaxant. An antisialagogue to lessen secretions, dexamethasone 0.15 mg/kg to reduce airway edema, and an orogastric tube for emptying of the stomach are often employed. The operating table is then turned to the endoscopist, or if the table is very small, the patient is repositioned without moving the table.

Maintenance of inhalational anesthetic usually involves high gas flows due to frequent disconnection of the circuit, reintubations, and the use of tools through the working channel of the bronchoscope. Many operators switch to an intravenous anesthesia technique (total intravenous anesthesia [TIVA]) with agents that allow for spontaneous ventilation and preservation of physiologic forces that prevent airway collapse. TIVA also reduces the exposure of the surgical team and all others to inhalation agent pollution of the OR environment. Dexmedetomidine is also an excellent medication when combined with adjuncts such as local anesthetics and/or low-dose propofol.

The choice between maintaining spontaneous and controlled ventilation depends on the clinical situation. Communication between the surgeon and anesthesia provider is critical to achieving an optimal outcome.

3 What are the surgical considerations that impact anesthetic management?

Bronchoscopy for removal of a foreign body is a shared airway procedure and may involve multiple episodes of airway extubation, complete airway obstruction, and brief compromises of ideal oxygenation and ventilation—the anesthesia provider and surgeon work integrally in a critical patient situation. Cooperation, communication, and mutual assistance are crucial to an acceptable outcome. The anesthesia provider may need to adjust their anesthetic regimen in consideration of the surgeon (eg, utilizing TIVA as opposed to maintenance inhalation agent technique) and be ready to assist with head and torso positioning during bronchoscopy. Likewise, the surgeon must be acutely cognizant of the requirements for oxygenation, ventilation, and depth of anesthesia.

4 What are the potential hazards and complications in regard to the airway?

Major airway hazards and complications are related to the characteristics of the foreign object and to the attempts for its retrieval.

An object that becomes lodged at the glottic opening or obstructs the trachea needs to be pushed distally into a less obstructing location. The most dreaded and difficult aspect of foreign body removal is successfully extracting the object past the narrowest portion of the upper airway, which is the glottic opening or cricoid cartilage in younger children and infants. Dropping of the object by the bronchoscopist can result in acute and total airway obstruction. Using the bronchoscope or a styletted tracheal tube to displace the foreign body into a mainstem bronchus may be lifesaving. Once the obstruction is moved distally, the team can then formulate an alternate approach for retrieval.

- Presenting symptoms of foreign body aspiration can range from mild to severe airway obstruction and are often nonspecific or seemingly innocuous.
- Inhalation induction and maintenance of TIVA with preservation of spontaneous ventilation is a common regimen in this situation.
- Constant communication and mutual assistance are vital to an efficient and successful removal procedure.
- Airway edema and irritability after endoscopy and foreign body removal attempts may lead to complications during extubation.
- *See Figure 108.1 and* ***Video 108.1*** *for additional details.*

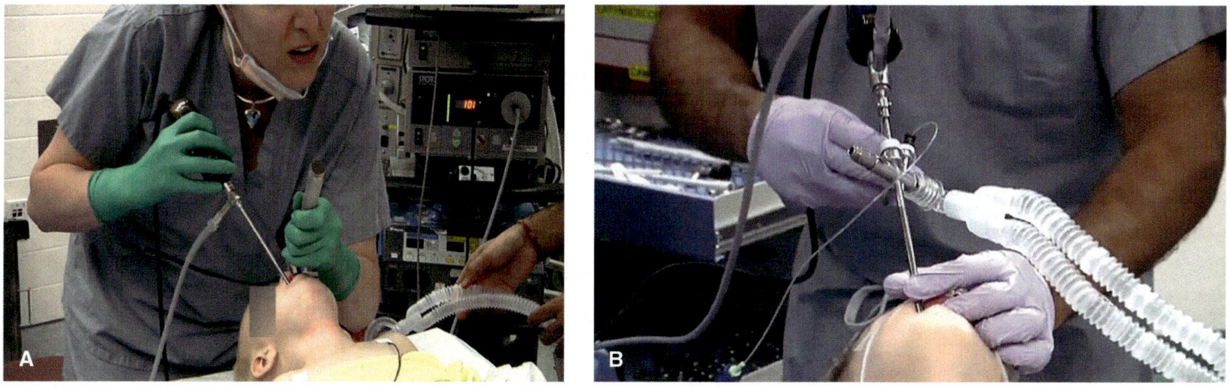

Figure 108.1. A: A rigid telescope is used with direct laryngoscopy to locate a tracheal foreign body. **B:** A rigid bronchoscope and telescope are used to locate a foreign body in the trachea. The anesthesia circuit is attached to the side port of the bronchoscope.

Suggested Readings

Aguirre Vázquez IR, Blanco Rodríguez G, Penchyna Grub J, Teyssier Morales G, Serrano Salas AL. Foreign bodies aspiration in pediatrics. 15-year experience. Analysis of 337 cases. *Cir Pediatr*. 2013;26:1–4.

Boufersaoui A, Smati L, Benhalla KN, et al. Foreign body aspiration in children: experience from 2624 patients. *Int J Pediatr Otorhinolaryngol*. 2013;77:1683–1688.

Chiu CY, Wong KS, Lai SH, Hsia SH, Wu CT. Factors predicting early diagnosis of foreign body aspiration in children. *Pediatr Emerg Care*. 2005;21:161–164.

Kendigelen P. The anesthetic consideration of tracheobronchial foreign body aspiration in children. *J Thorac Dis*. 2016;8(12):3803–3807.

Mahmoud M, Gunter J, Donnelly LF, et al. A comparison of dexmedetomidine with propofol for magnetic resonance imaging sleep studies in children. *Anesth Analg*. 2009;109:745–753.

109 Childhood Hemangiomas

Keith Haller

Clinical Scenario: A 4-year-old presents for resection of a large facial hemangioma overlying the left cheek, mandible, and submandibular area.

1 What are the anesthetic and airway management considerations for this case?

Vascular lesions include anomalies of arteries, veins, capillaries, or lymphatic vessels. They are classified into two groups: vascular tumors and vascular malformations. Infantile hemangiomas are the most common of the vascular tumors, and the majority (60%) appear on the head and the neck. Although some will spontaneously involute, large segmental (diffuse, dermatomal) hemangiomas and those involving the airway and vital areas of the face require intervention. "Beard distribution hemangiomas" and those involving the head and neck are associated with hemangiomas of the airway that have the potential to cause respiratory complications. Hemangiomas of the head and the neck can be associated with other syndromes, such as PHACES and Kassabach–Merritt syndromes, which can present additional anesthetic and airway challenges.

Many patients scheduled for endovascular interventions will have had diagnostic imaging examinations. CT and MRI can define the nature of the vascular lesion and are also useful to assess disease extension into the airway. Flexible fiberoptic laryngoscopy gives additional information regarding visualized airway involvement.

The preoperative physical examination and history should focus on signs and symptoms that might suggest airway involvement. A croupy cough and biphasic stridor in an infant may be indicative of a subglottic lesion. A history of difficult or noisy breathing, orthopnea, and dysphagia could be due to a hemangioma in the airway. In addition, location or size of the mass could impede mask ventilation or placement of an artificial airway, especially if the tongue or lips are extensively involved. If the mass is compressed by instrumentation or aggressive mask ventilation, significant bleeding may result. In spite of being a valid rescue device, bleeding can occur with the use of supraglottic airways (SGAs). In addition, induction of anesthesia with inhalational agents may exacerbate engorgement of the vascular malformation, which may lead to worsening airway obstruction.

2 How would you manage the airway in this case?

After preoxygenation and placement of standard American Society of Anesthesiologists monitors, inhalational induction with a mixture of nitrous oxide, sevoflurane, and oxygen can be initiated. Positioning the patient in the 30-degree head-up position can reduce vascular engorgement and airway obstruction. Once adequately anesthetized, IV access is established, and the patient should ideally receive an opioid to facilitate laryngoscopy. It is important to maintain spontaneous respirations and upper airway muscle tone to support the mask airway. Neuromuscular blockade should be avoided prior to intubation for this reason. Inadvertent soft tissue contact with instrumentation such as laryngoscope blades, endotracheal tube, stylets, or even SGAs can lead to bleeding, further complicating airway management.

We favor the use of a pediatric video laryngoscope (VL) (Glidescope, Verathon, Bothell, WA) for oral or nasal intubation. VL allows for a slow, gentle, and graded laryngoscopy. Additional information regarding unanticipated disease can be appreciated and recorded for later review.

When hemangiomas involve the lips or base of the tongue, it can be difficult to manipulate a laryngoscope and tracheal tube in the mouth simultaneously. In this scenario, the anesthesia provider can use a flexible intubating scope (FIS) in conjunction with a VL—the VL image may be used to direct the FIS into the larynx. The VL can be left in place or removed, and the tracheal tube then inserted. A careful tracheal tube–flexible scope pairing, which eliminates size differences and minimizes hang-up, should be sought. When there is a concern that vascular malformations are distorting the architecture of the airway, an advanced method for securing the airway utilizes a pediatric zero-degree rigid bronchoscope. Using a suspended Lindholm laryngoscope, the patient can be intubated over a rigid bronchoscope passed through the vocal cords under direct vision. Both of these methods facilitate the assessment and visualization of subglottic hemangiomas. Subglottic lesions may require jet ventilation for surgical interventions in the setting of segmental airway disease. The airway in this patient population can prove extremely challenging. The appropriate ear, nose, and throat personnel and invasive equipment should be on standby even in nonhead and neck surgery.

3 What are the surgical considerations that impact anesthetic management?

Surgeries involving or in proximity to major neurovascular structures may require intraoperative neuromonitoring, and the anesthetic should be tailored appropriately. A NIM endotracheal tube may be requested in these scenarios.

Treatment options for these patients range from endovascular interventions with sclerotherapy to laser treatments and open surgical excision. Frequently, these patients are scheduled for an endovascular intervention with open excision planned for the following day. The sclerosing agent or embolization material can have untoward effects, including hypoglycemia, venous thromboembolism, and cardiovascular collapse. There may be marked swelling of the vascular lesion associated with intense pain, requiring significant postoperative analgesia. In addition, swelling of lesions of the face, lips, and mouth can impede mask ventilation and make airway management significantly more difficult on extubation and in the OR the following day. Preoperative and intraoperative steroid administration may help to decrease postoperative swelling. Due to the vascular nature of these lesions, there can be significant bleeding with manipulation. Although modern surgical techniques have reduced this, blood should be available. Preoperative labs should include complete blood count and coagulation profiles, especially in the case of arteriovenous malformations and in consumptive coagulopathy as seen in Kassabach–Merritt syndrome.

4 Are there special considerations for the emergence or the end of the case?

Patients receiving sclerotherapy or embolization to structures in close proximity to the airway can experience swelling and airway obstruction. Extubation and/or rescue mask ventilation may be difficult. In addition, these lesions may become painful and exquisitely tender. Patients should receive intraoperative opioids and other pain adjuncts for adequate pain relief on emergence. Patients with large lesions receiving large doses of interventional sclerosants should be assessed for electrolyte abnormalities prior to emergence, such as hypoglycemia and metabolic acidosis. With long procedures where there is a concern for significant peritracheal edema, our clinical practice is to visually survey the glottis prior to extubation using a VL. A leak test can be performed under direct visualization and a decision to delay extubation may be made.

- Maintaining spontaneous respirations prior to intubation helps to prevent airway obstruction.
- Gentle VL can be used to assess the airway and allow limited trauma to friable vascular tissue.
- VL can be useful in vascular anomalies by providing new diagnostic findings to guide strategic therapeutic interventions.
- Significant untoward effects of instrumentation, sclerotherapy, and embolization therapy should be anticipated.
- *See Figure 109.1 and* ***Video 109.1*** *for additional details.*

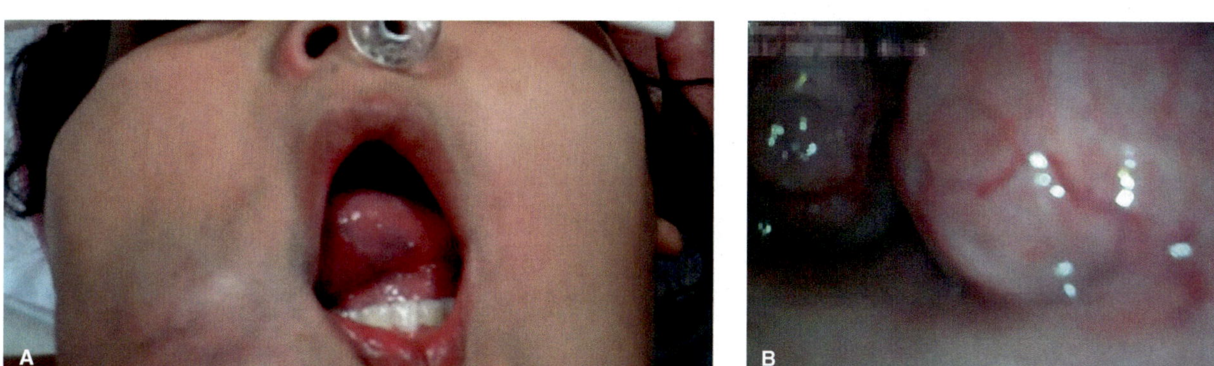

Figure 109.1. A: A child with a large lymphatic malformation of the head and neck that involves the underside of the tongue. **B:** On attempts at intubation, the same patient is found to have similarly enlarged tonsils that interfere with tracheal intubation.

Acknowledgments

We gratefully acknowledge the contributions of previous edition authors, Jonathan B. Lesser and Franco Resta-Flarer, as portions of those chapters have been retained in this revision.

Suggested Readings

De Ravin E, Barrette LX, Lu J, et al. Clinical practice guidelines on management of infantile hemangioma: a systematic quality appraisal using the AGREE II instrument. *Pediatr Hematol Oncol.* 2022;39(8):724–735.

Jacobs IN, Cahill AM. Special considerations in vascular anomalies: airway management. *Clin Plast Surg.* 2011;38:121–131.

O'Donnell TM, Alexander RE, Lando T, et al. Segmental hemangiomas of the upper airway. *Laryngoscope.* 2009;119(11):2242–2247.

Orlow SJ, Isakoff MS, Blei F. Increased risk of symptomatic hemangiomas of the airway in association with cutaneous hemangiomas in the "beard" distribution. *J Pediatr.* 1997;131:643–646.

Invasive Airway Access in Small Children

110

Morten Bøttger • Michael S. Kristensen

Clinical Scenario: A 9-day-old boy is referred to a tertiary hospital for ear, nose, and throat (ENT) assessment of stridor, present since birth, following a normal pregnancy and uncomplicated birth. He has difficulty with feedings and has moderate to severe accessory muscle retractions. He has no apparent dysmorphic features.

1 What are the anesthetic/airway management considerations for this case?

The patient's symptoms are suspicious for an upper airway stenosis (most frequently laryngomalacia, vocal cord paralysis, or subglottic stenosis). As the airway pathology is still unknown, conventional induction and mask ventilation is not recommended. Furthermore, the ENT team requests a *dynamic* assessment of the airway, which requires maintenance of spontaneous ventilation.

Maintaining spontaneous ventilation during airway assessment is a core airway management technique in neonates and small children. Many anesthesiologists prefer a sevoflurane-based induction for preservation of spontaneous ventilation. However, the use of inhalational anesthetics in a "narrow airway setting" comes with drawbacks. Induction speed and predictability may be affected by the degree of airway stenosis, and open airway administration of sevoflurane can contaminate the surroundings.

Propofol provides a predictable, titratable, and odor-free induction. Placing an intravenous line before induction is usually feasible in neonates and should be prioritized in difficult airway settings. In small children (<6 years), a bolus of propofol 2 to 3 mg/kg induces anesthesia and usually maintains spontaneous ventilation. A dose of fentanyl (1 mcg/kg IV) provides analgesia for suspension laryngoscopy. General anesthesia can be maintained by propofol infusion (10 mg/kg/h).

Following induction of anesthesia, video laryngoscopy can be performed to visualize the vocal cords and apply local anesthesia (lidocaine 4 mg/kg) to the glottis and proximal trachea. Before retraction of the video laryngoscope, a nasopharyngeal airway can be passed through the nose. Visual guidance aids positioning of the nasal airway just above the tip of the epiglottis.

2 How would you manage the airway in this case?

Prior to the case, members of both the ENT surgery and pediatric anesthesia teams should discuss a surgical and anesthetic plan. Diagnosing the origin of the stridor with an atraumatic approach is paramount in this case. Assessment of narrow airways in neonates poses the risk of edema, further compromising the airway. The neonatal intensive care unit should be aware of the patient, as ICU care may be required postoperatively.

Following induction of general anesthesia with propofol, video laryngoscopy revealed severe subglottic stenosis in this particular case (Figure 110.1). Due to the concern that a rigid bronchoscopy might cause edema and worsen airway obstruction, it is important to confirm that intubation is possible as a rescue technique should it become necessary.

During video laryngoscopy, the airway can be probed with a Portex Tracheal Tube Guide to examine intubation conditions. It is important to note that tracheal intubation can still fail despite reassuring information obtained from the tracheal tube guide. In this case, the attempt to intubate with an uncuffed endotracheal tube (ETT) (Portex Siliconized 2.0) was a failure, even with an attempt to stiffen the tube by sliding the tube over the tracheal tube guide.

The next step in this difficult airway plan was a surgical airway. In the case of subglottic stenosis, planning the tracheotomy site requires visual confirmation that the cartilaginous stenosis does not involve the planned stoma site. Ultrasonography of the neck can help locate the normal tracheal diameter from the stenotic area.

In this case, an supraglottic airway was placed next to provide a method of spontaneous ventilation with oxygenation. Following infiltration of the pretracheal soft tissues with local anesthetic, the tracheotomy was completed via a vertical incision with bilateral stay-sutures (Figure 110.2). The patient's spontaneous breathing was maintained throughout the procedure.

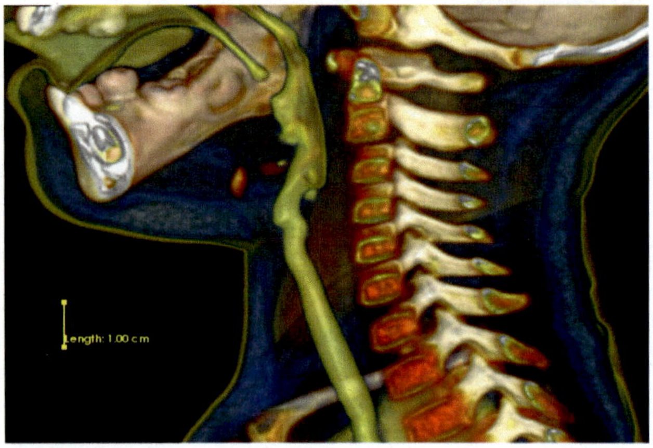

Figure 110.1. The colorized imaging of a child's airway shows the relative difficulty in isolating the larynx or trachea.

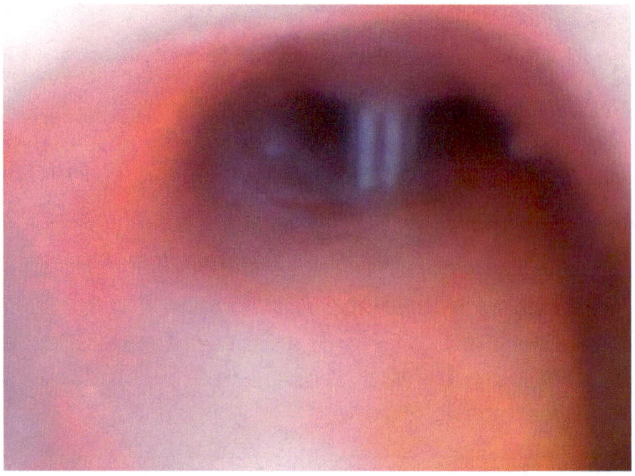

Figure 110.2. In a piglet model, a transcricothyroid catheter over the needles inadvertently punctures the posterior laryngeal wall.

3 What are the potential hazards and complications regarding the airway?

In this particular case, the surgeon had enough time to complete the needed tracheotomy before it became an emergency situation. Extreme caution should be taken to monitor airway edema, which can quickly change the airway structure and ability to intubate. Sedation should be carefully titrated to maintain spontaneous ventilation, which is crucial in a difficult pediatric airway.

Front of Neck Airway Access (FONA) in small children is challenging due to the unique anatomical features of the pediatric airway. Adult emergency(e)-FONA targets the cricothyroid membrane, which is a spacious and easily identifiable anatomic landmark in adults. In neonates, the cricothyroid membrane measures only roughly 2.5 × 3 mm with the distal border being the cricoid cartilage, the narrowest part of the normal neonatal airway. Therefore, tracheal access is advised rather than cricothyroid membrane access.

In children, percutaneous cannulation of the trachea is difficult because of the small diameter and pliable cartilaginous elements of the airway. Trans- or paratracheal placement of needle and/or catheter are known complication. During attempts to jet ventilate through a misplaced needle or catheter, severe tissue emphysema may result, making a subsequent surgical tracheotomy more difficult or even impossible. If transtracheal jet ventilation is attempted during complete upper airway obstruction, severe barotrauma to the lungs may occur.

The surgical tracheotomy is a definitive airway. In extreme emergency situations, some authors argue that a modified surgical technique provides about 95% success rate in animal models. The steps include: (1) Palpating and stabilizing the larynx, and making a vertical midline incision, (2) applying lateral traction to both sides of the skin incision, exposing the laryngeal and tracheal structures, (3) anterior luxation of proximal trachea with towel forceps, (4) performing a vertical slit-type cut through the proximal two to three tracheal rings, and (5) intubation with a cuffed tracheal tube.

It is important to emphasize that no consensus exists in solving this complex clinical condition in small children. It should be emphasized that the true unanticipated cannot-intubate–cannot-oxygenate scenarios leading to the need for an eFONA in children, in elective cases, is *extremely rare*. Focus should be on training anesthesiologists in basic and advanced airway skills to *prevent* the need for eFONA.

- Advanced airway management is a team effort, especially in the pediatric population.
- Maintain high levels of basic and advanced airway management skills, aiming at the *prevention* of a surgical airway.
- Performing a surgical airway in children should be the absolute last resort—irrespective of technique chosen.
- eFONA in small children (<6 years) should be a *tracheal maneuver*, bypassing both the narrow cricothyroid membrane and cricoid cartilage.
- *See* ***Video 110.1*** *for additional details.*

Suggested Readings

Both CP, Diem B, Alonso E, et al. Rabbit training model for establishing an emergency front of neck airway in children. *Br J Anaesth.* 2021;126(4):896–902.

Disma N, Virag K, Riva T, et al. Difficult tracheal intubation in neonates and infants. NEonate and Children audiT of Anaesthesia pRactice IN Europe (NECTARINE): a prospective European multicentre observational study. *Br J Anaesth.* 2021; 126(6):1173–1181.

Holm-Knudsen RJ, Rasmussen LS, Charabi B, Bøttger M, Kristensen MS. Emergency airway access in children—transtracheal cannulas and tracheotomy assessed in a porcine model. *Paediatr Anaesth.* 2012;(22):1159–1165.

Ulmer F, Lennertz J, Greif R, Bütikofer L, Theiler L, Riva T. Emergency front of neck access in children: a new learning approach in a rabbit model. *Br J Anaesth.* 2020;125(1):e61–e68.

111 Flexible Bronchoscopy in a Small Child

Paul Baker

Clinical Scenario: A 2-year-old boy has suffered three episodes of pneumonia, requiring intensive care of one occasion. The pediatric pulmonologist wishes to proceed with a diagnostic CT scan followed by diagnostic flexible bronchoscopy.

1 What are the anesthetic/airway management considerations for this case?

The child would undergo one anesthetic for two procedures in separate locations (CT scanner and operating room [OR]), with consequent airway, monitoring, and transport considerations. The CT scan and flexible bronchoscopy have different airway management requirements. While flexible bronchoscopy is ideally performed through a supraglottic airway (SGA), the CT scan necessitates breath-holding at a pressure (30 cm H_2O) greater than the leak pressure of most SGAs. Hence, most patients are intubated with a cuffed tracheal tube for the CT scan.

2 How would you manage the airway in this case?

During the preoperative assessment, particular attention should be paid to the child's current respiratory status. Additional comorbidities can include chronic lung disease, asthma, cardiac anomalies, underlying immunodeficiencies, neurologic disorders (including gastroesophageal reflux and aspiration), airway anomalies, or history of prior thoracic surgeries. The current proposed procedure is elective. Children who are systemically unwell with fevers, wheezing, or a productive cough should have their procedures postponed until resolution of these symptoms (ideally 2 or more weeks later). This helps to decrease the risk of airway complications.

Premedication with oral Midazolam can be used for preoperative sedation. Induction of anesthesia can be either inhalational induction or intravenous Propofol, if an intravenous catheter is already in situ. The goal of induction is to foster a calm environment to avoid crying and agitation. Excessive crying can increase oral secretions, which increase the risk of laryngospasm or breath-holding. A dose of IV propofol (once IV access has been established) and topical lidocaine spray provide excellent intubating conditions without the use of muscle relaxants. Propofol (2 to 3 mg/kg) helps to obtund laryngeal reflexes, improving intubating conditions. The larynx and tracheobronchial tree are anesthetized with 2% lidocaine (3 mg/kg) using a mucosal atomizer device (MADgic Laryngo-Tracheal Mucosal Atomization Device, Wolf Tory medical, Inc. Salt Lake City, Utah, USA). This important step requires a forceful push on the local anesthetic syringe to facilitate spread of local anesthetic throughout the airway. Topicalization of the airway is essential for flexible bronchoscopy to minimize coughing, breath-holding, laryngospasm, and bronchospasm. For the breath-hold required during the CT scan, apnea can be achieved with an additional dose of Propofol, and the anesthetic circuit is closed to 30 cm H_2O pressure to maximize the quality of CT imaging. This pressure exceeds the leak pressure of most SGAs, rendering these devices inappropriate for this type of airway management, so a cuffed tracheal tube should be used during the CT scan.

On arrival in the OR, the tracheal tube is removed from the anesthetized patient and replaced with an appropriately sized cLMA (LMA North America, Inc., San Diego, CA) (suitable for infants and children 10 to 20 kg) in order to maximize the function of the flexible bronchoscope. The cLMA provides a conduit for flexible bronchoscopy, and the child can breathe spontaneously during the procedure via a bronchoscopy elbow.

3 What are the potential hazards/complications in regard to the airway?

Maintaining oxygenation and avoiding airway trauma are the key objectives of any type of airway management. This child has an increased risk of complications during airway management, including hypoxia, bronchospasm, laryngospasm, and obstruction of the SGA. Gastric distension and regurgitation with aspiration can occur secondary to excessive bag mask ventilation or positive pressure ventilation through a SGA. Without adequate preoxygenation, hypoxia can occur almost immediately after the onset of apnea and withdrawal of facemask oxygenation. Prolonged intubation attempts can be traumatic and run the risk of patient awareness. Airway pressure control during breath-holds should be monitored to avoid excessive peak airway pressure of 80 cm H_2O, which can cause barotrauma. During transport, careful monitoring of ventilation, oxygenation, and depth of anesthesia is required. Care should also be taken to avoid inadvertent extubation during transport.

The child can breathe spontaneously through a cLMA during flexible bronchoscopy. Positive pressure ventilation should be avoided because of the risk of exceeding cuff leak pressure and inflating the stomach. Adequate depth of anesthesia and topicalization of the airway are essential to avoid light anesthesia with consequent coughing, breath-holding, laryngospasm, or bronchospasm. Excessively deep anesthesia can cause apnea and cardiovascular compromise. The cLMA can be associated with malpositioning, aspiration, and airway obstruction by the epiglottis or other airway structures. Smaller SGAs have been associated with poorer views with the flexible bronchoscope.

Postoperative care can be problematic. SGAs are best removed when the patient is deeply anesthetized to avoid laryngospasm or postobstructive pulmonary edema. Laryngospasm is the leading cause of respiratory-related cardiac arrest in pediatric anesthesia. If laryngospasm occurs, it is treated in a stepwise fashion with continuous positive airway pressure (CPAP), 100% oxygen, deepening of anesthetic, administration of succinylcholine, and reintubation if necessary. If stridor develops in the postoperative recovery phase, treatment includes oxygen, CPAP, racemic epinephrine, steroids, and helium.

4 What distinct airway devices (eg, specialized tracheal tube, rigid bronchoscope, bronchial blocker) might be used in this case, and what are the special considerations?

Since the introduction of the cLMA, anesthesia for flexible bronchoscopy in children has diversified, expanding diagnostic and therapeutic capabilities. Using a cLMA also allows dynamic inspection of the airway and reduces bacteremia. Some single-use polyvinyl chloride SGAs are associated with increased resistance to bronchoscope passage and are therefore not fit for this purpose. This problem does not apply to silicone SGAs. The alternative use of an endotracheal tube for bronchoscopy restricts the maximum size of the bronchoscope that can be used. It is also important to note that local anesthetic with sedation for flexible bronchoscopy is not tolerated by children.

- Flexible bronchoscopy for children is usually an elective procedure; therefore, careful preoperative assessment followed by appropriate treatment to optimize the child's medical status should occur prior to anesthesia.
- A silicone SGA is the ideal airway device to maintain spontaneous ventilation for flexible bronchoscopy in children, but risks include airway obstruction, aspiration, and inadequate ventilation.
- Anesthesia for flexible bronchoscopy requires topicalization of the airway and adequate depth of anesthesia to blunt airway reflexes such as cough, laryngospasm, bronchospasm, and breath-holding.
- *See Figure 111.1 and* ***Video 111.1*** *for additional details.*

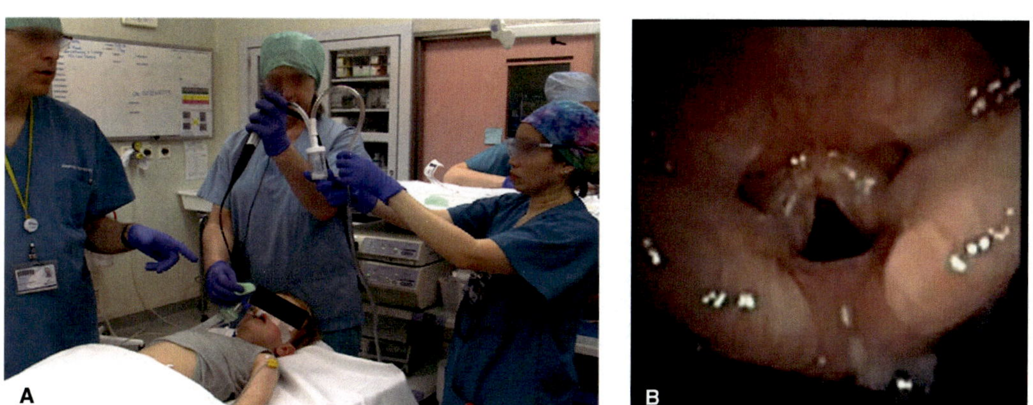

Figure 111.1. **A:** Flexible bronchoscopic exam with sampling in a small child. **B:** The use of a supraglottic airway for introduction of the bronchoscope allows the clinician to see the entire larynx in addition to the lower airway structures.

Suggested Readings

Aouad MT, Yazbeck-Karam VG, Mallat CE, Esso JJ, Siddik-Sayyid SM, Kaddoum RN. The effect of adjuvant drugs on the quality of tracheal intubation without muscle relaxants in children: a systematic review of randomized trials. *Paediatr Anesth.* 2012; 22(7):616–626.

Baker PA, Brunette KE, Byrnes CA, Thompson JM. A prospective randomized trial comparing supraglottic airways for flexible bronchoscopy in children. *Paediatr Anesth.* 2010;20(9):831–838.

Cumin D, Baker PA, Anderson BJ. Incidence of post-induction hypoxemia in children and the effect of induction gas composition. *Paediatr Anaesth.* 2021;31(7):763–769.

Roberts MH, Gildersleve CD. Lignocaine topicalization of the pediatric airway. *Paediatr Anaesth.* 2016;26(4):337–344.

von Ungern-Sternberg BS, Boda K, Chambers NA, et al. Risk assessment for respiratory complications in paediatric anaesthesia: a prospective cohort study. *Lancet.* 2010;376(9743):773–783.

Gender-Affirming Surgery for Correction of Thyroid Prominence

112

Mariel Poole • Michael Alperovich

Clinical Scenario: A 56-year-old Transgender female presents for gender-affirming surgery to correct the thyroid prominence.

1 What are the anesthetic/airway management considerations for this case?

Health care access for the transgender community has increased in the past decade. Appropriate pronoun use and addressing the patient with a gender-appropriate name are both important first steps in establishing trust in the physician–patient interaction. While sex and gender may be used as interchangeable terms, in the transgender population there are important distinctions. Sex is what was assigned at birth and is determined by the sexual organs and chromosomal composition. However, gender is based on how the person identifies themselves. A patient's gender can be male, female, nonbinary, genderfluid, genderqueer, intersex, or gender nonconforming. Many patients who present for gender-affirming surgery or facial feminization surgery have gender dysphoria, a DSM-5 diagnosis relating to issues in overall well-being arising from inconsistency between one's sex and gender.

In the United States, passage of the Affordable Care Act included protections against discrimination in health care on the basis of gender identity. Federal policy changes opened access to gender-affirming surgery for the transgender community and were associated with a large increase in facial feminization surgery nationally. Many transgender individuals pursue medical care (including hormonal therapy) and surgery to achieve an external physical appearance that is more harmonious with their gender identity. For patients to feel safe and to maintain trust with their physician, perioperatively, it is imperative to document and use the individual's preferred name and pronouns. Often, there may be a delay in amending a patient's legal name, leading to formal documentation or identification that differs from how a patient self-identifies.

Preoperatively, the patient should be asked about transition history, hormone therapy, prior surgeries, and an organ inventory must be taken. Given the historic barriers to access to care, patients should be asked about any care received from an unlicensed medical professional, as nonapproved fillers or other injectables can have devastating consequences. As per WPATH (World Professional Association for Transgender Health) guidelines, facial feminization surgery is deferred until completion of at least 1 year of hormonal therapy. Endocrinologists differ on whether hormonal therapy is withheld perioperatively, and the use of hormones perioperatively should be clarified. Prior reports have documented an increased risk of venous thrombosis, cardiovascular disease, and insulin resistance in patients receiving supplemental hormonal therapy.

The transgender female should be questioned specifically about nicotine use as smoking in combination with estrogen hormones can increase the risk of venous thrombosis. Historically, a higher prevalence of HIV in the transgender community has been associated with greater use of antiretroviral medication for either treatment of HIV or pre-exposure prophylaxis. Many of these prescriptions, particularly the nonnucleoside reverse transcriptase inhibitors and protease inhibitors, are metabolized by cytochrome P-450 enzymes. HIV medications may affect the metabolism or interact with medications that are part of the anesthetic plan.

In addition to routine airway considerations, transgender patients and, specifically, transgender females may have had prior voice-altering surgery that may affect airway management. These procedures include laser reduction glottoplasty, cricothyroid approximation, and endoscopic vocal cord shortening and retrodisplacement of the anterior commissure (VFSRAC). As these procedures act to weaken the vocal cords, intubation can be challenging. Chondrolaryngoplasty can itself cause vocal cord damage, tracheal damage, and dysphagia complicating airway management.

2 How would you manage the airway in this case?

Chondrolaryngoplasty can be performed under various forms of anesthesia, including local with sedation, general endotracheal anesthesia, or our preferred method of general anesthesia using a flexible fiberoptic laryngoscope with a supraglottic airway (SGA). Local anesthesia with sedation can be successful, but disadvantages include poor patient cooperation that can create unfavorable surgical conditions. Endotracheal intubation eliminates the risk of inconsistent patient cooperation and provides advantageous surgical conditions. However, endotracheal intubation limits the ability to use fiberoptic laryngoscopy to identify the level of the vocal cord attachments.

As with all cases involving anesthesia, a thorough preoperative airway examination is essential for safe airway management. Assessment of mouth opening, Mallampati score, neck range of motion, and thyromental distance should be assessed. Regular rescue airway equipment should be available. Assuming favorable conditions, the ideal plan is general anesthesia with an SGA. Proper SGA placement is confirmed with capnography, chest rise, and bilateral chest sounds on auscultation. Ideally, the patient is kept spontaneously breathing on total intravenous anesthesia (TIVA) in preparation for fiberoptic laryngoscopy, which will be discussed later in this chapter.

3 What are the surgical considerations that impact anesthetic management?

The thyroid prominence, or Adam's apple, is a male physical characteristic. Chondrolaryngoplasty, also known as thyroid cartilage reduction, thyroid chondroplasty, laryngeal chondroplasty, and laryngochondroplasty, is a surgical procedure most often performed for transgender female patients desiring a less prominent Adam's apple. This procedure is sometimes referred to as a tracheal shave although this is a misnomer as it involves a reduction in the thyroid cartilage and not the trachea.

The Adam's apple or laryngeal prominence is formed by the fusion of the anterior borders of the two laminae of the thyroid cartilage. In genetic males, they diverge at an angle of approximately 90 degrees, whereas in genetic females, the angle is more obtuse at approximately 120 degrees. The more acute angle in the transgender female population creates a more prominent thyroid cartilage. The goal of chondrolaryngoplasty is to reduce the anterior projecting thyroid cartilage thereby decreasing the anterior projection of the cartilage.

Beyond the standard risks of surgery, this procedure can cause injury to the anterior commissure tendon or the anterior junction point of the true vocal cords. Injury to this tendon can cause irreversible effects on a patient's voice by lowering it. This complication can be very troubling for a transgender female who wants to maintain a higher-pitched voice. Therefore, an anesthetic plan that incorporates an SGA with fiberoptic laryngoscopy can identify the level of the anterior commissure tendon and decrease the risk of injury to this tendon. After marking the position of the tendon along the external surface of the thyroid cartilage, surgical reduction can be limited to the thyroid cartilage above this point to prevent injury to the vocal cords.

Finally, any surgery near the airway requires appropriate safety measures to reduce the risk of airway fire. Effective communication between the surgeon and anesthesiologist is important, and FiO_2 should be reduced to below 30% to decrease the risk of fire with electrocautery use.

4 What distinct airway device (eg, specialized tracheal tube, rigid bronchoscope, bronchial blocker) might be used in this case, and what are the special considerations?

As briefly described above, general anesthesia with an SGA would be the most appropriate plan for this case. After proper placement of the SGA and confirmation that the patient is being maintained on adequate anesthetic, a fiberoptic connector is attached to the SGA in preparation for flexible bronchoscope insertion. Once the surgical field is prepped and draped, a 2-cm incision in the cervicomental fold is marked to conceal the scar in a natural crease. Local anesthetic is injected, the skin incised, the midline cervical fascia divided, and the sternothyroid and thyrohyoid muscles are retracted laterally to expose the thyroid cartilage.

Through continuous dialogue with the surgeon, the anesthesiologist carefully advances the fiberoptic scope through the SGA, allowing for visualization of the anterior commissure of the larynx. It should be noted that a surgeon's retractors may displace the airway anteriorly, making for a more challenging view with the fibrotic scope. Once a view of the anterior commissure is obtained, the surgeon advances a 25-gauge needle midline through the cartilage. The fiberoptic display is used to evaluate the position of the needle relative to the location of the anterior commissure. The needle is replaced as necessary to a position just cranial to the vocal cord attachment. With the inferior limit of thyroid cartilage resection marked by the needle, the surgeon can safely remove maximal cartilage above the needle for the ideal therapeutic result. At the portion of cartilage directly attached to the anterior commissure, at least 2 mm of cartilage is necessary for adequate structural support.

In some instances, the anterior-most projection of the thyroid cartilage can be located below the anterior commissure. In these instances, patients are counseled that a slightly less ideal final result is acceptable to reduce the risk of lowering the patient's voice. At the conclusion of the thyroid cartilage reduction, the fiberoptic scope is used to confirm the integrity of the anterior commissure tendon attachment.

- Gender-affirming procedures for the transgender population have increased in numbers, and facial feminization procedures present unique and complex airway management challenges.
- Risk of injury to the anterior commissure tendon of the vocal cord during this procedure can alter the pitch of a patient's voice and lead to a potentially devastating complication of a lower voice in a transgender female.
- Chondrolaryngoplasty or thyroid cartilage reduction is ideally performed under general anesthesia using an SGA with flexible fiberoptic laryngoscopy to identify the position of the anterior commissure tendon both before and immediately after the procedure.
- Regular and open communication between the anesthesia and surgical teams is essential to confirm anatomic landmarks, reduce fire risk, and minimize risk of injury to the vocal cords.
- *See Figure 112.1 and* ***Video 112.1*** *for additional details.*

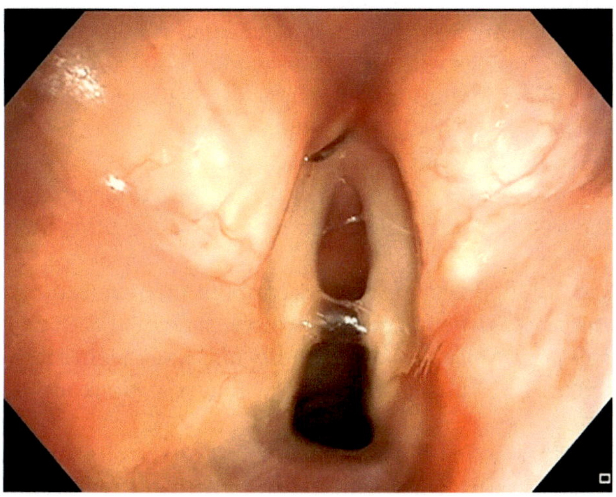

Figure 112.1. Surface anatomy localization of the anterior commissure has been achieved with the visualization of a probing needle. The patient is under general anesthesia and managed with a supraglottic airway.

Suggested Readings

Grundler S, Stacey MR. Thyroplasty under general anesthesia using a laryngeal mask airway and fiberoptic bronchoscope. *Can J Anaesth*. 1999;46(5 Pt 1):460–463.

Spiegel JH, Rodriguez G. Chondrolaryngoplasty under general anesthesia using a flexible fiberoptic laryngoscope and laryngeal mask airway. *Arch Otolaryngol Head Neck Surg*. 2008;134(7):704–708.

Sturm A, Chaiet SR. Chondrolaryngoplasty-thyroid cartilage reduction. *Facial Plast Surg Clin North Am*. 2019;27(2):267–272.

Tollinche LE, Van Rooyen C, Afonso A, Fischer GW, Yeoh CB. Considerations for transgender patients perioperatively. *Anesthesiol Clin*. 2020;38(2):311–326.

113 Gender-Affirming Voice Surgery

Mariel Poole • Nwanmegha Young

Clinical Scenario: A 56-year-old transgender female presents for gender-affirming voice surgery.

1 What are the anesthetic/airway management considerations for this case?

As discussed in the chapter on "gender-affirming surgery for correction of thyroid prominence," sex and gender are distinct terms. Sex refers to the sex of the individual designated at birth based on chromosomal make-up and sexual organs at birth. Gender is derived from how the patient identifies. A patient's well-being can be greatly compromised when gender is not harmonious with sex. Transgender females are biologically male, but identify as female. This incongruence in gender identity and sex assigned at birth can lead to a gender dysphoria leading to significant psychological burden. Individuals with gender dysphoria seek medical and surgical care to have their physical appearance be congruent with their gender identity.

A male's voice is typically much deeper than a female's. Many transgender females will undergo treatments to feminize their voice, lessening dysphoria related to their voice and facilitating society accepting them more readily by their true gender.

A thorough preoperative interview is necessary. Individuals must be asked about their transition history, hormone therapy, and prior surgeries. Many transgender patients are on hormone therapy that increases the risk of thrombus, cardiovascular disease, and insulin resistance. This community also has a higher rate of prescription use for either the treatment or prevention of HIV, which may interact with medications administered for anesthesia.

Any prior surgeries should be discussed, especially any that might have an effect on the airway. Chondrolaryngoplasty has the potential to cause vocal cord damage, tracheal damage, and dysphagia resulting in more challenging airway management. Gender-affirming voice surgery itself and other voice-correcting interventions act to weaken the vocal cords and can make airway manipulation difficult.

2 How would you manage the airway in this case?

Voice feminization is achieved through voice therapy, surgery, or a combination of both. Surgery aims to correct pitch, while voice therapy assists patients with non–pitch-related aspects of voice femininity. There are three main surgical options for vocal feminization: laser reduction glottoplasty, cricothyroid approximation, and endoscopic vocal cord shortening and retrodisplacement of the anterior commissure (VFSRAC). All of these methods aim to increase tension and decrease length or reduce mass of the vocal cords, resulting in a higher pitch in voice.

Laryngeal surgery necessitates that the surgeon and the anesthesiologist share the airway. This requires an in-depth preoperative discussion between the surgeon and anesthesiologist to determine the plans for airway management, ventilation technique, neuromuscular blockade utilization, reduction of fire risk, and ideal operating room table orientation.

Airway management is guided by the type of phonosurgery. As always, emergency airway equipment should be readily available. Total intravenous anesthesia (TIVA) may be utilized if the procedure necessitates an open airway, as is the case in cricothyroid approximation surgery. Intravenous infusions of remifentanil and propofol are often used.

Laser reduction glottoplasty and VFSRAC require general anesthesia with an endotracheal tube. Laser reduction glottoplasty is performed with a carbon dioxide laser, so a laser resistant endotracheal tube must be used. VFSRAC requires general anesthesia with a reinforced endotracheal tube.

3 What distinct airway device (eg, specialized tracheal tube, rigid bronchoscope, bronchial blocker) might be used in this case, and what are the special considerations?

The type of phonosurgery planned dictates airway management and anesthetic plan. Cricothyroid approximation may be performed under local anesthesia with an open airway. In laser reduction glottoplasty, a laser-resistant endotracheal tube is used. These endotracheal tube cuffs should be filled with saline tinted with methylene blue to indicate an event of cuff rupture. Effective communication between the surgeon and anesthesiologist is important regarding laser usage, and FiO_2 should be reduced to below 30% to decrease risk of airway fire.

VFSRAC is an endoscopic surgery necessitating general anesthesia with a reinforced endotracheal tube preferably. The surgery is performed through a narrow, 2-cm endoscopic tube that is inserted through the mouth. In brief, the anterior third of the vocal cords and the area of the larynx immediately inferior to them are roughened with the anterior third of the vocal folds and then sutured together with permanent sutures. Healing retrodisplaces the anterior commissure of the larynx resulting in a higher-pitched voice.

4 Are there special considerations for the emergence or the end of the case?

Phonosurgery aims to weaken the vocal cords, resulting in a higher-pitched voice. The surgery can cause damage to the vocal cords, including paralysis. Vocal cord paralysis is a devastating complication that could lead to aspiration upon extubation or even loss of a patent airway. The surgery itself decreases the glottic opening, resulting in a more difficult airway upon extubation. Reintubation after extubation for airway rescue could prove more difficult, and the anesthesiologist should be readily prepared for such an event. As always, emergency airway equipment should be available.

- Special attention should be given when addressing the transgender population to use preferred pronouns and gender-appropriate names.
- Gender-affirming surgery strives to increase the patient's voice pitch, and voice therapy assists with non–pitch-related aspects of voice femininity.
- Multiple approaches exist for gender-affirming voice surgery, and airway management is dictated by the type of surgery being performed.
- Phonosurgery requires close communication between surgeon and anesthesiologist.

Suggested Readings

Nolan IT, Morrison SD, Arowojolu O, et al. The role of voice therapy and phonosurgery in transgender vocal feminization. *J Craniofac Surg*. 2019;30(5):1368–1375.

Song TE, Jiang N. Transgender phonosurgery: a systematic review and meta-analysis. *Otolaryngol Head Neck Surg*. 2017;156:803–808.

Tollinche LE, Van Rooyen C, Afonso A, Fischer GW, Yeoh CB. Considerations for transgender patients perioperatively. *Anesthesiol Clin*. 2020;38(2):311–326.

114 Vocal Cord Augmentation

Eric L. Vu • Ashutosh Wali

Clinical Scenario: A 35-year-old woman had a unilateral vocal cord paralysis for less than 1 year. She now presents for vocal cord augmentation with the injection of voice gel.

1 What are the anesthetic and airway management considerations for this case?

Vocal cord augmentation is performed to improve symptoms of vocal fatigue, hoarseness, dyspnea, or dysphagia due to glottal incompetence. Common indications include vocal fold paralysis, paresis, atrophy, or scarring. First described by Brünings in 1911, this procedure is performed by the otolaryngologist in either the office or the OR. Airway management is dictated by the surgical approach.

If the procedure is performed by a percutaneous approach, local anesthesia is applied by the surgeon, and sedation with monitored anesthesia care (MAC) is typically sufficient. Airway management may only involve a nasal cannula with continuous capnography. A titratable and rapidly reversible sedation technique can be utilized in order to allow the patient to cooperate in the evaluation of phonation quality.

The procedure may also be performed transorally, in which case, general anesthesia (GA) is required. Although nonintubation techniques have been described, routine intubation with a smaller-sized tracheal tube (TT) is most commonly used. Fortunately, due to the quick nature of this procedure (typically ~10 minutes), problems with ventilation related to small TT size are uncommon.

With a general anesthetic technique, a short-acting neuromuscular blocking agent is recommended. It is not unreasonable to perform a rapid sequence induction (RSI) in these patients, as the risk of pulmonary aspiration has been described. Glycopyrrolate may be given to reduce secretions and improve visualization during tracheal intubation and the surgical procedure. Dexamethasone administration can also be considered to reduce airway edema. After the procedure, the surgeon may apply a local anesthetic to the laryngeal structures to reduce the risk of laryngospasm.

2 How would you manage the airway in this case?

Commonly, vocal cord augmentation is performed with the patient sedated under MAC. Electrocautery is rarely used, so there is no contraindication to using nasal oxygen. The goal of sedation is to keep the patient comfortable, but cooperative for voice evaluation. A variety of sedative regimens have been described, including titrated fentanyl, midazolam, or propofol. Dexmedetomidine with or without remifentanil infusions may also be good options, particularly if the patient is at high risk for upper airway obstruction. There is no one best technique as long as the patient's airway patency, oxygenation, and ventilation are closely monitored.

A superior laryngeal and/or a transcricothyroid membrane block may be performed for patient comfort. These blocks can be performed by the anesthesiologist or otolaryngologist. Alternatively, an atomized lidocaine technique can be used for local anesthesia of the airway.

If GA is necessary, the authors' preference is to perform a RSI with a hypnotic and short or intermediate-acting neuromuscular blocker, followed by intubation with a 6.0-mm or 6.5-mm microlaryngeal TT (a smaller size is utilized to avoid displacement of the injected biomaterial by the TT). The patient may also be given 0.2 mg of glycopyrrolate and 8 to 10 mg of dexamethasone to reduce secretions and edema, respectively. In the rare case of airway compromise, advanced airway equipment and a tracheotomy tray should be immediately available. In the postanesthesia care unit, the patient should be closely monitored for complications including laryngospasm, airway obstruction, or negative pressure pulmonary edema.

3 What are the surgical considerations that impact anesthetic management?

In vocal cord augmentation surgery, the otolaryngologist medializes a paralyzed vocal cord by injection of a biomaterial into the deep vocal fold layers. Temporary biomaterials will last 4 to 6 months and include bovine gelatin, collagen-based products, carboxymethylcellulose, and hyaluronic acid gel. Longer-lasting implants (9 to 12 months) include autologous fat, polytetrafluoroethylene, and calcium hydroxylapatite.

Vocal cord augmentation can be performed by percutaneous translaryngeal injection under nasoendoscopy guidance. After laryngeal anesthesia has been performed, the nasal passages are prepared with a vasoconstrictor (oxymetazoline or phenylephrine) and a topical anesthetic. A flexible nasopharyngoscope is passed, and the vocal cords are visualized. A 25G or 27G needle is passed midline through the cricothyroid membrane and directed toward the paralyzed vocal cord. The needle pierces the cord, and the injection is performed. The surgeon may request that the patient speak, and watches for apposition of the working vocal cord against the now medialized one.

Although studies have shown that the trend of performing vocal cord augmentation in the awake patient has risen from 11% to 43% from 2003 to 2008, this procedure may still be performed under GA due to surgeon or patient preference. Occasionally, there is a need for additional procedures such as direct laryngoscopy, microlaryngoscopic surgery, or autologous fat harvest. The surgeon may also request GA in cases where the procedure may be technically difficult and extreme precision is required. In such an event, a transoral approach may be utilized. Complete muscle relaxation is typically preferred during the injection.

In a 5-year retrospective analysis of 36 patients, 73.1% of patients were satisfied with their voice, with no significant difference between the use of autologous fat or calcium hydroxylapatite. With persistent vocal cord paralysis despite injections and vocal exercises, the patient may require an Isshiki thyroplasty as the next option for treatment.

4 What are the potential hazards and complications in regard to the airway?

Complications after vocal cord augmentation are rare. The anesthesia provider should be prepared to address airway obstruction, bleeding from laryngeal or perilaryngeal structures, aspiration, and laryngospasm. Postoperatively, some patients complain of dyspnea, which can occur with overinjection of the vocal folds. These patients should be closely monitored. Initial treatment includes humidified oxygen and oral or intravenous steroids. If symptoms worsen, the patient may require tracheal reintubation. Airway edema typically resolves with time. In rare cases, the patient may require revision surgery.

After vocal cord augmentation surgery, foreign bodies and allergic reactions from the injected compounds can occur. Vocal fold granuloma formation is extremely rare but has been reported and could theoretically affect future tracheal intubation. However, in most cases, there is no issue securing a protected airway in patients after this procedure. There has been a reported case of a severe systemic reaction within 30 minutes after vocal cord injection. Treatment of anaphylactoid or anaphylactic reactions should be initiated with epinephrine, diphenhydramine, and dexamethasone. If there are signs of airway compromise, tracheal intubation and at least 24 hours of observation is recommended.

- Vocal cord augmentation is performed to improve symptoms due to glottal incompetence.
- The anesthetic and airway management varies from sedation with MAC to GA.
- Patients should be monitored after surgery for life-threatening airway compromise.
- Postoperatively, patients usually have very minor pain or dysphagia that can be treated with acetaminophen or nonsteroidal anti-inflammatory drugs.
- *See Figure 114.1 and* ***Video 114.1*** *for additional details.*

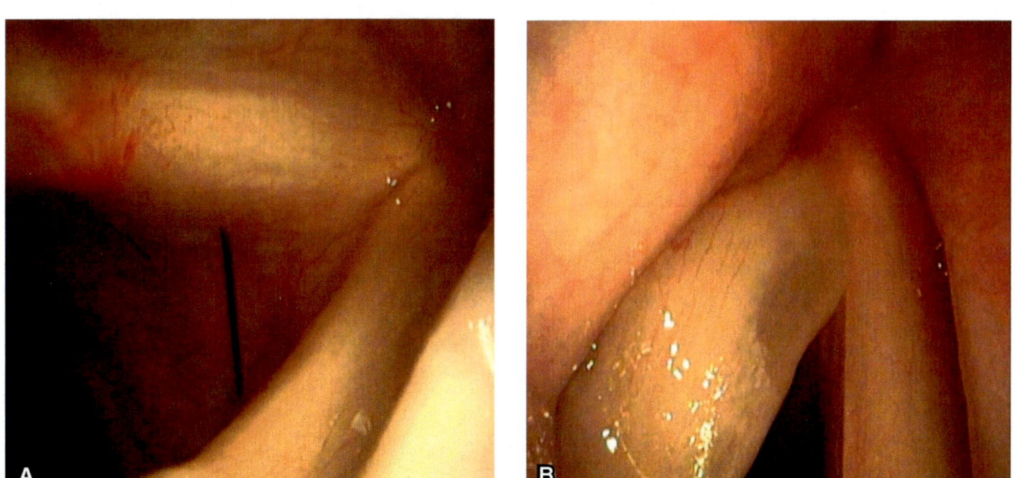

Figure 114.1. A: A percutaneously placed needle is positioned to inject vocal cord gel. **B:** Gel has been injected into the paralyzed left vocal cord in an effort to get opposition against the right-sided cord during adduction.

Suggested Readings

Cohen JC, Reisacher W, Malone M, Sulica L. Severe systemic reaction from calcium hydroxylapatite vocal fold filler. *Laryngoscope*. 2013;123(9):2237–2239.

Giraldez-Rodriguez LA, Johns M 3rd. Glottal insufficiency with aspiration risk in dysphagia. *Otolaryngol Clin North Am*. 2013; 46(6):1113–1121.

Sanderson JD, Simpson CB. Laryngeal complications after lipoinjection for vocal fold augmentation. *Laryngoscope*. 2009;119(8): 1652–1657.

Sulica L, Rosen CA, Postma GN, et al. Current practice in injection augmentation of the vocal folds: indications, treatment principles, techniques, and complications. *Laryngoscope*. 2010;120(2):319–325.

Zeleník K, Formánek M, Walderová R, Formánková D, Komínek P. Five-year results of vocal fold augmentation using autologous fat or calcium hydroxylapatite. *Eur Arch Otorhinolaryngol*. 2021;278(4):1139–1144.

PART B LOWER AIRWAY

SECTION I INTERVENTIONAL PULMONOLOGY

Flexible Bronchoscopy 115

Brooks V. Udelsman • Vincent J. Mase Jr

1 Describe in detail the device or technique.

Device

The first flexible bronchoscope (FB) became commercially available in 1968. The original FB consisted of a long, flexible optical device connected to a light source that transmitted images through fiberoptic bundles to an eyepiece. In modern video bronchoscopy, the eyepiece has been replaced with a camera and image processor that allows for projection on a monitor. FBs are available through several commercial manufactures and include both single-use devices that are discarded and multiuse devices that require sterilization after each procedure. Self-contained single-use devices are particularly useful for emergent floor procedures or in intensive care units where obtaining a video tower can be time consuming.

The FB is composed of (1) a control handle, (2) a flexible shaft, (3) a distal tip. Suctioning is performed through a working channel. This working channel also allows the passage of specialized instruments and wires depending on the indication for the procedure. The control handle includes a suction button, lever, and a port for the working channel. The control handle is held in the operator's dominant hand, while the nondominant hand stabilizes the flexible shaft and endotracheal tube (ETT). The operator's index finger rests on the suction button that can be pressed and held down for selective activation. The operator's thumb controls the lever, which flexes or extends the tip of the FB. The tip of the FB flexes 130 degrees but only extends 110 degrees. The working port is capped with a one-way valve through which instruments can be passed. A saline or air-filled syringe can be connected to the working port to flush the working channel if it is occluded by thick airway secretions or blood.

When in use, the control handle represents a focal point of rotation for the scope. By rotating the operator's hand, wrist, and arm, the upright FB can achieve 360 degrees of rotation at the tip of the instrument. However, translation of this movement to the tip of the instrument is dependent on the midportion of the flexible shaft remaining straight. The more bent the flexible shaft, the less rotation is translated to the tip. Bending of the shaft is a common pitfall and will result in suboptimal views of the bronchial anatomy. Keeping the shaft straight is paramount to effective bronchoscopy and maintaining 1:1 control of the scope. This often requires the operator to stand on a step stool. Some FBs come with a wheel at the connection between the handle and the flexible shaft, which can be turned for 360 degrees of rotation without movement of the operator's arm.

The size of the FB is measured by the outer diameter (OD) of the shaft. Larger diameter scopes (4.9 mm to 6.3 mm) have a working channel which facilitates suctioning of the airway and passage of devices used in interventional bronchoscopic procedures. These scopes require at least an 8.0-Fr ETT to maintain adequate ventilation of the patient. More commonly, a 3.8-mm OD scope is used, which fits through a double lumen endotracheal tube (DLT) or through a 7.5 ETT when placed concomitantly with a 9-Fr Arndt bronchial blocker (BB) or with a 7-Fr EZ-blocker. For the Fuji Univent blocker, an 8.0 ETT is required with this scope. When placing a 7-Fr BB through a 6.0 ETT, the pediatric FB (2.8-mm OD) is required. However, it is best practice to check before intubating the patient if the FB fits through the airway management device. Smaller FBs have a narrower working channel, which makes it difficult to suction the airway.

Technique

Flexible bronchoscopy can be performed under general anesthesia, conscious sedation, or in the awake patient. Severe hypoxia is a relative contraindication to bronchoscopy, and during the procedure, the average arterial partial pressure of oxygen drops by 20 mm Hg. When performed under general anesthesia, local anesthetic is unnecessary. In the awake patient, topicalization of the vocal cords and carina is critical. For details on airway topicalization, see Chapter 11: Preparation for Awake Intubation. To avoid desaturation, conventional nasal cannula or high-flow nasal cannula may be applied. Awake bronchoscopy should be performed cautiously in patients with underlying oxygen requirement or limited reserve. In these patients, a mild drop in oxygen saturation can rapidly escalate to life-threatening hypoxia. Moderate sedation can aid in effective bronchoscopy and reduce patient discomfort. Depending on the required sedation depth, this is accomplished with boluses of fentanyl and midazolam or with infusions of propofol, dexmedetomidine, remifentanil, and other sedative drug combinations. Vocal cords topicalization can temporarily increase risk of aspiration and patients should remain *nil per os* for 1 to 3 hours after local anesthetic is applied. A bedside nursing swallow evaluation is often performed prior to reinstitution of regular diet.

Before introducing the FB, proper functioning of the light source, suction, and eye piece/monitor should be confirmed. The FB should be "white-balanced" as described by the specific device manufacturer. A silicone-based lubricant should be applied to the shaft, and the lens at the tip cleaned with alcohol and defogger. The FB is inserted via the nose, mouth, or airway management device (ie, oral airway, laryngeal mask airway, ETT, DLT, tracheostomy) to access the lower airway. To maintain ventilation during the procedure, a dual-port adapter (ventilation and bronchoscopy port) is used. The set ventilator flows need to be higher than usual, as frequent suctioning impedes adequate ventilation.

Once the scope is in the trachea, a normal orientation should be established. The cartilaginous rings should be in the "12 o'clock" (anterior) position, and the longitudinally running stripes of the membranous airway in the "6 o'clock" (posterior) position. By maintaining this orientation, the left airway remains on the left side of the screen and the right airway on the right side of the screen.

Both a thorough understanding of the normal and the pathologic appearance of the tracheobronchial tree and proper technique are essential for effective bronchoscopy. The carina is the first anatomic landmark identified and typically comes into view with one-third to one-half of the FB has entered the airway. The carina is sharply angled with two round openings representing the left and right mainstem bronchi. If the carina is not identified, the FB should be partially withdrawn. Most likely the scope and possibly the ETT are too deep and are resting on the right mainstem bronchus. The right mainstem bifurcates 1.5 to 2.5 cm into the right upper lobe (RUL) bronchus and the bronchus intermedius (BI), representing the right secondary carina. Identifying the RUL bronchus confirms the right/left orientation. To enter the RUL bronchus, the shaft is turned 90 degrees clockwise (right) and the lever is pushed down (thumb down) while the FB is advanced. The RUL bronchus is recognized by the typical trifurcated appearance ("Mercedes Benz" sign) (Figure 115.1A). With the posterior airway striae oriented in the 6 o'clock position, the segmental airways can be identified (striae run into posterior, anterior is above posterior, and apical off to right). The FB is then extended (lever neutral) and withdrawn back into the right mainstem bronchus. With the shaft straight, the FB is advanced into the BI that ends in a trifurcation (Figure 115.1B). Going from medial to lateral, there is a reversed large "D" (right middle lobe bronchus), a circle (basilar segments of the right lower lobe bronchus), and a small forward-facing "D" (superior segment bronchus of the right lower lobe). Upon further advancement into the basilar segments, just under the right middle lobe, is the entrance into the medial segmental bronchus of the right lower lobe, followed by a linear trifurcation representing the anterior, lateral, and posterior segmental bronchi of the right lower lobe.

After inspecting the right-sided airway, the FB is withdrawn into the trachea slightly above the primary carina. The shaft is rotated counterclockwise (left) and the left mainstem bronchus is entered. After advancing the FB 4 to 5 cm, the left secondary carina is encountered (two openings) (Figure 115.1C). The striae of the posterior or membranous airway identify the left lower lobe bronchus and the anterior opening represents the left upper lobe bronchus. Each lobar bronchus (left upper and left lower lobe bronchi) separates into segmental airways. In the left lower lobe, the most posterior opening is the superior segment, and the other openings represent basilar segmental airways (anterior, lateral, and posterior). In the left upper lobe, lingular segments arise from an early bifurcation or tertiary carina. The lingular airway is identified by the relationship to the posterior airway. If the posterior striae are in the 6 o'clock position, then the lingula is in the 3 o'clock position.

At the conclusion of the procedure, normal saline should be suctioned through the working channel to clean the FB. Otherwise, the working channel becomes chronically plugged with secretions, debris, or blood clots. Complications of bronchoscopy are rare and most commonly include bronchospasm, laryngospasm, and hoarseness. Major complications such as airway perforation, pneumothorax, and severe airway hemorrhage are extremely rare but should be ruled out in the appropriate clinical setting.

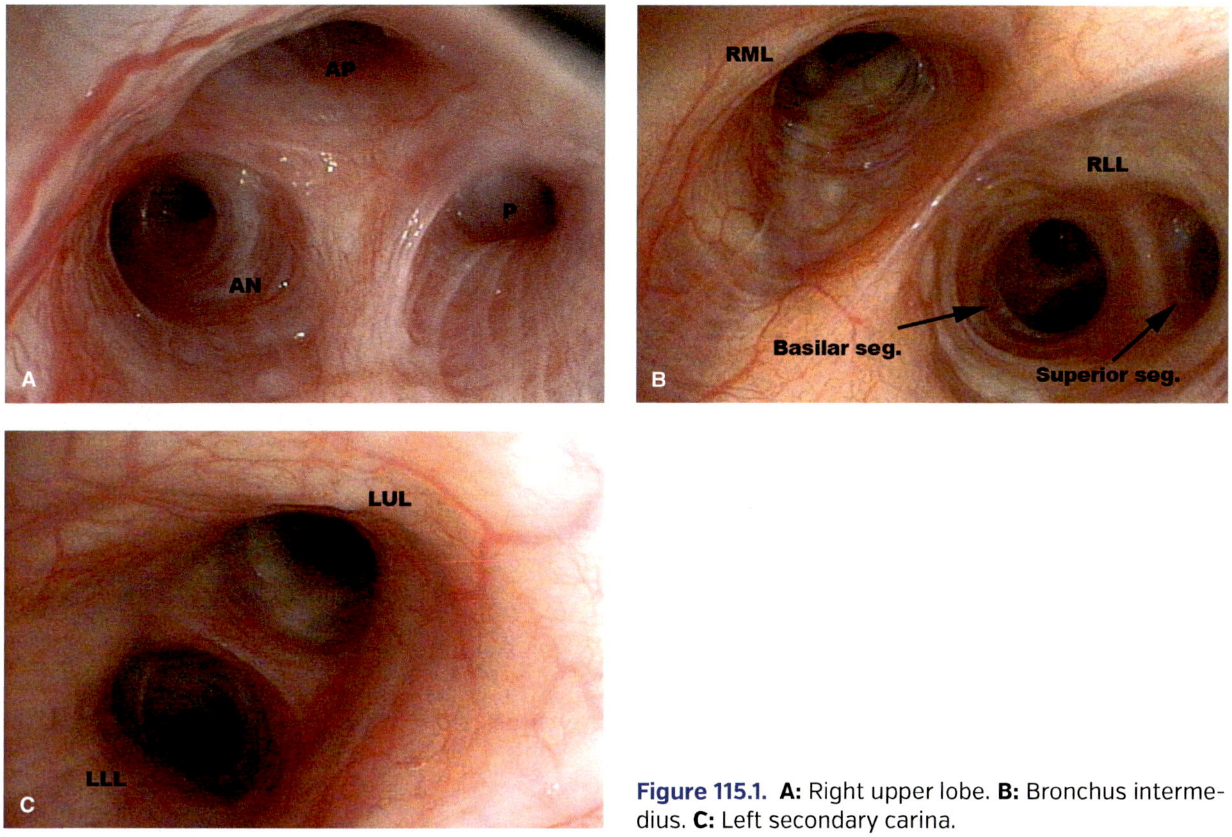

Figure 115.1. **A:** Right upper lobe. **B:** Bronchus intermedius. **C:** Left secondary carina.

2 Tricks for the Difficult Bronchoscopy

At times, bronchoscopy can be challenging because of secretions, blood, or aspirated material. In such instances it may be preferable to place a large single lumen tube and use a large bore FB to clear the airway prior to placing a lung isolation device. Blind suctioning with a soft ETT suction device can also aid in effective clearance of the airway prior to insertion of the FB. The FB should not be forced through strictures or used blindly, given the risk of airway and parenchymal injury.

During particularly challenging cases, short periods of apnea may be helpful to prevent secretions from moving in and out of view with ventilation. With particularly tenacious secretions or clots, it is preferable to suction until the FB becomes impacted (the working channel full), withdraw the FB while holding down continuously the flush button, and flush the working port outside the patient (thereby permanently cleaning the airway of that debris), rather than flushing into the airway. On extremely rare occasions, there is too much debris to suction, and the airway is not identifiable for intubation. In this case, the suction port can be hooked to oxygen rather than suction (anesthesia workstation's auxiliary oxygen outlet set to 2 to 3 L/min and connected to the FB's suction port). The gentle, intermittent (few second bursts) insufflation of oxygen pushes fluid and debris away just enough to visualize and confirm the endotracheal position. However, this maneuver can easily induce a pneumothorax. Therefore, it should only be performed in extreme circumstances.

- A thorough understanding of components of the FB and appreciation of tracheobronchial anatomy are of utmost importance for the thoracic anesthesiologist.
- Proper airway orientation during bronchoscopy consists of placing the cartilaginous rings toward the "12 o'clock" position, and the striae in the "6 o'clock" position.
- Identifying the primary carina and RUL bronchus confirms the right/left orientation.
- Large bore ETTs and bronchoscopes can aid in the control of copious and viscous airway secretions.
- *See Figure 115.2 and* ***Video 115.1*** *for additional details.*

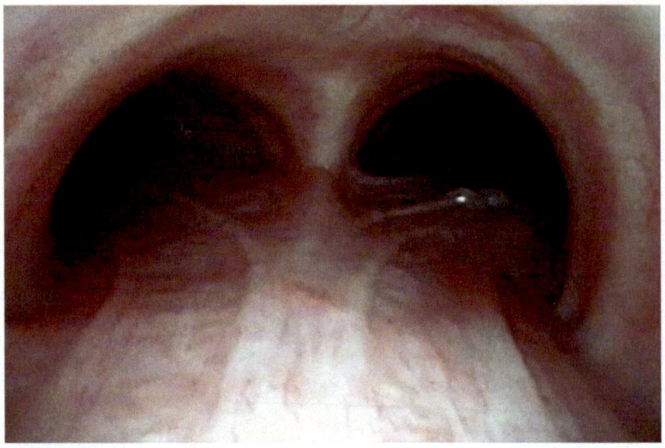

Figure 115.2. Normal tracheal carina.

Suggested Readings

Campos JH. Update on tracheobronchial anatomy and flexible fiberoptic bronchoscopy in thoracic anesthesia. *Curr Opin Anaesthesiol.* 2009;22(1):4–10.

Casal RF, Ost DE, Eapen GA. Flexible bronchoscopy. *Clin Chest Med.* 2013;34(3):341–352.

Du Rand IA, Blaikley J, Booton R, et al; British Thoracic Society Bronchoscopy Guideline Group. British Thoracic Society guideline for diagnostic flexible bronchoscopy in adults: accredited by NICE. *Thorax.* 2013;68(8):786–787.

Miller RJ, Casal RF, Lazarus DR, Ost DE, Eapen GA. Flexible bronchoscopy. *Clin Chest Med.* 2018;39(1):1–16.

Pelaia C, Bruni A, Garofalo E, et al. Oxygenation strategies during flexible bronchoscopy: a review of the literature. *Respir Res.* 2021;22(1):253.

Endobronchial Ultrasound Bronchoscopy

116

Basem B. Abdelmalak • Joseph Cicenia

Clinical Scenario: A 63-year-old man is presenting for bronchoscopy with endobronchial ultrasound (EBUS) and transbronchial biopsy of a left lower lobe mass. His pulmonary function tests are FEV_1 50% and DLCO 55%.

1 What are the anesthetic and airway management considerations for this case?

Preoperative assessment is conducted in the customary fashion with special attention dedicated to airway evaluation, symptoms of respiratory compromise (hoarseness, stridor, and/or dysphagia), and review of the pulmonologist's evaluation of the size and location of the mass.

Premedication with sedatives and anxiolytics should be considered carefully because of the limited respiratory reserve of this patient. At the authors' institution, general anesthesia is preferred over conscious sedation (for reasons discussed below). A total intravenous anesthetic (TIVA) technique, usually an infusion of propofol, is preferred over an inhalational anesthetic technique. TIVA ensures continuous delivery of the anesthetic and prevents pollution of the OR by inhalational anesthetics caused by circuit leaks. Furthermore, frequent suctioning by the proceduralist can remove inhalational agents from the airway. When propofol infusion is used, a concomitant narcotic infusion is usually not necessary as the procedure is not very painful. In addition, a narcotic infusion, such as remifentanil, may lead to hypotension and/or bradycardia, which would necessitate unnecessary and avoidable administration of fluids and/or vasopressors. However, more recent studies suggest that this procedure can be safely performed using moderate sedation without impacting the quality of procedural oncologic outcomes. Ultimately, the type of anesthesia administered should be dependent on the patient's comorbidities and the familiarity and comfort of both the proceduralist and the anesthesiologist with the chosen technique.

Muscle relaxants are used in these procedures to facilitate endotracheal tube (ETT) or supraglottic airway (SGA) insertion. Muscle relaxants also improve overall lung compliance by eliminating the chest wall component and thus making positive-pressure ventilation easier, and more effective. Moreover, they provide a motionless patient, which is advantageous for the proceduralist. It allows for precise node and/or lesion biopsy and therefore improves the diagnostic yield of the procedure. Unexpected patient movements, such as coughing if not paralyzed (which is very difficult to abolish with the application of local anesthetics alone), can have deleterious consequences.

When general anesthesia utilizing a TIVA technique is used, the authors recommend employing a hypnosis/depth of anesthesia monitor such as Bispectral Index (BIS) Monitor (Covidien, Boulder, CO) to prevent intraoperative awareness.

2 How would you manage the airway in this case?

The incidence of difficult airway in this patient population should be no different than in the general surgical population. Patients with known difficult airways, or with signs and symptoms suggestive of the same, should be managed accordingly. Patients with difficult airways and advanced pulmonary pathology with home oxygen dependency are unable to tolerate apnea even for a very brief period. Therefore, awake intubation with spontaneous ventilation and supplemental oxygen should be considered. Awake intubation should also be considered in patients who are scheduled for biopsy of a symptomatic large anterior mediastinal mass.

3 What are the surgical considerations that impact anesthetic management?

EBUS requires the use of a larger-diameter FB, and requires longer procedure times than traditional bronchoscopic examinations. For these reasons, these procedures may not be well tolerated by patients if performed under moderate sedation. Additionally, a high degree of precision is required when small nodes or lesions in proximity to the great vessels are targeted. Hence, general anesthesia with complete muscle relaxation is needed and preferred.

4 What are the potential hazards and complications in regard to the airway?

Postoperative hypercarbia and hypoxemia resolve in most instances spontaneously. At times, noninvasive ventilation with a mask delivering continuous positive airway pressure, or bilevel positive airway pressure is required. Also, postoperative cough is usually self-limited. Minor or major bleeding (depending on the source of bleeding, biopsy site, and type of biopsy performed) can occur. The development of a pneumothorax or pneumomediastinum may require placement of a thoracostomy tube. Respiratory failure, requiring intubation, is a possibility, in particular in patients with limited pulmonary reserve.

5 What distinct airway device (eg, specialized tracheal tube, rigid bronchoscope, BB) might be used in this case, and what are the special considerations?

Intubation with a large internal diameter ETT, at least a size 8.5-mm ID, facilitates ventilation around the relatively large-diameter FB. It can be cut short to facilitate the maneuverability of the EBUS FB and decrease the resistance to its insertion and removal through the ETT. That said, when a risk of major bleeding is considered, the tube is not shortened, as the full-length tube can be helpful to selectively intubate a main stem bronchus and achieve lung isolation.

In cases where the intended biopsy site is subglottic (paratracheal), an SGA (eg, laryngeal mask airway, I-gel) can be effective. The SGA allows bronchoscopic access to the high paratracheal nodes (required in staging procedures) and offers a means of ventilation. The SGA provides an alternative when a large-diameter ETT cannot be inserted (patients who are small or who have small tracheal diameters). However, the SGA does not guarantee reliable protection against aspiration. Use of a swivel connector/adaptor with either the ETT or SGA will allow uninterrupted ventilation during flexible bronchoscopy.

6 Are there special considerations for the emergence or the end of the case?

At the authors' institution, we use 100 mcg of fentanyl bolus with induction to minimize postoperative cough. Patients typically go home immediately following a short recovery (~45 minutes). This compares favorably with that of invasive thoracic surgery, which requires postoperative hospital and even ICU admission.

The key to favorable outcomes lies in deep understanding of the underlying lung pathology, open two-way communication between the anesthesiologist and pulmonologist, understanding the nature of the procedure, and above all, vigilance and preparedness.

- Advanced diagnostic bronchoscopy is evolving and widely spreading as it offers a minimally invasive alternative to some invasive thoracic procedures.
- Special attention should be given to airway evaluation and symptoms suggesting compromise: hoarseness, stridor, and/or dysphagia.
- General anesthesia with TIVA and muscle relaxation or moderate sedation are acceptable anesthetic choices.
- Considering their advantages and limitations, both ETT and SGA have been used successfully for these procedures, with authors' preference for ETT.
- *See Figure 116.1 and* ▶ ***Video 116.1*** *for additional details.*

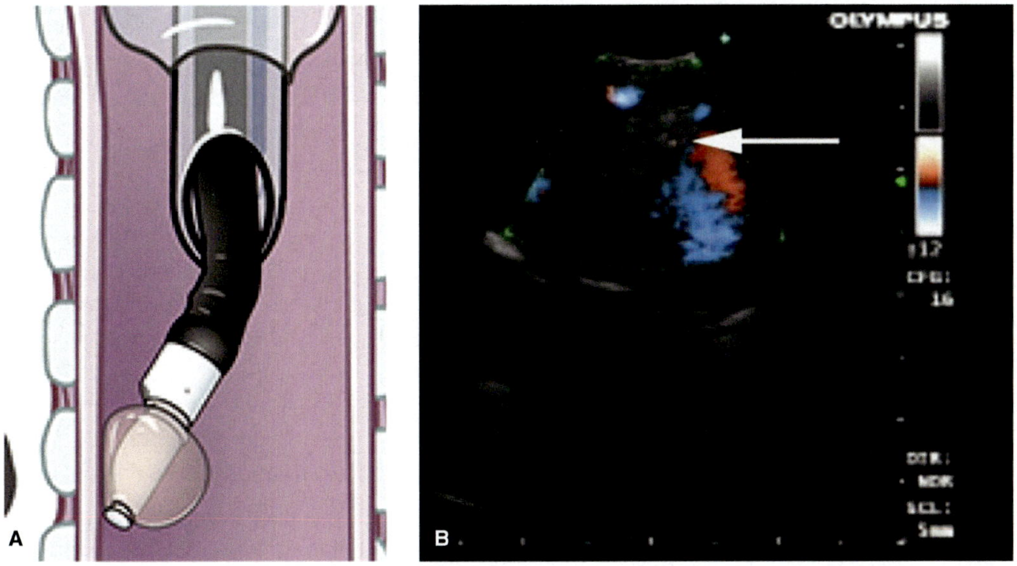

Figure 116.1. **A:** The endobronchial ultrasound probe is seen emerging from the ETT and budding the bronchial wall to allow for scanning and transbronchial biopsy. **B:** Endobronchial ultrasound. The *arrow* indicates a lymph node, and the *color map* identifies a blood vessel.

Suggested Readings

Abdelmalak BB, Gildea TR, Doyle DJ. Anesthesia for bronchoscopy. *Curr Pharm Des.* 2012;18(38):6314–6324.

Abdelmalak B, Sarkiss M. Anesthesia for diagnostic bronchoscopic procedures. In: Abdelmalak B, Doyle DJ, eds. *Anesthesia for Otolaryngologic Surgery*. Cambridge University Press; 2013:297–308.

Fernandes MGO, Santos VF, Martins N, et al. Endobronchial ultrasound under moderate sedation versus general anesthesia. *J Clin Med.* 2018;7(11):421.

117 Airway Management for Robotic Bronchoscopy

Or Kalchiem-Dekel • Alessia Pedoto

Clinical Scenario: A 56-year-old male underwent nondiagnostic electromagnetic navigation bronchoscopy for an incidental 1.3-cm left lower lobe lung nodule. He is now referred for a repeat biopsy via robotic-assisted bronchoscopy. He is a former 1-pack per day smoker. His pulmonary function tests show an FEV_1 of 66% of predicted and a DLCO of 52% of predicted.

1 What are the anesthetic/airway management considerations for this case?

Robotic-assisted bronchoscopy is an emerging platform for the sampling of parenchymal lung lesions. In contrast to percutaneous lung biopsy, robotic-assisted bronchoscopy allows sampling of multiple unilateral or bilateral lesions and, when clinically indicated, can be combined with mediastinal lymph node staging with linear endobronchial ultrasound (EBUS) bronchoscopy, while providing a superb safety profile in terms of pneumothorax and bleeding risks.

Robotic-assisted bronchoscopy is generally performed as an ambulatory outpatient procedure in a dedicated procedure suite by either an interventional pulmonologist or a thoracic surgeon. General anesthesia and endotracheal intubation are required for optimal procedure performance. Standard preoperative evaluation can usually be accomplished in the immediate preoperative period unless the patient is considered to be at an increased anesthesia risk and requires a formal consult. A thorough physical exam of the airway will allow planning for the intubation. In case of anticipated difficulty, such as Mallampati class 3 or higher or a history of neck surgery or radiation, a video laryngoscope in addition to the fiberoptic bronchoscope may be necessary to secure the airway in the sitting position.

2 How would you manage the airway in this case?

Robotic-assisted bronchoscopy is ideally performed under general anesthesia with neuromuscular blockade. A large endotracheal tube (8.5- to 9.0-mm inner diameter) is recommended to allow adequate ventilation, prevent atelectasis, and accommodate the EBUS bronchoscope if mediastinal staging is planned. A certain ventilatory protocol is required in order to minimize atelectasis in the lung periphery and "CT-to-body divergence" (Figure 117.1). By keeping the lungs expanded, the ventilation protocol aims at imitating the preoperative CT conditions. The ventilatory protocol consists of utilizing a tidal volume of 10 mL/kg ideal body weight, positive end expiratory pressure (PEEP) value of 10 cm H_2O or 15 cm H_2O if the lower lung lobes are evaluated, and a target FiO_2 of 30%, as tolerated by the patient.

Possible complications include hemodynamic instability, due to chest hyperinflation and decreased venous return, or pneumothorax in patients with emphysema or as a result of the sampling procedure. In high-risk patients, continuous invasive or noninvasive hemodynamic monitoring may be required. Pneumothorax should be anticipated by maintaining a high index of suspicion if intraoperative high peak inspiratory pressures or hypoxemia are encountered. Secretions may be significant in current smokers or in patients who recently quit, requiring frequent suctioning. This can interfere with the sampling by promoting lung atelectasis.

3 What are the surgical considerations that impact anesthetic management?

Robotic-assisted bronchoscopy is a recent addition to the armamentarium of endoscopic technologies used to localize, navigate into, sample, and potentially treat peripheral lung nodules. These tools are collectively termed *guided bronchoscopy*. Guided bronchoscopy techniques offer a higher diagnostic yield for peripheral lesions (50% to 80%) when compared with traditional bronchoscopy (20% to 50%), while maintaining an excellent safety profile; namely, 1% to 2% risk of pneumothorax. Image-guided percutaneous biopsy remains the primary alternative approach for the sampling of peripheral lung lesions; however, it is associated with 20% to 30% risk of pneumothorax and 8% need for chest tube placement.

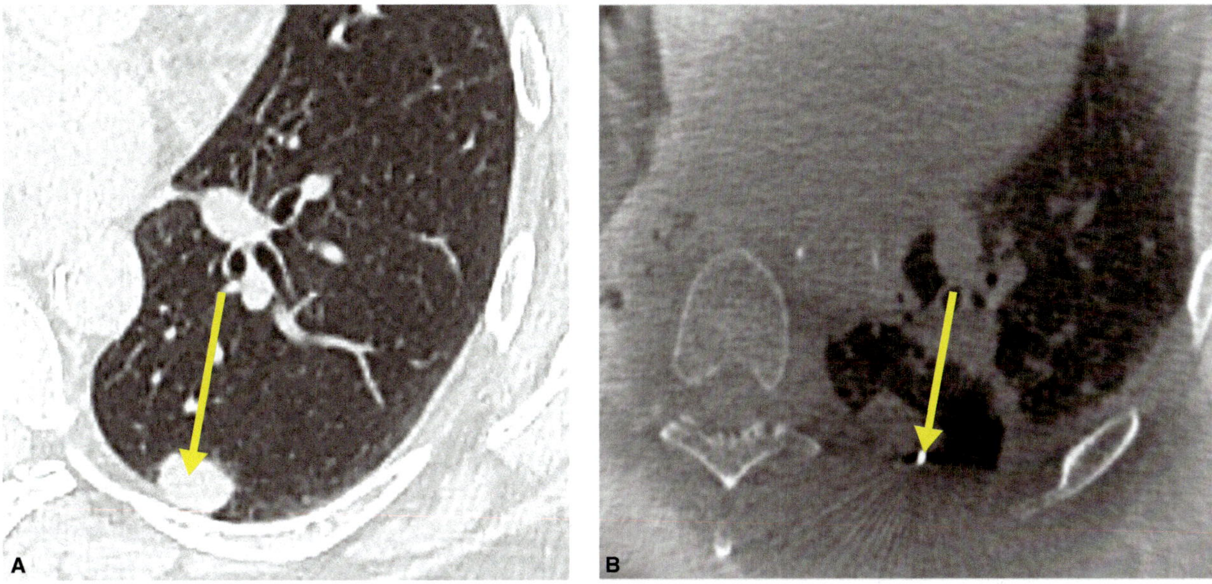

Figure 117.1. CT-to-body divergence. In **Panel A**, the lesion identified on the high-definition CT. **Panel B:** on the day of surgery, the lung is not as inflated, changing the position of the lesion. The *yellow arrow* identifies the path of the needle, based on the CT mapping.

Any guided bronchoscopy procedure, robotic-assisted bronchoscopy included, can be "deconstructed" into four stages:

1. *Planning:* A thin-slice CT is obtained prior to the procedure to identify the lesion and the bronchial tree anatomy. Three-dimensional reconstruction of the CT is performed using proprietary software to devise a "roadmap" to the target lesion.
2. *Registration and Navigation:* The real-time airway view is registered with the virtual roadmap for synchronization and the bronchoscope is navigated to the target based on the combined real time and virtual views. Successful navigation relies on airway anatomy (patent vs narrowed), target location (central vs peripheral), and the presence or absence of a leading airway ("bronchus sign"). CT-to-body divergence refers to dyssynchronization between the preoperative CT and actual navigational process.
3. *Intraoperative confirmation:* Intraoperative imaging is utilized to assess tool-to-lesion relationship. Frequently used imaging tools include radial-probe EBUS, 2D fluoroscopy, and stationary or mobile cone-beam CT, which often requires a breath hold maneuver for optimal imaging quality.
4. *Tissue acquisition:* Sampling is performed using a variety of tools. In some instances, a breath hold maneuver will be required for precise sampling. Across multiple studies, the lesion size emerged as the major determinant of a diagnostic sampling. The smaller the lesion, the more difficult to successfully sample it is.

Two robotic-assisted bronchoscopy platforms are currently available:

1. Monarch™ (Johnson & Johnson, New Burnswick, NJ)—this platform relies on electromagnetic technology for 3D localization of the bronchoscope and its tools in the thorax. The electromagnetic field is created by a generator and sensed via reference transducers placed on the patient, which allows to triangulate the lesion. The steerable bronchoscope is devised as a "mother–daughter" system with a 6-mm proximal "mother" bronchoscope that is wedged in a proximal airway while the 4.4-mm "daughter" bronchoscope is navigated into the lung periphery and the tools are deployed via a 2.1-mm working channel. Sampling is performed under direct vision. Metal bodies can interfere with the electromagnetic field and should be avoided. For example, electrocardiogram leads should be placed away from the field and metallic endotracheal tube holder should be avoided. Pacemakers or automated implantable cardioverter-defbrillator may also affect the integrity of the electromagnetic field.
2. Ion™ Endoluminal Platform (Intuitive Surgical, Sunnyvale, CA)—this platform utilizes shape-sensing technology to allow catheter localization within the 3D space of the thorax. A 3.5-mm catheter with a 2.0-mm working channel is navigated into the periphery while occupied by a vision probe. Once the target has been reached, the vision probe is removed, and the sampling is performed without direct visualization.

4 What are the potential hazards/complications in regard to the airway?

The most clinically significant complications include pneumothorax (1.5% to 3.8%) and serious bleeding (0.1% to 2.5%). Compared to image-guided percutaneous biopsy, the bronchoscopy-associated pneumothorax rate is significantly lower, while the bleeding rate is comparable. The ability to biopsy multiple sites, ipsilateral or bilateral, during the same session, the option of mediastinal staging, and the lower complication rate represent several advantages of robotic-assisted bronchoscopy over image-guided biopsies; however, its diagnostic yield remains inferior to image-guided biopsy.

5 Are there special considerations for the emergence or the end of the case?

At the end of the procedure, patients are usually taken to PACU for recovery. A chest radiograph is often obtained to exclude a pneumothorax. Subclinical pneumothoraxes, especially in asymptomatic patients, often do not require decompression. Patients can still be discharged after meeting criteria. Significant size or symptomatic pneumothorax may require drainage via needle aspiration, thoracic vent, or tube thoracostomy. Outpatient versus inpatient management following thoracic aspiration is dictated by patient- and facility-associated clinical and logistic considerations. Postbronchoscopy bronchospasm and/or cough are common and respond well to nebulized inhaled bronchodilators.

- Robotic-assisted bronchoscopy is an emerging modality for the diagnosis of peripheral lung lesions.
- Procedures are performed under general anesthesia with neuromuscular blockade.
- Relatively high tidal volumes and PEEP are required to attenuate lung atelectasis during the procedure.
- Pneumothorax is the most common significant complication; however, risk remains low compared with other lung biopsy modalities.
- *See Figure 117.2 and* ***Video 117.1*** *for additional details.*

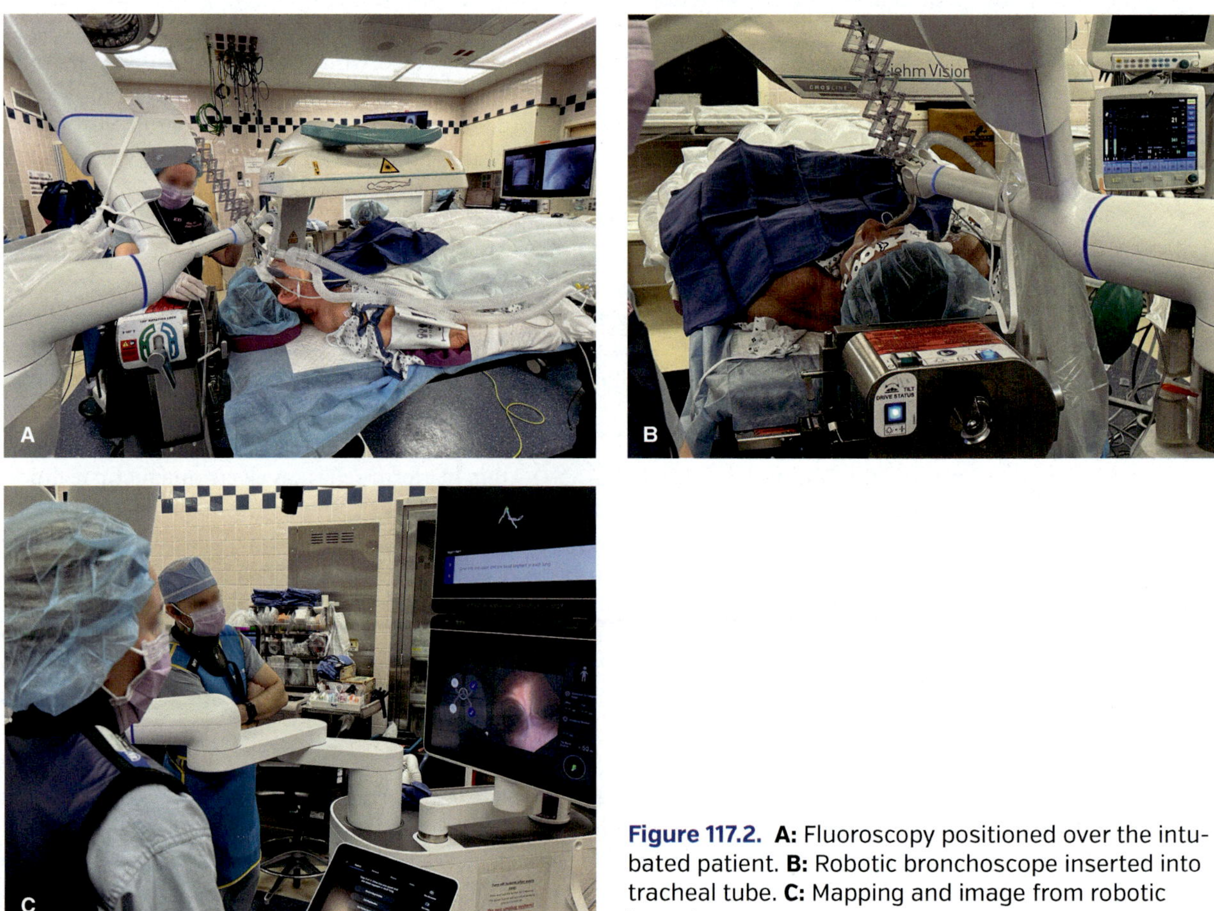

Figure 117.2. A: Fluoroscopy positioned over the intubated patient. **B:** Robotic bronchoscope inserted into tracheal tube. **C:** Mapping and image from robotic bronchoscope.

Suggested Readings

Bhadra K, Setser RM, Condra W, Pritchett MA. Lung navigation ventilation protocol to optimize biopsy of peripheral lung lesions. *J Bronchology Interv Pulmonol.* 2022;29(1):7–17.

DiBardino DM, Yarmus LB, Semaan RW. Transthoracic needle biopsy of the lung. *J Thorac Dis.* 2015;7(Suppl 4):S304–S316.

Folch E, Mittal A, Oberg C. Robotic bronchoscopy and future directions of interventional pulmonology. *Curr Opin Pulm Med.* 2022;28(1):37–44.

Kalchiem-Dekel O, Connolly JG, Lin IH, et al. Shape-sensing robotic-assisted bronchoscopy in the diagnosis of pulmonary parenchymal lesions. *Chest.* 2022;161(2):572–582.

Ost DE, Ernst A, Lei X, et al; AQuIRE Bronchoscopy Registry. Diagnostic yield and complications of bronchoscopy for peripheral lung lesions. Results of the AQuIRE Registry. *Am J Respir Crit Care Med.* 2016;193(1):68–77.

118 Airway Management for Bronchial Thermoplasty

John B. Pawlowski • Ruma Bose

Clinical Scenario: A 45-year-old woman with a 30-year history of asthma is scheduled for bronchial thermoplasty (BT). She has recently experienced an increase in the severity of her disease, requiring multiple hospitalizations and escalation of medical therapy.

1 What are the anesthetic and airway management considerations for this case?

BT represents the treatment for severe forms of asthma, resistant to maximal medical therapy. It consists of delivering radiofrequency energy to the bronchial mucosa, with the ultimate goal to decrease the amount of smooth muscle. The increased level of heat produced initially injures the epithelium, blood vessels, nerves, and smooth muscle. Although the other components of the bronchial wall have the capacity to regenerate, it has been demonstrated that smooth muscle is replaced by connective tissue.

The major consideration for patients scheduled for BT is that all have severe and refractory forms of asthma. All patients are treated with inhaled beta-2 agonists and corticosteroids, and many may also be taking long-acting beta agonists, leukotriene inhibitors, theophylline, and omalizumab. Often, these patients can benefit from nebulized beta agonists just before or immediately after the BT treatment. It is important to recognize that the BT treatment may produce significant inflammation of the airways, stimulate mucus production, and provoke airway irritability and coughing. Therefore, patients should be forewarned that they might feel worse before they feel better.

Contraindications to BT are represented by the presence of an implantable electronic device and severe comorbid conditions. An active respiratory infection and/or an asthma exacerbation are valid reasons to cancel the procedure.

2 How would you manage the airway in this case?

The airway should be managed as any flexible bronchoscopic procedure of considerable duration. These procedures usually last for 1 to 2 hours. General anesthesia with a laryngeal mask airway (LMA) is a commonly used technique. However, this procedure can also be performed under moderate to deep sedation. Spontaneous ventilation or pressure-support ventilation can be employed during the procedure. A total intravenous anesthetic (TIVA) with propofol (100 to 200 μg/kg/min) and remifentanil (0.1 μg/kg/min) is an example of common anesthetic combinations typically utilized. In order to minimize the risk of airway fire, during the times radiofrequency energy is employed, the Fio_2 should be reduced to below 30%.

3 What are the surgical considerations that impact anesthetic management?

The goal of BT is to reduce the mass of airway smooth muscle from lobar and segmental bronchi via thermal energy (65 °C). The process leads to the development of structural changes in the bronchial wall, with decreases in mucous gland hyperplasia and alterations in autonomic tone. BT is usually scheduled in three sessions, approximately 3 weeks apart. In order to prevent undertreating or overtreating the patient, the procedure is performed in a consistent sequence of airway intervention. In the first session, the right lower lobe segments are treated. The second session involves treatment of the left lower lobe. In the last session both upper lobes are treated. Inflammation and obliteration of the entrance into the right middle lobe can result in lobar collapse, a phenomenon known as the "right middle lobe syndrome."

The BT catheter device needs to be positioned with precision, to avoid both gaps and overlapping treatment. For this reason, deep sedation or general anesthesia is required. The distal airways are treated initially and the radiofrequency probe is gradually withdrawn into the more proximal airways. Lidocaine spray to the airway mucosa and glycopyrrolate administered intravenously (to decrease secretions) can facilitate proper location of the BT probe (**Video 118.1**).

4 Are there special considerations for the emergence at the end of the case?

Patients often feel short of breath and experience coughing episodes after the BT treatments. Albuterol and lidocaine nebulizers can help alleviate these symptoms. Short courses of parenteral corticosteroids are also indicated. Occasionally, collapse or mucus plugging of the treated lobe has been reported. This situation may require a repeat bronchoscopy.

- All patients scheduled for this procedure have severe asthma, refractory to medical management.
- BT is delivered in three sessions, each 3 weeks apart. A recent upper respiratory tract infection or an asthma exacerbation is a valid reason to postpone a session of BT.
- Usually, TIVA with an LMA is used to provide adequate conditions for BT treatment.
- The immediate postoperative period is difficult, due to reactive airways, bronchospasm, and bronchial secretions with possible mucus plugging.
- *See Figure 118.1 for additional details.*

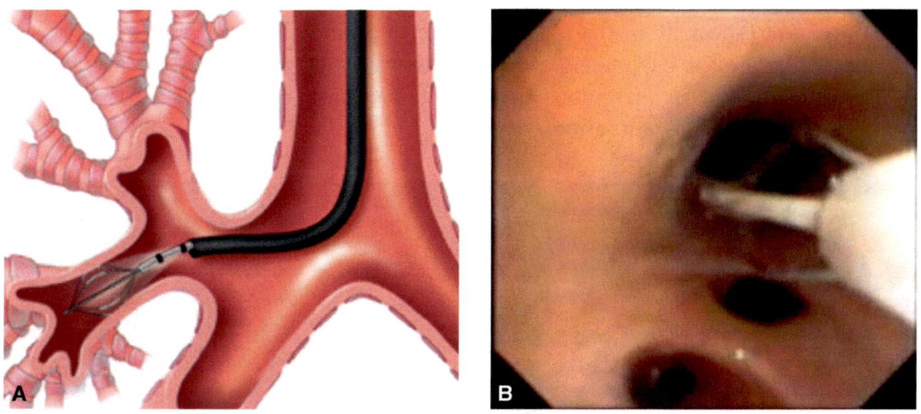

Figure 118.1. A: Illustration of the bronchial thermoplasty probe placed in right upper lobe. **B:** Bronchial thermoplasty probe placed in right lower lobe.

Suggested Readings

Castro M, Rubin AS, Laviolette M, et al. Effectiveness and safety of bronchial thermoplasty in the treatment of severe asthma: a multicenter, randomized, double-blind, sham-controlled clinical trial. *Am J Respir Crit Care Med.* 2010;181(2):116–124.

Pavord ID, Cox G, Thomson NC, et al; RISA Trial Study Group. Safety and efficacy of bronchial thermoplasty in symptomatic, severe asthma. *Am J Repir Crit Care Med.* 2007;176(12):1185–1191.

Wahidi MM, Kraft M. Bronchial thermoplasty for severe asthma. *Am J Respir Crit Care Med.* 2012;185(7):709–714.

119 Airway Management for Cryobiopsy

Bryan Husta • Alessia Pedoto

Clinical Scenario: A 75-year-old female is scheduled for a flexible bronchoscopy and a transbronchial cryobiopsy (TBCB) of a newly diagnosed lung mass. She had one episode of hemoptysis 1 week ago.

1 What are the anesthetic/airway management considerations for this case?

Cryobiopsy is an outpatient procedure, usually done under general anesthesia (GA) by the interventional pulmonologists to gather larger and more preserved samples of lung tissue for diagnostic and staging purposes (Figure 119.1). Either a flexible bronchoscope through an endotracheal tube (ETT) or a rigid bronchoscope can be used for the purpose. The anesthetic plan should be customized to each patient after a detailed discussion with the pulmonologist, especially in the presence of active hemoptysis. Depending on the patient's comorbidities (active hemoptysis, severe chronic obstructive pulmonary disease (COPD), coronary, and cerebrovascular disease) and the technique used (rigid vs flexible bronchoscopy), continuous hemodynamic monitoring, arterial blood gas analysis, and jet ventilation may be needed.

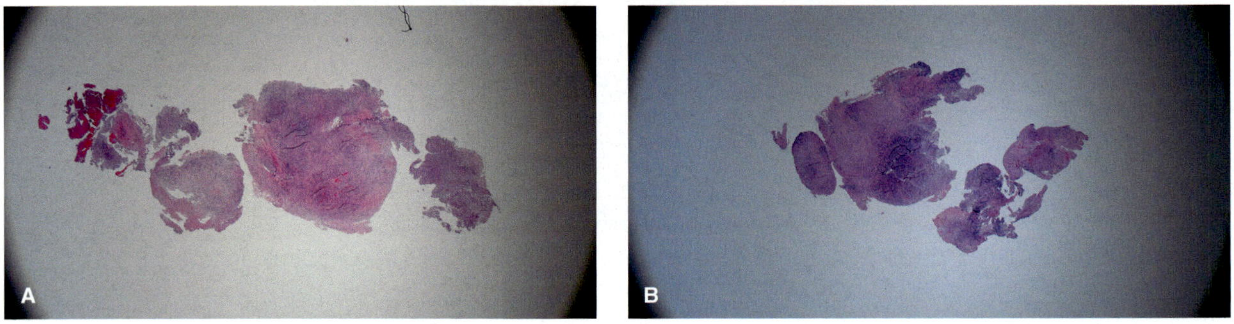

Figure 119.1. Sample size after cryobiopsy (**A**), after forceps (**B**).

In stable patients and for elective procedures, patients may be evaluated in the immediate preoperative period. A thorough history and physical exam may help risk stratify the patient and should suffice.

While anticoagulants and antiplatelets should be stopped in the preoperative period, low-dose acetylsalicylic acid can be continued. Renal function, coagulation, and platelets should be known on the day of the procedure. Pulmonary function tests (PFTs), if available, can help identifying the severity of lung disease, while echocardiography can assess the presence of pulmonary hypertension, two factors that can respectively increase the risk of pneumothorax (PNX) and bleeding. Pulmonary hypertension (PAP >50 mm Hg), coagulopathy (INR >1.5; partial thromboplastin time above range or platelets <100K), any contraindications to stop anticoagulation, severe cardiac disease or severe COPD (forced vital capacity <50%, diffusing capacity of the lungs for carbon monoxide <35%, oxygen saturation <90%) are relative contraindications to the procedure.

2 How would you manage the airway in this case?

Depending on the surgical approach, a supraglottic device, a large ETT, or a rigid bronchoscope will be used to secure the airway.

Flexible bronchoscopy is usually done after the induction of GA to assess the airway. The use of a supraglottic airway device allows the full exam of the trachea, from the vocal cords to the subsegmental bronchi. Muscle paralysis is recommended to prevent coughing or movements which would change the radiographic landmarks used to reach the affected tissue during the cryobiopsy.

If the procedure is done via **flexible bronchoscopy**, a large ETT (8.5 F) is recommended to accommodate the bronchoscope, the occlusion balloon device, and facilitate mechanical ventilation. Endotracheal intubation provides a secure airway in case of bleeding. Hypoxemia may occur when the occlusion balloon is inflated in the area of the biopsy. The procedure should be stopped in case of severe hypoxemia during mechanical ventilation, uncontrolled hemorrhage, new arrhythmias, or hemodynamic instability.

If the risk of airway bleeding is high, or in the presence of active hemoptysis, cryobiopsy is usually done via a combination of **rigid** and **flexible bronchoscopy**. Muscle paralysis will facilitate the placement of the rigid bronchoscope and the use of jet ventilation. Total intravenous anesthesia (TIVA) is recommended due to the leak of the system. The use of bispectral index monitoring (BIS) should be considered to titrate the anesthetic and prevent recall.

3 What are the surgical considerations that impact anesthetic management?

TBCB has been introduced as a promising alternative to surgical lung biopsy in the diagnostic approach of interstitial lung pathology, due to the ability to obtain a significantly larger sample size with reduced crush artifact when compared to the traditional transbronchial forceps biopsies (TBFB).

The tissue is acquired by using a metallic probe that is rapidly cooled to −79 °C via either liquid nitrous oxide or liquid carbon dioxide, causing adhesion of the tissue to the probe. Specimens are withdrawn with the bronchoscope and the cryoprobe *en boc*, thawed into normal saline and then transferred to formalin for processing.

These cases are usually performed as an outpatient procedure under GA. An endobronchial ultrasound (EBUS) probe placed in the affected area, either through a large ETT or a rigid bronchoscope can be used to identify significant blood vessels at the biopsy site. A rigid bronchoscope seems to offer additional advantages when attempting to decrease the rate of hemorrhage.

The affected area and the proper placement of the cryoprobe are localized via real-time x-ray and compared to the CT imaging. Major vasculature is identified via EBUS. The scout EBUS images are saved and displayed side by side to guide the biopsy. Prior to sampling, either a 6- or 8-F arterial balloon embolectomy catheter or a 9-F commercially available bronchial blocker is positioned proximal to the cryoprobe at the intended site of biopsy, with the goal of occluding small segmental portions of the distal airway. Radiographically opaque contrast may be employed for the balloon inflation to confirm via fluoroscopy the proper occlusion of the biopsied airway. Prior to taking the biopsy, the cryoprobe position is confirmed in real time as at 1 to 2 cm from the pleura to avoid PNX. Freezing periods should be short (5 to 7 seconds). Once the frozen probe is pulled, the balloon should be immediately inflated to tamponade any bleeding. The ability to safely use high FiO_2 concentrations during the procedure is particularly advantageous in patients with poor lung function.

4 What are the potential hazards/complications in regard to the airway?

The most common complications during cryobiopsy include airway bleeding (14.2%) and PNX (9.4%).

Bleeding

Bleeding is usually controlled by inflating the balloon of the occlusion catheter for 1 to 2 minutes. In the presence of heavy bleeding not resolving after balloon compression, 60 to 210 cc of cold saline (4 °C) or epinephrine 1:100,000 can be instilled in 2-mL aliquots up to a maximum dose of 0.6 mg. The use of intravenous tranexamic acid (TXA) prior to the start of cryobiopsy in patients at high risk for bleeding has been reported, however, this is not routine practice. If bleeding still persists, postoperative intubation, mechanical ventilation, and continued hemostasis via blocker may be necessary.

Pneumothorax

The risk of **PNX** is decreased by placing the probe at least 1 cm away from the pleura. Continuous x-ray imaging guides the probe placement for biopsy, ensuring adequate distance from the pleura. Patients with severe emphysema are at increased risk and may require chest tube placement in the postoperative period.

Hypoxemia and Infection

Hypoxemia (incidence <5%) and **infection** (incidence <2%) are relatively rare complications but can occur in the perioperative period.

5 What distinct airway device (eg, specialized tracheal tube, rigid bronchoscope, bronchial blocker) might be used in this case, and what are the special considerations?

Depending on the sampling technique, different airway devices may be needed.

Cryobiopsy Through a Flexible Bronchoscope

An 8.0 or an 8.5 ETT is needed to accommodate the flexible bronchoscope and a bronchial blocker, often placed outside the ETT to increase the working space and facilitate mechanical ventilation. The blocker is placed through the vocal cords prior to intubation and secured in position by the cuff of the ETT. Univent™ (Teleflex) tubes are commercially available single-lumen tubes with a small separate lumen accommodating a hollow nonlatex blocker that extends 8 to 10 cm beyond the tip. The tube stiffness, the large outer diameter paired with a relatively small inner one, should be considered as potential causes of airway trauma and make the Univent™ tube a less desirable choice for airway management in these cases. In addition, mechanical ventilation may be difficult if a therapeutic bronchoscope is deployed within the lumen of the tube, therefore, Univent™ tubes are not routinely used.

Cryobiopsy Through a Rigid Bronchoscope

Cryobiopsy through a rigid bronchoscope is done in patients at high risk for bleeding, such as the ones on anticoagulants, with uremia, or thrombocytopenia. Jet ventilation is commonly used for rigid bronchoscopy, although standard mechanical ventilation may also be employed. The occlusion catheter is placed at the sample site via flexible bronchoscopy and its position confirmed via fluoroscopy.

Independently from the technique used, a thorough discussion should occur between the anesthesia and the interventional pulmonology team prior to the start of the procedure to formulate the best plan for the patient. Patients need to be fully paralyzed to prevent coughing and motion during the procedure, which would change the location of the specimen on the radiographic images. TIVA should be considered for any case where an air leak is expected. BIS should be used to monitor the depth of the anesthetic and prevent recall.

6 Are there special considerations for the emergence or the end of the case?

1. **Hypoxemia** or **bronchospasm** are relatively common short-term complications after bronchoscopy. The use of nebulizers and brief sessions of incentive spirometry while in post-anesthesia care unit (PACU) usually resolve the symptoms.
2. **Airway bleeding**: If severe and not responding to occlusion balloon treatment, it may require postoperative mechanical ventilation, and balloon compression with an endobronchial blocker. Paralysis may be needed to avoid coughing and dislodging the clot. Intravenous TXA has been used in high-risk patients prior to the start of the procedure with good results. The use of inhaled TXA has been described to treat massive hemoptysis. However, its routine use is not common clinical practice.
3. **PNX** should be excluded in PACU by chest x-ray. If subclinical, patients may still be discharged home after proper monitoring and meeting criteria. Oxygen via nasal cannula can expedite the reabsorption of the pneumothorax by displacing nitrogen in the pleural cavity (Graham's law). Chest tube placement and patient admission may be necessary if the size is significant, or in the presence of respiratory symptoms. Pneumostats™ valves have been used as ambulatory devices to allow patient discharge. A follow-up appointment is needed for their removal.

- Cryobiopsy is a promising diagnostic technique for interstitial lung disease.
- Bleeding is the most common complication, requiring the use of a bronchial blocker to tamponade the area after the sample is taken.
- This procedure is usually performed under GA and muscle paralysis to facilitate sampling conditions.
- Sampling can be taken via flexible or rigid bronchoscopy.
- *See Figure 119.2,* **Video 119.1**, *and* **Video 119.2** *for additional details.*

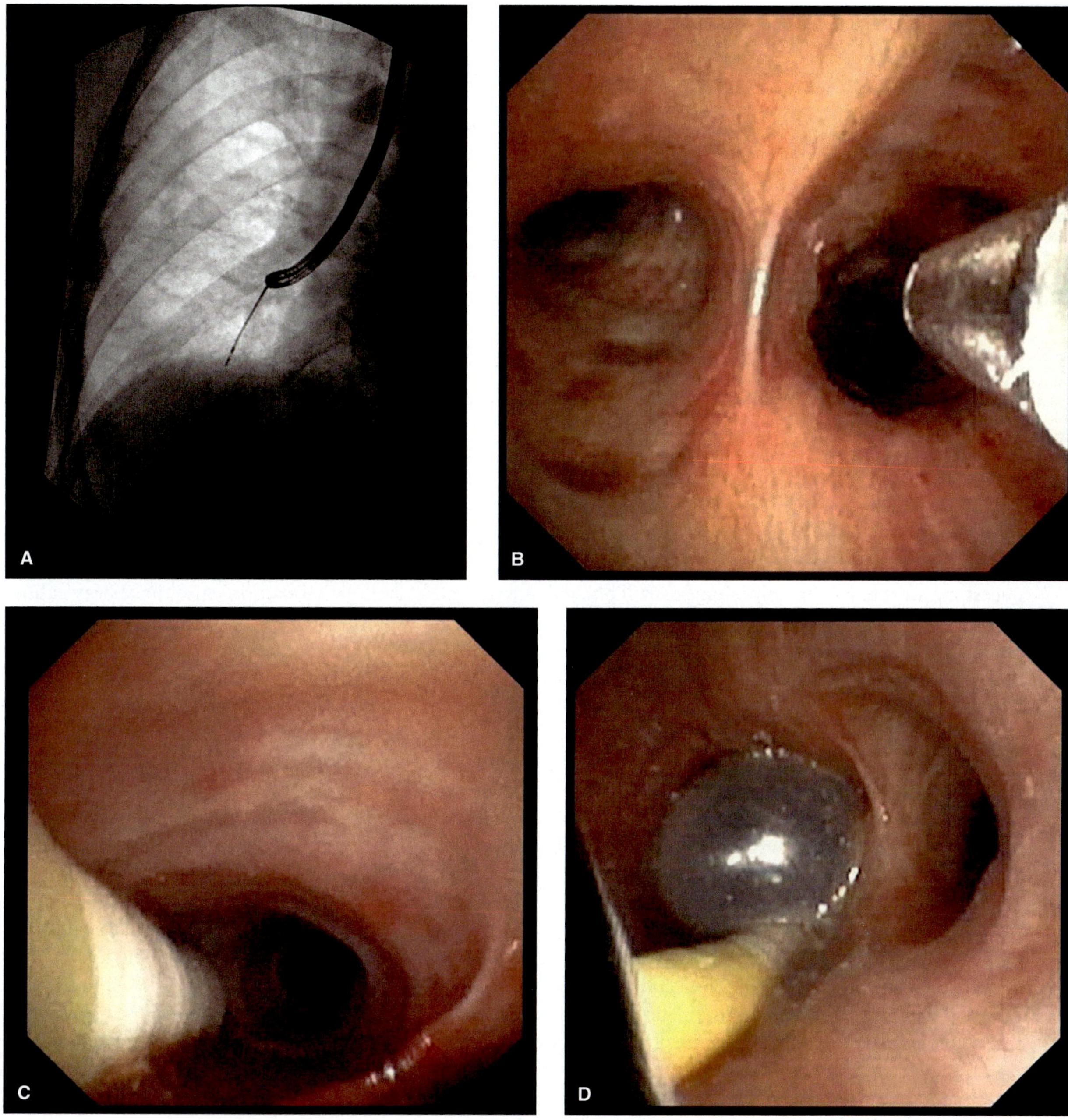

Figure 119.2. Fluoroscopic (**A**) and bronchoscopic image of the cryoprobe (**B**) at the sample area. The Fogarty catheter is placed inside the ETT (**C**) and inflated (**D**) after the specimen is taken.

Suggested Readings

Dhillon SS, Harryanto H, Randhawa S, Rosell A, Salamonsen M. Transbronchial lung cryobiopsy: a meticulous technique. *J Bronchol Intervent Pulmonol.* 2020;27(2):e19.

DiBardino DM, Haas AR, Lanfranco AR, Litzky LA, Sterman D, Bessich JL. High complication rate after introduction of transbronchial cryobiopsy into clinical practice at an academic medical center. *Ann Am Thorac Soc.* 2017;14(6):851–857.

Hetzel J, Maldonado F, Ravaglia C, et al. Transbronchial cryobiopsies for the diagnosis of diffuse parenchymal lung diseases: expert statement from the Cryobiopsy Working Group on safety and utility and a call for standardization of the procedure. *Respiration.* 2018;95(3):188–200.

Lentz RJ, Argento AC, Colby TV, Rickman OB, Maldonado F. Transbronchial cryobiopsy for diffuse parenchymal lung disease: a state-of-the-art review of procedural techniques, current evidence, and future challenges. *J Thorac Dis.* 2017;9(7):2186–2203.

Sethi J, Ali MS, Mohananey D, Nanchal R, Maldonado F, Musani A. Are transbronchial cryobiopsies ready for prime time?: a systematic review and meta-analysis. *J Bronchology Interv Pulmonol.* 2019;26:22–32.

120 Airway Management for Nonsurgical Endobronchial Tumor Resection

Alessia Pedoto

Clinical Scenario: A 72-year-old male with a large left main stem endobronchial tumor with postobstructive pneumonia and recent hemoptysis is presenting to the OR for endobronchial tumor resection.

1 What are the anesthetic/airway management considerations for this case?

Malignant airway obstruction can be characterized by the extent of the tumor burden and its relationship to the central airways. Tumors can present extrinsic to the airway, potentially leading to collapse from external forces, or as intrinsic to the airway and lead to obstruction by pure endoluminal obstruction. The vast majority of tumors are mixed obstructions with components of both intrinsic and extrinsic airway compromise. The relationship of the tumor to the airway can be preoperatively evaluated through the use of computed tomography or intraoperatively using endobronchial ultrasound. This relationship will determine the modalities used by the bronchoscopist to relieve the obstruction. Generally, obstruction of at least 50% of the airway is necessary for it to be clinically significant. This said, anything that can further compromise the airway caliber, such as bleeding, mucous plug, or airway debris, can convert a noncritical airway obstruction to a medical emergency. As such, hemostasis in the airway is essential throughout the case. This often necessitates the use of thermal modalities prior to debridement in order to devascularize the tumor. With respect to the extent of the tumor, it is often classified by the reduction in caliber of the residual airway compared to that above and beyond the obstruction. The final consideration prior to embarking on a debulking procedure is the ability to establish flow to functional lung distal to the obstruction. Hypoxic vasoconstriction may occur in cases of prolonged obstruction leading to decreased blood flow. Alternatively, large tumors may at once obstruct the airway and compress the vasculature resulting in minimal blood flow to the lung beyond the obstruction. This is quite important as reestablishing patency to a hypoperfused lung may result in worsening of ventilation–perfusion matching in turn exacerbating the hypoxia.

Endobronchial tumor destruction may be accomplished using several modalities. Thermal modalities include argon plasma coagulation, electrosurgery, Nd:YAG laser photo resection, photodynamic therapy, brachytherapy, or cryotherapy. Mechanical destruction can be accomplished by "coring out" the tumor from the airway using the bevel of the rigid endoscope. In the setting of hemoptysis and postobstructive pneumonia, the modality used will depend on the urgency of procedure, the severity of the bleeding, and the characteristics of the tumor. Modalities such as photodynamic therapy, brachytherapy, and cryotherapy have a delayed effect and generally require a second procedure in 24 to 48 hours to debride the airway of necrotic tissue. These procedures should be used with caution in patients with a critical airway, as tissue sloughing can result in an airway emergency.

2 How would you manage the airway in this case?

The goals of airway management in this patient are to minimize the risk of exacerbating the airway obstruction, to avoid hypoxemia/hypoventilation, and to minimize the exposure of the team to volatile anesthetics throughout the use of the high-frequency jet ventilator during rigid bronchoscopy.

In general, airway management is performed by the bronchoscopist. After hyperoxygenation and induction with total intravenous anesthesia and paralytics, the rigid bronchoscope is advanced into the trachea. Inhalants may be used prior to intubation with the rigid bronchoscope and continued throughout the case if using a closed system. Many rigid bronchoscopists prefer to use an open system and jet ventilation due to large system leaks, particularly when instrumenting the airway. During the use of thermal modalities it is essential to reduce the FiO_2 to a maximum of 40% to avoid an airway fire. This requires close communication between the bronchoscopist and the anesthesiologist to ensure appropriate time to exhaust higher levels of oxygen from the system. During debridement, it is often necessary to hold ventilation briefly during evacuation of tumor from the airway to minimize the risk of propelling debris distally. Devitalization of tumor tissue is very important to minimize the risk of bleeding during the procedure. In the advent of bleeding, it is essential to perform intermittent pulmonary toilet to evacuate blood and clot from the patent airways to maximize oxygenation and ventilation. In addition, should the bleeding become severe, the bronchoscopist may consider performing single lung ventilation by advancing the rigid bronchoscope into the nonbleeding mainstem bronchus. This will allow for pulmonary toilet as well as clot formation/tamponade of the bleeding airway.

Should the patient desaturate at any point during the case, bag-assisted ventilation may be performed while holding the jet ventilation. Also, a side port to allow for supplement O_2 entrainment may be attached to the rigid bronchoscope. Pending reversal of anesthesia, one may consider bag-mask ventilation, placing a laryngeal mask airway, or alternatively bronchoscopic intubation with an endotracheal tube. The endotracheal tube should be positioned proximal to a stent if placed during the procedure to minimize the risk of accidental displacement of the stent during extubation.

3 What are the potential hazards/complications in regard to the airway?

The major risks in the setting of malignant airway obstruction complicated by postobstructive pneumonia and bleeding include: (1) bleeding, (2) distal occlusion of airway by tumor debris, (3) airway fire, (4) gas embolism, (5) pneumothorax, and (6) airway perforation. The use of thermal modalities in bronchoscopy has greatly improved the survival of patients with airway obstruction. The complication rate associated with airway fires has been reported to be approximately 3 per 1000 cases. It is absolutely essential that the intraoperative FiO_2 be maintained at 40% or less to avoid this potentially devastating emergency. In addition, mitigating the risk of any bleeding by performing regular pulmonary toilet, considering single-lung ventilation as described above, and giving the patient breaks periodically to perform bag ventilation via the rigid bronchoscope is crucial. In situations where the tumor is highly vascularized, it is important to consider the risk of gas embolism. There has been concern regarding the development of gas emboli when argon plasma coagulation is employed for hemostasis. It is most likely that this occurs when the probe is in contact with the lesion rather at a safe distance from the lesion as described in the directions for use. The final consideration is the potential of airway occlusion by debris showered distally by ventilation. In almost all cases, ventilation may be safely held for a brief time to evacuate tumor from the airway.

As these procedures should ideally be performed with a rigid bronchoscope with jet ventilation, total intravenous anesthesia should be used to avoid any exposure of the team to volatile anesthetics. The other potential complications include airway perforation by the bevel of the rigid bronchoscope or a stent (if used), airway bleeding, and pneumothorax. Friability of tissues is increased in the setting of both tumor and infection. As such, it is essential that the rigid bronchoscope remain in line with the airway at all times due to the potential for the bevel to perforate the airway at the site of the tumor. Appropriate stent sizing based on inspiratory CT images is essential to minimize the risk of airway perforation due to the stent's excessive radial force. Finally, there does exist a risk of barotrauma with jet ventilation in particular if the exhalation is blocked.

4 Are there special considerations for the emergence or the end of the case?

Disruption of stents by endotracheal tubes and other devices postoperatively if placed during the procedure, can create life-threatening obstruction of the central airways. The use of endotracheal tubes and laryngeal masks following extubation with the rigid bronchoscope should be assessed on a case-by-case basis with the operating bronchoscopist. The other consideration is coughing, particularly if a stent was placed. It is very important to perform pulmonary toilet and suppress cough to reduce risk of stent displacement and further bleeding.

- The goal of airway management in this patient is to minimize the risk of exacerbating the airway obstruction, avoid hypoxemia/hypoventilation, and to minimize the exposure of the team to volatile anesthetics.
- The major risks in the setting of malignant airway include: (1) bleeding, (2) distal occlusion of airway by tumor debris, (3) airway fire, (4) gas embolism, (5) pneumothorax, and (6) airway perforation.
- The risk of airway perforation may be mitigated by ensuring the rigid bronchoscope is always in line with the airway and by avoiding excessive radial force, particularly in areas with extensive necrotic tumor.
- Postoperative forceful coughing should be avoided as it can disrupt hemostasis achieved during the procedure and displace a stent.
- *See Figures 120.1 and 120.2 for additional details.*

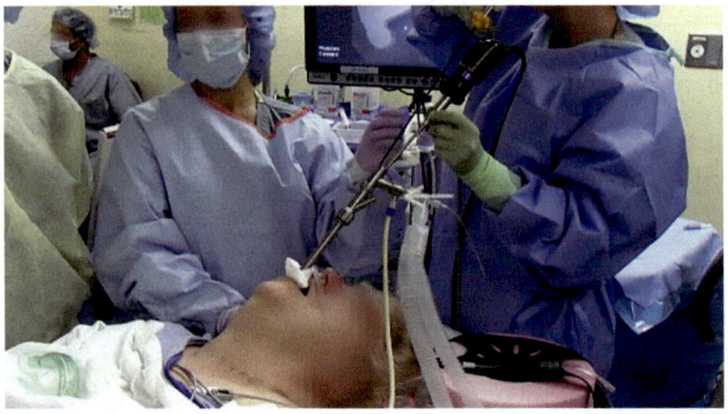

Figure 120.1. An instrument and camera used through a rigid bronchoscope during jet ventilation. See **Video 120.1** for additional details.

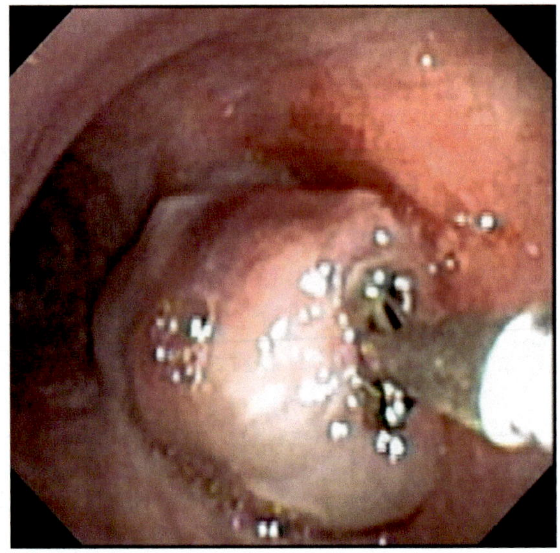

Figure 120.2. Endobronchial tumor retrieved with a grasper via rigid bronchoscopy. See **Video 120.2** for additional details.

Suggested Readings

Cavaliere S, Dumon JF. Laser bronchoscopy. In: Bolliger CT, Mathur PN, eds. *Interventional Bronchoscopy*. Karger; 2000:108–119.

Corey R, Hia KM. Major and massive hemoptysis: Reassessment of conservative management. *Am J Med Sci*. 1987;294(5):301–309.

Perrin G, Colt HG, Martin C, Mak M, Dumon JF, Gouin F. Safety of interventional rigid bronchoscopy using intravenous anesthesia and spontaneous assisted ventilation. *Chest*. 1992;102(5):1526–1530.

Pue CA, Pacht ER. Complications of fiberoptic bronchoscopy at a university hospital. *Chest*. 1995;107:430–432.

Studer W, Bolliger CT, Biro P. Anesthesia for interventional bronchoscopy. In: Bolliger CT, Mathur PN, eds. *Interventional Bronchoscopy*. Vol 30. Karger; 2000:44–54.

Thompson A, Fleischmann KE, Smilowitz NR, et al. 2024 AHA/ACC/ACS/ASNC/HRS/SCA/SCCT/SCMR/SVM guideline for perioperative cardiovascular management for noncardiac surgery: A report of the American College of Cardiology/American Heart Association Joint Committee on clinical practice guidelines. *Circulation*. 2024;150:e351–e442.

Interventional Management of Tracheal Stenosis

121

Gaetane C. Michaud

Clinical Scenario: A 68-year-old male with known tracheal stenosis presents to the OR for a rigid and flexible bronchoscopic evaluation and placement of a tracheal stent. His symptoms of severe stridor, hoarseness, and shortness of breath have been getting worse in the past months.

1 What are the anesthetic/airway management considerations for this case?

Tracheal stenosis can be a debilitating condition that more commonly results from trauma, tracheostomy, and prolonged intubation with an endotracheal tube. Symptomatic patients typically present with two primary types of stenosis that include web stenosis and complex stenosis. Web stenoses are typically circumferential subglottic membranes obstructing the airway that do not involve the tracheal cartilage rings. Complex stenoses can have a web component but are often fibrotic in nature and can involve the cartilage. Flexible bronchoscopy can be utilized to diagnose and characterize lesions, but is rarely used alone to treat stenoses that require intervention beyond balloon dilation. Rigid bronchoscopy is more often utilized for minimally invasive management of complex tracheal stenosis in that laser photo or electrocautery resection, dilation, and silicone stent placement can be accomplished in the same setting under airway control. Thermal resection using an Nd:YAG laser or electrocautery and serial dilation may be performed by the methods described by Metha and Tremblay. Radial incisions are made in the membranous portions of the stenosis at 3 and 9 o'clock, followed by serial dilations with rigid bronchoscopes of increasing size or a Controlled Radial Expansion (CRE) balloon. Following submaximal dilation, a silicone tracheal stent is placed through the rigid bronchoscope to maintain patency of the lumen.

2 How would you manage the airway in this case?

The goal of airway management in this patient is to minimize the risk of thermal injury to the airway, avoid hypoxemia, and to minimize the exposure of the team to volatile anesthetics throughout the use of the high-frequency jet ventilator during the rigid bronchoscopy. In general, airway management is performed by the bronchoscopist. After preoxygenation and induction with total intravenous anesthesia and paralytics, the rigid bronchoscope is advanced through the vocal cords and positioned just above the stenosis. The flexible bronchoscope is typically passed through rigid bronchoscope and beyond the stenosis to evaluate the distal airways and determine the length and complexity of the stenosis. Depending on the caliber of the airway at the level of the stenosis, it is often advisable to use a pediatric flexible bronchoscope to minimize impact on ventilation. Inhalants may be used prior to intubation with the rigid scope and continued throughout the case if using a closed system. Many rigid bronchoscopists prefer to use an open system and jet ventilation due to large system leaks, particularly when instrumenting the airway. If thermal modalities are employed to incise the membranous portion, an FiO_2 limit of 40% is recommended during the use of the laser/electrocautery to avoid an airway fire. During balloon dilation and/or insertion of a stent to maximally dilate the airway, ventilation may be interrupted briefly due to airway occlusion by the device. Should the patient desaturate at any point during the case, bag-assisted ventilation may be performed while holding the jet ventilation. Also, a side port to allow for supplement O_2 entrainment may be attached to the rigid bronchoscope. Pending reversal of anesthesia, one may consider bag-mask ventilation, laryngeal mask, or alternatively bronchoscopic intubation with an endotracheal tube. The endotracheal tube should be positioned proximal to the stent to minimize the risk of accidental displacement of the stent during extubation (**Video 121.1**).

3 What are the potential hazards/complications in regard to the airway?

Total intravenous anesthesia should be used during jet ventilation to avoid any exposure of the team to volatile anesthetics. The other potential complications include airway perforation by the bevel of the rigid bronchoscope or the stent, airway bleeding, and pneumothorax. It is essential that the rigid bronchoscope remain in line with the airway at all times due to the potential for the bevel to perforate the airway, particularly the posterior membrane. It is also important to avoid overdilation of the stenotic airway with either the balloon or rigid bronchoscope due to the risk of airway perforation due to excessive radial force. Appropriate stent sizing following dilation is essential to minimize risk of airway perforation due to the stent's excessive radial force. Finally, there does exist a risk of barotrauma with jet ventilation in particular if the exhalation is blocked.

The use of thermal modalities such as Nd:YAG lasers or electrocautery are valuable tools in mucosal sparing photoresection of the membranous components of complex stenosis. The complication rate associated with airway fires has been reported to be approximately 3 per 1000 cases. It is absolutely essential that the intraoperative FiO_2 be maintained at 40% or less to avoid this potentially devastating emergency. In addition, it is important to minimize the depth of incision to avoid injury to the airway cartilage.

4 Are there special considerations for the emergence or the end of the case?

The utility of stents in the airways is based on their positioning. Disruption of stents by endotracheal tubes and other devices postoperatively can reduce the efficacy of a procedure and create life-threatening obstructions of the central airways. The use of endotracheal tubes and laryngeal masks following extubation with the rigid bronchoscope should be assessed on a case-by-case basis with the operating bronchoscopist.

- Tracheal stenosis can be a debilitating condition that commonly results from trauma, tracheostomy, and prolonged intubation with an endotracheal tube.
- Rigid bronchoscopic techniques for tracheal stenosis, whereby airway management is performed by the bronchoscopist, may include laser resection or electrosurgery, dilation, and stent placement.
- Airway fires are a major emergency to avoid during laser bronchoscopy and it is essential that the intraoperative FiO_2 be maintained at 40%.
- Disruption of stents by endotracheal tubes and other devices postoperatively can create life-threatening obstructions of the central airways, and extubation should be assessed on a case-by-case basis.
- *See Figure 121.1 for additional details.*

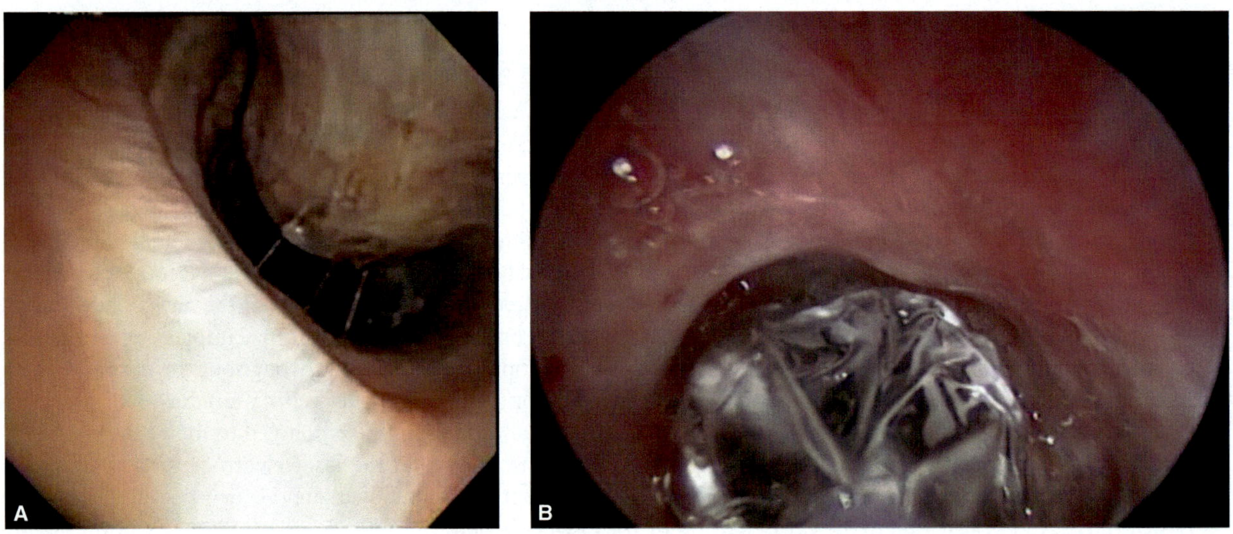

Figure 121.1. **A:** Stenotic lesion of the trachea. **B:** Tracheal lesion undergoing balloon dilation.

Suggested Readings

Brichet A, Verkindre C, Dupont J, et al. Multidisciplinary approach to management of postintubation tracheal stenosis. *Eur Respir J.* 1999;13(4):888–893.

Cavaliere S, Dumon JF. Laser bronchoscopy. In: Bolliger CT, Mathur PN, eds. *Interventional Bronchoscopy.* Karger; 2000:108–119.

Dumon JF. A dedicated tracheobronchial stent. *Chest.* 1990;97:328–332.

Mehta AC, Lee FY, Cordasco EM, Kirby T, Eliachar I, De Boer G. Concentric tracheal and subglottic stenosis. Management using the Nd:YAG laser for mucosal sparing followed by gentle dilation. *Chest.* 1993;104:673–677.

Perrin G, Colt HG, Martin C, Mak M, Dumon JF, Gouin F. Safety of interventional rigid bronchoscopy using intravenous anesthesia and spontaneous assisted ventilation. *Chest.* 1992;102(5):1526–1530.

Pue CA, Pacht ER. Complications of fiberoptic bronchoscopy at a university hospital. *Chest.* 1995;107:430–432.

Studer W, Bolliger CT, Biro P. Anesthesia for interventional bronchoscopy. In: Bolliger CT, PN M, eds. *Interventional Bronchoscopy.* Vol 30. Karger; 2000:43–54.

Interventional Management of Tracheomalacia

122

Gaetane C. Michaud

Clinical Scenario: A 62-year-old male with severe tracheomalacia presents to the OR for bronchoscopic evaluation and stent placement. He has a chronic, productive, "seal-barking" cough, severe shortness of breath with minimal exertion and limited exercise capacity.

1 What are the anesthetic/airway management considerations for this case?

Tracheomalacia (or tracheobronchomalacia) is a condition characterized as a weakness in the intrinsic structural integrity of the central airways. Oftentimes this "weakness" is attributed to a reduction or atrophy of the longitudinal elastic fibers of the pars membranacea or more general impairment of the integrity of the cartilage supporting the airway. The net result is excessive dynamic airway collapse upon expiration. Work by Boiselle defined collapse of greater than 70% to be clinically significant. Multiple comorbidities have been associated with tracheobronchomalacia (TBM) including chronic obstructive pulmonary disease (COPD) and gastroesophageal reflux disease. Morbid obesity has been shown to be synergistic with COPD leading to very severe malacia. This leads to a wide degree of patient presentations that include dyspnea, productive cough, recurrent infections, and respiratory failure. In general, TBM is considered a clinical diagnosis based on CT evidence of significant collapse that is then confirmed by flexible bronchoscopy. Respiratory maneuvers are performed both during imaging as well as bronchoscopy to simulate increased respiratory effort. It is essential to minimize sedation as opioids and benzodiazepines can negatively impact airway tone, exaggerating the dynamic collapse.

To determine the functional extent of a patient's disease and evaluate if airway stabilization results in improvement of respiratory symptoms, a stent can be temporarily implanted in the patient's airways. Patients demonstrating significant clinical improvement during their stent trial may be considered candidates for surgical airway stabilization, tracheoplasty. If the disease extends into the subsegmental airways, then central airway stabilization via stenting is unlikely to be beneficial.

2 How would you manage the airway in this case?

The goal of airway management in this patient is to minimize the intraoperative functional airway collapse, to decrease cough during the procedure, and to minimize the exposure of the team to volatile anesthetics throughout the use of the high-frequency jet ventilator during the rigid bronchoscopy. In general, airway management is performed by the bronchoscopist. After hyperoxygenation and induction with total intravenous anesthesia and paralytics, the rigid bronchoscope is advanced into the trachea. Inhalants may be used prior to intubation with the rigid bronchoscope and continued throughout the case if using a closed system. Many rigid bronchoscopists prefer to use an open system and jet ventilation due to large system leaks, particularly when instrumenting the airway. As no thermal modalities are employed during this procedure, there are no FiO_2 limitations or concerns for airway fire. During stent insertion, ventilation is interrupted briefly as the stent occludes the rigid bronchoscope and consequently the airway. Should the patient desaturate at any point during the case, bag-assisted ventilation may be performed while holding the jet ventilation. Also, a side port to allow for supplemental O_2 entrainment may be attached to the rigid bronchoscope. After rigid bronchoscope removal while emerging, in order to efficiently ventilate the patient, one may consider bag-mask ventilation, placing a laryngeal mask airway, or alternatively bronchoscopically intubating with an endotracheal tube. The endotracheal tube should be positioned proximal to the stent to minimize the risk of accidental stent displacement during extubation.

3 What are the potential hazards/complications in regard to the airway?

Total intravenous anesthesia should be used during jet ventilation to avoid any exposure of the team to volatile anesthetics. In a review by Ali and Austin, the safe use of topical, inhaled, and general anesthetics in the setting of tracheobronchomalacia is described. Of note, it has also been reported that anesthesia can exacerbate underlying tracheomalacia and result in progressive hypercapnic respiratory failure.

The other potential complications include airway perforation by the bevel of the rigid bronchoscope or the stent, airway bleeding, and pneumothorax. It is essential that the rigid bronchoscope remain in line with the airway at all times due to the potential for the bevel to perforate the airway, particularly the posterior membrane. Appropriate stent sizing based on inspiratory CT images is essential to minimize risk of airway perforation due to the stent's excessive radial force. Finally, there does exist a risk of barotrauma during jet ventilation, in particular if the exhalation is blocked.

4 Are there special considerations for the emergence or the end of the case?

The utility of airway stents is based on their positioning. Disruption of stents by endotracheal tubes and other devices postoperatively can reduce the efficacy of a procedure as well as create life-threatening obstructions of the central airways. Therefore, the use of endotracheal tubes and laryngeal mask airways following rigid bronchoscope removal should be assessed on a case-by-case basis and discussed with the proceduralist.

- TBM is a condition characterized by weakness of the intrinsic structural integrity of the central airways.
- The goal of airway management is to minimize intraoperative dynamic airway collapse.
- Total intravenous anesthesia should be used during jet ventilation to avoid any exposure of the team to volatile anesthetics.
- Disruption of stents by endotracheal tubes and other devices postoperatively can create life-threatening obstructions of the central airways.
- *See Figures 122.1 and 122.2 for additional details.*

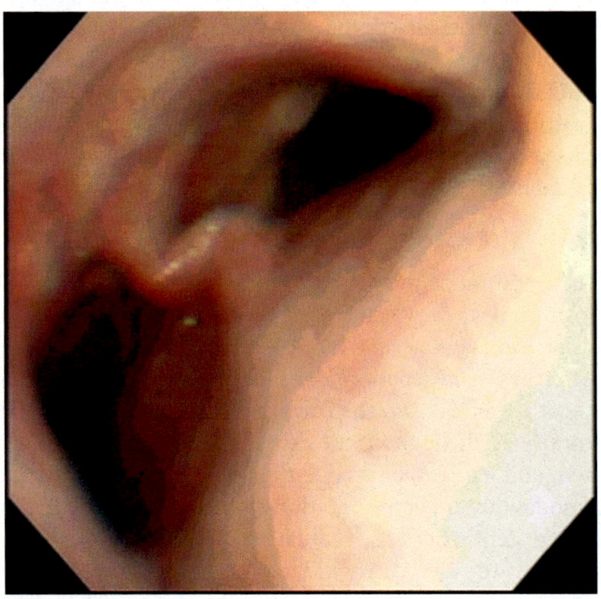

Figure 122.1. View of carina in a patient with airway collapse due to tracheobronchomalacia. See **Video 122.1.**

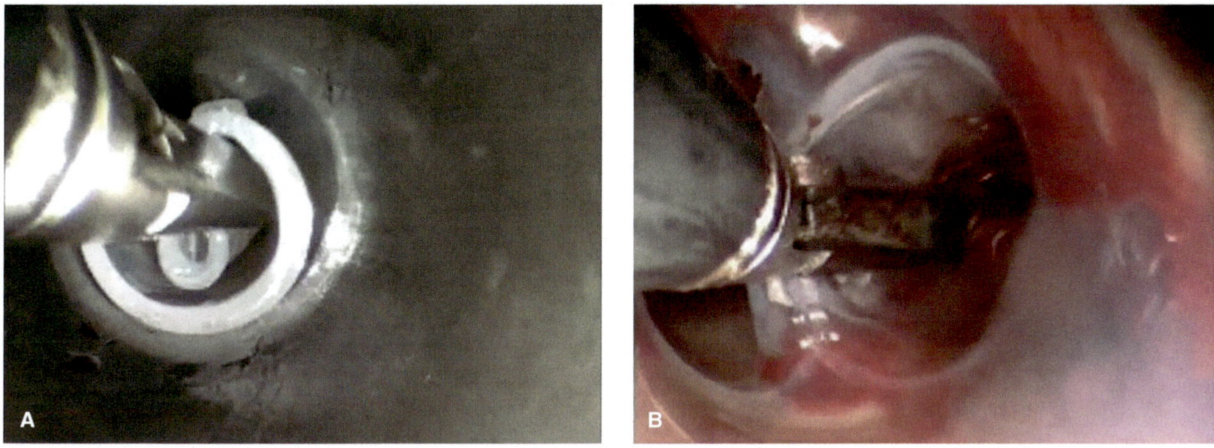

Figure 122.2. **A:** Limbs of the stent are crimped and loaded into the rigid bronchoscope. **B:** Bibronchocarinal stent is deployed at the carina.

Suggested Readings

Austin J, Ali T. Tracheomalacia and bronchomalacia in children: pathophysiology, assessment, treatment, and aesthesia management. *Paediatr Anaesth.* 2003;13:3–11.

Carden KA, Boiselle PM, Waltz DA, Ernst A. Tracheomalacia and tracheobronchomalacia in children and adults: an in-depth review. *Chest.* 2005;127(3):984–1005.

Collard P, Freitag L, Reynaert MS, Rodenstein DO, Francis C. Respiratory failure due to tracheobronchomalacia. *Thorax.* 1996; 51:224–226.

Katoh H, Saitoh S, Takiguchi M, Yamasaki Y, Yamamoto M. A case of tracheomalacia during isoflurane anesthesia. *Anesth Analg.* 1995;80:1051–1053.

Perrin G, Colt HG, Martin C, Mak M, Dumon JF, Gouin F. Safety of interventional rigid bronchoscopy using intravenous anesthesia and spontaneous assisted ventilation. *Chest.* 1992;102(5):1526–1530.

123 Bilateral Lung Lavage

Kyle Bramley

Clinical Scenario: A 30-year-old man with pulmonary alveolar proteinosis (PAP) presents for bilateral whole-lung lavage (WLL). He is otherwise healthy.

1 What are the anesthetic and airway management considerations for this case?

PAP is a rare lung disease characterized by the accumulation of surfactant-like material in the alveoli with ensuing restrictive pulmonary function and impaired diffusion capacity. It is most commonly autoimmune, but can be related to infections, heavy metal exposure, or hematologic malignancies.

WLL is the mainstay treatment for PAP. This is a procedure in which the lung is lavaged with large amounts of normal saline (NS). The therapeutic effect of this procedure is the result of the mechanical emptying of alveoli and improvement in oxygenation and ventilation. Most patients have a dramatic clinical improvement after a lavage, though some patients will need repeat procedures.

WLL is a complex procedure that involves a multidisciplinary team. It is performed under general anesthesia and requires lung isolation with a double lumen tube (DLT).

WLL is sometimes performed unilaterally, with staged procedures several weeks apart, or can be performed bilaterally during the same anesthetic.

2 How would you manage the airway in this case?

Following preoxygenation and anesthesia induction, a left-sided DLT is inserted and the appropriate position is verified using the standard technique. After placing the patient in semilateral decubitus, with the lung to be lavaged up, the DLT's position is rechecked. The adequacy of the seal is verified using the air-bubble test. This is performed while ventilating one lumen and maintaining the clamp on the other lumen, and immersing both lumens in water. An airway pressure of 40 cm H_2O is applied to the ventilated lumen. The absence of air bubbles arising from the nonventilated lumen confirms an adequate seal.

The lumen of the lung to be lavaged is maintained clamped, and enough time is allowed to promote complete lung collapse. Instillation of warmed NS boluses (0.5 to 1 L) via a closed circuit is started. Currently, no standardized closed systems are available on the market. The majority of these circuits are constructed at the time of the procedure using bifurcated tubing and collection devices (Figure 123.1). After passive recovery of the opaque fluid through a closed drainage system, the next washing cycle begins.

Gravity is used to facilitate inflow of NS by suspending the prewarmed saline bags approximately 50 cm above the carina. A rapid infusion device can be used for the same purpose, with particular attention being paid to the instillation pressure. High pressures may cause barotrauma.

In order to facilitate fluid drainage, mechanical percussion is performed. This can be performed by a team member with manual chest percussion or a pneumatic oscillation vest clearance system. Alternating between various positional maneuvers (Trendelenburg and reverse Trendelenburg) can facilitate fluid inflow and outflow.

During this time, ventilator parameters (airway pressures and tidal volume) are closely monitored to assess for potential leakage of fluid from the nonventilated lung into the ventilated lung. If available, continuous (breath-by-breath) compliance monitoring can be used to detect leakage.

Close inspection of the ventilated lumen of the DLT is performed throughout the procedure to rule out the presence of fluid: unintended inflow of NS into the ventilated lung during instillation or leakage of drained milky fluid from the nonventilated lung into the ventilated lung. Meticulous charting of the instilled NS amount versus the output is extremely important.

The procedure is repeated until the recovered fluid is clear. This may take several hours and as much as 20 L of NS per lung.

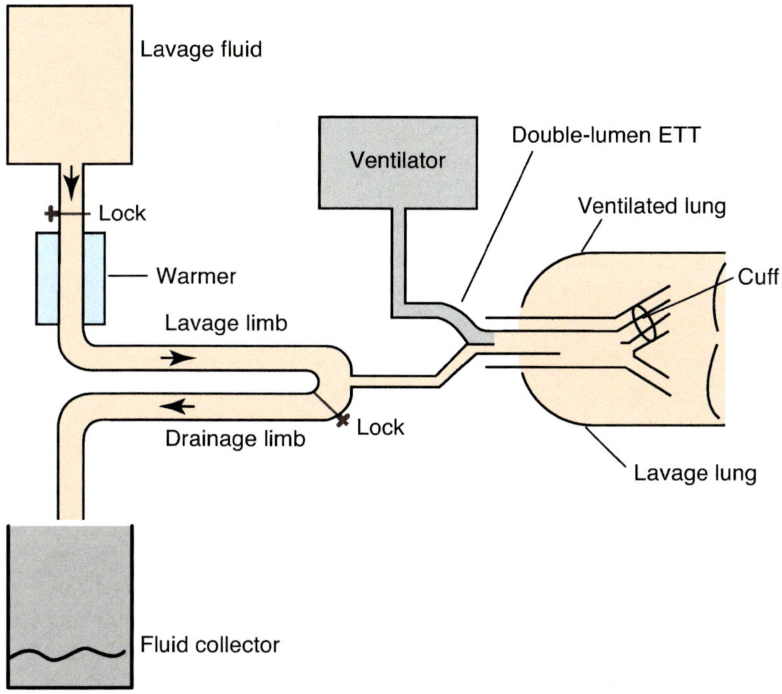

Figure 123.1. WLL equipment and setup. The WLL circuit is as follows: the lavage fluid is hung in multiliter bags from an IV pole and run through a warmer. A lock is located between the lavage fluid and warmer to control the volumes and timing of the lavage fluid being instilled. One Lung is ventilated while the other is being lavaged. The lavage and drainage limbs are in continuity with the lavage lung only. There is a lock in the drainage limb to control the timing of drainage into the fluid collector. (Modified from Michaud G, Reddy C, Ernst A. Whole-lung lavage for pulmonary alveolar proteinosis. *Chest*. 2009;136(6):1678–1681. Copyright © 2009 The American College of Chest Physicians. With permission.)

At the completion of one-lung lavage, thorough suctioning of both lungs is performed, two-lung ventilation is resumed, and recruitment maneuvers are employed to restore lung expansion. If BLL is desired, the patient is repositioned on the other side and the same protocol is performed for the contralateral lung. At the end of the BLL, two-lung ventilation is resumed until extubation criteria are met (**Video 123.1**).

3 What are the potential hazards and complications in regard to airway management?

WLL is performed in patients with marginal respiratory reserve. Worsening of the preexisting depressed lung function and development of hypoxemic respiratory failure is a constant threat during the procedure.

Following induction of general anesthesia, the time to safely secure the airway is very short. Thorough preoxygenation is of paramount importance.

WLL requires lung isolation. Therefore, during the procedure, oxygenation relies on only one lung, the gas exchange of which is already impaired by the intra-alveolar material. Bronchial blockers are not an option for lung isolation. Their very small lumen does not allow fluid inflow into the isolated lung. DLTs are the only realistic option for lung isolation, the left DLT being more commonly employed than the right. The shape and the overall design of the right DLT preclude a watertight seal and increase the chances for leakage. Another reason for avoiding the use of a right DLT is the possibility for right upper lobe bronchus blockage by the tube or bronchial cuff. As a result, the entire right upper lobe would not be lavaged or ventilated.

In patients with severely impaired lung reserve, single-lung ventilation may not be tolerated and cases of WLL with extracorporeal membrane oxygenation support have been performed.

As previously noted, another complication of the WLL procedure is leakage of fluid into the contralateral, ventilated lung. This is secondary to DLT dislodgement in the setting of vigorous chest percussions and multiple positional changes. Treatment includes rapid endobronchial suctioning and repositioning of the DLT. Temporary ventilation of the lavaged lung may be necessary if there is severe hypoxemia.

4 Are there special considerations for the emergence at the end of the case?

Thorough suctioning via the FB is performed at the end of the procedure. If extubation criteria are not met, the DLT is changed to a single-lumen endotracheal tube. Use of positive end expiratory pressure is indicated to promote reexpansion of the lavaged lungs. Extubation to continuous positive airway pressure may improve oxygenation after the procedure.

Depending on the severity of illness and the procedure, patients can be discharged home, admitted for observation, or admitted to the ICU for management of respiratory failure.

- WLL is a complex procedure that involves a multidisciplinary team.
- WLL requires single-lung ventilation.
- Worsening of the preexisting depressed lung function and development of hypoxemic respiratory failure is a constant concerns during the procedure.
- *See Figure 123.2 for additional details.*

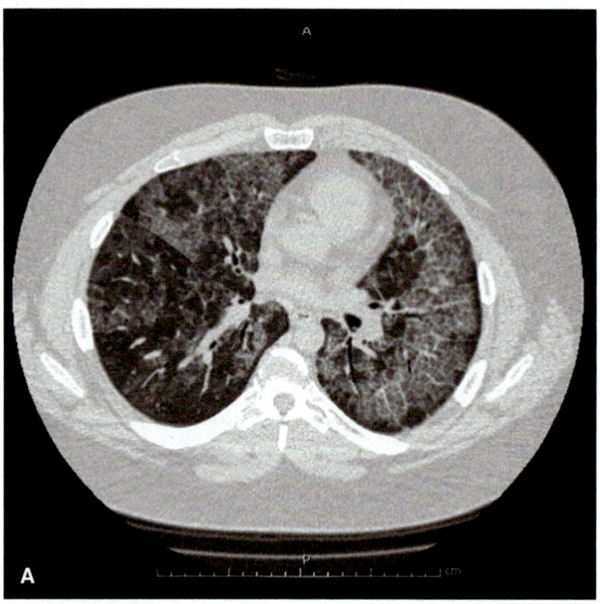

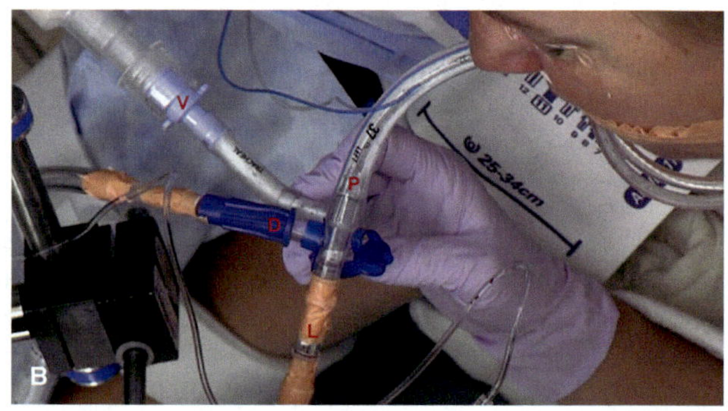

Figure 123.2. **A:** Computed tomography scan showing the "crazy paving" pattern commonly seen in PAP. Characterized by interlobular and intralobular septal thickening with ground glass. **B:** Patient (P), ventilator (V), lavage (L), and drainage (D) circuit limbs joined at the tracheal tube connector.

Suggested Readings

Ben-Abraham R, Greenfeld A, Rozenman J, Ben-Dov I. Pulmonary alveolar proteinosis: step-by-step perioperative care of whole lung lavage procedure. *Heart Lung.* 2002;31(1):43–49.

Doerschuk C. Pulmonary alveolar proteinosis–is host defense awry? *N Engl J Med.* 2007;356(6):547–549.

Gay P, Wallaert B, Nowak S, et al; Froudarakis ME; Groupe d'Endoscopie Thoracique de Langue Française. Efficacy of whole-lung lavage in pulmonary alveolar proteinosis: a multicenter international study of GELF. *Respiration.* 2017;93(3):198–206.

Michaud G, Chakravarthy R, Ernst A. Whole-lung lavage for pulmonary alveolar proteinosis. *Chest.* 2009;136:1678–1681.

Webb ST, Evans AJR, Varley AJ, Klein AA. Anaesthesia for serial whole-lung lavage in a patient with severe pulmonary alveolar proteinosis: a case report. *J Med Case Rep.* 2008;2:360.

Medical Thoracoscopy for Pleural Biopsy

124

Viji Kurup • Alessia Pedoto

Clinical Scenario: A 67-year-old woman with a large right pleural effusion and a pleural plaque presents for a thoracoscopic pleural fluid drainage and pleural biopsy. Currently she is significantly dyspneic. Her medical history is significant for severe chronic obstructive lung disease. Her pulmonary function tests (PFTs) are FEV_1 42% and diffusing capacity of the lungs for carbon monoxide 40%.

1 What are the anesthetic and airway management considerations for this case?

Pleural effusions can be secondary to congestive heart failure, pneumonia, malignancy (commonly lung cancer, breast cancer, and lymphoma), and pulmonary embolism. Patients can be either asymptomatic, or present with dyspnea, chest pain, or cough, like with large pleural effusions. Diagnosis can be made by physical exam, identifying decreased or absent breath sounds, and confirmed either by an abnormal chest x-ray or CT scan, demonstrating blunting of the lateral costophrenic angle for small effusions or complete opacification of one hemithorax for large ones, or via ultrasound exam.

Treatment of the underlying pathology is key. Surgical candidates are usually patients with recurrent effusions. Thoracocentesis, chest tube placement, decortication, or pleurodesis (fusion of the visceral and parietal pleura to prevent recurrence of symptomatic effusions) are among the different surgical options.

Most of the anesthetic considerations for these cases are related to the underlying disease. In the presence of significant respiratory compromise secondary to large pleural effusions, a decision should be made whether the effusion needs to be tapped under local anesthesia to improve symptoms and decrease the anesthetic risks.

2 How would you manage the airway in this case?

Depending on the operator (surgeon vs interventional pulmonologist) and the patient's comorbidities, medical pleuroscopy can be done either with local, regional, or sedation or general anesthesia. Local anesthesia can be used for thoracentesis in patients who are severely symptomatic. In urgent situations, this can be done at the bedside or prior to the start of the anesthetic. A semisitting position with the head elevated at 30 degrees will improve ventilation by optimizing pulmonary mechanics. Regional anesthesia with sedation or general anesthesia with or without lung isolation are other available options.

Regional anesthesia with IV sedation is a very successful alternative to general anesthesia, especially in patients at high risk. Patients can position themselves in the lateral decubitus prior to starting sedation either with propofol or dexmedetomidine infusion. After the US exam of the chest, the entry port for the thoracoscope is marked (Figure 124.1), identifying the proper dermatome for the peripheral nerve or paravertebral block, which are usually done via US guidance. Erector spinae, midpoint transverse process to pleura nerve block or serratus plane block can be performed with good dermatomal coverage. A single injection of a large volume of local anesthetic has been demonstrated to spread three levels above and below the injection site (Figure 124.2). Paravertebral blocks or thoracic epidural catheters are alternative options.

General anesthesia with a supraglottic device is an alternative in patients who are not at high risk for aspiration and do not require lung isolation, or as a rescue for failed blocks.

3 What are the surgical considerations that impact anesthetic management?

Medical thoracoscopy or pleuroscopy refers to thoracoscopic procedures aimed at examining the pleural cavity, either to drain fluid or to perform a biopsy or pleurodesis. Parapneumonic effusions, empyemas, and malignant effusions are the usual indications for this procedure. "Organization" of the pleural infection can result in the formation of an inelastic, fibrous pleural peel which impairs lung reexpansion. To complicate matters further, there can be loculations within the effusion, which make it resistant to drainage with a single chest tube. Intrapleural fibrinolytics, medical thoracoscopy, video-assisted thoracoscopic surgery (VATS) or, in resistant cases, open surgical decortication are potential surgical options.

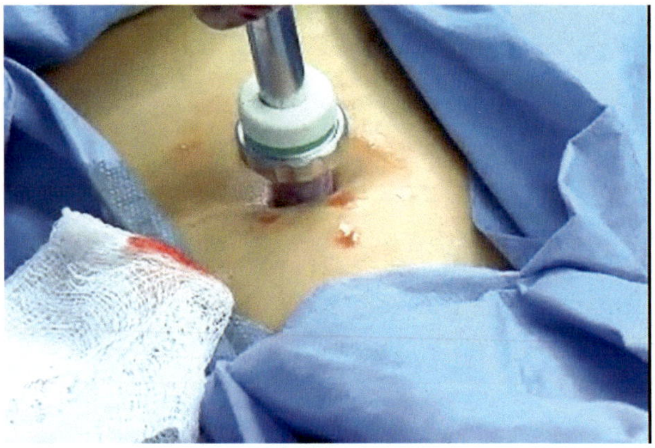

Figure 124.1. Thoracic port has been placed.

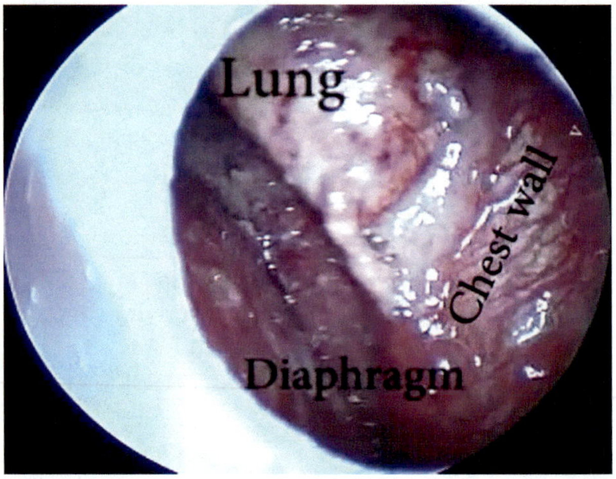

Figure 124.2. Thoracoscopic view of collapsed lung, chest wall, and diaphragm.

When performing a medical thoracoscopy, the trocar entry site in the chest is best chosen by ultrasonographic identification of the largest fluid collection. Usually, upon entry, the fluid is aspirated, and the thoracic cavity is explored for the presence of loculations or, in this case, biopsy of the pleural plaque. Subsequently, a chest drain is placed under visual guidance.

4 What distinct airway device (eg, specialized tracheal tube, rigid bronchoscope, and BB) might be used in this case, and what are the special considerations?

The specific airway device needed depends on the condition of the patient and the actual planned procedure. Thoracoscopy can be done under local, regional, or general anesthesia. When performed under local or regional anesthesia, consideration should be given to patient positioning (symptomatic patients benefit from 30-degree head-up tilt) as well as to oxygen supplementation (nasal cannula or face mask). If lung isolation is not needed, a supraglottic airway device can be safely used. When lung isolation is required, as for VATS lung decortication, a double lumen tube or a bronchial blocker (BB) through an endotracheal tube are acceptable options. In the presence of a large pleural effusion, the lung is already collapsed by the surrounding fluid, facilitating lung isolation.

- Medical thoracoscopy is usually done for pleural effusions and may involve multiple procedures.
- Patients may be significantly symptomatic, warranting a careful preoperative evaluation to formulate the best anesthetic plan.
- Surgeons or pulmonologists with the proper expertise should perform this procedure. Local, regional, or general anesthesia are safe and available options.
- Preoperative communication among the surgeon, patient, and anesthesiologist is important to formulate the best anesthetic plan for each individual patient.
- *See Figure 124.3 and* ***Video 124.1*** *for additional details.*

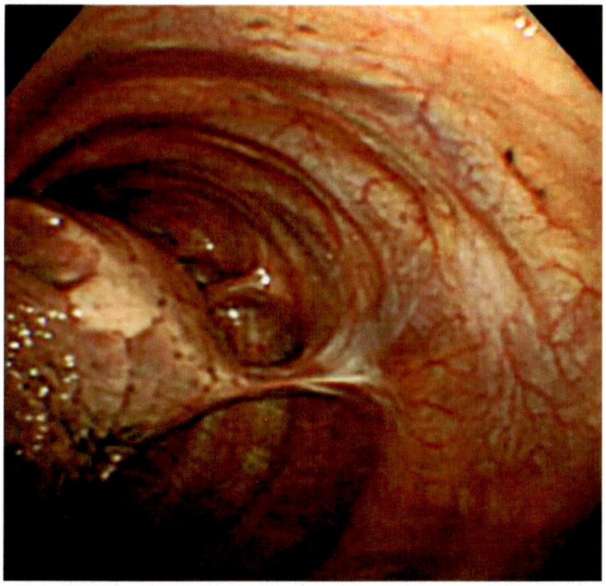

Figure 124.3. Thoracoscopic view of a collapsed lung with pleural adhesions.

Suggested Readings

Avarsala SK, Lentz RJ, Maldonado F. Medical thoracoscopy. *Clin Chest Med.* 2021;42:751–766.

Kostroglou A, Kapetanakis EI, Rougeris L, Froudarakis ME, Sidiropolou T. Review of the physiology and anesthetic considerations for pleuroscopy/medical thoracoscopy. *Respiration.* 2022;101:195–209.

Pedoto A, Kalchiem-Deckel O, Baselice S, Husta B, Rosemblatt M. Ultrasound guided midpoint transverse process to pleura nerve block for medical thoracoscopy: a case report. *A A Pract.* 2020;14(8):e01240.

Sharp A, Mudda G, Braehler MR, Gesthalter YB. Erector spinae block. A novel anesthetic approach for pleuroscopy. *J Bronchol Interv Pulmonol.* 2022;29:109.

125 Left-Sided Double-Lumen Tube

Loreta Grecu

1 Describe in detail the device or technique.

Double-lumen tubes (DLTs) are airway devices used for lung isolation and one-lung ventilation (OLV). The left-sided double-lumen tube (LDLT) is utilized in both left- and right-sided surgeries.

Modern disposable DLTs are constructed from polyvinyl chloride. Their design represents two endotracheal tubes (ETTs) "molded" together, each with a separate cuff. One of the tubes is longer and made for endobronchial positioning. It is called the "bronchial lumen" and has the "bronchial cuff." The blue color of this cuff allows for easier recognition during flexible bronchoscope (FB). The shorter tube is the "tracheal lumen" with its "tracheal cuff." The names of each lumen derive from their optimal position in the airway. The tracheal lumen tip should be positioned in the distal trachea, and the bronchial lumen tip of the LDLT should be above the secondary carina in the left bronchus. The LDLT has a stylet in the bronchial lumen and a fixed curvature, which allows placement in the left bronchus. The two lumens have large diameters, allowing for low resistance to gas flow, faster lung deflation, and easy suctioning. Each lumen can be connected to a separate ventilator, but more commonly, they are connected to the same breathing circuit via a "Y" piece.

To institute lung isolation, both cuffs are inflated, thereby protecting against contamination from the other lung. To establish OLV, after both cuffs are inflated, one lumen is clamped, ceasing ventilation to that lung.

To avoid possible complications, choosing the appropriate DLT size is important. The general rule is to choose the tube that fits into the mainstem bronchus and allows a small air leak while the cuff is deflated. Some believe that sizes 35F and 37F are suitable for women, while sizes 39F and 41F are for men. Others suggest measuring the tracheal, left bronchial, and even cricoid cartilage transverse diameters on an ultrasound or by using CT scanning.

Before placement, the tube and the stylet require good lubrication. DLTs can be placed using direct laryngoscopy (DL), a FB, or other video laryngoscopic devices. When performing DL, a Macintosh blade is more suitable as it provides the largest area to pass the tube. There are two techniques used for positioning DLTs via DL. The blind technique is performed by turning the DLT 90 degrees toward the left after the bronchial cuff passes through the vocal cords (VC). To decrease the risk of tracheobronchial injury, most clinicians prefer removing the stylet at the time of rotation, though it can be kept in place to facilitate endobronchial passage. Another technique is to position the LDLT in the trachea using a standard DL and then guide the tube in the left mainstem using the FB. Neither of these techniques is superior to the other. When the DLT cannot be advanced into the left mainstem, the practitioner needs to evaluate for causes of extrinsic bronchial compression (descending thoracic aortic aneurysm, mass). If no etiology is identified, then rotating the patient's head to the right may aid in proper positioning of the LDLT. Alternatively, a smaller LDLT can be used.

DLT position requires confirmation by auscultation and bronchoscopy. After both cuffs are inflated, auscultation of both lung fields should reveal equal breath sounds. If the LDLT is in correct position, when the bronchial lumen is clamped, breath sounds should only be heard over the right chest, whereas when the tracheal lumen is clamped, breath sounds should only be heard over the left chest. However, auscultation can be misleading.

Therefore, an FB exam is required to confirm proper DLT position. The FB is initially placed into the tracheal lumen. At the carinal level, the right mainstem bronchus is visualized (shortly past the carina is the takeoff of the right upper lobe). Depending on the DLT brand, the ideal position of the bronchial cuff is either at carinal level or in the left bronchus slightly below the carina into the left bronchus. The FB is then placed into the bronchial lumen. The secondary carina should be visible and patent. Correct DLT position is established only after examining both lumens.

DLT malpositions result in a variety of complications that clinicians need to understand, recognize, and treat. LDLT migration into the upper or lower lobe results in increased airway pressures, desaturations, or pneumothorax (when the left lung is ventilated), or inadequate deflation (when the left lung is collapsed). When the right or both lungs are ventilated, herniation of the bronchial cuff above the carina leads to increased airway pressures. In situations of DLT malposition, the FB is placed through the bronchial lumen, and the anatomy is identified. If the left side anatomy is visualized (bifurcation), then the FB is placed through the tracheal lumen, and the tube is pulled back until carina is seen. If right-sided anatomy is visualized (trifurcation), then the bronchial lumen is pulled back into the trachea, the FB is then directed into the left mainstem, and the DLT is advanced into correct position. Tube manipulations should be performed with both cuffs deflated.

2 Where or when is this device or technique used in airway management?

The DLT is the most utilized device for lung isolation and OLV. Absolute indications for lung isolation include video assisted thoracoscopic surgery, lung lavage, bronchopleural fistula, bronchial disruption, and contamination prevention (infection, hemorrhage). Relative indications for OLV are classified as high priority (upper lobectomy, pneumonectomy, minimally invasive cardiac surgery, thoracic aortic aneurysm repair) and low priority (esophageal surgery, middle, and lower lobectomy).

3 What distinguishes this device or technique from similar airway management methods?

DLTs are considered the gold standard lung-isolation device. As compared to the bronchial blockers, DLTs have decreased likelihood of displacement and require shorter times to place. DLTs allow suctioning of both lungs, administration of continuous positive airway pressure to the nondependent lung, and alternating OLV. Disadvantages include the larger size (making them more challenging to insert), and limited use for postoperative ventilation.

Because the left bronchus is longer, the LDLT has a higher safety margin for occluding the upper lobe bronchus as compared to a right DLT. Therefore, it is more commonly used in both left- and right-sided surgeries.

Author Caveats

Optimal management of DLTs relies on understanding the ABC of lung isolation: **A**natomy, **B**ronchoscopy, **C**hest imaging. Correct and rapid positioning of LDLT is determined by the operator's experience in utilizing this device. Recognizing bronchial anatomy via FB is essential for successful DLT placement. Chest imaging is important in identifying airway abnormalities and in choosing the optimal size of the lung isolation device.

- LDLT is the preferred device for lung isolation.
- LDLT has a higher safety margin and is less likely to dislodge during surgery.
- Knowledge of tracheobronchial anatomy and of bronchoscopic technique is paramount for successful placement of an LDLT.
- *See Figures 125.1 and 125.2 as well as* ***Videos 125.1*** *and* ***125.2*** *for additional details.*

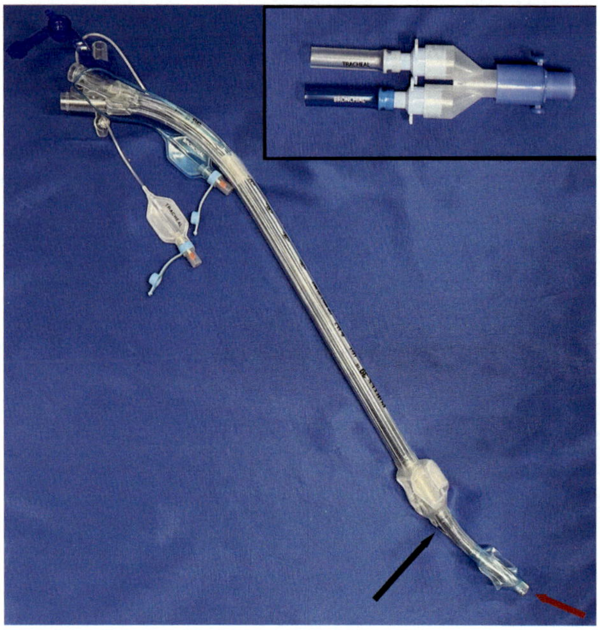

Figure 125.1. Typical left-sided double-lumen tube. Tracheal lumen (*black arrow*). Bronchial lumen (*red arrow*). Anesthesia circuit connector (*insert*).

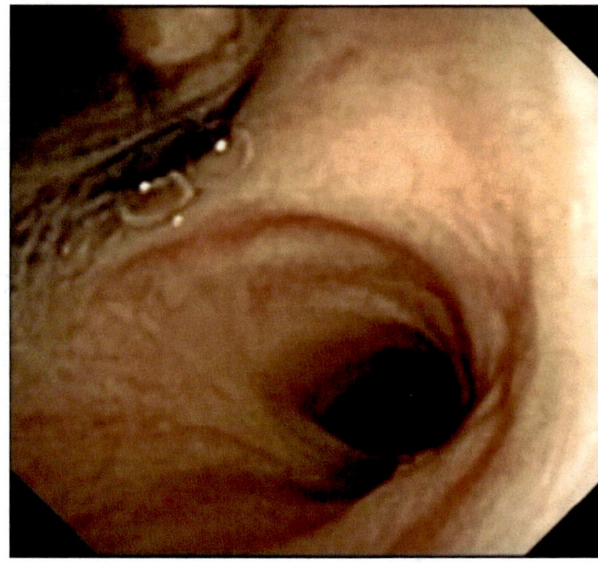

Figure 125.2. The cuff of the left-sided bronchial lumen is seen in the left main stem bronchus at the level of the carina.

Suggested Readings

Clayton-Smith A, Bennett K, Alston RP, et al. A comparison of the efficacy and adverse effects of double-lumen endobronchial tubes and bronchial blockers in thoracic surgery: a systematic review and meta-analysis of randomized controlled trials. *J Cardiothorac Vasc Anesth.* 2015;29(4):955–966.

Hao D, Saddawi-Konefka D, Low S, Alfille P, Baker A. Placement of a double-lumen endotracheal tube. *N Engl J Med.* 2021;385:e52.

Langiano N, Fiorelli S, Deana C, et al. Airway management in anesthesia for thoracic surgery: a "real life" observational study. *J Thorac Dis.* 2019;11(8):3257–3269.

Pedoto A. How to choose the double-lumen tube size and side: the eternal debate. *Anesthesiol Clin.* 2012;30:671–681.

Seo JH, Bae JY, Kim HJ, Hong DM, Jeon Y, Bahk JH. Misplacement of left-sided double-lumen tubes into the right mainstem bronchus: incidence, risk factors and blind repositioning techniques. *BMC Anesthesiol.* 2015;15:157.

Zhang C, Qin X, Zhou W, et al. Prediction of left double-lumen tube size by measurement of cricoid cartilage transverse diameter by ultrasound and CT multi-planar reconstruction. *Front Med (Lausanne).* 2021;8:657612.

Right-Sided Double-Lumen Tube

126

Loreta Grecu

Clinical Scenario: A 53-year-old man presents for a left pneumonectomy for a 5-cm centrally located mass in the left lung with possible involvement of the left mainstem bronchus.

1 What are the anesthetic and airway management considerations for this case?

The most important surgical and anesthetic consideration for this case is the possible tumor involvement of the left mainstem bronchus. Therefore, a bronchoscopy prior to lung isolation is indicated, as it will guide both the surgeon and the anesthesiologist toward a definitive plan. If, during bronchoscopy, left endobronchial involvement is identified, a right-sided double-lumen tube (RDLT) is the preferred airway device for lung isolation. If the left bronchus is free of tumor, then any lung isolation device can be used with certain precautions.

While bronchial blockers (BBs) or left-sided double-lumen tube DLTs (LDLTs) are possible alternatives, in this case, the devices would be placed in the operative field. Therefore, lung isolation may be lost when the devices require removal from the left mainstem. Moreover, in situations of left bronchial involvement, the device may impinge on the tumor, causing injury.

2 How would you manage the airway in this case?

The initial bronchoscopy can be performed after the patient is asleep using an oral airway and a FB. If a large surgical FB is required (to perform biopsies), then it is probably easier to initially place a single-lumen ETT or an SGA. When the bronchoscopy is completed, the ETT is exchanged for an RDLT (see Chapter 140: Single Lumen To Double Lumen Tube Exchange).

The RDLT has a similar construction as the LDLT, with the exception that the curvature facilitates entrance into the right mainstem. Due to the different anatomy of the right bronchus, the bronchial lumen of the RDLT has a ventilating slot specially designed for the right upper lobe (RUL) bronchus takeoff.

Insertion of an RDLT is performed in a similar manner as the LDLT (see Chapter 125: Left-Sided Double-Lumen Tube). After the bronchial cuff passes through the vocal cords, the tube is rotated clockwise while advancing it into the right mainstem.

Optimal position confirmation is performed by auscultation and using the FB. Alternatively, and less commonly, fluoroscopy may be utilized to aid with proper placement. However, perfect placement is more difficult to obtain as compared to LDLT, due to the need to align the RUL bronchus takeoff with the ventilating slot. Confirmation of proper positioning of an RDLT is performed by initially placing the FB through the tracheal lumen. The carina with an unobstructed left mainstem should be visualized. The bronchial cuff (blue) should be seen into the right mainstem. Subsequently, the FB is placed through the bronchial lumen, and upon its exit, the right middle and lower lobes should be visualized unobstructed. When withdrawing the FB, the RUL takeoff should also be identified through the special ventilation slot of the RDLT. Since the lumen is narrow, visualization of the usual RUL bronchus trifurcation may be impaired, but the entrance should be observed. The RDLT placement should be verified immediately after intubation, after patient positioning in lateral decubitus, and at any time desaturations or lung-isolation problems occur.

3 What are the surgical considerations that impact anesthetic management?

If the initial bronchoscopy demonstrates left endobronchial tumor involvement, the most important next step is to determine if a sleeve or a regular pneumonectomy will be performed. If the surgeon considers that a left bronchial stump can be created with tumor-free margins, then a regular pneumonectomy is required. In this case, placement of an RDLT allows the surgeon to proceed uninterrupted and without concern for damaging the isolating device's cuff.

In the event that the tumor involves the bronchus close to the carina, a sleeve pneumonectomy with carinal reconstruction is required. This procedure is more complex and carries a higher operative risk. The surgical approach may be a right thoracotomy. In this scenario, airway management requires a thorough plan crafted by the anesthesiologist in collaboration with the surgeon. For detailed airway management options, see Chapter 147: Left Mainstem Bronchus Resection Via Right Thoracotomy.

4 What are the potential hazards and complications in regard to the airway?

In general, DLTs cause more airway trauma than ETTs or BBs because of their larger size.

The risk of malpositioning is greater with an RDLT than with an LDLT. When the distance between the carina and the distal margin of the RUL orifice measured by CT scan is more than 23 mm, the malposition risk is decreased. In addition, a modified RDLT with a larger lateral orifice may alleviate some of the placement difficulties. For this patient undergoing a left pneumonectomy, the RDLT tracheal lumen is clamped, allowing collapse of the left lung, and the bronchial lumen ventilates the right lung. A possible misalignment between the RUL bronchus takeoff and the RDLT ventilation slot may result in inadequate ventilation of the RUL with subsequent desaturation. In other situations when right lung collapse is required, RDLT malposition results in inadequate RUL collapse with suboptimal surgical exposure. RDLT migration may occur either after patient positioning or during lung manipulation. An RDLT position reassessment using the FB should be performed as soon as the issue arises. Anatomy recognition is essential in order to expeditiously solve the problem.

- In patients with left bronchial tumor involvement, the RDLT is the preferred lung-isolation device.
- When using an RDLT, alignment of the ventilation slot with the RUL bronchus takeoff is required.
- Proper RDLT placement should be evaluated after intubation, after patient positioning, and at any time when desaturations occur or lung isolation is problematic.
- Practitioners should place RDLTs for elective cases, to become accustomed with the device.
- *See Figures 126.1 and 126.2 as well as* ***Video 126.1*** *for additional details.*

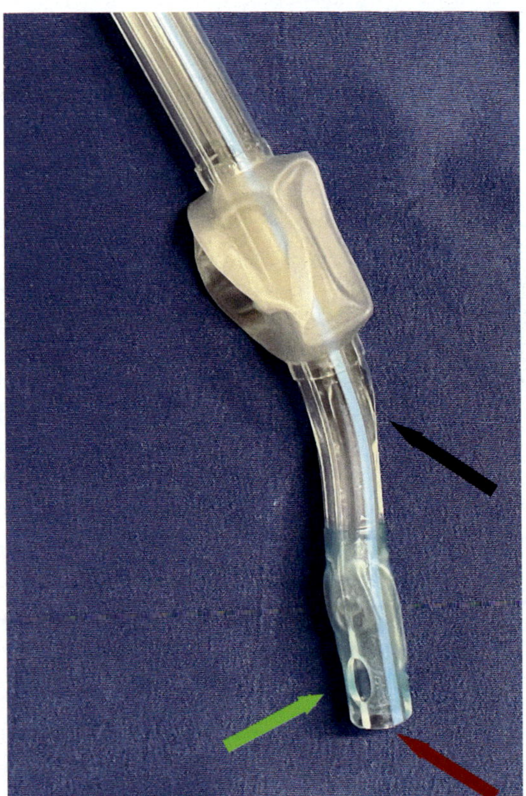

Figure 126.1. Distal-end right-sided double-lumen tube. Tracheal lumen (*black arrow*). Bronchial lumen (*red arrow*). Murphy eye (*green arrow*).

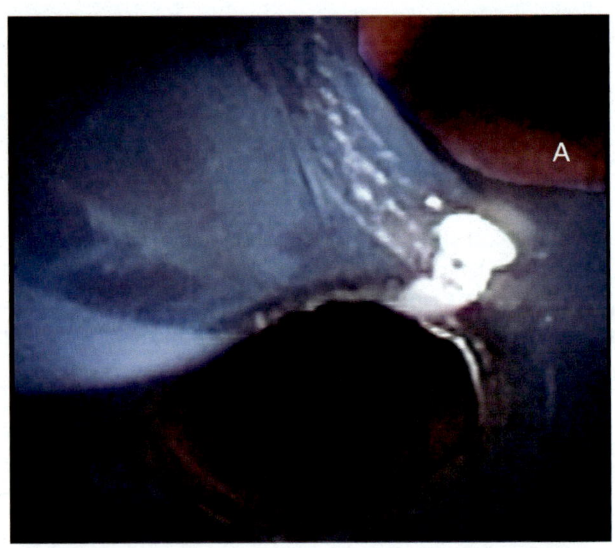

Figure 126.2. Right upper lobe seen through the Murphy eye of a well-positioned right-sided double-lumen tube (*A*).

Suggested Readings

Brodsky JB. Con: a bronchial blocker is not a substitute for a double-lumen endobronchial tube. *J Cardiothorac Vasc Anesth.* 2015;29(1):237–239.

Bussières JS, Lacasse Y, Côté D, et al. Modified right-sided Broncho-Cath double lumen tube improves endobronchial positioning: a randomized study. *Can J Anaesth.* 2007;54(4):276–282.

Ehrenfeld JM, Walsh JL, Sandberg WS. Right- and left-sided Mallinckrodt double-lumen tubes have identical clinical performance. *Anesth Analg.* 2008;106(6):1847–1852.

Kim JH, Park SH, Han SH, Nahm FS, Jung CK, Kim KM. The distance between the carina and the distal margin of the right upper lobe orifice measured by computerized tomography as a guide to right-sided double-lumen endobronchial tube use. *Anaesthesia.* 2013;68(7):700–705.

Yu W, Wang Z, Gao D, et al. A method for addressing right upper lobe obstruction with right-sided double-lumen endobronchial tubes during surgery: a randomized controlled trial. *BMC Anesthesiol.* 2018;18(1):130.

127 Silicone Double-Lumen Tubes

Peter Slinger

1 Describe in detail the device.

Silicone double-lumen tubes (DLTs), similar to the polyvinyl chloride (PVC) DLTs, have two lumens: a tracheal and a bronchial one. The most important difference is that the distal bronchial portion of the silicone DLT has a wire coil embedded in the wall to maintain patency and the appropriate configuration. In addition, silicone DLTs are more flexible and may be easier to position in a distorted bronchus. Also, the flexible distal bronchial lumen and the bevel of the bronchial orifice of the Silbroncho™ DLT facilitate a tube exchange when replacing an endotracheal tube with a DLT (Figure 127.1). Silicone DLTs are made by several manufacturers and are currently available as left- and right-sided silicone DLTs, in sizes 33, 35, 37, 39 Fr.

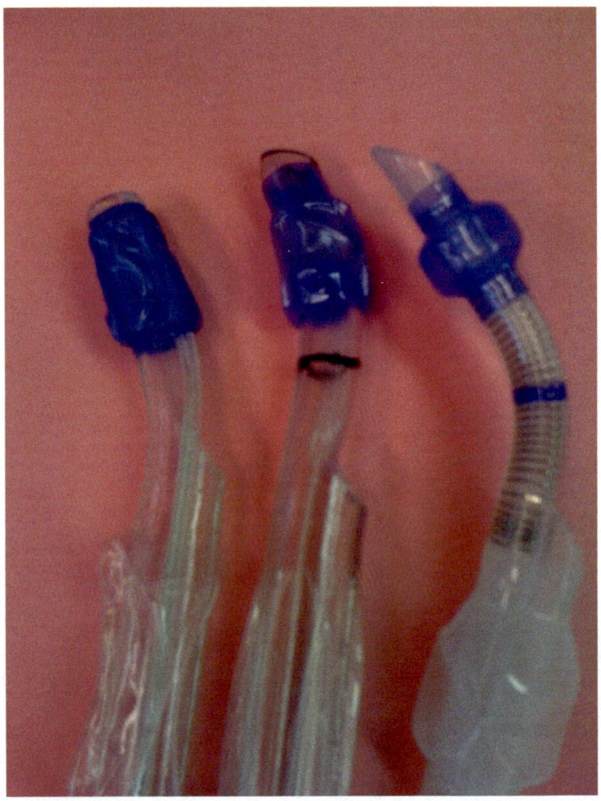

Figure 127.1. A comparison of the distal bronchial lumens of three commercial double-lumen tubes (DLTs). On the left is the Rusch polyvinyl chloride DLT (Teleflex, Athlone, Ireland), which has no bevel on the distal orifice. In the middle is the Mallinckrodt polyvinyl chloride DLT (Covidien, Dublin, Ireland), which has a short bevel on the bronchial orifice. On the right is the Silbroncho silicone DLT (Fuji Systems, Tokyo, Japan), which has a longer bevel.

2 When is this device used?

The silicone DLTs, having a more flexible bronchial lumen, are particularly useful in situations of abnormal anatomy of the lower airways, in particular in those airways with an altered carinal angle. One example is represented by patients with previous lung resection surgery. This causes a lung volume loss of the operated side, which in turn, distorts the carinal angle. Difficulties may be encountered when attempting to place a PVC DLT in a patient with previous major lung resection surgery (lobectomy). In addition, a partial or complete obstruction of the bronchial orifice of a PVC DLT by the medial wall of the bronchus may occur. This obstruction may be further worsened after the patient is turned into lateral decubitus for surgery. Another example is patients with large descending aortic artery aneurysms, which impinge on the left main stem bronchus and change the carinal angle. Silicone DLTs, with their more flexible bronchial lumen, can be particularly useful for such situations.

3 What distinguishes this device from similar airway management methods?

The majority of disposable DLTs are made of PVC. However, this is a relatively stiff material, and these tubes may not easily conform to the shape of an abnormal airway. Unlike the commonly used PVC DLTs, the silicone DLTs are manufactured of silicone, which confers them more flexibility. In addition, the wire coil embedded in the wall of the distal bronchial lumen assures flexibility and maintains luminal patency. However, silicone DLTs have a slightly thicker wall than PVC DLTs, so the internal diameter of each lumen may be slightly smaller (approx. 0.5 mm) than that of a PVC DLT of the same French caliber. A pediatric bronchoscope that passes narrowly through the lumens of a 35-Fr PVC DLT may not pass through the lumens of a 35-Fr silicone DLT.

- Before placing a silicone 35-Fr DLT in vivo, check that the well-lubricated FB passes through the lumens.
- There is often a cost differential, with silicone DLTs being more expensive than most PVC DLTs. This will depend on the manufacturer, supplier, and purchasing arrangements. At the author's institution, silicone DLTs are approximately twice as expensive as PVC DLTs.
- *See Figure 127.2 for additional details.*

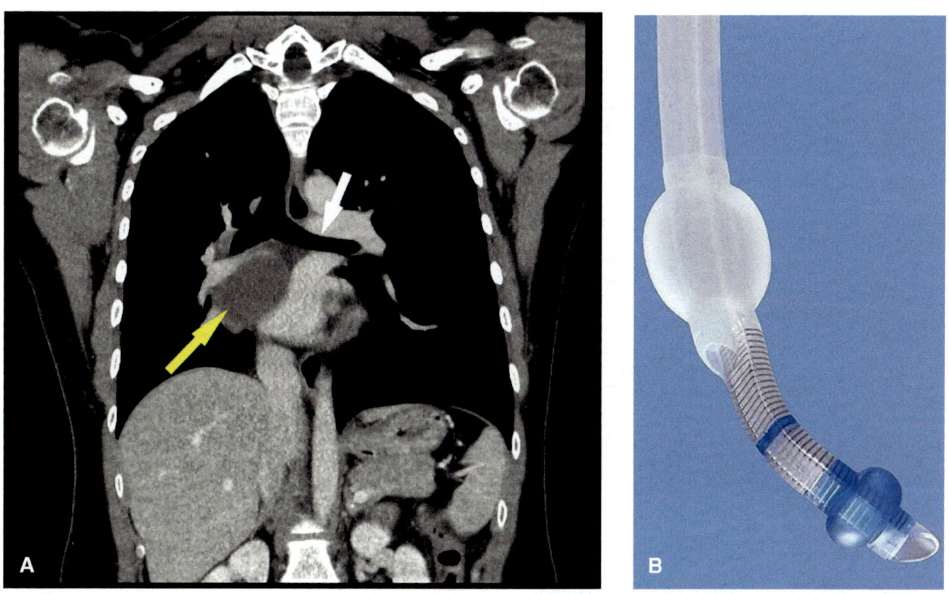

Figure 127.2. **A:** Coronal CT scan of a patient with a right-sided mediastinal cyst (*yellow arrow*) and a previous partial left upper lobe resection resulting in an increase in the angulation of the left mainstem bronchus (*white arrow*). **B:** The distal bronchial and tracheal orifices of a left-sided silicone double-lumen tube (Silbroncho, Fuji Systems, Tokyo, Japan). The distal bronchial lumen has embedded wire loops in the wall to increase stability and retain flexibility.

Suggested Readings

Gamez R, Slinger P. A simulator study of tube exchange with three different designs of double-lumen tube. *Anesth Analg*. 2014; 119:449–453.

Lee JS, Kil TY, Chung JY. Comparison of a silicon double-lumen endobronchial tube (Silbroncho®) with a polyvinyl chloride tube (Broncho-Cath®) in right-side thoracic surgery. *Korean J Anesthesiol*. 2005;48:509–513.

Slinger P, Campos J. Anesthesia for thoracic surgery. In: Gropper M, ed. *Miller's Anesthesia*. 9th ed. Elsevier; 2020:1648–1716.e8.

128 Anchor Double Lumen Endotracheal Tube

S. Zach Frabitore • Theresa A. Gelzinis • Kyuho Lee

1 Describe in detail the device.

The Anchor Double Lumen Endotracheal Tube (DLT) (Flexicare, United Kingdom, Insung, Medical, Korea) is an innovative approach to single-lung isolation and ventilation. The main advantages of this device include a design that improves blind first-pass success and that minimizes the risk of tracheobronchial injuries. The Anchor DLT is available as right- and left-sided tubes and includes sizes 33 to 41 French. Unlike the standard polyvinylchloride DLT, the Anchor DLT is composed of medical grade silicone, which provides flexibility with the possibility of reducing the incidence of tracheobronchial injuries and a wire-reinforced endobronchial tip, ensuring patency of the endobronchial lumen. The Anchor DLT is constructed with three cuffs, a tracheal balloon that is reinforced to minimize damage from the teeth during intubation, an endobronchial balloon, and a carinal balloon, located on the opposite side of the endobronchial cuff, that is used as a diverting balloon (Figure 128.1). When the carinal balloon is inflated, it prevents the endobronchial lumen from entering the opposite bronchus and prevents the DLT from being inserted too deep (Figure 128.2). Another unique feature of this tube is the method of isolating the lung. Although the connector device is similar in structure to the standard DLT one, the isolating mechanism consists of an on/off plunger instead of a clamp or twisting a valve that is necessary with other commercially available DLTs (Figure 128.3).

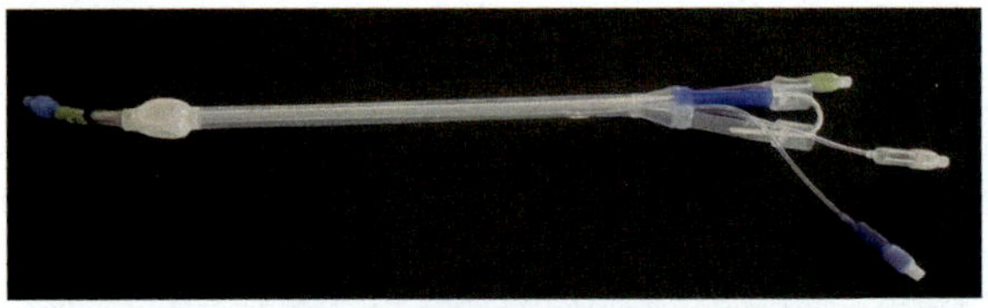

Figure 128.1. Anchor Double Lumen Tube.

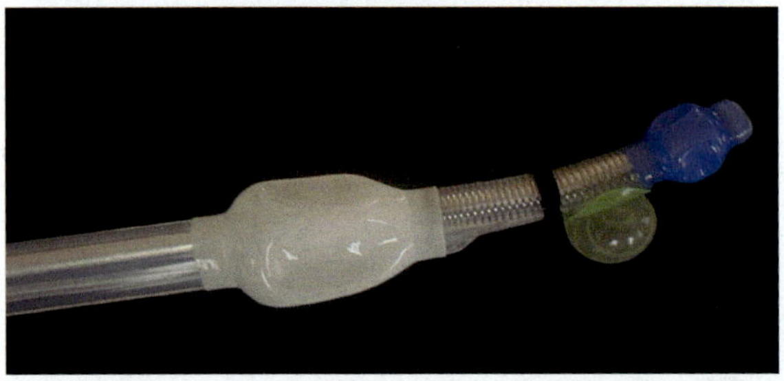

Figure 128.2. The Anchor DLT's carinal balloon prevents both the bronchial lumen from entering the contralateral side and too deep an insertion.

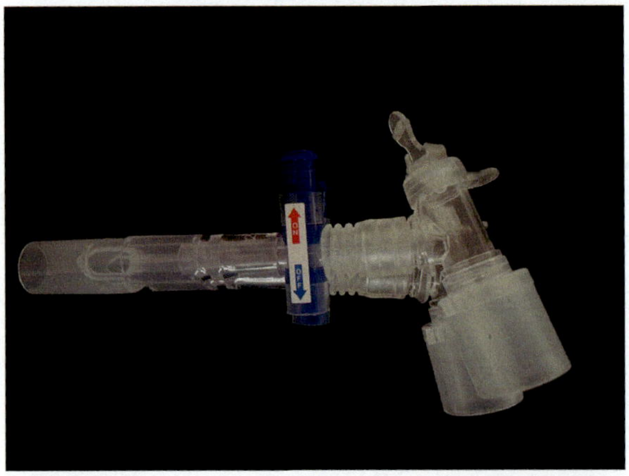

Figure 128.3. The Anchor DLT has an integrated "on/off" plunger that obstructs each lumen as needed.

The insertion technique is similar to that of a standard DLT. After preoxygenation and induction, the Anchor DLT is inserted with the endobronchial cuff pointed upward. After the endobronchial cuff is inserted into the trachea, the stylet is removed and the tube is rotated 90 degrees toward the desired bronchus and the carinal balloon is inflated with 8 to 10 cc of air. The tube is then inserted until resistance is felt. The carinal balloon is then deflated and both the tracheal and bronchial balloons are inflated. The position can then be confirmed using flexible bronchoscopy (**Video 128.1**).

2 Where or when is this device used?

The Anchor DLT can be used in any situation where one-lung ventilation is required. Indications for the use of the Anchor DLT include patients requiring lung isolation due to infection or hemorrhage in the contralateral lung, to lavage one lung in the treatment of pulmonary alveolar proteinosis, to avoid ventilating a lung with a bronchopleural fistula or to prevent the rupture of pulmonary blebs, and for lung separation for procedures where one lung ventilation is required, such as lung resection, esophagectomy, robotic mitral valve repair, and thoracic aortic aneurysm resection.

3 What distinguishes this device from similar airway management devices?

The four distinguishing features of this device are the tube composition, the reinforced tracheal balloon, the carinal balloon, and the plunger mechanism to isolate the lung. The silicone composition may reduce the incidence of tracheobronchial injuries, and the reinforced tracheal cuff may reduce cuff damage to the balloon during insertion. The carinal balloon assists in placement by diverting the endobronchial lumen toward the desired bronchus and by optimizing tube depth by preventing excessive tube insertion. These features may increase the chance of first-pass success, especially with providers who are not as proficient with DLT placement. The last feature is the method for lung isolation. The plunger device is simple to use and color coded to easily determine whether and which lung is isolated.

Since this is a relatively new device, there is a paucity of literature about its use. A study by Kim et al., compared the Anchor left-sided double-lumen tubes to conventional left-sided double-lumen tubes in regard to insertion to the optimal depth in 190 patients undergoing thoracic surgical procedures. They reported that although the incidence of right mainstem intubations was similar between the two groups, the target depth was reached in the majority of patients in the Anchor DLT group. A case report by Seo et al., described the use of the Anchor DLT after failure to place a standard DLT, in a patient receiving lung transplantation with significant pulmonary secretions. The authors blindly placed a standard DLT and could not ventilate or isolate the lung due to the secretions. They reintubated the patient with the Anchor DLT and were able to properly position the tube without the use of flexible bronchoscopy. The indications and advantages of the Anchor DLT will be elicited with further experience with this tube.

Suggested Readings

Kim N, Byon HH, Kim GE, et al. A randomized controlled trial comparing novel triple-cuffed double-lumen endobronchial tubes for lung isolation. *J Clin Med*. 2020;9:977.

Seo Y, Kim N, Paik HC, Park D, Oh YJ. Successful blind lung isolation with the use of a novel double-lumen endobronchial tube in a patient undergoing lung transplantation with massive pulmonary secretion: a case report. *Medicine (Baltimore)*. 2019; 98:e16869.

129

Double-Lumen Tube Placement Using the Glidescope

Felice Eugenio Agrò • Giuseppe Pascarella

1 Describe in detail the technique.

Double-lumen tube (DLT) intubation via direct laryngoscopy (DL) may fail due to poor visualization of the glottic opening. In this case, the use of a Glidescope video laryngoscope may secure the airway. The technique of Glidescope DLT intubation is similar to the regular one. As suggested by the manufacturer, it is performed in a four-step technique, which combines direct vision of the patient and indirect vision of the glottis on the Glidescope monitor. The four steps are:

1. **Look in the mouth of the patient and introduce the Glidescope blade (GB).** Use the nondominant hand to open the mouth and use the dominant hand to insert the GB in the oral cavity. The blade is inserted midline and carefully advanced until it completely passes the posterior portion of the tongue, and the tip is positioned in the vallecula.
2. **Look at the screen to identify the epiglottis.** To obtain the best glottic view, manipulate the device gently, advancing or withdrawing the blade, in combination with tilting movements to view the blade in the vallecula or on the posterior face of the epiglottis. At this point, elevate the tip of the blade to see the glottic opening and to obtain more space to intubate. Generally minimal lift force is needed. When the tip is adequately positioned, the glottis is displayed in the center of the monitor.
3. **Look again in the mouth to insert the DLT.** Insert the DLT in the oral cavity and carefully advance it until its tip is near the tip of the GB. By performing this maneuver while looking in the mouth of the patient and not at the monitor, the risk of pharyngeal soft-tissue damage is reduced.
4. **Look back at the monitor to intubate.** View the tip of the DLT near the tip of the GB, and the glottis. At this point, advance the DLT toward the vocal cords. A new manipulation of the blade may be needed to facilitate the insertion of the DLT. Finally, gradually withdraw the stylet (about 5 cm) while the DLT passes through the vocal cords and then completely remove it. After the DLT passes through the cords, continue advancing it with a concomitant rotation toward the main bronchus desired to be intubated.

2 Where or when is this technique used in airway management?

The Glidescope design is ideal for a patient with an anterior larynx. Currently, it is used for DLT and single-lumen tube intubations as a rescue device when DL fails, or as a first choice, both in case of predicted or unpredicted difficult airways by experienced operators. It may be used with the patient's head in sniffing or neutral position as well. As a consequence, it is ideal for patients with reduced or contraindicated neck movements, and it is also helpful in obese patients. Moreover, it may be used in patients with secretions or bloody airways (trauma), because it embeds an antifogging heat lamp. A portable version has been produced, allowing Glidescope's use in out-of-OR scenarios. Finally, the Glidescope has an important teaching role for routine and difficult intubations due to the ability to see and record the intubation sequence.

3 What distinguishes this technique from similar airway management methods?

As compared to the traditional laryngoscope, the Glidescope presents various differences both in usage technique and in design.

First of all, it is inserted midline in the oral cavity and displacement of the tongue is not required. The head can be placed in sniffing or in neutral position. Furthermore, for a successful intubation, Glidescope does not require the alignment of the three axes (oral, pharyngeal, and laryngeal). In fact, the eyes of the operator are transferred to the tip of the blade by the camera, making it possible to see "around the corner." Often, in DL the epiglottis partially covers the laryngeal aperture. By using the Glidescope, the epiglottis aligns itself to the tip of the blade, offering an improved glottic view. This implies that the lift force needed to visualize the glottis is lower compared to DL. Considering the GB's design (60-degree angulation), the tube should always be used with a stylet, curved according to the blade angulation. Generally, the use of Glidescope improves the Cormack-Lehane (C-L) view by 1 degree compared to DL.

The four-step technique employed for DLT intubation using the Glidescope may seem more complex, but it has a steep learning curve. Moreover, Glidescope's use reduces the risk of laryngeal and upper airway trauma, as all maneuvers are performed under direct or indirect vision. Due to the antifog lamp, the presence of secretions and blood does not limit vision.

Compared to DL (in the hands of an experienced operator), the Glidescope technique is faster, has a lower failure rate, requires less intubation attempts, and decreases the incidence and severity of sore throat, hoarseness, and dysphagia.

However, the Glidescope has a limited utility in patients with a reduced mouth opening (<3 cm).

Thanks to its different features (disposable blades, portability), the Glidescope is one of the more effective devices among the different available video laryngoscopes.

Author Caveats

Based on the author's experience, the suggestions below improve the manufacturer-recommended four-step technique.

Introduce the tube in the lateral part of the mouth until the 90-degree angle reaches the lips (generally corresponding to the visualization of the tube tip on the screen). At this point, rotate the tube anteriorly (move the tube from the lateral insertion site toward midline) to align its tip with the GB tip. When the alignment is obtained, advance the tube toward the vocal cords with a cloche maneuver (moving the tube toward the head of the patient).

The Glidescope should always be used with a stylet. A dedicated rigid stylet (Gliderite) is available for both single-lumen tube and DLT. This stylet has been designed according to the angulation of the GB. When the Gliderite is inserted in the tube, bending or manipulation is not needed. The angulation assured by the Gliderite allows the alignment of the tip of the tube and of the blade after the insertion.

If the Gliderite is not available, the stylet of the DLT may be used, bending the tip to at least 90 degrees (hockey stick shape). This angulation complements the angle of the GB, facilitating intubation. To obtain the correct angulation, we suggest placing the styletted DLT and the GB on the same plane and bending the tip following the blade's curvature.

After the tube tip is oriented toward the glottis, stop advancing and withdraw the stylet. The stylet should be withdrawn at least 5 cm. When using the Gliderite, withdrawing the stylet is easy because it is designed to allow this maneuver by elevating the thumb of the hand that is holding the tube. When using a normal stylet, withdrawing may be difficult, as it has been bent at an acute angle.

- The Glidescope facilitates DLT intubation in both ordinary and difficult airways.
- Glidescope intubation always requires the use of a stylet, which should have the same angulation of the GB.
- Gliderite is a manufacturer-designed precurved stylet that allows for an easier and faster DLT Glidescope intubation.
- *See Figure 129.1 and* ***Video 129.1*** *for additional details.*

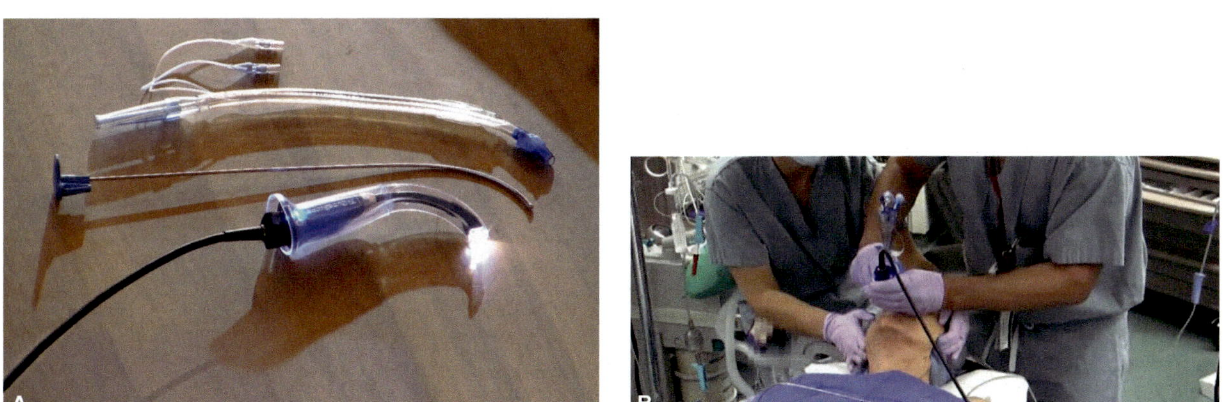

Figure 129.1. A: Double-lumen tube, rigid stylet, and Glidescope. **B:** A double-lumen tube being placed using a Glidescope.

Suggested Readings

Agrò FE, Doyle DJ, Vennari M. Use of GlideScope® in adults: an overview. *Minerva Anestesiol.* 2015;81(3):342–351.

Bussieres JS, Martel F, Somma J, Morin M, Gagné N. A customized stylet for GlideScope® insertion of double lumen tubes. *Can J Anaesth.* 2012;59(4):424–425.

El-Tahan MR. Videolaryngoscopes for placement of double lumen tubes: is it time to say goodbye to direct view? *Saudi J Anaesth.* 2016;10(2):218–227.

Hsu HT, Chou SH, Wu PJ, et al. Comparison of the GlideScope® videolaryngoscope and the Macintosh laryngoscope for double-lumen tube intubation. *Anaesthesia.* 2012;67(4):411–415.

Huang P, Zhou R, Lu Z, Hang Y, Wang S, Huang Z. GlideScope® versus C-MAC®(D) videolaryngoscope versus Macintosh laryngoscope for double lumen endotracheal intubation in patients with predicted normal airways: a randomized, controlled, prospective trial. *BMC Anesthesiol.* 2020;20(1):119.

Double-Lumen Tube Placement Using the McGrath Blade

130

Lena N. Glowka • Katherine A. Michelini

1 Describe in detail the device or technique.

The McGrath MAC is a type of video laryngoscope with a MacIntosh-type curved blade. It can be used as conventional direct laryngoscopy alone or in conjunction with video laryngoscopy. This device has a small digital camera, located adjacent to the blade tip, that is projected onto a small screen on top of the blade handle. Using the camera feature of this blade can assist in improving the overall Cormack–Lehane laryngeal view. The technique of using the McGrath blade to place a double-lumen tube (DLT) closely resembles that of direct laryngoscopy using a traditional MacIntosh blade. The patient should first be placed in the optimal position for direct laryngoscopy. After adequate opening of the patient's mouth, the McGrath blade should be inserted into the right side of the mouth, and the blade should then be used to sweep the tongue to the left side of the mouth. Once the blade tip is advanced into the vallecula, a lifting motion should reveal the glottic opening. When using the video laryngoscope feature of the McGrath blade, the operator should first look directly at the patient and the blade and then to the screen for confirmation of the manual movements. Once a view of the vocal cords is obtained, focus should be placed on advancing the bronchial cuff of the DLT (with the bronchial concave curve facing anteriorly) through the mouth and into the posterior pharynx under direct vision. The operator can then either advance the bronchial cuff through the vocal cords under direct vision or, if the view of the glottic opening is inadequate, use the video screen to advance the bronchial cuff through the vocal cords. The DLT is then rotated 90 degrees (either left or right, depending on the sidedness of the DLT being used) and advanced until resistance is met. At this point, the McGrath blade is removed, the tracheal cuff is inflated, and adequate ventilation of both lungs is verified with inspection, auscultation, and confirmation of sustained end tidal CO_2.

2 Where or when is the device used in airway management?

Double-lumen endotracheal tubes remain the gold standard airway devices utilized for lung isolation during thoracic surgeries. Occasionally, the placement of a DLT may prove difficult even in the most experienced of hands due to its larger overall diameter and more rigid shape compared with a single-lumen endotracheal tube. Traditionally, the technique of choice for placing a DLT has been direct laryngoscopy using a curved MacIntosh blade. Video laryngoscopes have emerged as an important tool in airway management and can be a useful tool to assist with the placement of a DLT in an anticipated or unanticipated difficult airway. The McGrath offers additional advantages over other video laryngoscopes for DLT placement as discussed in the section that follows.

3 What distinguishes this device or technique from similar airway management methods?

The McGrath enhances DLT placement by improving the view of the glottic opening and allowing for direct visualization of the bronchial cuff passing the vocal cords. This improved visualization is particularly useful in airways that cannot be managed with direct laryngoscopy alone. Compared to video laryngoscopy using a hyperangulated curved blade, the McGrath video laryngoscope paired with a MAC 3 or 4 blade creates more space in the mouth for manipulation of the DLT and does not require reshaping of the DLT stylet. Similarly, compared with the Glidescope blade, the McGrath blade has a lower profile, thus offering more "real estate" in the mouth.

Author caveats

The use of the McGrath video laryngoscope with a MAC 3 or 4 blade can be a helpful tool for placement of a DLT in an airway that is anticipated to be a difficult direct laryngoscopy.

The McGrath video laryngoscope, which can also be used as a direct laryngoscope, may be an optimal choice of laryngoscope for airways with copious secretions or blood, which may obscure the view obtained with the camera.

The use of the hyperangulated McGrath blade still affords more mouth space and a slimmer blade profile than the Glidescope blade, but will require reshaping of the DLT to match the hyperangulation and allow the DLT to pass through the cords.

- The McGrath video laryngoscope can provide improved visualization of the glottic opening over a traditional direct laryngoscope with a MacIntosh blade.
- The McGrath paired with a MAC 3 or 4 blade provides adequate room in the mouth for manipulation of the DLT during placement.
- The DLT, which comes preshaped with a stylet, does not need to be molded to the shape of a hyperangulated blade when using the McGrath with a MAC blade.
- *See Figure 130.1 and* ***Video 130.1*** *for additional details.*

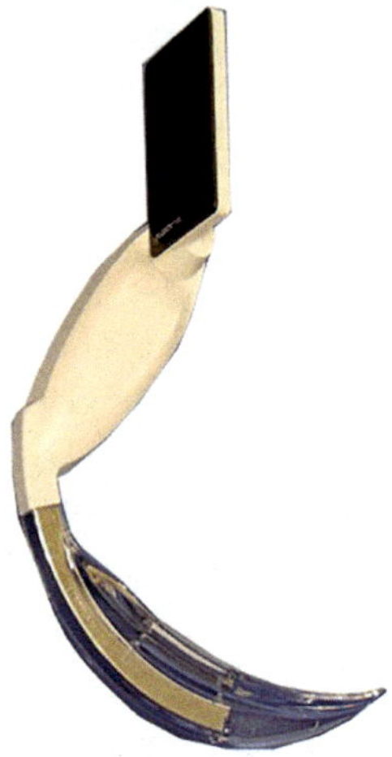

Figure 130.1. The McGrath Mac Laryngoscope. (© 2025 Medtronic. All rights reserved. Used with the permission of Medtronic.)

Suggested Readings

Falzon D, Alston RP, Coley E, Montgomery K. Lung isolation for thoracic surgery: from inception to evidence-based. *J Cardiothorac Vasc Anesth*. 2017;31(2):678–693.

Hao D, Saddawi-Konefka D, Low S, Alfille P, Baker K. Placement of a double-lumen endotracheal tube. *N Engl J Med*. 2021;385(16):e52.

Karczewska K, Bialka S, Smereka J, et al. Efficacy and safety of video-laryngoscopy versus direct laryngoscopy for double-lumen endotracheal intubation: a systematic review and meta-analysis. *J Clin Med*. 2021;10(23):5524.

Double-Lumen Tube with Incorporated Fiberoptic Bronchoscopy

131

Javier H. Campos • Satoshi Hanada

1 Describe in detail the device or technique.

VivaSight Double-Lumen Tube

Lung separation techniques are used to provide one-lung ventilation (OLV) in patients undergoing thoracic, mediastinal, cardiac, vascular, or esophageal procedures. The left-sided double-lumen tube (DLT) is the most common device used for lung separation because of its greater margin of safety when compared to a right-sided DLT. In the past 10 years, DLTs have undergone some modifications to improve their efficiency. Some manufacturers have shortened and modified the endobronchial lumen tip to improve insertion while advancing the DLT through the glottis. Others have used a reinforced wire in the inner wall of the endobronchial lumen tip to prevent kinking as the DLT enters the left mainstem bronchus. ET View Medical has designed a new device called the VivaSight DLT with an integrated high-resolution camera. This camera is embedded at the end of the endotracheal lumen, so that when connected to a screen monitor via a cable, it allows a continuous view of the tracheal carina. In addition, this DLT device has an integrated flushing system that allows for in situ camera lens cleaning. Figure 131.1A displays the VivaSight DLT, and Figure 131.1B displays the embedded camera with optic illumination.

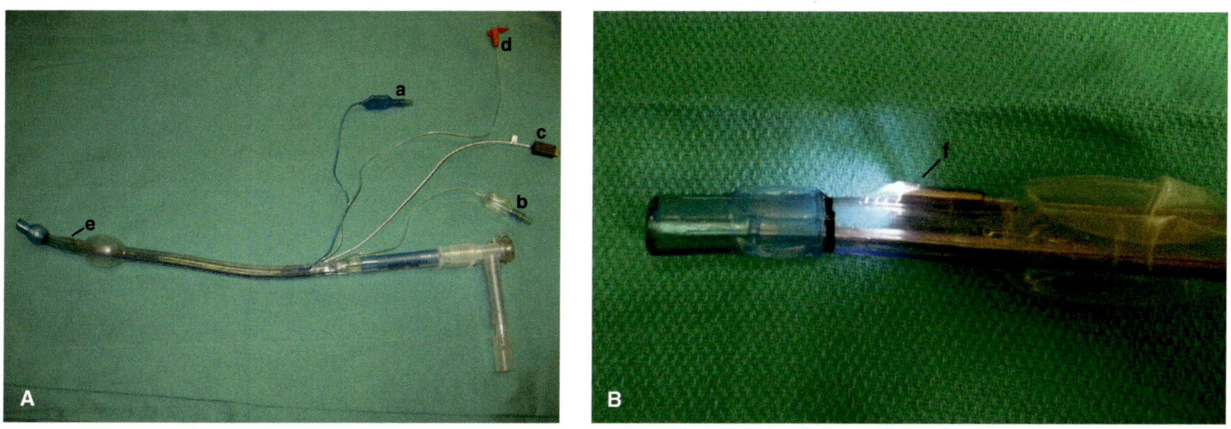

Figure 131.1. A: The VivaSight double-lumen tube (DLT) with incorporated camera. *a*, Bronchial lumen cuff balloon; *b*, tracheal lumen cuff balloon; *c*, video connection; *d*, flushing port; *e*, position of camera and exit of flushing port. **B:** *f*, camera and light source.

In principle, the VivaSight DLT is similar to any disposable DLT, and has all the features of a standard DLT. Placement during intubation is the same as for a standard DLT using direct laryngoscopy and direct visualization of the vocal cords. After the VivaSight DLT is advanced through the vocal cords, the camera cable is connected to the screen monitor to observe the passage of the endobronchial tip in the left mainstem bronchus. To achieve optimal DLT position, a flexible bronchoscopic examination should be performed.

At the present time, only the left-sided VivaSight DLT is available in sizes 37Fr, 39Fr, and 41Fr. One of the advantages of the VivaSight DLT is that it allows for a continuous display of the tracheal carina. If the DLT is in the correct position, the camera allows visualization of the tracheal carina and the outer edge of the inflated endobronchial balloon. The device provides a continuous display of the position of the DLT and, perhaps, allows for faster detection of DLT malpositions by direct observation on the monitor screen.

The VivaSight DLT has some limitations. First, accumulation of secretions may obscure the view. Using the suction channel and flushing it with normal saline will, in part, alleviate the problem. Also, applying defogger solution to the tip of the integrated light source will improve the view. Second, there is a need to connect to a screen monitor. Therefore, careful attention must be given to the connection of the VivaSight DLT and the screen to avoid mishaps (such as pulling the DLT out of position accidentally because of the cable connections). Third, the practitioner should be aware that connecting the camera for prolonged periods of time may lead to melting the portion of the tube near the light source. Finally, the view of the integrated camera in the DLT allows only viewing of the tracheal carina; this camera device cannot be used to inspect or confirm the takeoff of the right upper lobe bronchus. **Video 131.1** displays the screen monitor device connected to the VivaSight DLT.

2 Where or when is this device or technique used in airway management?

The VivaSight DLT indications are identical to the ones used for a standard DLT during lung separation techniques and OLV. The main advantage of the VivaSight DLT is the continuous observation of the distal balloon (endobronchial cuff) through the screen monitor, so that malpositions can be easily detected and corrected.

3 What distinguishes this device or technique from similar airway management methods?

The main difference with the VivaSight DLT is that it incorporates an internal camera which, when connected to an external screen monitor, allows for a continuous confirmation of the tube position. Because the position of the internal camera is integrated at the end of the endotracheal lumen, it only allows a view distal to the tube (ie, visualization of tracheal carina, entrance of the endobronchial lumen into the left mainstem bronchus, and an outer edge of the fully inflated endobronchial balloon).

Although the optimal position of the VivaSight DLT requires the use of the flexible bronchoscope (FB) to perform a complete inspection through the endotracheal and endobronchial lumen, the advantage of the VivaSight DLT is the continuous visualization of the optimal position of the DLT when the camera is connected to the screen monitor. When the patient is in lateral decubitus position and a malposition is detected, there is no need to pass an FB; as long as the DLT is connected to the screen monitor, repositioning the tube becomes very easy. The VivaSight DLT reduces the need for bronchoscopy during airway manipulation. In addition, time duration of intubation with visual confirmation of tube position is significantly reduced with the VivaSight DLT when compared to conventional DLT.

- The VivaSight DLT has an integrated high-resolution camera incorporated at the distal end of the endotracheal lumen that, when connected to a screen monitor, allows continuous visualization of the tracheal carina and positioning of the DLT.
- The VivaSight provides continuous airway monitoring with uninterrupted visualization during lung-isolation procedures.
- The VivaSight DLT facilitates immediate corrections of DLT malpositions at the level of the tracheal carina.
- In order to maintain good visualization with the VivaSight camera, it is recommended that a defogging solution be used prior to insertion.
- *See Figure 131.2 for additional details.*

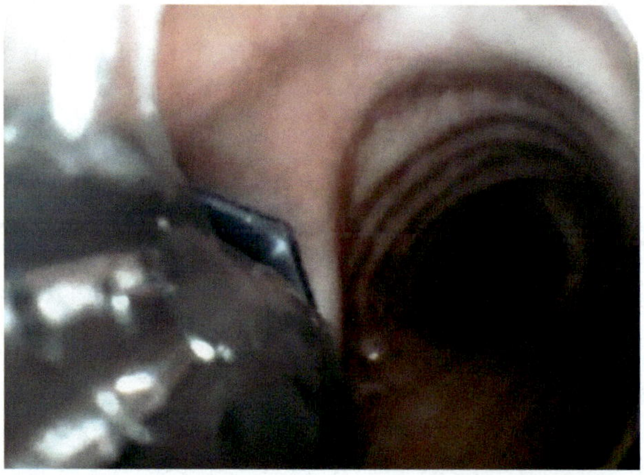

Figure 131.2. Image from integrated camera of left-sided bronchial lumen and cuff correctly positioned.

Suggested Readings

Campos JH. Separation of the lung: double-lumen endotracheal tubes and endobronchial blocker. In: Cohen E, ed. *Cohen's Comprehensive Thoracic Anesthesia*. 1st ed. 2021:213–239.

Levy-Faber D, Malyanker Y, Nir RR, Best LA, Barak M. Comparison of VivaSight double-lumen tube with a conventional double-lumen tube in adult patients undergoing video-assisted thoracoscopic surgery. *Anaesthesia*. 2015;70:1259–1263.

Onifade A, Lemon-Riggs D, Smith A, et al. Comparing the rate of fiberoptic bronchoscopy use with a video double lumen tube versus a conventional double lumen tube—a randomized controlled trial. *J Thorac Dis*. 2020;12:6533–6541.

132 Single-Lumen Tubes with Incorporated Video Camera

Manuel Granell Gil

1 Describe in detail the device.

One-lung ventilation in thoracic surgery aims to collapse the lung, thus providing adequate surgical exposure. To achieve lung isolation and one-lung ventilation, double-lumen tubes (DLTs) or bronchial blockers (BBs) are mainly used.

Most of these types of interventions can be performed with lung isolation using BBs, which can be introduced through an endotracheal tube guided by flexible bronchoscope (FB). A new single-lumen (SL) endotracheal tube with an embedded high-resolution camera at the distal tip (VivaSight SL) has been developed. The tube has a cable connection from the camera to a monitor, that allows continuous imaging of the airway. In addition, the VivaSight SL has an integrated flushing system that allows for in situ camera lens cleaning. These single-lumen VivaSight SL endotracheal tubes are available in sizes 7.0-, 7.5-, and 8.0-mm internal diameters.

2 Where or when is this device used?

The endotracheal tube with embedded camera facilitates tracheal intubation and insertion of the BBs as well as continuous monitoring of the BB's correct position during patient repositioning and/or the entire surgery, usually without the need to use FB. In 2009, a study was published on the use of this device for the insertion of a BB in patients undergoing left lung lobectomy. The study identified a 100% success rate in the insertion of the BB at the first attempt and a 6.2% displacement rate, with great ease of repositioning without the need to use the FB.

Another indication is its use in patients with known or expected difficult upper airways, and in morbidly obese patients. The ETT with embedded camera can be introduced directly using a direct laryngoscope/video laryngoscope or thought a laryngeal mask airway. In a study of 50 patients with a normal airway, intubation was performed through the Fastrach mask and it was successful on first attempt in 94% of cases, and on the second attempt in 4% of the cases. In addition, intubation was achieved faster than with FB, and no intubation-associated injuries were observed, probably because direct vision of the glottis prevented the injuries associated with blind intubation.

Finally, its usefulness has also been described for intubating patients without the need for a laryngoscope using an oral intubating airway as initial guide.

3 What distinguishes this device from similar airway management methods?

The endotracheal VivaSight SL is similar with a regular endotracheal polyvinyl chloride tube with the only difference that it has the embedded camera at its tip which, connected to a monitor, allows continuous visualization of the airway.

See Figure 132.1 and **Video 132.1** *for additional details.*

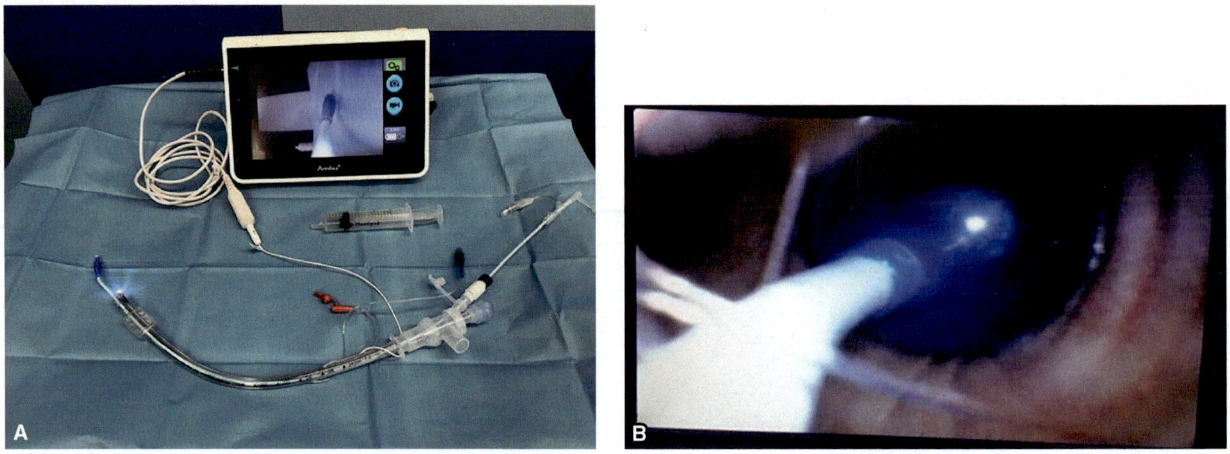

Figure 132.1. A: VivaSight SL tracheal tube with Uniblocker. **B:** Cuff of the Uniblocker positions in the Right Mainstem Bronchus, as seen on the ViviSight SL monitor.

Suggested Readings

Barak M, Assalia A, Mahajna A, Bishara B, Braginski A, Kluger Y. The use of VivaSight TM single lumen endotracheal tube in morbidly obese patients undergoing laparoscopic sleeve gastrectomy. *BCM Anesthesiology*. 2014;14:31.

Campos J. Chapter 16: Lung isolation. In: Slinger P, ed. *Principles and Practice of Anesthesia for Thoracic Surgery*. Springer; 2011: 227–246.

Gaitini LA, Yanovski B, Mustafa S, Hagberg CA, Mora PC, Vaida SJ. A feasibility study using the VivaSight Single Lumen™ to intubate the trachea through the Fastrach laryngeal mask airway: a preliminary report of 50 cases. *Anesth Analg*. 2013; 116(3):604–608.

Giglio M, Oreste D, Oreste N. Usefulness of ETView TVT endotracheal tube for correct positioning of bronchial blockers in left lobectomy: an easy and safe combination. *Minerva Anestesiol*. 2009;75(1–2):1–4.

Granell Gil M, Solís Albamonte P, Córdova Hernández C, Cobo I, Guijarro R, de Andrés Ibañez JA. Intubation in two patients with difficult airway management and tracheal stenosis after tracheostomy in thoracic surgery. *Rev Esp Anestesiol Reanim (Engl Ed)*. 2018;65(6):347–350.

133 Univent Tubes

Jan Ehrenwerth

1 Describe in detail the device or technique.

- The Univent™ tube consists of a standard single-lumen endotracheal tube with a small secondary lumen that has an integrated bronchial blocker. The bronchial blocker is initially withdrawn into the endotracheal tube during intubation. The bronchial blocker can then be extended 8 to 10 cm beyond the tip to selectively block the right or left mainstem bronchus. The blocker may also be used to selectively isolate an individual lobe of the right or left lung.
- The bronchial blocker consists of a small cuff on a relatively stiff hollow shaft. The blocker has a separate pilot balloon for inflating the blocker's cuff. The small hole in the shaft allows deflation of the lung that is being blocked. The stiff shaft (so-called torque control) allows the blocker to be rotated into either the right or left mainstem bronchus.
- An flexible bronchoscope (FB) is required for proper placement of the blocker. After the patient is intubated with the blocker withdrawn into its channel, the bronchoscope is then passed through the main lumen of the Univent™ tube. Next, the blocker is extended into the desired bronchus under direct vision. The blocker's cuff is inflated under direct vision to assure that the bronchus is occluded, and the cuff is not herniated over the carina.

There are several advantages of the Univent™ tube. Since the bronchial blocker is incorporated into the tube, it is not necessary to obtain a separate blocker. The Univent™ tube also comes in seven different sizes. These range (in half-size increments) from a 6.0 to a 9.0 internal diameter. With the Univent™ tube either mainstem bronchus or even an individual lobe can be blocked.

Advantages of the Univent™ over a double-lumen tube include use in difficult intubations, rapid sequence inductions, and when it is desirable to leave the patient intubated postoperatively. Also, if the trachea or a mainstem bronchus is distorted by something like a descending aortic aneurysm, it may be impossible to place a double-lumen tube. However, placing a blocker may be possible in this situation.

There are several disadvantages to the Univent™ tube. First, when the blocker is withdrawn into the channel and then extended after intubation, the cuff on the blocker can rupture. This could lead to pieces of the cuff lodging in the trachea or a bronchus. It is therefore important to inspect the blocker after it is removed from the patient.

Since the channel in the shaft of the blocker is small, it can take a long time for the blocked lung to collapse. In the event that the blocked bronchus needs to be suctioned, the cuff would have to be deflated, and the FB or a suction catheter would need to be used. In order to block lung expansion in this situation, ventilation would need to be stopped prior to deflating the cuff of the bronchial blocker. The main disadvantage of this device is its large outer diameter. Hence, in today's clinical practice, its use has dramatically decreased.

The Univent™ tube can be used with continuous positive airway pressure (CPAP); however, it does not come with an adaptor to accomplish this task. Additional disadvantages of the blocker include dislodgement with patient movement, need for a FB to accurately place the blocker, more expensive than a double-lumen tube, and inability to block the right lung when the right upper lobe bronchus arises from the trachea. Finally, the Univent™ similar to other bronchial blockers, cannot be used when doing lung lavage for pulmonary alveolar proteinosis.

2 Where or when is this device or technique used in airway management?

The Univent™ endotracheal tube is used for lung isolation when it is desirable to selectively block the right or left mainstem bronchus. Most commonly, these tubes are used to facilitate surgical procedures in the thoracic cavity. These include video-assisted or open thoracotomy for resection of a lung lobe or pneumonectomy. The Univent endotracheal tube (ETT) can also be useful for surgery involving the esophagus or descending thoracic aorta. Other indications include protecting one lung from being contaminated by the other lung, in cases such as unilateral hemoptysis or infection. It is also useful in patients with a giant unilateral lung cyst or bleb, or in patients with a bronchopleural-cutaneous fistula.

However, one of the main indications for using the Univent™ ETT is in patients who are difficult to intubate. It is usually easier to place a single-lumen tube in these patients as opposed to a double-lumen endotracheal tube. This is also true in patients who require a rapid sequence intubation. Finally, in patients who will need postoperative ventilation, the Univent™ tube is more convenient, since a double-lumen tube would need to be exchanged for a single-lumen tube at the end of the case.

3 What distinguishes this device or technique from similar airway management methods?

The Univent™ tube is different from other bronchial blockers like the Arndt™ or Cohen™ in that the blocker is incorporated into the additional channel in the tube. All of the other blockers are sold as a stand-alone device, and must be used with an additional ETT. Also, the relatively stiff shaft of the blocker, allows it to be rotated, which facilitates placement into the desired bronchus. This is the so-called "torque control" feature.

Author Caveats

One of the major problems with the blocker is that it moves out of position when the patient is turned into the lateral position. One trick is to place the blocker past the orifice of the main stem bronchus with the cuff deflated. After the patient is turned into position, reinsert the FB down the main channel of the tube, and under direct vision, withdraw the blocker into the correct position. Now the cuff can be inflated and it can be verified that the bronchus is occluded.

Another caveat is to know the size of the FB before deciding on the size of the Univent™ tube that will be used. Because the outside diameter (OD) of the Univent™ tube is larger than a standard single-lumen endotracheal tube, it is desirable to use the smallest size tube that the FB will comfortably fit through. For instance, an 8.0 internal diameter (ID) Univent™ has an O.D. of 13.5 mm. This is the same OD as a number 10.0 single-lumen ET tube.

Since both the right and left mainstem bronchi have less cartilage than the trachea, it is important to not overinflate the cuff of the blocker, which could damage the bronchus. Also, as with any bronchial blocker, barotrauma and pneumothorax are potential complications.

Placing the Univent just below the cords, allows more room to manipulate the blocker. If the blocker will not pass into the desired bronchus, the FB can be inserted into the Univent ET and the entire tube threaded over the FB into the desired bronchus. The blocker is then extended, and the Univent tube withdrawn into the trachea. If this technique is used, care must be exercised not to damage the bronchus.

See Figure 133.1 and **Video 133.1** *for additional details.*

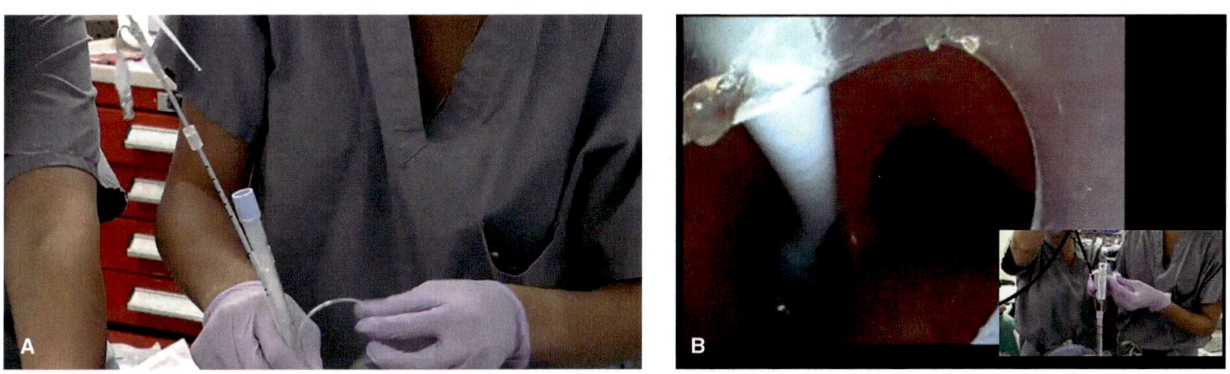

Figure 133.1. A: Bronchial blocker seen emerging from a Univent tracheal tube. **B:** Cuff of bronchial blocker seen in left mainstem bronchus as viewed with a flexible bronchoscope.

Suggested Readings

Brodsky JB. Lung separation and the difficult airway. *BJA*. 2009;103(suppl 1):i66–i75.

Campos JH. An update on bronchial blockers during lung separation techniques in adults. *Anesth Analg*. 2003;97:1266–1274.

Neustein SM. The use of bronchial blockers for providing one lung ventilation. *J Cardiothorac Vasc Anesth*. 2009;23:860–868.

134 Fuji Uniblocker Bronchial Blocker

Shamsuddin Akhtar

1 Describe in detail the device or technique.

The Fuji Uniblocker BB is a lung isolation device that is inserted into the bronchus of the lung that will not be ventilated. The Fuji Uniblocker's shaft is made of wire mesh coated with polyurethane, ensuring that any manipulation is translated to its tip. It has a curvature, like a hockey stick, which facilitates entrance into the desired bronchus. The shaft has a 2-mm lumen through the center. This allows lung deflation during one lung ventilation (OLV). In addition, suction can be applied to the lumen to speed lung collapse. Alternatively, application of continuous positive airway pressure or oxygen insufflation to the nonventilated lung improves oxygenation during OLV. The Fuji Uniblocker comes with two stylets, one at the tip and another at the distal end of the blocker placed through the central lumen of the catheter. The stylet at the tip is designed to maintain the bronchial blocker (BB) shape during transportation and needs to be removed prior to placement. The distal end stylet helps guide the BB into the desired bronchus. After proper placement, the stylet is removed and discarded. The Fuji Uniblocker is available in two sizes: a 5Fr and a 9Fr. A 5Fr BB is used for children and can be placed through a 4.5 endotracheal tube (ETT). This blocker has an outer diameter of 1.7 mm and a shaft length of 40 cm (effective length 32.5 cm). A 5Fr cuff's length is 8 mm, and maximal cuff volume is 3 mL. The 9Fr Fuji Uniblocker is most used in adults and requires at least an 8.0 ETT for placement. The 9Fr BB is 65 cm in length (effective length 50 cm), has an outer diameter of 3 mm, and is latex free. The blocker has a high-volume balloon made of silicone, which impairs the diffusion of gas into or out of the cuff. For a 9Fr Fuji Uniblocker, the cuff's length is 22 mm, and the maximum recommended inflation volume is 8 mL (Table 134.1). The balloon should only be inflated with air and under direct vision using the flexible bronchoscope (FB).

TABLE 134.1 Characteristics of the Cohen Flexitip Endobronchial Blocker, the Arndt Blocker, and the Fuji Uniblocker

	Fuji Uniblocker	Arndt Blocker	Cohen Blocker	EZ-Blocker
Available sizes	5Fr, 9Fr	5Fr, 7Fr, 9Fr	9Fr	7Fr
Balloon shape	Spherical	Spherical (S) Elliptical (E)	Spherical	Two Spherical (left and right)
Maximal balloon volume	3 cc for 5Fr 8 cc for 9Fr	2 cc for 5Fr 6 cc for 7Fr 8 cc for 9Fr (S) 12 cc for 9Fr (E)	8 cc	6.9 cc for left 9.1 for right
Central channel	2.0 mm for 9Fr	1.4 mm for 9Fr	1.6 mm	4 very small channels
Guidance mechanism	Preshaped curvature	Nylon guide-loop	Wheel device Preangled tip	Y-shaped distal ends
Smallest ETT required	4.5 ETT for 5Fr 8.0 ETT for 9Fr	4.5 ETT for 5Fr 6.0 ETT for 7Fr 7.5 ETT for 9Fr	8.0 ETT	7.0 ETT

Before insertion, the blocker's balloon should be tested for leaks, and then fully deflated. It is desirable to lubricate (preferably with silicone) both the blocker cuff and the FB to facilitate insertion and passage through the single-lumen ETT. A FB no larger than 4.0 mm outer diameter should be utilized in order to facilitate the simultaneous passage of the BB and the scope through the ETT. The Fuji Uniblocker is equipped with torque control, which allows guidance of the blocker into the desired bronchus. The Fuji Uniblocker is also equipped with a swivel connector that enables rotation of the ventilator circuit if the patient is moved and allows easy insertion of both the blocker and FB. In addition, at the completion of OLV, the connector facilitates easy removal of the BB without disconnecting the breathing circuit.

As with other blockers, the Fuji Uniblocker is advanced through an ETT side by side with the FB, under continuous visualization. When the Fuji Uniblocker is placed in the right mainstem, the edge of the blocker's inflated balloon should be viewed 5 mm below the tracheal carina. However, on the left side, the cuff should be seen at least 5 to 10 mm below the tracheal carina. Any BB manipulation requires prior cuff deflation.

2 Where or when is this device or technique used in airway management?

Fuji Uniblocker is just one of the devices that can be used in clinical situations when OLV is required. It is particularly useful when managing patients with difficult airways requiring OLV, where a single lumen ETT can be placed, followed by a BB. It can also be utilized in patients who are mechanically ventilated and have an appropriately sized ETT in situ (equal or larger than 8.0 mm). The Fuji Uniblocker is also a good lung-isolation device in a tracheostomized patient or in situations requiring selective lobar blockade.

3 What distinguishes this device or technique from similar airway management methods?

The Fuji Uniblocker is unique in two ways. One, it has a bronchial cuff made of silicone, which is impermeable to gases. With a maximal inflation volume of 8 mL of air, the blocker's transmitted pressure is reliably less than 30 mm Hg. This pressure is thought to be safe for the bronchial mucosa. Second, the Fuji Uniblocker has a torque control, designed to optimize control of the blocker's movements. Thus, placement of the blocker is less cumbersome. In one study, the Arndt BB required repositioning more frequently than the Cohen BB or the Fuji Uniblocker.

Author Caveats

As compared to DLTs, BBs take more time to place and require a longer duration for full-lung collapse. The Fuji Uniblocker is no exception. An incomplete balloon seal or a dislodged BB most likely causes incomplete lung isolation. Migration of the bronchial balloon into the trachea leads to difficulty in ventilation and increased airway pressures. Evaluating the BB position with the FB can help resolve all these complications. A rare complication is represented by air trapping, which can occur when the blocker is displaced into a tracheal position, and successive, stacked tidal volumes are forced in the airway distal to the blocker. Air trapping leads to a profound decrease in preload and possible cardiac arrest. This complication needs to be immediately recognized and treated by deflating the balloon and repositioning the blocker correctly.

- To place a 9F (3-mm) Fuji Uniblocker BB, requires a minimum 8.0 ETT.
- The Fuji Uniblocker balloon is made of silicone, which is impermeable to gases and limits the bronchial mucosal pressure to less than 30 mm Hg.
- The Fuji Uniblocker has a torque control, built into the shaft of the blocker, designed to optimize the blocker's movements.
- *See Figure 134.1 and 134.2 for additional details.*

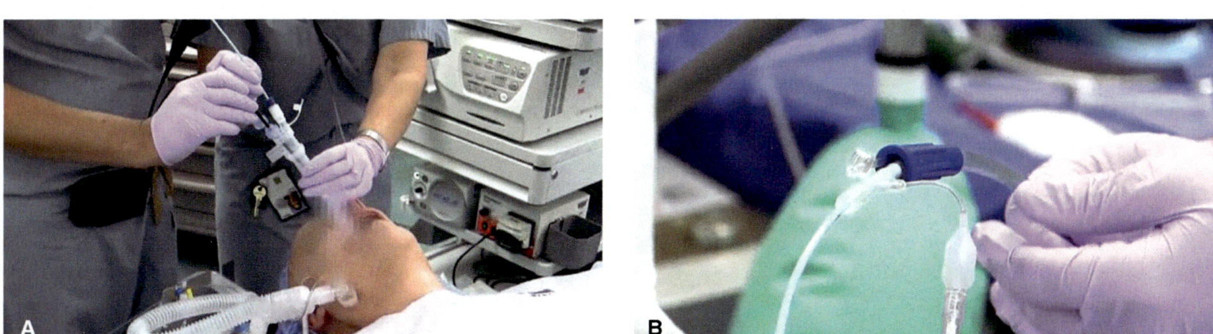

Figure 134.1. **A:** Fuji Uniblocker being positioned within a single-lumen tracheal tube under the guidance of a flexible bronchoscope. See **Video 134.1** for additional details. **B:** Suction being applied to the Fuji Uniblocker lumen to hasten lung deflation.

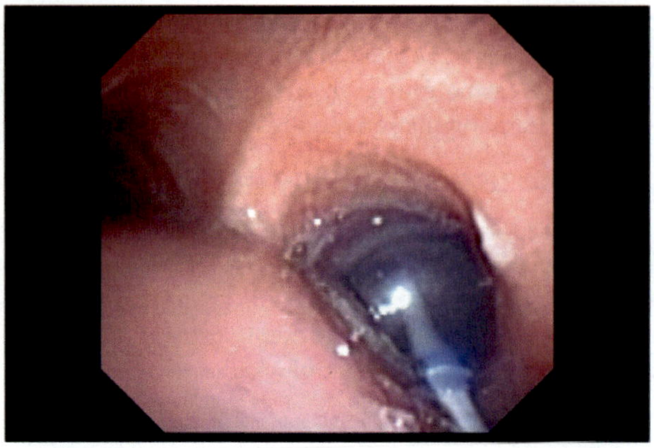

Figure 134.2. Cuff of the Fuji Uniblocker in the right main stem bronchus.

Suggested Readings

Campos J. Lung isolation. In: Slinger P, ed. *Principles and Practice of Anesthesia for Thoracic Surgery*. Springer; 2011:227–246.

Campos J, Musselman ED, Hanada S, Ueda K. Lung isolation techniques in patients with early-stage or long-term tracheostomy: a case series report of 70 cases and recommendations. *J Cardiothorac Vasc Anesth*. 2019;33(2):433–439.

Narayanaswamy M, McRae K, Slinger P, et al. Choosing a lung isolation device for thoracic surgery: a randomized trial of three bronchial blockers versus double-lumen tubes. *Anesth Analg*. 2009;108(4):1097–1101.

Sandberg WS. Endobronchial blocker dislodgement leading to pulseless electrical activity. *Anesth Analg*. 2005;100:1728–1730.

Shaw AD, Grichnik K, Barbeito A, Campos J. Lung separation techniques. In: Barbeito A, Shaw AD, Grichnik K, eds. *Thoracic Anesthesia*. McGraw Hill; 2012:83–104.

Arndt Bronchial Blocker

135

Sherif Assaad • Albert C. Perrino Jr

1 Describe in detail the device or technique.

The Arndt wire-guided endobronchial blocker was first introduced into clinical practice in 1999. The endobronchial blocker set is composed of a multiport airway adapter and the endobronchial blocker catheter (EBB).

The multiport airway adapter has three ports; one for attachment to the ventilatory circuit, one through which the EBB is inserted, and the third which provides a single central diaphragm port for insertion of the flexible bronchoscope (FB). The central diaphragm of the bronchoscopy port prevents air leak during mechanical ventilation when the bronchoscope is in use, while the EBB port has an adjustable gasket to snug the EBB tightly and prevent gas leak. When the EBB is removed, a significant airway leak will occur.

The EBB contains an internal lumen extending throughout its length that allows deflation of the nonventilated lung either passively or actively by applying suction through an adapter that is included in the set. Through another included adapter, this port can also be used to apply CPAP when indicated. For placement of the EBB, a nylon wire comes preloaded in the lumen of the catheter and extends out of the distal end of the lumen exposing a closed loop. The FB is passed through this loop and thereby, is used to guide the blocker into the desired lung to be deflated. This guide-loop nylon wire is pulled out after insertion of the EBB to allow deflation of the lung. The newer 9F Arndt blockers' nylon wire was modified to increase its stiffness such that it can be reinserted into the lumen. This feature permits bronchoscopic guided repositioning during the case if necessary.

The catheter is available in 3 sizes: 5F, 7F, and 9F. The 5F catheter can be inserted in 4.5 mm or larger internal diameter endotracheal tubes (ETTs), the 7F can be used with as small as a 6.0 mm internal diameter ETT, while for the 9F catheters, the smallest internal diameter ETT that can be used is 7.5 mm. The speed of gas exiting the nonventilated lung is directly proportional to the size of the catheter.

The EBB has a high-volume low-pressure balloon at its end. It is manufactured in two shapes, spherical and elliptical. The spherical balloon is typically 1 to 2 cm in length and is designed for blocking the right main stem bronchus while the elliptical balloon is longer and is designed for blocking the left main bronchus. The inflation volume of the balloon varies according to the size of the blocker. The 5F balloon is inflated with 0.5 to 2.0 cc, the 7F is inflated with 2.0 to 6.0 cc, the 9F spherical balloon is inflated with 4.0 to 8.0 cc while the 9F elliptical balloon is inflated with 6.0 to 12.0 cc. One should attempt to use the least volume to block the desired bronchus.

Technique of Insertion

Generously lubricate the bronchoscope, the EBB and the inside of the ETT with silicone-based lubricant. Our preferred approach is to first insert the catheter through the EBB port of the Arndt multiport airway adapter until the guide loop comes into view., Insert the FB through the central diaphragm of the adapter and pass it through the guide loop. The guide loop can be left loose over the FB or cinched into the FB by screwing the guide-loop port and pulling back on the snare. The adapter is then connected to the ETT and the ventilation circuit is connected to the ventilation port of the adapter. Both the FB and the EBB are advanced together till the carina is visualized. The FB is then advanced into the main bronchus that is required to be deflated. The guide-loop snare is loosened to allow the blocker to be advanced into the bronchus. The balloon is then inflated to ensure that it fills the endobronchial lumen and does not herniate into the main stem trachea. The blocker port of the adapter is then tightened to avoid air leak during mechanical ventilation and migration of the EBB.

2 Where or when is this device or technique used in airway management?

In patients with difficult airway, a single-lumen ETT can be inserted and the endobronchial blocker can be inserted after to achieve one-lung ventilation (OLV). In patients with tracheostomy, the multiport adapter is connected to the Shiley tracheostomy, and the EBB is inserted with the FB into the bronchus required to be deflated.

To achieve lobar blockade in patients who could not tolerate OLV, for example, operating on the contralateral side after a pneumonectomy or lung resection. The use of the double-blocker technique, for example, in patients in which the takeoff of the right upper lobe is very proximal in the right main stem bronchus or in patients in which the takeoff of the right upper lobe may take place from the distal trachea.

In patients requiring ventilation with small ETT or in pediatric patients, the internal diameter of the ETT might not allow the passage of both FB and EBB together, and hence, a new technique of extraluminal insertion of the Arndt-Blocker has been described. In this approach, the tip of the shaft of the EBB is bent to 30 to 45 degrees to facilitate steering of the blocker. The blocker is inserted first prior to the ETT. The EBB positioning can be modified subsequently using the FB passed through the ETT. In a study of adult patients undergoing thoracic surgery, the insertion of the extraluminal blocker was faster compared to the intraluminal insertion. There was no difference in the quality of lung isolation or the requirement for repositioning.

3 What distinguishes this device or technique from similar airway management methods?

The device is distinguished from other bronchial blockers by:

- The presence of the nylon guide-loop allows the FB to navigate the EBB under direct vision into the lung or portion of the lung that needs to be deflated in an easier and reliable manner.
- The spherical and elliptical-shaped balloons that are designed to suit the difference in morphology between the right and left main bronchi.
- The ability to reinsert the guide-loop nylon into the lumen to help repositioning of the blocker.
- The presence of 5F blocker that allows it to be used in pediatric patients.
- The ability to use this blocker for selective lobar blockade or double-blocker technique.
- Although the speed of lung deflation with EBB is slower, the quality of the OLV is similar to the other bronchial blockers or the double-lumen tubes. The Arndt EBB required more frequent repositioning during the OLV period.

Author Caveats

For right main stem deflation, the guide-loop is often not required to be used with the FB, as the blocker more frequently will pass into the right main stem without navigation. For left main stem bronchus or other portions of the lung that need to be deflated, snaring the guide loop tight around the tip of the FB and advancing both together minimizes hang-up at the carina. For left main stem bronchus or other portions of the lung that need to be deflated, we recommend using the 9F EBB to reinsert the guide-loop nylon into the lumen in case repositioning of the blocker is required during the case.

- The available small-sized catheter (5F) allows its use in pediatric patients.
- The nylon guide-loop helps the Arndt BB navigate into the left mainstem or other distant bronchi.
- The Arndt BB requires more frequent repositioning, especially when placed on the right side.
- *See Figure 135.1 and* ***Video 135.1*** *for additional details.*

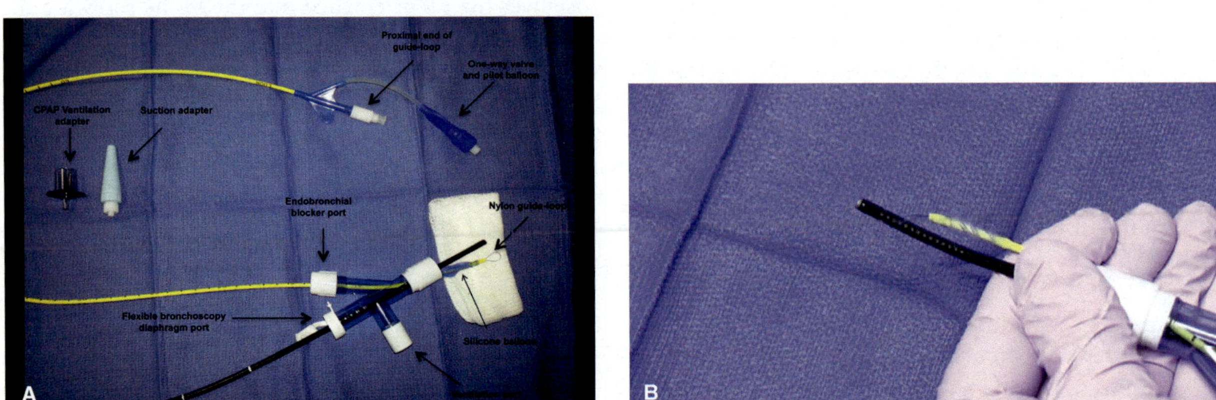

Figure 135.1. **A:** The elements of the Arndt Bronchial Blocker. **B:** Nylon loop of the Arndt Bronchial Blocker positioned over a flexible bronchoscope.

Suggested Readings

Dumans-Nizard V, Liu N, Laloë PA, Fischler M. A comparison of the deflecting-tip bronchial blocker with a wire-guided blocker or left-sided double-lumen tube. *J Cardiothorac Vasc Anesth.* 2009;23(4):501–505.

Narayanaswamy M, McRae K, Slinger P, et al. choosing a lung isolation device for thoracic surgery: a randomized trial of three bronchial blockers versus double-lumen tubes. *Anesth Analg.* 2009;108:1097–1101.

Neustein S. The use of bronchial blockers for providing one-lung ventilation. *J Cardiothorac Vasc Anesth.* 2009;23(6):860–868.

Templeton TW, Morris BN, Goenaga-Diaz EJ, et al. A prospective comparison of intraluminal and extraluminal placement of the 9-French Arndt bronchial blocker in adult thoracic surgery patients. *J Cardiothorac Vasc Anesth.* 2017;31(4):1335–1340.

Yao W, Qiu J, Wan L, Zhang C. A modified method of extraluminal placement of the 9 Fr Arndt bronchial blocker guided by Airtraq videolaryngoscopy in adult thoracic surgery. *J Cardiothorac Vasc Anesth.* 2019;33(4):1173–1175.

136

Cohen Bronchial Blocker

Javier H. Campos

1 Describe in detail the device or technique.

The Cohen blocker is an independent endobronchial blocker that is available only in size 9F and 65 cm length with an inner lumen measuring 1.4 mm in diameter. This device comes with a spherically shaped balloon that is considered a high-volume, low-pressure cuff. Near the distal end of the blocker, there are side holes incorporated to facilitate lung deflation. The characteristic of the Cohen blocker is that it relies on a wheel-turning device located in the most proximal part of the unit that allows deflection of the tip of the blocker into the desired bronchus. This device has been purposely preangled at the distal tip to facilitate insertion into a target bronchus. Also, there is a torque grip located at the 55-cm mark to allow the rotation of the blocker. At the distal tip of the blocker, above the balloon, there is an arrow that indicates in which direction the tip deflects. The Cohen blocker also comes with a multiport adaptor that facilitates an airtight seal. In addition, this blocker comes with a cone-shaped device that is attached to the proximal end, and when connected to suction, it expedites lung collapse.

Figure 136.1 shows the Cohen flexitip bronchial blocker (BB). Before insertion, the blocker balloon must be tested by fully inflating it prior to insertion to ensure that the balloon inflates and deflates properly. The Cohen blocker is advanced through a single-lumen endotracheal tube (ETT) of at least 8.0-mm internal diameter (ID).

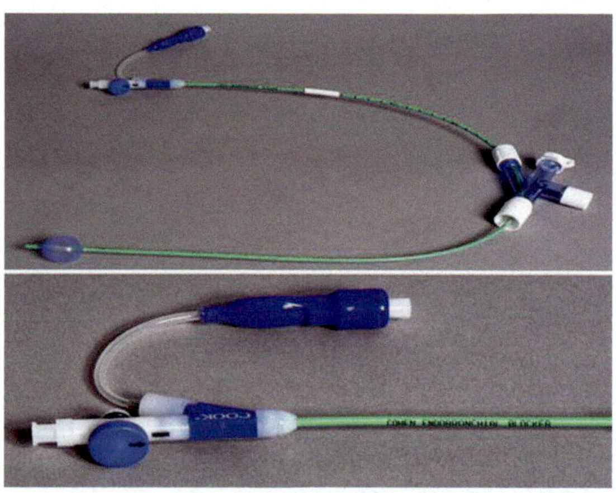

Figure 136.1. The Cohen Flexitip Endobronchial Blocker along with the multiport connector. Also the bottom picture shows the proximal end of the blocker with the twisting wheel device.

This blocker needs to be lubricated to facilitate insertion and passage through the single-lumen ETT. The deployment of the Cohen blocker involves placing the BB through the ETT and using the flexible bronchoscope (FB) to observe the passage of the blocker into the mainstem bronchus. Figure 136.2 shows a single-lumen ETT and the passage of the Cohen blocker.

Visualization with a FB of the optimal position of a Cohen blocker in the right mainstem bronchus is by observing the outer surface of the fully inflated balloon (4 to 8 mL of air) placed at least 10 mm below the tracheal carina. Figure 136.3 shows the optimal placement of the Cohen blocker into the right mainstem bronchus as seen with the FB.

Intubation of the left mainstem bronchus can be facilitated by allowing the tip of the single-lumen ETT to be near the entrance of the left bronchus, then twisting the Cohen blocker to the left side. After the blocker is seen inside the left bronchus, the single-lumen ETT is withdrawn a few centimeters so the tip of the tube is at least 3 cm above the tracheal carina. The optimal position is achieved when the blocker balloon's outer surface is seen with the FB at least 10 mm below the tracheal carina inside the left mainstem bronchus.

In some cases, the placement of the Cohen blocker in the left mainstem bronchus can be difficult. This fact is mainly due to the sharp angle of the bronchus in relationship to the trachea. In these cases, turning the

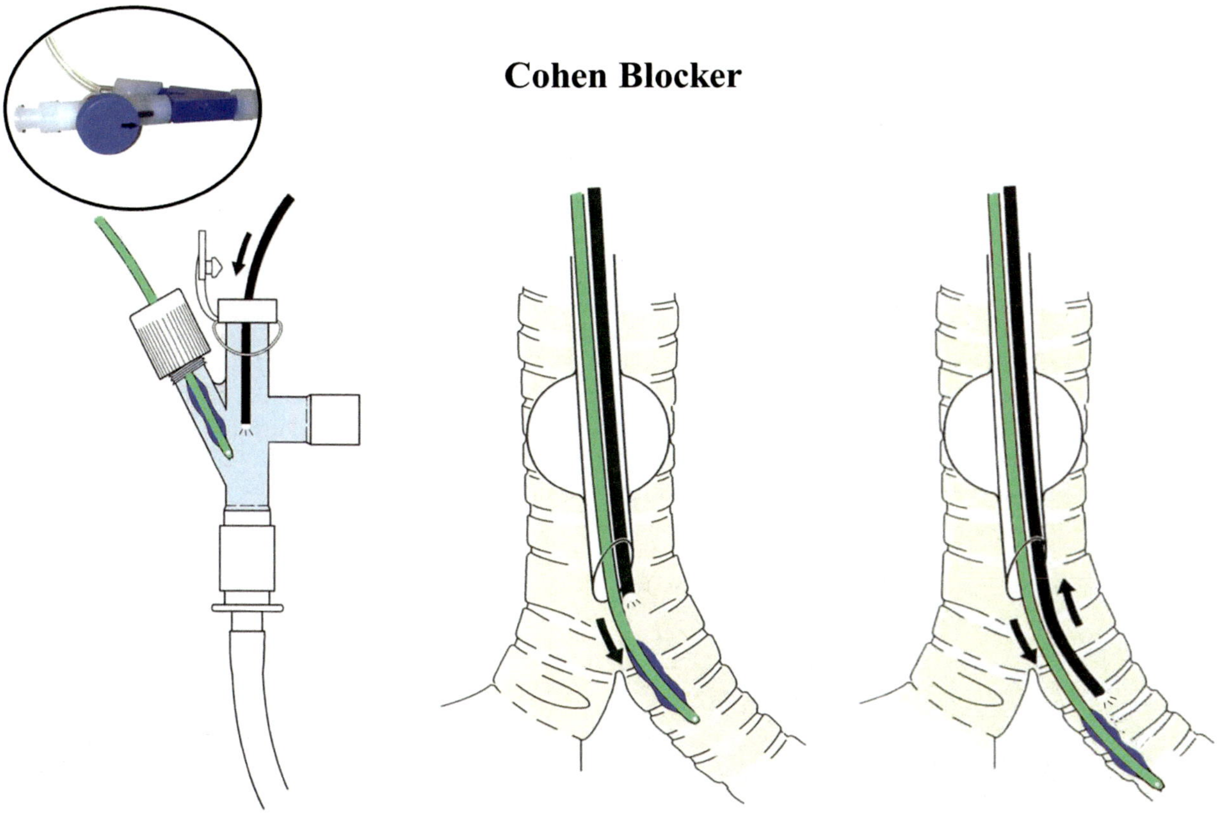

Figure 136.2. Placement of the Cohen Blocker through a single-lumen endotracheal tube (ETT) into the left mainstem bronchus. The twisting wheel device is displayed in the circle.

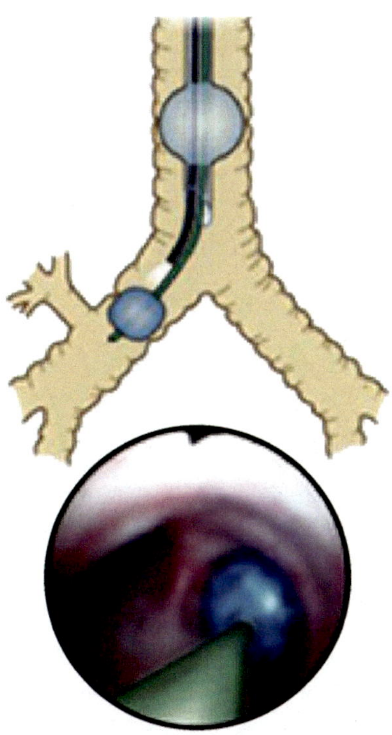

Figure 136.3. Placement of the Cohen Flexitip Endobronchial Blocker into the entrance of the right mainstem bronchus when seen with the fiberoptic bronchoscope.

patient into a right lateral decubitus position (with the left side up) will push the left bronchus into a midline position in relationship to the trachea. At this point, the Cohen blocker can be easily advanced under these circumstances under direct visualization with a FB.

2 Where or when is this device or technique used in airway management?

The Cohen blocker is an independent BB that is used to achieve one lung ventilation (OLV). It involves blockade of a mainstem bronchus to allow lung collapse distal to the occlusion. Its main uses are in procedures which require OLV, such as thoracic and esophageal surgery or open descending thoracic aneurysm repair. The use of a Cohen blocker is particularly advantageous in patients who present for surgeries requiring OLV and have a difficult airway that requires an awake oral or nasal intubation with a single-lumen ETT. After the ETT is safely placed with the patient awake, general anesthesia can be induced, and the blocker can be deployed in the desired bronchus, thus providing OLV conditions. Also, the Cohen blocker is commonly used in patients who have a tracheostomy in place and require OLV. The multiport adaptor can be easily connected to the cuffed Shiley disposable tracheostomy cannula as shown in Figure 136.4. Another important use of this device is in patients who have undergone thoracic surgery with OLV and need mechanical ventilation in the postoperative period. In such cases, removal of the BB and its adapter allows the existing single-lumen ETT to be left in place.

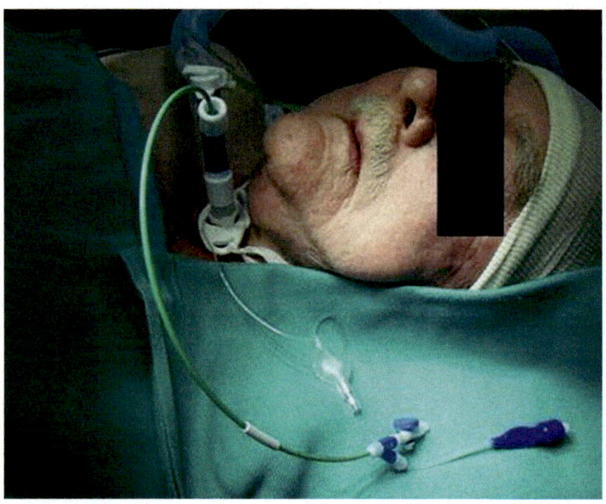

Figure 136.4. Cohen Flexitip Endobronchial Blocker placed via a multiport adapter in a patient with a preexisting tracheostomy.

3 What distinguishes this device or technique from similar airway management methods?

There are several advantages and disadvantages of the Cohen flexitip BB.

An advantage of the Cohen blocker is the fact that it is relatively soft in comparison to the stiffer blockers, such as the Fuji Uniblocker. In addition, the Cohen blocker does not require guidance via a nylon wire as does the Arndt blocker. Instead, it relies on the steering wheel device that deflects the tip into the desired bronchus. The tip of the blocker is seen with the FB while it advances into the targeted bronchus. Due to the fact that the blocker tip is distal to the FB, direct guidance is easily observed. The use of a Cohen blocker also allows for an easy recognition of the tracheal anatomy with the FB if the tip of the single-lumen ETT is above the carina and the blocker balloon is fully deflated. Another advantage of the Cohen flexitip blocker is the possibility to achieve selective lobar blockade in patients with previous lobectomy who require lung resection on the contralateral lung. Selective lobar blockade will maintain or improve oxygenation.

Disadvantages of the Cohen blocker include its small suctioning channel that could delay lung collapse as well as the possibility of dislodgement or loss of seal of the bronchial balloon. Another disadvantage is represented by the steering wheel that facilitates deflection of the blocker tip into the main bronchus. For the novice user, with limited experience with this device, manipulating the steering mechanism can be problematic.

- The Cohen flexitip BB is commonly used in patients requiring OLV and who present with a difficult airway necessitating an awake intubation.
- The Cohen flexitip BB relies on twisting the wheel to deflect the distal tip into the desired bronchus to be blocked.
- The Cohen flexitip BB has a high-volume, low-pressure cuff property. In addition, it has central and side holes in the distal tip that when connected to suction expedite lung collapse.
- A unique characteristic of the Cohen flexitip BB is its easiness to use in patients who have an existing tracheostomy in place and require lung isolation.
- *See Figure 136.5 and* ***Video 136.1*** *for additional details.*

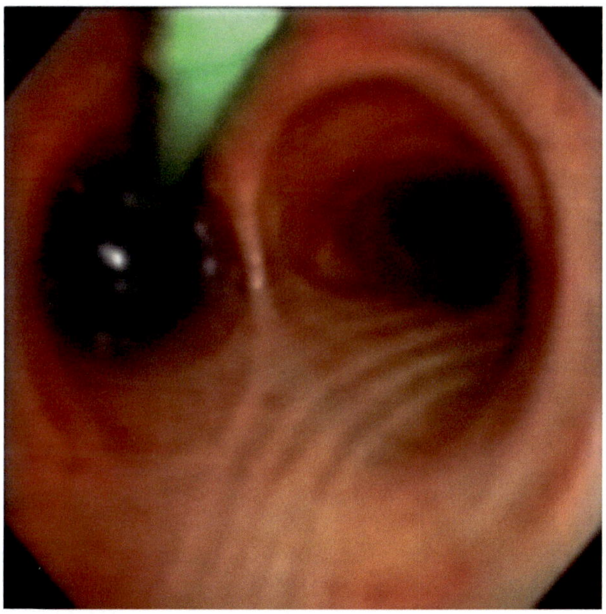

Figure 136.5. Cohen Flexitip Endobronchial Blocker in use.

Suggested Readings

Campos J. Lung isolation. In: Slinger P, ed. *Principles and Practice of Anesthesia for Thoracic Surgery.* 2nd ed. Springer; 2019:283–309.

Campos JH. Separation of the lung: double-lumen endotracheal tubes and endobronchial blocker. In: Cohen E, ed. *Cohen's Comprehensive Thoracic Anesthesia.* 1st ed. Elsevier Inc.; 2021:213–239.

Campos JH. Update on selective lobar blockade during pulmonary resections. *Curr Opin Anaesthesiol.* 2009;22:18–22.

Campos JH, Musselman ED, Hanada S, Ueda K. Lung isolation techniques in patients with early stage or long-term tracheostomy: a case series report of 70 cases and recommendations. *J Cardiothorac Vasc Anesth.* 2019;33:433–439.

Dumans-Nizard V, Liu N, Laloë PA, Fischler M. A comparison of the deflecting-tip bronchial blocker with a wire-guided blocker or left-sided double-lumen tube. *J Cardiothorac Vasc Anesth.* 2009;23:501–505.

137 EZ-Blocker

Katherine A. Michelini

1 Describe in detail the device or technique.

The EZ-blocker is a type of bronchial blocker used for one lung ventilation (OLV). It is a Y-shaped device with two symmetrical distal extensions that mirror the bifurcation of the trachea. Both ends are 4 cm long and are designed with an inflatable polyurethane spherical cuff and a central lumen. To facilitate identification, the central lumens and corresponding pilot balloons are color coded: one blue and the other yellow, yet both spherical cuffs are blue. Upon evaluating the EZ-blocker placement with flexible bronchoscope (FB), one balloon appears blue and the other one appears green (from the combination of the yellow central lumen with the overlaying blue cuff). The minimal occlusive volume for use in the left bronchus is 6.7 ± 1.16 mL and 8.0 ± 1.1 mL for use in the right bronchus. However, the best method to assess adequate cuff filling is direct evaluation with FB. The central lumens can also be used for oxygen administration, suction, or continuous positive airway pressure administration to the nonventilated lung. The device is manufactured in one size: 7F outer diameter and 750 mm in length. The required minimal inner diameter of the single-lumen endotracheal tube (ETT) is 7 mm.

The EZ-blocker has a three-way EZ-multiport adapter. The blocker is advanced through its designated port of the adapter. The bifurcated cuffs are naturally directed toward the left and right mainstem bronchi. The second port serves for FB control, and the third port is attached to the ETT and connected to the ventilator.

The device can be introduced blindly or under FB guidance. When the device is placed blindly, it should be advanced until slight resistance is met. This should correspond to the contact of the blocker bifurcation with the carina. However, flexible bronchoscopy is required to identify the position of the left and right cuffs.

2 Where or when is this device or technique used in airway management?

The EZ-blocker can serve as an alternative to any other BB in cases where expected or unexpected difficult intubation conditions preclude the use of a double lumen tube (DLT). In addition, the use of blockers avoids the need for tube exchange in patients who require postoperative mechanical ventilation. The device can be useful in emergency situations when immediate OLV is required and a 7.0 ETT is in situ. As compared to other BB, the use of this device is particularly suitable in cases of sequential OLV. A good example is bilateral thoracoscopic sympathectomy, as this device does not require repositioning from one bronchus to the other. One specific utility of the EZ-blocker is during minimally invasive esophagectomy in the prone position. Since the blocker is anchored to the carina, dislodgement requiring repositioning (extremely difficult in prone position) is avoided and the use of a DLT (high risk of kinking and bronchial injury in prone position) is unnecessary. Similarly, the blocker is frequently utilized during minimally invasive cardiac surgical procedures and procedures that require right lung deflation. The EZ-blocker has also been successfully utilized for bilateral apneic oxygenation during tracheal resection surgery.

Selective lobar blockade is unfeasible with the EZ-blocker, as the Y-shaped distal end makes it nearly impossible to advance the catheter beyond the left or right mainstem bronchi.

3 What distinguishes this device or technique from similar airway management methods?

The polyurethane cuff is a "high-pressure–low-volume cuff." Previous work with other BBs has demonstrated that only 10% to 20% of the intracuff pressure is transmitted to the bronchial mucosa. However, it is important not to exceed the maximum volume required to create a seal (in the left mainstem bronchus, 6.7-mL air generates intracuff pressures of 39.8 mm Hg, while in the right mainstem bronchus, 8.0-mL air generates intracuff pressures of 84.6 mm Hg).

When compared with the Cohen Flex-Tip blocker, fewer malpositionings occur with the EZ-blocker, due to its Y-shaped distal end that adds stability. Initial placement has also been shown to be easier.

Compared to the DLT, the EZ-blocker has a lower incidence of tracheobronchial hematomas. However, no difference in vocal cord injury was noted, but patients who received an EZ-blocker experienced less sore throat and hoarseness.

As with other BBs, there is no separate access to the ventilated lung during the procedure. Because strict lung separation and aspiration of the distal airways are difficult to achieve, this device is not recommended for use in lung transplantation or procedures with high risk of contralateral contamination.

Author Caveats

When the device is inserted blindly, the majority of malpositionings are related to both extensions entering the right mainstem bronchus. To permit the Y-shaped distal part to deploy properly, a minimum of 4 cm between the distal end of the ETT and the carina is required. In cases where the ETT is too close to the carina to allow deployment, temporary retraction of the ETT (even above the vocal cords) can facilitate deployment of the EZ blocker. Placement under FB guidance avoids this problem. Additionally, if the two distal ends are inserted in a *horizontal plane*, the likelihood of both entering the right mainstem bronchus is reduced.

Since the right mainstem bronchus is larger compared to the left one, more air is necessary for the right bronchial cuff to achieve the minimal occlusive volume. There is no relationship between the angle of the tracheal bifurcation and the volume necessary to occlude the bronchus.

In case of proximal branching of the right upper lobe, it is difficult to balance the proximal position of the cuff required to block this lobe with the risk of cuff herniation, and this increases the risk of tracheal herniation of the cuff. Labeling of the cuffs (left and right) after bronchoscopic control avoids confusion during the use of the device. It is obvious that both cuffs should never be inflated simultaneously, as this generates complete airway obstruction. Care should be taken to insert the BB through the central lumen of the ETT and not through the Murphy eye.

Due to concerns regarding cuff pressures and the associated risk of mucosal injury, it is important to inflate with the minimal volume necessary to occlude the bronchus. Clinically, the minimal volume is determined during two-lung ventilation in pressure-controlled mode. The appropriate cuff is slowly inflated until the delivered tidal volume is half of its initial value. Alternatively, the central lumen of the deflated lung is connected to the CO_2 sensor. With a well-isolated lung, no CO_2 should be detected. Additionally, cuff inflation can be directly observed using the FB, which is the preferred method.

Although the shaft of the EZ-blocker has two narrow lumens that open distal to the cuffs, accomplishing lung deflation through them is tedious. A better approach is to deflate both bronchial cuffs, disconnect the patient from the ventilator until lung collapse is achieved, then inflate the cuff of the lung desired to be isolated and initiate OLV. This technique allows for a rapid and qualitative lung collapse.

- The EZ-blocker is a Y-shaped symmetrical BB (Figure 137.1).
- The EZ-blocker is easy to position and has a lower incidence of dislodgements.
- The EZ-blocker has a high cuff pressure. To decrease the risk of mucosal injury, minimal occlusive volume assessment is mandatory.
- *See Figure 137.2 and* **Video 137.1** *for additional details.*

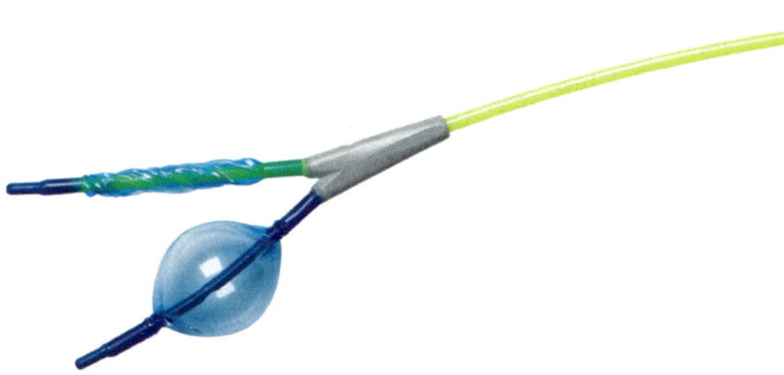

Figure 137.1. Bifurcation of the EZ-blocker right and left (inflated) arms.

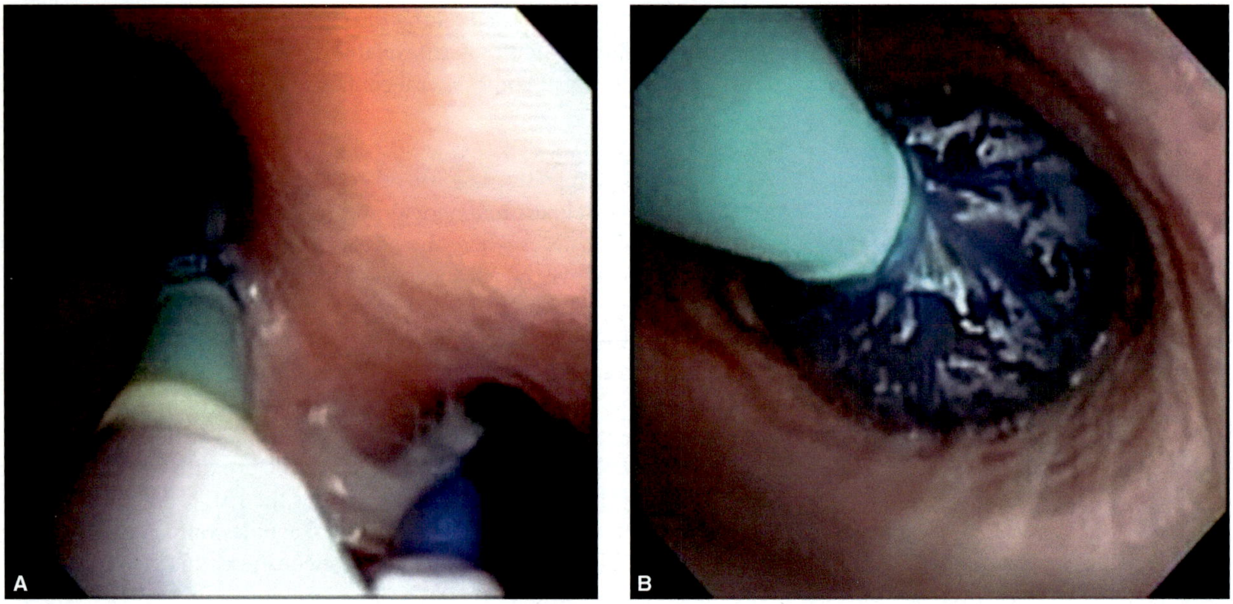

Figure 137.2. **A:** Flexible bronchoscope view of the EZ-blocker correctly positioned over the carina. **B:** The inflated cuff of the right-sided EZ-blocker arm.

Acknowledgments

We gratefully acknowledge the contributions of previous edition author, Arne Neyrinck, as portions of those chapters have been retained in this revision.

Suggested Readings

Kus A, Hosten T, Gurkan Y, Gul Akgul A, Solak M, Toker K. A comparison of the EZ-blocker with a Cohen Flex-tip blocker for one-lung ventilation. *J Cardiothorac Vasc Anesth*. 2014;28(4):896–869.

Mourisse J, Liesveld J, Verhagen A, et al. Efficiency, efficacy, and safety of EZ-blocker compared with left-sided double-lumen tube for one-lung ventilation. *Anesthesiology*. 2013;118:550–561.

Mungroop HE, WaiP T, Morei MN, Loef BG, Epema AH. Lung isolation with a new Y-shaped endobronchial blocking device, the EZ-Blocker. *Br J Anaesth*. 2010;104:119–120.

Rispoli M, Rossella Nespoli M, De Simone MG, Maria Mattiacci D, Buono S, Corcione A. EZ-Blocker in tracheal surgery. *J Cardiothorac Vasc Anesth*. 2015;29:e89–e90.

Ruetzler K, Grubhofer G, Schmid W, et al. Randomized clinical trial comparing double-lumen tube and EZ-Blocker for single-lung ventilation. *Br J Anaesth*. 2011;106:896–902.

Tang J, Merritt RE, Essandoh M. Entrapment of an EZ-blocker in the Murphy eye of an endotracheal tube. *J Cardiothorac Vasc Anesth*. 2019;33:2873–2874.

Endobronchial Tubes and Endobronchial Intubation

138

Arthur R. Formanek III • Philip M. Hartigan

1 Describe in detail the device or technique.

Endobronchial tube (EBT) is a general term for a ventilating tube positioned in a mainstem bronchus rather than the trachea. As such, they enable lung isolation and single-lung ventilation. Double-lumen tubes may be considered EBTs, but these are described separately in Chapters 125: Left-Sided Double-Lumen Tube and 126: Right-Sided Double-Lumen Tube. We shall limit this discussion to single-lumen tubes advanced to an endobronchial position, as well as indications, advantages, limitations, and technical points. While proprietary EBTs exist, any long, cuffed tube deliberately advanced into a mainstem bronchus may serve as an EBT (Figure 138.1).

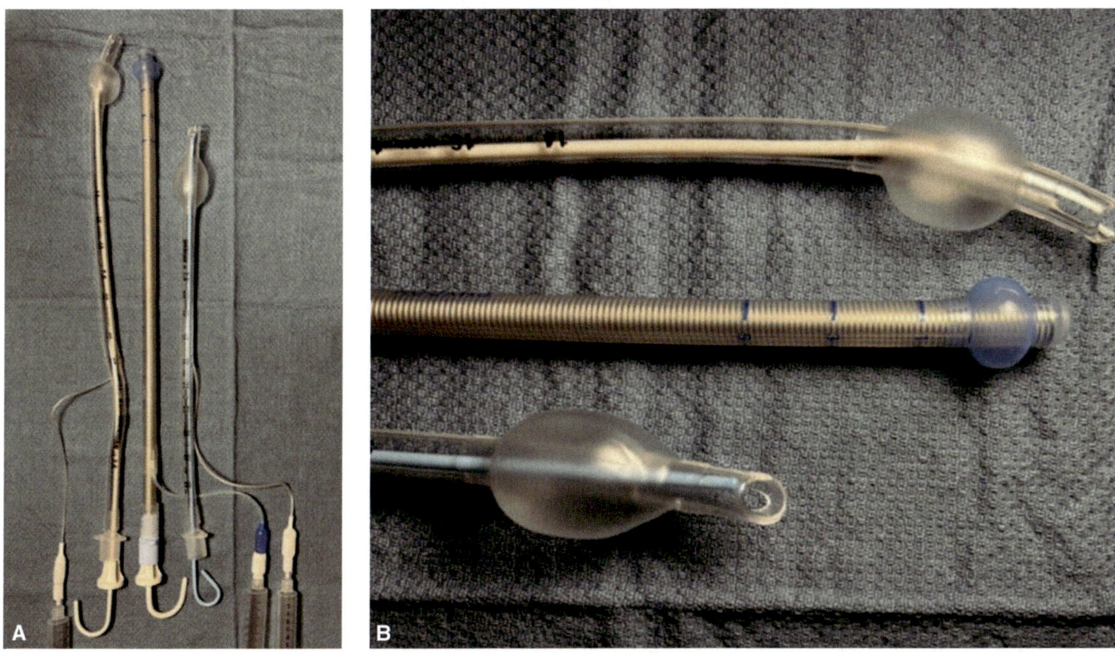

Figure 138.1. A: Examples of tubes used for endobronchial intubation with different lengths and different cuff-to-tip distances. Top to bottom: 7.5 mm OD Nasal RAE endotracheal tube, which has been straightened (Sheridan Preformed nasal Tube, Teleflex, Morrisville, NC); 7.5 mm OD Phycon (Phycon Wire Reinforced ETT with Cuff (Fuji Systems Corp, Fukushima, Japan); 7.5 mm OD Endotracheal Tube (Sheridan/HVT ETT, Teleflex, Morrisville, NC). **B:** Close-up view of the distal ends of the tubes displayed in **A**.

However, standard commercially available EBTs are longer and have a shorter, more spherical cuff as compared to regular ETTs. The short cuff of an EBT, which allows it not to protrude over the carina, comes at a cost. For cuffs to have a low-pressure/high-volume profile, it is required that a large surface area of the cuff be in contact with the airway mucosa, thereby distributing the pressure over a larger area. However, short cuffs distribute the pressure over a smaller area, and thus require higher pressures to achieve an air seal. Also, small tubes within large lumens may require overinflation to achieve an air seal. Mucosal ischemic injury may result from excessive cuff pressure, a prolonged period of inflation, and low mucosal arteriolar perfusion pressure. If such risk is suspected, intermittent inflation "vacations" are recommended (brief periods of apnea with cuff deflation).

While proprietary EBTs have sufficient length, they may be so flexible that despite fixing the tube at the incisors, the tip may back out of the bronchus into an endotracheal position and assume a greater curvature within the pharynx. In order to prevent this issue, some commercially available EBTs (WRETT, Ambu Fuji Systems Solutions) are made of silicone rubber and have wire-reinforced walls. This provides added stability of the tube during manipulation and warmth. The cuff of these tubes can provide adequate seal in both a bronchial as well as a tracheal position. The commercially available adult sizes of these EBTs are 5.5, 6.5, and 7.5.

Endobronchial intubation can be performed quickly and simply in most situations when emergent lung isolation is required, including in locations where a double lumen tube (DLT) may not be immediately available. For example, an intubated patient who develops massive hemoptysis or airway collapse may be converted to endobronchial intubation without exchanging tubes (assuming sufficient length of endotracheal tube [ETT] in place). This may be performed blindly for right endobronchial intubations, but for left endobronchial intubations, one must generally guide the tube over a bronchoscope. Blind left mainstem intubation may be achieved by rotating an ETT 180 degrees such that the bevel favors the left, and simultaneously turning the head to the right while advancing the tube. In either case, bronchoscopic evaluation is advised to confirm position and assess depth relative to the secondary carina.

The principal limitations of an EBT are that one cannot ventilate the opposite bronchus or bronchoscopically visualize the carina and opposite bronchus to directly assess tube position. Confirmation of appropriate depth and cuff position must be performed radiographically, or deduced from depth of insertion at the incisors, auscultation, or from the distance to the secondary carina when looking through the lumen of the tube itself. In adults, the distance from the lower border of the larynx to carina is 10 to 12 cm, depending on the height of the patient. Vocal cords are approximately 2 cm above the lower border of the larynx. Thus 12 to 14 cm is the typical distance between vocal cords and carina in adults. However, the distance from the upper incisors to the vocal cords will vary depending on pharyngeal anatomy and neck position. Generally, an EBT needs to be at least 30 cm to reach an endobronchial position, or more, depending upon the amount of curvature that the EBT takes within the mouth and the cuff design. Nasal right angle endotracheal tube (RAE) ETTs when straightened out and passed orally have sufficient length to become EBTs, but the tendency of the curvature to reassert itself may lead to the cuff backing out of the bronchus despite firmly affixing the tube at the incisors. Other disadvantages of an EBT are that the cuff may obstruct the right upper lobe during right endobronchial intubations. This is mitigated by the short cuff length of some proprietary EBTs.

2 Where or when is this device used?

There is overlap in the indications for EBTs and DLTs, but generally, EBTs should be considered when a DLT is either unavailable or there is need for a large lumen for effective suctioning. Patients with very difficult anatomy for intubation with a DLT, or who have a deviated trachea, shifted carina, or retracted bronchus, may be isolated more easily with an endobronchial intubation instead of a DLT. Specific situations where the use of an EBT may be considered include the following:

- Massive hemoptysis
- Traumatic bronchial disruption from deceleration injury
- Acute bronchopleural fistula with large air leak
- Rescue maneuver to stent open a collapsed airway (eg, mediastinal mass syndrome)
- Tracheal resection/reconstruction surgery
- Pediatric thoracic surgery where an appropriate-sized DLT is not available
- Lung isolation where a DLT is either unavailable or problematic due to anatomy

In massive hemoptysis from an endobronchial biopsy or tumor, contralateral endobronchial intubation allows effective suctioning of blood, isolation from further contamination, and single-lung ventilation. Alternatively, endobronchial intubation may be performed to the bleeding bronchus, positioning the cuff to tamponade the source of hemorrhage. The larger lumen of a single-lumen EBT is an advantage over DLTs for suctioning blood and organized clots. When a massive air leak from a bronchial disruption or large acute bronchopleural fistula precludes effective ventilation with an endotracheal tube, endobronchial intubation to the opposite bronchus may be lifesaving. Driving the EBT over a bronchoscope under direct vision would be advised to prevent inadvertent further disruption of the affected bronchus.

Extrinsic compression of the distal trachea and one or both mainstem bronchi from a mediastinal mass can occur with induction or at any time after general anesthesia induction. Advancing a single-lumen tube beyond the level of extrinsic compression to stent open the airway is one of several suggested rescue maneuvers.

In tracheal resection/reconstruction surgery, there may be times when the endotracheal tube needs to be advanced to an endobronchial position while the trachea is divided and opened. There may also be a need for a distally positioned tube following anastomosis, to protect the anastomosis from positive pressure ventilation or direct pressure from the cuff of a conventional tube. EBTs may be useful in such situations. Cross-field ventilation, jet ventilation, or extracorporeal oxygenation may be used in concert with, or instead of, EBT in such cases.

3 What distinguishes this device from similar airway management methods?

Standard ETTs have such a long cuff and long distance from cuff-to-tip that when used as an EBT, there is danger that the tip may extend beyond the secondary carina, or that the cuff is half above the carina and half within the bronchus. In addition, the length of standard ETTs may not be sufficient for endobronchial intubations. Do-it-yourself techniques for creating tube extensions have been described but are not endorsed by these authors. It should be noted that 8.5 mm outer diameter (OD) standard ETTs may not fit within the smaller lumen of the left mainstem of a normal-sized adult.

Suggested Readings

Kubota H, Kubota Y, Toyoda Y, Ishida H, Asada A, Matsuura H. Selective blind endobronchial intubation in children and adults. *Anesthesiology*. 1987;67:587–589.

Lin W-L, Cheng C-H. Predicting optimal insertion depth of a left-sided double-lumen endotracheal tube. *J Cardiothorac Vasc Anesth*. 2016;30(4):942–946.

139 Double-Lumen Tube to Single-Lumen Tube Exchange

Jan Ehrenwerth

Clinical Scenario: A 43-year-old man has undergone a 10-hour en bloc resection of the right upper lobe and first rib. Three years ago, the patient underwent a thyroidectomy and right neck dissection. He received radiation therapy 6 months ago, and since then has felt a significant stiffness in his neck. He is morbidly obese and has obstructive sleep apnea. For this procedure, a double-lumen tube (DLT) was placed awake using an flexible bronchoscope (FB). At the end of the procedure, the patient has a rapid shallow breathing pattern. The decision is made to keep the patient intubated and transfer him to the ICU.

1 What are the anesthetic and airway management considerations for this case?

This case presents a major challenge for the anesthesiologist. Not only is the patient morbidly obese and a known difficult intubation, but he also has had radiation therapy to his neck and undergone a lengthy surgical procedure. The prolonged surgery can result in significant swelling of the oropharyngeal soft tissues. It would be desirable to extubate this patient at the end of the case; however, his medical history and current breathing pattern make him a poor candidate for extubation.

A trial extubation can be attempted. However, failing to reintubate him and losing the airway is a real possibility. In addition, with this patient's history, it may be impossible to perform an emergency tracheotomy.

2 How would you manage the airway in this case?

Since this patient will be left intubated, it is desirable to change the double-lumen tube (DLT) to a single-lumen endotracheal tube (ETT). An attempt should be made to assess the airway. This can be performed by trying to visualize the larynx using direct laryngoscopy and following the path of the DLT. The patient will require anesthesia and muscle relaxation to facilitate visualization of the larynx and to avoid a sympathetic response to laryngoscopy. If this technique is not successful, a video laryngoscope can be utilized.

The degree of swelling can be determined visually. If there is massive swelling, the practitioner needs to decide whether or not to attempt the exchange of the DLT to an ETT. This is a risk/benefit decision. Since nursing personnel may not be familiar with a DLT, sending the patient to the ICU with this tube incurs a risk. However, this must be balanced against the risk of being unable to exchange the DLT and completely losing the airway. As the patient has the airway secured, the anesthesiologist must have a high degree of certainty that the DLT can be successfully changed to an ETT.

If, during direct laryngoscopy, the larynx can be visualized, then an assistant can remove the DLT, while the anesthesiologist watches and then immediately places the ETT. There is a small chance that once the DLT is removed, the anesthesiologist may lose sight of the larynx. Therefore, it is prudent to first insert an airway exchange catheter (AEC). This can be done in two ways. If the larynx is easily visualized, the AEC can be placed alongside the DLT, after the tracheal and bronchial cuffs are deflated. The DLT is removed, and if the anesthesiologist is not able to place the ETT directly, then the tube can be threaded over the AEC. However, the AEC may be dislodged when the DLT is removed. Also, the anesthesiologist may not have actually placed the AEC in the trachea before removing the DLT.

The more utilized method is placing the AEC into the DLT. There are several important things to remember when using this strategy. First, the AEC must be placed down the bronchial lumen of the DLT and needs to be twice the length of the tube that is being removed. Therefore, a special AEC, typically 100 cm in length and labeled "for use with a DLT," should be utilized. In the opposite case, where an ETT is being exchanged for a DLT, then a shorter (about 80 cm) AEC can be used.

3 What are the potential hazards and complications in regard to the airway?

The major hazard of exchanging the DLT for an ETT is losing the airway. In order to safely perform this exchange, the diameter of the AEC should be close to the internal diameter of the bronchial lumen. This must be confirmed before the tube exchange is attempted. If the AEC is too small, it can be dislodged during the exchange, or the new tube may not follow it into the trachea. The AEC should be lubricated (preferably with silicon) before it is placed into the bronchial lumen.

The AEC can cause perforation of the tracheobronchial tree resulting in a pneumothorax, which has been reported in 1.5% of attempted tube exchanges. Therefore, the AEC should never be forced once resistance is met. The catheter has markings on it, so the insertion depth can be monitored and should not be placed into the trachea beyond 25 cm at the teeth.

Placing a tube over the AEC does not always go smoothly. The ETT may meet resistance at the glottic level. This can be overcome by rotating the tube clockwise or counterclockwise while trying to advance it. Another recommendation is to use a laryngoscope or video laryngoscope to elevate the tongue and soft tissues, which can help the tube pass from the pharynx into the larynx. After the AEC is withdrawn from the single or DLT, the catheter must be carefully inspected to ensure that tip was not broken off during the procedure.

4 What distinct airway device might be used in this case, and what are the special considerations?

An FB can be used to accomplish the tube exchange. The FB is preloaded with a single-lumen ETT and placed alongside the DLT. The tracheal cuff of the DLT is deflated, and the FB is then advanced beyond the cuff. The DLT can then be removed, and the single-lumen ETT advanced into the trachea. This is a technically difficult maneuver, as the FB may be dislodged when the DLT is removed.

More commonly, an AEC is used for the tube exchange. AECs have a lumen that allows jet ventilation. This is useful in situations where the tube does not follow the AEC and ventilation is necessary. The jet ventilator must be assembled and ready to use beforehand. The inflation pressure is set to 25 to 50 psi on the regulator. A short inspiratory time is used, and the chest wall observed for movement. The expiratory time should be long enough for the patient to completely exhale. The anesthesiologist needs to remember that exhalation is passive, and the vocal cords must be relaxed in order to prevent barotrauma. The AEC should not be positioned in a bronchus, as this could lead to barotrauma.

When leaving a patient intubated after thoracic surgery, the anesthesiologist must carefully evaluate the risks and benefits of exchanging a DLT for a single-lumen ETT. If there is any doubt about the ability to exchange the tube, then the patient should be taken to the ICU with the DLT in place.

- Careful assessment of the airway prior to attempting a tube exchange is necessary.
- The proper size and length of the AEC should be verified prior to removing the DLT.
- Always perform the safest maneuver first and have a backup plan.
- Never risk losing the airway when the patient has a secure airway with a DLT.
- *See Figure 139.1 and* ***Video 139.1*** *for additional details.*

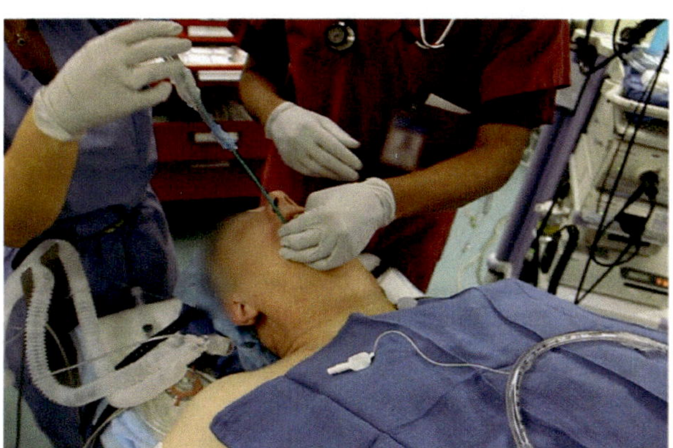

Figure 139.1. A double-lumen tube has been removed using a specialized tube exchanger. A single-lumen tracheal tube will be advanced over the exchange catheter.

Suggested Readings

Brodsky JB. Lung separation and the difficult airway. *Br J Anaesth.* 2009;103(1):i66–i75.

Fetterman D, Dubovoy A, Reay M. Unforeseen esophageal misplacement of airway exchange catheter leading to gastric perforation. *Anesthesiology.* 2006;104:1111–1112.

McLean S, Lanam CR, Benedict BS, Kirkpatrick N, Kheterpal S, Ramachandran SK. Airway exchange failure and complications with the use of the Cook Airway Exchange Catheter: a single center cohort study of 1177 patients. *Anesth Analg.* 2013; 117:1325–1327.

Thomas V, Neustein SM. Tracheal laceration after the use of an airway exchange catheter for double-lumen tube placement. *J Cardiothorac Vasc Anesth.* 2007;21:718–719.

Single Lumen Tube to Double Lumen Tube Exchange

140

Felice Eugenio Agrò • Sabrina Migliorelli

1 Describe in detail the device or technique.

Difficult airway management is a challenging aspect of daily anesthetic practice and is even more challenging when the surgery demands placement of a double-lumen tube (DLT). Intubating with a DLT can be more difficult than intubation with a single-lumen endotracheal tube. The larger size, the rigidity, and the shape of the DLT without a bevel at the tip of the tube can obscure the view of the glottis. In practice, in patients with an anticipated difficult airway, endotracheal tube can be placed with various techniques during an awake fiberoptic bronchoscopy or after induction of general anesthesia. One suggested strategy is to intubate the trachea with a single-lumen endotracheal tube and then to exchange the single-lumen tube (SLT) for a DLT over an airway exchange catheter (AEC), aided by visualization with a video laryngoscope.

Changeover of the SLT to a DLT through a tube exchanger catheter is a major challenge and needs technical skills.

For an AEC to work, it must have a hollow center channel and universal adapter to insufflate oxygen. The exchange catheter must have a flexible tip distally to avoid airway lacerations, be long in length, and have outer markings to control the depth of insertion while in use. For a DLT, the exchange catheter should be at least 83 cm long. A 14-Fr AEC can be used to facilitate insertion of 39- and 41-Fr DLTs. For a 35- or 37-Fr DLT, an 11-Fr AEC can be used. A sniffing position will facilitate tube exchange. After the AEC is lubricated, it is advanced through a single-lumen endotracheal tube. The airway catheter should not be inserted deeper the 24 cm from the lips to avoid incidental rupture or laceration of the trachea. After cuff deflation, the single-lumen endotracheal tube is withdrawn, then the endobronchial lumen of the DLT is advanced over the exchange catheter (Figure 140.1).

It is optimal to use a video laryngoscope during the tube exchange to guide the DLT through the glottis under direct vision (Figure 140.2). Proper final position of the DLT is then achieved with auscultation, presence of end-tidal carbon dioxide ($ETCO_2$) waveform, and a fiberoptic bronchoscopy examination through the DLT's tracheal tube.

2 Where or when is the device used in airway management?

Lung separation techniques are designed to facilitate surgical exposure and provide one-lung ventilation (OLV) in patients undergoing thoracic, mediastinal, vascular, esophageal, or selective spine surgery. Lung separation can be achieved with two different techniques. The first involves the double-lumen DLT technique. This device is made of disposable polyvinyl, chloride material, or silicone material. The DLT is a bifurcated tube with both an endotracheal and an endobronchial lumen and can be used to achieve the separation of either the right or left lung. The second technique involves using a bronchial blocker (BB) to block the mainstream bronchus to allow lung collapse distal to the occlusion. Both DLTs and BBs are termed difficult (to insert) tubes because they have an increased outside diameter (OD), which makes them relatively harder to put into a hole of a given size, and an increased overall rigidity, which impairs optimal shaping of the tube.

According to recent surveys in the United Kingdom, Italy, the Middle East, and a survey conducted by the European Association of Cardiothoracic Anesthesiologists, DLTs are preferred by a large majority of thoracic anesthesiologists (more than 90%).

The most common indications for lung separation and OLV are for providing a still operative field and surgical exposure or for lung isolation, for prevention of contamination to the contralateral lung from bleeding or pus material, and during the application of differential lung ventilation or for continuing of the airway gas exchange, such as bronchopleural fistula, and during a lung lavage.

In patients who require OLV and present with a difficult airway, the primary initial goal is to establish an airway with a single-lumen endotracheal tube. Occasionally, a patient who requires a difficult tube will also have a difficult airway.

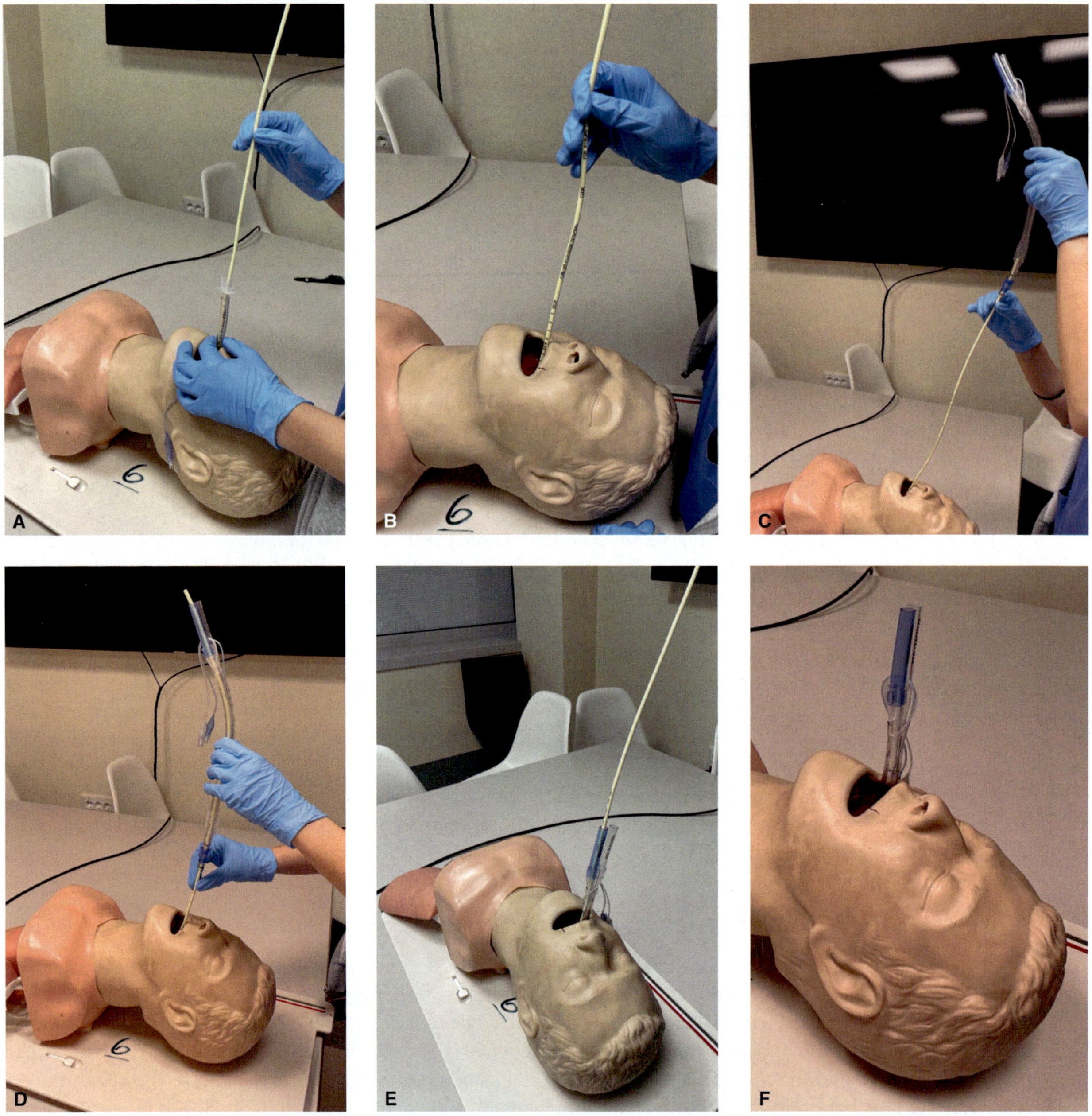

Figure 140.1. Sequence of steps for single-lumen to double-lumen tube (SLT and DLT) exchange, through the external view. **A:** The airway exchange catheter is in the single-lumen tube (SLT); **B:** The SLT is withdrawn and the airway exchange catheter remains in the respiratory tree; **C, D:** The DLT is advanced over the exchange catheter through the endobronchial lumen; **E, F:** The DLT is in place.

3 What distinguishes this device or technique from similar airway management methods?

Successful lung isolation can be achieved by using one (or two simultaneous) BB. BB is structurally similar to the AEC used for the tube exchange with the difference of having a thin polyurethane cuff at the distal end and a fixing system to connect it to the SLT at the proximal end.

Use BB instead of DLT offers the advantage of being placed through a conventional SLT. However, it absolutely requires fiberoptic guidance. In emergency situations, securing the airways is a priority, and this is performed easier and faster with an SLT for all anesthesiologists. Moreover, in patients with abnormal airway anatomy (postlaryngeal/pharyngeal surgery, tracheotomy or abnormal anatomy, eg, porcine trachea), predicted difficult intubation or at risk of vocal cord injuries (eg, singers) as well as in children, BBs are most suitable for lung separation as far as the chest wall and lungs compliances are normal. Likewise, if postoperative

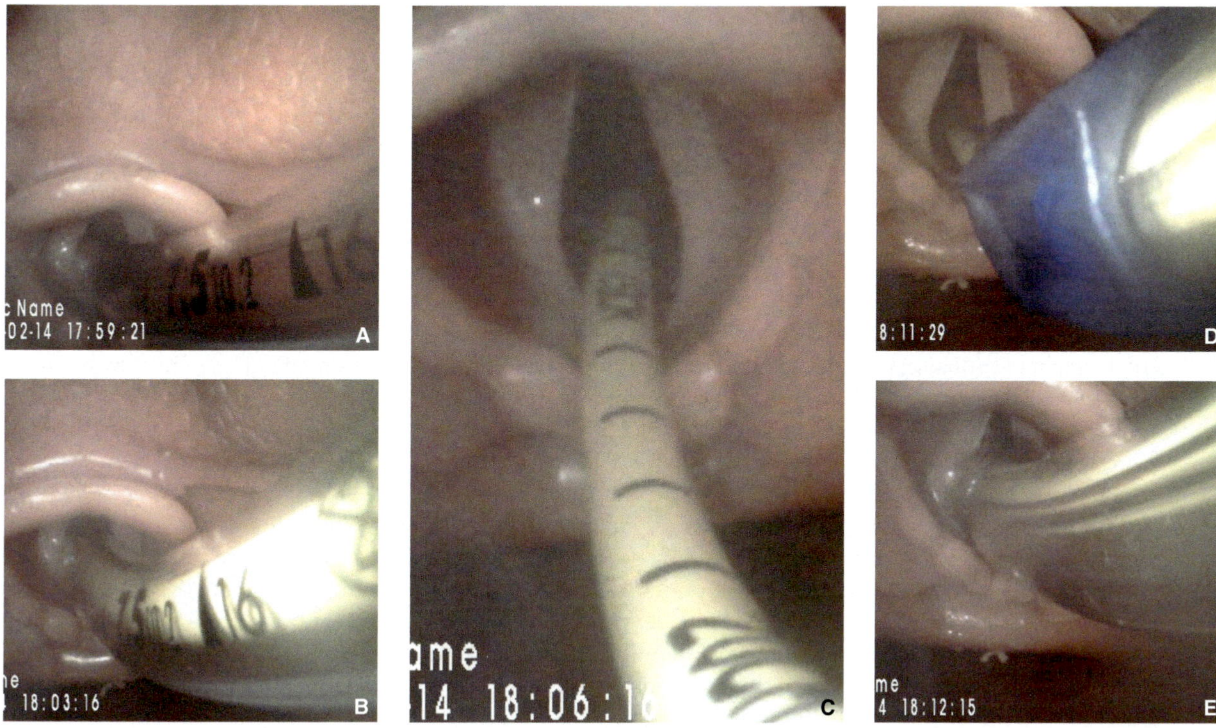

Figure 140.2. Sequence of steps for single-lumen to double-lumen tube (SLT and DLT) exchange, through the internal view of the glottis. **A:** The SLT is in place, between the vocal cords; **B:** The airway exchange catheter is in the SLT; **C:** The airway exchange catheter remains in the respiratory tree, after removing the SLT; **D:** The DLT is over the exchange catheter through the endobronchial lumen, it is possible to see the blue endobronchial cuff that will be cuffed in the left bronchus; **E:** The DLT is in place.

ventilation is needed, the use of a BB is a good choice, avoiding the dangerous replacement of the DLT by an SLT with an AEC. Eventually, BBs remain the only option in children and in patients who have undergone pneumonectomy and those requiring selective lobar exclusion (eg, severe lung disease).

Transient symptoms such as sore throat (10% to 45%), voice hoarseness (15% to 25%) and irritative cough have been more frequently reported in the literature postoperatively with DLTs than with SLTs combined with BBs. Likewise, a higher incidence of mucosal damage and hematoma has been observed within the larynx and the trachea-bronchial tree following the utilization of DLTs versus BBs.

On the other hand, with BB, small suction channel does not allow drainage of fluids; inadvertent resection of the guide wire and stapling the distal tip of the BB have been reported that required surgical reexploration. Intraoperative displacement or loss of seal and difficulties in repositioning are more frequent with BB than with DLT. Near-fatal hypoxic complications may also result from dislodgment of the inflated BB balloon into the trachea, leading to complete airway obstruction or severe gas trapping into the lungs associated with cardiovascular collapse.

Author Caveats

DLTs can be placed directly either with direct or video laryngoscopy, in order to facilitate passage of the tube over the airway guide past supraglottic tissues. Based on the author's experience, although visualizing the glottis with a video laryngoscope is usually straightforward, direct DLT intubation with a video laryngoscope is often difficult and tricky in a patient with a difficult airway. When a DLT fails to pass the laryngeal inlet, it is usually because the tip of the tube has engaged the right vocal cord or arytenoid; the correct maneuver is a 90-degree counterclockwise rotation of the tube, which rotates the tip from a 3 o'clock to a 12 o'clock position. The risk of a tube falling to pass the laryngeal inlet is minimized by using a relatively small tube and a relatively large airway guide or a specific intubation stylet designed for DLT placement with a GlideScope, the GlideRite DLT Stylet to facilitate intubation.

The size of the airway guide and the size of the difficult tube must be determined. The best chance of any tube reliably following an airway guide into the trachea occurs when the airway guide has a relatively large outer diameter (OD) and the tube has a relatively small internal diameter (ID). The suggestion to use concentrically arranged airway guides (4.0 and 7.0 mm OD) is unique and should help to minimize any discrepancy between the OD of the airway guide and the ID of the tube.

The airway guide should never be inserted against resistance, although the tips of the commercially made tube exchangers and flexible bronchoscope (FB) are somewhat rounded and blunt. The risk of perforation is also related to the depth of insertion of the airway guide. For this reason, during insertion of the airway guide, the clinician must always be aware of the depth of insertion. Excessive depth of insertion (ie, subcarinal or >26 cm) increases the risk of tracheobronchial tree perforation and barotrauma with jet ventilation.

In addition, a jet ventilator should be immediately available in case the new tube does not follow the airway guide into the trachea, and the jet ventilator should be preset at 25 psi by the use of an additional in-line regulator. Use of a jet ventilator with an additional in-line regulator allows for a breath-by-breath increase in tidal volume if clinically judged to be necessary. in addition, the upper airway should be made maximally patent during jet ventilation by putting the patient in an optimal "sniffing" position, use of bilateral jaw thrust and oropharyngeal airways, and by avoiding jet ventilation during phonation. The safe use of an airway guide for ventilation may allow time for the safe use of an alternative reintubation strategy, such as the use of an FB or a surgical airway.

Finally, if the combination of airway guide and tube creates a sufficiently large annular space between them, then the annular space can be used for capnographic and clinical confirmation that tracheal reintubation has occurred. This can be accomplished by passing the airway guide through the self-sealing diaphragm of a bronchoscopy elbow and ventilating around the airway guide, but within the lumen of the tube. The great benefit of this procedure is that the clinician does not need to remove the airway guide and give up its known intratracheal location to find out if tracheal reintubation has occurred.

There are other different clinical situations in which the AEC is useful, for example in changing of DLT for an SLT at the end of complicated or prolonged surgery in a patient that requires mechanical ventilation in the postoperative period, as in the large esophageal surgery, in order to avoid the incidence of airway compression damage, edema, or hematoma due to a DLT.

AEC could also play an important role as part of an extubation strategy when managing difficult airways that may require reintubation. It is included in all the guidelines on tracheal extubation. This may occur after certain surgeries, such as head and neck surgery, in patients whom tracheal intubation has been difficult or in patients with prolonged tracheal intubation in critical care. AECs are placed prior to extubation and retained in situ after extubation and they act as a conduit for an endotracheal tube, if reintubation is required.

- In patients who require OLV and present with a difficult airway, the primary initial goal is to establish an airway with a single-lumen endotracheal tube.
- Proper use of airway guides could improve the successful use of "difficult tubes" (such as DLTs) in patients with difficult airways.
- It is optimal to use a video laryngoscope during the tube exchange to guide the DLT through the glottis under direct vision.
- Be careful not to lose the airway when changing tubes.
- *See* ◉ ***Video 140.1*** *for additional details.*

Suggested Readings

Benumof JL. Difficult tubes and difficult airways. *J Cardiothorac Vasc Anesth.* 1998;12:131–132.

Brodsky JB. Lung separation and the difficult airway. *Br J Anaesth.* 2009;103:i66–i75.

Campos JH. Lung isolation in patients with difficult airway in thoracic anesthesia. In: Cohen E, ed. *Comprehensive Thoracic Anesthesia*. Elsevier; 2021:240–248.

Campos JH. Lung isolation techniques for patients with difficult airway. *Curr Opin Anaesthesiol.* 2010;23:12–17.

Gamez R, Slinger P. A simulator study of tube exchange with three different designs of double-lumen tubes. *Anesth Analg.* 2014; 119:449–453.

Tracheoplasty for Tracheobronchial Malacia

141

John B. Pawlowski

Clinical Scenario: A 60-year-old man with morbid obesity presents for right thoracotomy for tracheoplasty. He has obstructive sleep apnea and a long-standing history of persistent cough and decreased exercise tolerance. He was diagnosed with tracheobronchial malacia (TBM) and had undergone several stent placements with moderate improvement of his symptoms.

1 What are the anesthetic and airway management considerations for this case?

TBM is a softening of the intrathoracic or extrathoracic portions of the trachea and/or bronchus. The softening of the intrathoracic airway leads to collapse of the airway during exhalation (see Chapter 122: Interventional Management of Tracheomalacia). Patients with TBM often present with symptoms of dyspnea, cough, retention of secretions, and recurrent infections. While conventional spirometry shows varying results, an expiratory chest x-ray or expiratory CT scan reveals severe collapse of the large airways. A dynamic CT with an expiratory phase best demonstrates TBM. These patients may also have significant smoking history or cardiovascular comorbidities.

The anesthetic considerations regarding a tracheoplasty surgery are the need for lung isolation, continuous hemodynamic monitoring, and reliable extubation at the conclusion of the case. A FB is of critical importance during this case as it is utilized during initial placement of the endotracheal tube and for repeated tube repositioning, as well as for pulmonary toilet. Adequate postoperative pain control is an important determinant of extubation at the completion of the case. Therefore, a thoracic epidural is recommended in such procedures.

2 How would you manage the airway in this case?

A tracheoplasty procedure requires access to the posterior aspect of the tracheobronchial tree, which is accomplished via a right thoracotomy approach extending to the posterior thorax. This procedure can also be performed using robotic assistance via a right-sided approach. The airway management requires a standard endotracheal tube (8.0 or 8.5 mm) with bronchial blocker. The ETT is advanced to the mid-tracheal position. The bronchial blocker is positioned using FB, such that the bronchial cuff can both occlude the right upper lobe and the bronchus intermedius. This allows the surgeon to suture the mesh to the posterior airway. Left lung ventilation is initiated at the beginning of the procedure by inflating the bronchial blocker cuff. Active suction is needed to deflate the right lung and is applied to the lumen of the bronchial blocker.

Patients with TBM have abundant, thick secretions. In order for the patient to adequately tolerate OLV, a constant pulmonary toilet is required throughout the entire case. As the surgeon completes portions of the tracheal repair, the tube is temporarily withdrawn into the proximal trachea. This maneuver permits the surgeon to assess the caliber of the repaired airway and to verify that the tube is not sutured to the patient's airway. During these times of tube reposition, there are multiple and prolonged episodes of apnea. Therefore, inhalation anesthetic levels can decrease significantly. Adding a total intravenous anesthetic (TIVA) infusion may be required to assure analgesia, hypnosis, and amnesia. When the airway repair is completed, the tube is finally advanced to the midtrachea. The bronchial blocker cuff is deflated, and the patient undergoes two-lung ventilation. At the conclusion of the case, the standard ETT, usually size 8.0 or 8.5, allows the surgeon to perform a bronchoscopy.

Alternatively, the airway can be managed with a specially crafted left-sided endobronchial tube. This tube is produced from a left DLT, usually one size smaller than normally used for the patient. The tracheal lumen and cuff are removed by a scalpel by the surgeon; therefore, this lumen will not be utilized for ventilation. Essentially, this DLT is transformed into an endobronchial tube, which allows the surgeon to suture the mesh to the posterior airway without fearing the puncture of the tracheal cuff. This tube is placed into the left mainstem bronchus via direct laryngoscopy. The position is verified using the FB. Left lung ventilation is initiated at the beginning of the procedure by clamping the tracheal lumen and inflating the bronchial cuff. When the airway repair is complete, the tube is withdrawn into the trachea, with the bronchial cuff functioning as a tracheal cuff, the tracheal lumen remaining clamped, and the patient being ventilated on two lungs. At this point, the endobronchial tube transforms into a single-lumen ETT. Similarly, this airway can also be managed with a wire-reinforced endobronchial tube placed in the left mainstem bronchus. The disadvantage of this technique is that one cannot directly visualize or suction the right mainstem bronchus. However, when the surgery is completed, the tube is retracted into a tracheal position, and the cuff will be able to provide an adequate seal.

3 What are the surgical considerations that impact anesthetic management?

The posterior approach to the trachea and bronchi using a right thoracotomy incision leaves the surgeon a large distance from the airways. A long incision, long instruments, and a tedious dissection are needed to approach the posterior aspect of the airways. The posterior longitudinal fibrous wall of the trachea and bronchi is plicated, and a Y-shaped Dacron mesh is sewn over it. This reinforced posterior wall creates extra support and prevents airway collapse during expiration. Retraction can dislodge the position of the endobronchial tube and can also impede the venous return to the heart, causing hypotension. Secretions often obstruct the tube, requiring frequent bronchoscopic suctioning of the airways.

4 Are there special considerations for the emergence at the end of the case?

To minimize positive pressure on fresh anastomoses and decrease the risk of dehiscence and ventilator-associated infection, it is preferable that the patient is breathing spontaneously and extubated at the conclusion of the case. The patient should be placed in a sitting or a reverse Trendelenburg position, on 100% Fio_2, and with the pharynx well suctioned. Complete reversal of neuromuscular blockade should be assured, and appropriate muscle strength and responses to commands should be confirmed. Prior to extubation, the patient needs to demonstrate adequate tidal volumes and respiratory rates with acceptable levels of CO_2. A preoperative conversation with the patient regarding the critical role of their cooperation during the extubation process can add tremendous success to the conclusion of this complex procedure.

However, although reintubation can cause mucosal damage and can even break the suture lines of the tracheoplasty, the anesthesiologist must be ready to emergently reinstrument the airway, if respiratory failure develops. Various airway devices (FB, Glidescope, etc.) need to be available in the OR until the patient has been safely transferred to the ICU. These devices allow direct visualization and help avoid "blind" advancement of the ETT during urgent reintubation.

- Patients with severe TBM suffer from dynamic collapse of the airway during exhalation; these patients have difficulty clearing their thick and abundant secretions.
- A standard endotracheal tube (8.0 or 8.5) is inserted in the midtrachea; left lung ventilation is required for the case and accomplished using a bronchial blocker placed in the right main stem bronchus.
- Periodic advancement and withdrawal of the endotracheal tube and requirements for apnea necessitate close communication between the anesthesiologist and the thoracic surgeon.
- Extubation at the conclusion of surgery is preferred; emergency reintubation can damage the suture lines of the tracheoplasty.
- *See Figure 141.1 for additional details.*

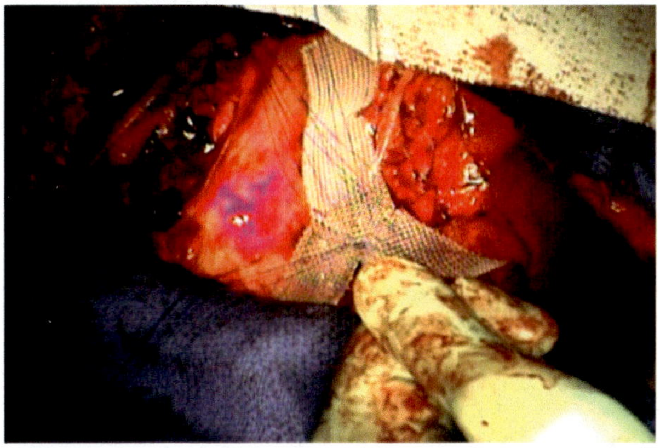

Figure 141.1. Image taken during tracheoplasty surgery identifying the fortifying mesh placed on the posterior wall of the tracheobronchial tree.

Acknowledgments

We gratefully acknowledge the contributions of previous edition author, Deborah S. Reynolds, as portions of those chapters have been retained in this revision.

Suggested Readings

Cho JH, Kim HJ, Kim J. External tracheal stabilization technique for acquired tracheomalacia using a tailored silicone tube. *Ann Thorac Surg*. 2012;94(4):1356–1358.

Damle SS, Mitchel JD. Surgery for tracheobronchomalacia. *Semin Cardiothorac Vasc Anesth*. 2012;16:203–208.

Gangadharan SP, Bakhos CT, Majid A, et al. Technical aspects and outcomes of tracheobronchoplasty for severe tracheobroncho-malacia. *Ann Thorac Surg*. 2011;91(5):1574–1581.

Lazzaro R, Patton B, Lee P, et al. First series of minimally-invasive robot-assisted tracheobronchoplasty with mesh for severe tracheobronchomalacia. *J Thorac Cardiovasc Surg*. 2019;157:791–800.

142 Tracheal Resection Surgery

D. John Doyle

Clinical Scenario: A 48-year-old male with a long-standing history of stridor and inability to exercise due to tracheal stenosis presents to the OR for tracheal resection surgery. The patient's past medical history is significant for obesity (BMI 45 kg/m^2) and obstructive sleep apnea on continuous positive airway pressure 10 cm H_2O at home. He has undergone several interventional procedures, including tracheal dilation and tracheal stent placement, but with suboptimal results.

1 What are the anesthetic and airway management considerations for this case?

The usual cause for acquired tracheal stenosis is prolonged endotracheal intubation, although gastroesophageal reflux disease and Wegener granulomatosis (now officially known as granulomatosis with polyangiitis) are sometimes responsible. Prolonged intubation, the use of an excessively sized endotracheal tube (ETT), or use of an ETT with an overpressurized cuff can lead to tracheal mucosal ischemia, followed by ulceration/inflammation, ultimately leading to tracheal fibrosis.

Anesthetic and airway management involves very close collaboration with the surgeon. The anesthetic goals for these cases represent performing a safe induction, facilitating surgical exposure, and providing conditions that allow extubation at the completion of the procedure.

Since the trachea is pathologically narrowed, initial placement of a small-bore tracheal tube (eg, Microlaryngeal tube [MLT] ETT size 4 or 5) is often needed. However, some surgeons desire the use of a special ETT which allows for neuromonitoring of the surrounding nerves. Other airway management techniques are also theoretically possible; these include jet ventilation via a special catheter or the use of spontaneous ventilation via an laryngeal mask airway (described in Chapter 80: Subglottic Jet Ventilation). In situations where the trachea is too narrow to allow passing of even an MLT, the use of extracorporeal membrane oxygenation (ECMO) or cardiopulmonary bypass to support ventilation during surgery should be strongly considered.

Since the airway will be open during the resection part of the procedure, total intravenous anesthesia is customarily provided. In addition, the considerations of obstructive sleep apnea and morbid obesity apply in this case.

2 How would you manage the airway in this case?

A review of available office reports, CT scans, and nasopharyngoscopy videos, in conjunction with a discussion with the surgeon, will provide some guidance as to the largest ETT that should pass by the stenosis/stent portion of the airway and still allow for adequate ventilation. In this case, a size 5 MLT ETT would probably suffice.

If this patient was judged to be difficult to intubate (eg, because of obesity), proceeding with awake intubation using a flexible bronchoscope (FB) or a video laryngoscope would be a reasonable option. Otherwise, general anesthesia induction can proceed in the usual manner. Rapid sequence induction is not ordinarily necessary in all obese patients. Note that patients with tracheal stenosis are usually not difficult to mask ventilate once general anesthesia and muscle relaxation have been established.

During laryngoscopy, a size 5 oral MLT ETT will be passed beyond the proposed tracheal resection site with the tip placed just above the carina. A pediatric FB can be helpful to confirm correct positioning. Anesthesia can be maintained with a propofol infusion (eg, starting at 100 to 150 μg/kg/min and then titrating) along with an opiate (eg, remifentanil infusion starting at 0.1 μg/kg/min) and a paralytic agent. In addition, a radial arterial line and a second large-bore intravenous line should be placed.

3 What are the surgical considerations that impact anesthetic management?

After positioning and prepping, the surgeon will start exposing the trachea. When exposure is adequate, a tracheal incision is then performed. Prior to this step, the patient is put on 100% oxygen, the ETT cuff is deflated, and the ETT is pulled back above the planned incision site, then left in place. A sterile wire-reinforced ETT (eg, size 5 or 6) is then inserted into the distal trachea by the surgeon and the breathing circuit attached (cross-field ventilation). When the end-to-end anastomosis portion of the procedure is near completion, the cross-field ETT is then removed, and the original tube is pushed back down the trachea under direct vision, followed by completion of the anastomosis.

4 What are the potential hazards and complications in regard to the airway?

Airway fire is a potential concern in such cases. While scissors and blades are usually used during the resection phase, the use of electrocautery is sometimes necessary and may necessitate lowering the delivered oxygen concentration.

5 What distinct airway device (eg, specialized tracheal tube, rigid bronchoscope, bronchial blocker) might be used in this case, and what are the special considerations?

A narrow-bore MLT ETT is often employed in the first phase of the case, followed by a narrow-bore wire-reinforced ETT for the cross-field placement portion (into the distal trachea). A pediatric FB can be helpful to confirm correct positioning of the ETT tip. A tube exchange catheter is sometimes left in place after extubation, in case reintubation becomes necessary.

6 Are there special considerations for the emergence at the end of the case?

At the end of the surgery, the patient is woken up gently, then extubated. The use of a remifentanil infusion during the case can be helpful to achieve this goal. Care must be taken to avoid neck extension, which stretches the anastomosis; consequently, some surgeons temporarily suture the patient's chin to the anterior chest wall to maintain neck flexion. Following extubation, the patient is admitted to the postanesthesia care unit (PACU), and subsequently to a specialized step-down unit. As noted above, a tube exchange catheter is occasionally left in place after extubation, in case reintubation becomes necessary.

- Patients with tracheal stenosis are usually not difficult to ventilate by mask.
- Intubation will usually require a narrow-bore ETT.
- Cross-field ventilation is usually performed during the "open airway" phase of the surgery.
- In expected tenuous airway management situations due to a very narrowed trachea, placing the patient electively on ECMO can be salutary.
- Gentle extubation with the neck placed in flexion is needed to avoid potential disruption of the anastomosis.
- *See Figures 142.1 and 142.2 for additional details.*

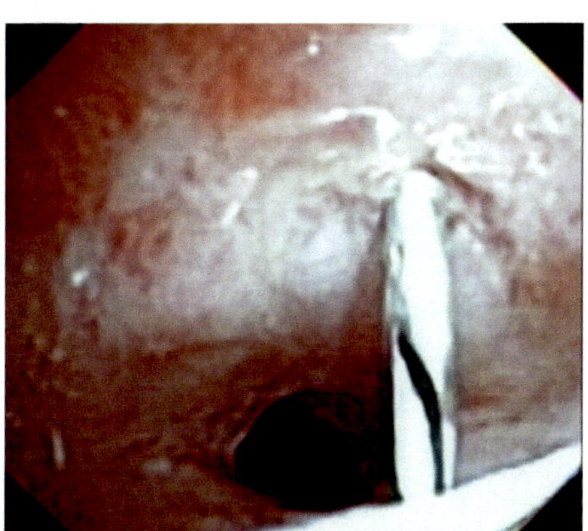

Figure 142.1. A transthoracic needle is placed under flexible bronchoscope guidance in order to identify the site of the tracheal stenosis. See **Video 142.1** for additional details.

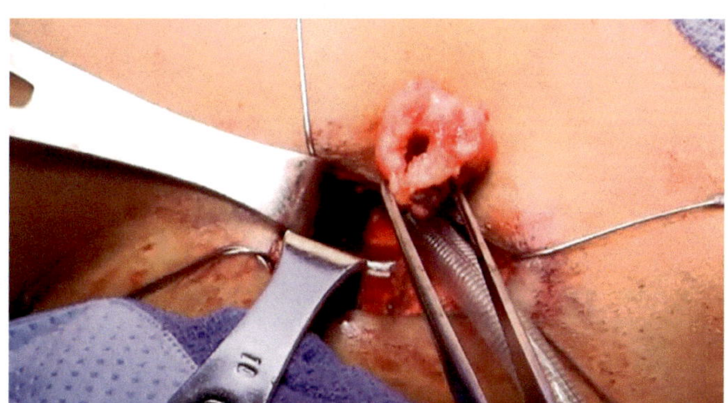

Figure 142.2. The stenotic section of the trachea is resected. See **Video 142.2** for additional details.

Suggested Readings

Apfelbaum JL, Hagberg CA, Connis RT, et al. 2022 American Society of Anesthesiologists Practice Guidelines for management of the difficult airway. *Anesthesiology*. 2022;136(1):31–81.

Heidegger T. Management of the difficult airway. *N Engl J Med*. 2021;384(19):1836–1847.

Hobai IA, Chhangani SV, Alfille PH. Anesthesia for tracheal resection and reconstruction. *Anesthesiol Clin*. 2012;30:709–730.

Puchalski J, Musani AI. Tracheobronchial stenosis: causes and advances in management. *Clin Chest Med*. 2013;34(3):557–567.

Tracheal Resection Using a Supraglottic Airway

143

Lena N. Glowka

Clinical Scenario: A 50-year-old woman with a history of postintubation tracheal stenosis presents to the OR for a tracheal resection. Her preoperative flexible bronchoscopy reveals a subglottic airway stenosis of 4 cm in length. The patient is edentulous and has a BMI of 27 kg/m^2.

1 What are the anesthetic and airway management considerations for this case?

The anesthetic management of the tracheal resection surgery can be challenging and requires advanced planning due to the substantial risk for disruption and discontinuation of the airway.

Unique to tracheal surgery is the focus on lower airway pathologies. Standard difficult airway algorithms do not take into consideration problems below the vocal cords. Induction of general anesthesia is completed after adequate preoxygenation. In the case of critical stenosis, inhalational induction while the patient is breathing spontaneously is generally considered the safest method. However, intravenous induction is an acceptable technique in milder cases of stenosis. In cases of tight stenosis, rigid bronchoscopy might be required to potentially dilate and secure the airway. The ability to mask ventilate should be ensured prior to administering neuromuscular blocking agents or securing the airway.

Maintenance of anesthesia is typically total intravenous anesthesia because the procedure includes sequential periods of apnea during surgical anastomosis.

Following intubation, the patient is positioned supine with an inflatable bag underneath the shoulders to extend the neck with the head stabilized by a gel roll. A cervical incision is the most common surgical approach. Before performing the end-to-end anastomosis, the anesthesiologist deflates the air bag and lifts the head. This maneuver produces cervical flexion to help reduce traction on the anastomosis. This position can make the head difficult to access for the remainder of the procedure.

When the trachea is incised, the distal trachea is intubated with a sterile endotracheal tube (ETT) and connected to a sterile breathing circuit across the surgical field. This technique is called cross-field ventilation. Lung inflation and end-tidal CO_2 should always be verified after placement of the ETT in the distal trachea. To perform the end-to-end tracheal anastomosis, intermittent apneic periods (2 to 3 minutes each) are required and the distal ETT is removed. Optimization of oxygenation and hyperventilation may be required between periods of apnea.

2 How would you manage the airway in this case?

Following the induction of general anesthesia and mask ventilation confirmation, an appropriately sized supraglottic airway (SGA) is inserted in the pharynx and positioned. Adequate mechanical ventilation through this device should be confirmed prior to proceeding. The use of an SGA has several advantages. First, direct manipulation of the lower airway by the ETT is avoided, reducing the risk of bleeding, injury, and potential rupture of the stenotic portion. Second, bronchoscopic evaluation through the SGA (using an flexible bronchoscopy) of the entire trachea is possible without retraction of the ETT. Third, it eliminates the risk of ETT cuff puncture with tracheal incision. Fourthly, reintubation at the end of the procedure is not necessary, and weaning from mechanical ventilation can be performed using the SGA.

In case an ETT is required due to loss of airway patency or inadequate mechanical ventilation, an intubation stylet can be introduced through select SGAs prior to removal. The use of an SGA is not recommended in patients who have an increased risk of aspiration or patients who cannot be appropriately ventilated through an SGA (eg, morbidly obese patients or those with upper airway obstruction).

3 What distinct airway device (eg, specialized tracheal tube, rigid bronchoscope, bronchial blocker) might be used in this case, and what are the special considerations?

Combinations of different techniques have been described to manage the airway during a tracheal resection. The proposed airway management plan should be discussed with the surgical team ahead of time. The chosen technique should be one with which the entire team is familiar. Most importantly, a backup airway management plan should be discussed in advance in the case of any unexpected complications or emergencies.

The classical airway technique for tracheal resection surgery is described in a separate chapter. An alternative to the distal surgical intubation is the use of jet ventilation through a catheter inserted in the proximal ETT and passed in the distal trachea.

The use of extracorporeal support (cardiopulmonary bypass or extracorporeal membrane oxygenation) for tracheal and, especially, carinal resections has been described. The use of extracorporeal support increases the risk of complications, so the use of this technique should therefore be reserved for patients with critically narrow airways or those who will not tolerate periods of apnea.

4 Are there special considerations for the emergence or the end of the case?

In the postoperative period, the neck is usually kept under flexion to reduce the tracheal-suture tension. This is normally achieved by placing sutures between the chin and the chest. Immediate emergence of anesthesia, extubation, and return to spontaneous ventilation is highly recommended when feasible. The plan for airway management during emergence from anesthesia is of equal importance to the one at induction. The surgeon should be available in the OR to perform emergency tracheotomy, if necessary.

Before emergence from anesthesia, the airway should be cleared of secretions and blood. Extubation can be performed with the patient either fully awake or under deep anesthesia. Intravenous anesthetics can be continued. However, a switch to inhalational anesthetics allows for a smoother awakening and avoids laryngospasm. The presence of an inflated ETT cuff or coughing during extubation can potentially cause disruption of the tracheal anastomosis or external sutures. To help prevent coughing and bucking during emergence, the addition of a low-dose remifentanil infusion can be helpful. Nebulized lidocaine can help further desensitize the trachea.

When an SGA is used in these cases, return of spontaneous ventilation can be achieved while the patient is still under adequate anesthesia. This also allows for an optimal assessment of the lower airway and any residual airway obstruction. In addition, the SGA device avoids direct trauma to the fresh sutures.

When extubating patients who carry an increased risk of requiring reintubation or have difficult airways, an intubation bougie or stylet can be inserted through the laryngeal mask airway (LMA) into the trachea to serve as a conduit or a temporary oxygenation device.

If airway obstruction occurs following extubation, one must differentiate between an obstruction at the level of the tracheal anastomosis or an insufficient patency of the vocal cords. In the case of vocal cord edema, the administration of nebulized epinephrine may be necessary.

- Induction and emergence from anesthesia for tracheal resection surgery requires careful planning.
- Adequate mask ventilation before airway instrumentation is recommended, especially in cases of critical tracheal stenosis.
- The use of an LMA throughout the procedure is feasible, avoids additional tracheal injury, and allows for a more controlled emergence.
- *See Figure 143.1 and* ***Video 143.1*** *for additional details.*

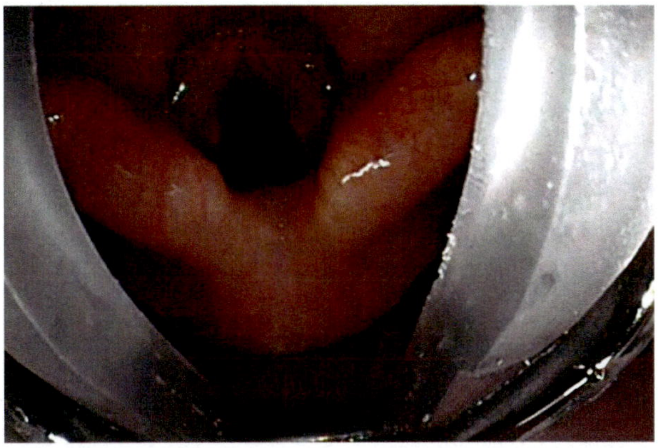

Figure 143.1. The larynx is visualized with a flexible bronchoscope through a laryngeal mask.

Acknowledgments

We gratefully acknowledge the contributions of previous edition author, Arne Neyrinck, as portions of those chapters have been retained in this revision.

Suggested Readings

Hobai IA, Chhangani SV, Alfille PH. Anesthesia for tracheal resection and reconstruction. *Anesthesiol Clin.* 2012;30(4):709–730.

Schieren M, Boehmer A, Dusse F, Koryllos A, Wappler F, Defosse J. New approaches to airway management in tracheal resections—a systematic review and meta-analysis. *J Cardiothorac Vasc Anesth.* 2017;31(4):1351–1358.

Smeltz AM, Bhatia M, Arora H, Long J, Kumar PA. Anesthesia for resection and reconstruction of the trachea and carina. *J Cardiothorac Vasc Anesth.* 2020;34(7):1902–1913.

144 Tracheal Stenosis in a Term Pregnant Patient

Adriana Herrera

Clinical Scenario: A 24-year-old, 40 weeks pregnant patient presents for elective C-section. The patient has a history of tracheal stenosis due to a past episode of prolonged intubation. She developed shortness of breath while exercising, and occasional stridor. These symptoms have worsened with the progression of her pregnancy. Currently, she requires a semi-upright position to sleep and has a constant audible stridor.

1 What are the anesthetic and airway management considerations for this case?

Tracheal stenosis is a rare and life-threatening problem that represents a major management challenge for anesthesiologists. More details regarding this disease can be found in Chapter 79: Subglottic Stenosis—Noncritical/Supraglottic Jet Ventilation. The airway changes occurring during pregnancy due to hormonal changes cause hyperemia and mucosal edema with an increased tendency of airway bleeding. A previously asymptomatic tracheal stenosis patient can develop symptoms in pregnancy due to these changes. Symptoms usually present when the airway is reduced to 30% of normal or to 5- to 6-mm diameter. Patients present with cough, difficulty clearing secretions, and dyspnea on exertion that progresses to dyspnea at rest, often with progressive stridor, wheezing, and even difficulty speaking. Progesterone-induced relaxation of the lower esophageal sphincter, delayed gastric emptying, and increased intragastric pressure from the gravid uterus contribute to increasing the aspiration risk.

On physical examination, an audible stridor, increased respiratory rate, use of accessory muscles, and difficulty speaking (voice quality, hoarseness, dyspnea with phonation) help determine the severity of the stenosis. However, patients with severe tracheal stenosis may be asymptomatic.

The evaluation of the severity of tracheal stenosis should include a flexible bronchoscopy, a CT scan, and/or an MRI. An airway ultrasound could be a useful tool in evaluating the subglottic diameter. Concern of radiation exposure exists. Abdominal lead shielding with a short radiation exposure during pregnancy after the first trimester decreases this risk significantly. Pulmonary function tests are not routinely recommended. The flow–volume loop presents a fixed upper airway obstruction.

2 How would you manage the airway in this case?

This situation has the potential of having a catastrophic outcome if the airway is lost. The anesthetic plan for airway management should be discussed clearly with the patient, family, and surgical team.

Even though spinal or epidural anesthesia would be an attractive option, since the airway would not be manipulated, the patient's inability to tolerate supine position, presence of a high neuraxial block, or other intraoperative complications may not make it the best alternative. Moreover, patients using their respiratory accessory muscles may present with respiratory failure after neuraxial anesthesia. C-section under general anesthesia is the safest choice.

If the procedure is elective, patients should fast for 8 hours preoperatively. H2 blockers and metoclopramide can be administered to reduce the aspiration risk. A semi-upright position with left uterine displacement is necessary. Use of glycopyrrolate to dry secretions and facilitate flexible bronchoscopy is recommended.

Immediately available airway equipment should include different types and sizes of blades, endotracheal tubes (cuffed, uncuffed, and armored), laryngeal mask airways, Glidescope blades, and flexible bronchoscopy (FB) in adult and pediatric sizes. Rigid bronchoscopy is usually reserved for evaluation, dilation, and stent placement. However, in emergency situations, it can be used to relieve airway obstruction. The ENT and neonatal teams should be at bedside for an emergent surgical airway and/or for fetal distress requiring emergent C-section.

Difficulties with ventilation and intubation should be anticipated. A thorough preoxygenation is of utmost importance. For a cooperative patient in an elective situation, awake flexible bronchoscopic intubation is the safest option. Sedation should be avoided if possible, as it incurs various risks such as hypoventilation, hypoxemia, respiratory distress, aspiration, and hemodynamic changes affecting the mother and/or the fetus. Anesthesia of the oropharynx is achieved with local anesthetics such as lidocaine 4%. Nasal intubation is not recommended, as these patients are more prone to bleeding due to mucosal engorgement. Subglottic anesthesia is achieved by spraying the vocal cords with lidocaine through a FB or via transtracheal block. The overall goal is to maintain spontaneous ventilation and hemodynamic stability with minimal sedation. In an uncooperative patient, an inhalational induction is a potential choice. However, the aspiration risk in a pregnant woman after the first trimester is increased. Rapid sequence induction is another possibility, but the potential of difficult ventilation and intubation is a major concern. Jet ventilation and high-flow nasal cannula have also been utilized for oxygenation. In extremely complex situations where the tracheal stenosis is so tight that it cannot tolerate airway interventions, initiating elective venovenous extracorporeal membrane oxygenation before anesthesia induction is a possibility.

Early communication between the surgical and anesthesiology teams is critical for patient safety. Assessment of these patients should be done early in pregnancy. Appropriate planning for either an elective or an emergency procedure decreases morbidity and mortality and improves maternal and neonatal outcomes.

3 What are the potential hazards and complications in regard to the airway?

Airway changes associated with increased estrogen levels include edema and hyperemia of the mucosa, increasing the risk of mucosal bleeding. These changes cause a decrease in the tracheal lumen with worsening respiratory symptoms. Hypoxemia occurs faster due to decreased functional residual capacity and increased oxygen requirements.

Airway loss is the most feared complication. Detailed planning and the availability of a rigid bronchoscope may be life-saving. Depending on the severity and location of the stenosis, and the type of surgical procedure, there are multiple ways to manage the airway (see Chapters 121: Interventional Management of Tracheal Stenosis and 142: Tracheal Resection Surgery). In extreme situations, extracorporeal membrane oxygenation or cardiopulmonary bypass guarantees oxygenation while securing the airway.

4 Are there special considerations for the emergence or the end of the case?

Planning extubation requires the same care and attention as intubation, because similar concerns exist.

The risk of aspiration is still present on extubation. Orogastric suctioning, elevated head position, and extubating the patient fully awake are recommended measures to mitigate this risk. Difficulties encountered during intubation lead to increased risk at extubation. Added edema and inflammation to the airway results in a smaller tracheal lumen, with subsequent respiratory distress on extubation. The possibility of a failed extubation, with a potential "cannot-ventilate, cannot-intubate" situation, should not be taken lightly, as it can change rapidly from a secure airway to a life-threatening situation. It may be more prudent to temporarily leave the patient intubated, allowing the airway edema to decrease. If additional imaging and/or surgical management of the tracheal stenosis is required, then leaving the patient intubated is highly desirable.

- Due to pregnancy-induced hormonal changes, worsening symptoms of tracheal stenosis may appear.
- Evaluation of the tracheal stenosis severity should include a flexible bronchoscopy, a CT scan, and/or an MRI. Airway ultrasound may be useful to evaluate the subglottic diameter.
- Early communication between the obstetric and anesthesiology teams is critical for patient safety. Consider involving Otolaryngology or Cardiothoracic surgical teams if indicated.
- Planning extubation requires the same care and attention as intubation, because similar concerns exist.
- In rare situations, worsening of symptoms and poor response to palliative management during pregnancy may result in preterm delivery with immediate surgical repair of the tracheal stenosis.
- *See Figure 144.1 for additional details.*

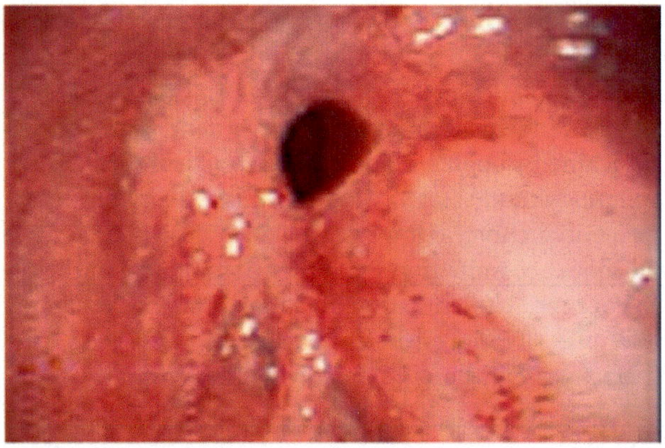

Figure 144.1. Tracheal stenosis in a pregnant patient.

Suggested Readings

Bahhady IJ, Ernst A. Risks of and recommendations for flexible bronchoscopy in pregnancy: a review. *Chest*. 2004;126(6): 1974–1981.

Fang S, Pai B H P. Successful management of subglottic stenosis in pregnancy. *BMJ Case Rep*. 2021;14(3):e236466.

Isono S, Kitamura Y, Asai T, Cook TM. Case scenario: perioperative airway management of a patient with tracheal stenosis. *Anesthesiology*. 2010;112:970–978.

Kuczkowski KM, Benumof JL. Subglottic tracheal stenosis in pregnancy: anaesthetic implications. *Anaesth Intensive Care*. 2003; 31(5):576–577.

Lakhal K, Delplace X, Cottier JP, et al. The feasibility of ultrasound to assess subglottic diameter. *Anesth Analg*. 2007;104(3):611–614.

Tracheoesophageal Fistula Repair

145

Jeffrey J. Schwartz • Andrew Dhanasopon

Clinical Scenario: A 61-year-old man presents to the OR for a tracheoesophageal fistula (TEF) repair via right thoracotomy. The patient has a history of COVID-19 pneumonia requiring prolonged intubation and placement of a tracheostomy, which was subsequently removed. Attempts at repairing the fistula by placing a tracheal stent have failed.

1 What are the anesthetic and airway management considerations for this case?

Acquired TEF is a rare but serious complication. The most common cause is malignancy, typically esophageal cancer that erodes through the anterior wall to the adjacent membranous trachea. The most common benign cause of TEF is pressure necrosis from endotracheal or tracheostomy tube balloon cuffs. In intubated patients, signs of TEF may include evidence of copious gastric secretions suctioned from the endotracheal tube, or clinical signs of aspiration pneumonitis or pneumonia. In nonventilated patients, symptoms of TEF include consistent coughing after swallowing and dysphagia.

Preoperative optimization includes minimizing aspiration events and preserving lung function with head-of-bed elevation, pulmonary toilet, and aggressive treatment of pneumonitis and pneumonia. In addition, as with any esophageal surgery, nutritional supplementation may be necessary via enteric tube (G-tube, jejunal feeding tube) or parenterally. When possible, it is prudent to wean patients off mechanical ventilation prior to TEF repair. Broadly, benign TEF is managed with an open surgical procedure, while malignant TEF is typically managed with stenting to preserve quality of life using the least invasive means.

Anesthetic and airway management considerations differ between the interventional bronchoscopic/endoscopic and the surgical approach. Since TEF is an unprotected connection between the gastrointestinal tract and the airway, aspiration of stomach contents, with potential pneumonitis, is a constant risk. RSI does not mitigate this risk. Positive-pressure ventilation from above the level of the TEF risks insufflation of air into the esophagus and stomach increasing the aspiration risk.

2 How would you manage the airway in this case?

Airway management depends on the interventional/surgical approach. A bronchoscopic approach requires either no endotracheal tube (ETT) or one that is positioned above the TEF to allow the interventionalist access to the TEF. If stenting of the esophagus and trachea is planned, then the trachea should be stented first because the esophageal stent may cause tracheal compression.

For an interventional approach, a rigid bronchoscopic technique is preferred. Alternatively, a large-diameter ETT can be placed, and the stenting can be done with a flexible bronchoscope. Regardless, the TEF remains unprotected and positive pressure ventilation (PPV) will insufflate air into the esophagus. A nasogastric tube can be placed to vent the gas and prevent stomach inflation. The minimum airway pressure necessary to maintain adequate ventilation should be used. Jet ventilation via the ventilating port of the rigid bronchoscope may allow adequate ventilation with lower airway pressures. If an ETT is used, a FB should be used to confirm that the tip of the ETT is above the fistula to allow the proceduralist access.

The surgical approach depends on the location of the TEF. High TEFs require an anterior cervical neck incision, while TEFs below the thoracic inlet are usually managed via right thoracotomy. If a cervical incision is planned for a high TEF near the cervicoesophageal junction, then a single-lumen ETT placed distal to the TEF is sufficient. It may be necessary to shorten the tip of the ETT by cutting it in order to ensure the tip is above the carina while the cuff is below the TEF.

For an open thoracotomy, the airway management depends on the location of the TEF. The most common site of a TEF is in the upper two-thirds of the trachea. This would best be managed with a left-sided double lumen tube (DLT) and right lung collapse. FB could assure that the fistula is not visualized below the tip of the tracheal lumen of the DLT. Therefore, the fistula would be situated above or beside the tracheal cuff, thus isolating the lungs from the esophagus.

If tracheal reconstruction is necessary to repair the TEF, the airway can be managed (see Chapter 142: Tracheal Resection Surgery) with a combination of cross-field ventilation and intubation of the distal trachea.

A carinal TEF, repaired via subcostal and cervical incisions, can be managed with bilateral ETTs placed in the main stem bronchi. This allows isolation of the TEF and ventilation of both lungs. This technique incurs the risk of occluding the right upper lobe bronchus and the risk of the laryngeal inlet not being large enough to admit two ETTs.

A right carinal TEF in a patient status post left pneumonectomy can be managed with a left-sided DLT placed into the right main stem bronchus, allowing isolation of the fistula, the ability to continually monitor the relative position of the cuff in relation to the TEF, and suctioning of regurgitated contents via the tracheal lumen.

A left main stem TEF can be managed with a right-sided DLT. As the surgical approach requires a right posterolateral thoracotomy, the right lung is ventilated intermittently with small tidal volumes.

There is no single best method to manage the airway in the presence of a TEF. Knowledge of the fistula anatomy as well as any associated pathology, combined with the goal of isolating the fistula, providing adequate ventilation, and meeting the surgical needs, should be used to individualize management. Good planning and communication with the surgeon are paramount.

Maintenance of spontaneous ventilation and avoidance of PPV until the TEF is isolated can be advantageous. An effective inhalation induction in a patient with already compromised pulmonary function and likely copious secretions can be a difficult task to achieve.

Rarely, venovenous extracorporeal membrane oxygenation may be considered if the repair requires tracheal reconstruction that cannot be managed with cross-field ventilation.

3 What are the potential hazards and complications in regards to the airway?

Depending on the location and size of the TEF, there may be no way to fully isolate the airway from the esophagus. Aspiration, gastric insufflation, and inadequate ventilation would continue to be a risk throughout the induction of anesthesia and during the surgery.

The ETT may accidentally be placed into the TEF if the anatomy is unclear or if the ETT is carelessly positioned. This needs to be recognized immediately, as ventilation into the TEF will inflate the stomach and not the lungs.

4 Are there special considerations for the emergence or the end of the case?

Immediate or early extubation is a very important consideration. There is an increased risk of anastomotic breakdown and tracheal stenosis if the patient remains intubated. Preexisting lung disease, malnutrition, muscle wasting, and anemia impair respiratory reserve and the ability to cough and clear sections. The patient's respiratory status may be tenuous after extubation.

- The major risks are pulmonary aspiration, inadequate ventilation, and gastric insufflation.
- Proper airway management requires integration of the TEF anatomy and surgical requirements into the overall plan.
- The goal of airway management should be to isolate the airway and gastrointestinal tract.
- *See Figures 145.1 and 145.2 for additional details.*

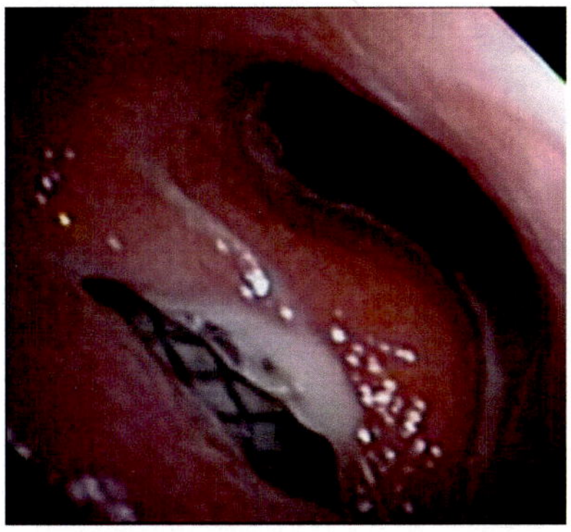

Figure 145.1. A previously inserted esophageal stent is visualized through a tracheoesophageal fistula. See Video 145.1 for additional details.

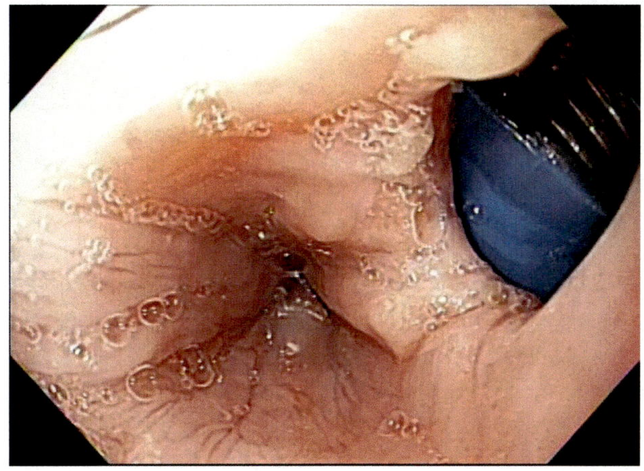

Figure 145.2. A reinforced tracheal tube is visualized using an esophageal flexible scope via a tracheoesophageal fistula. See Video 145.2 for additional details.

Suggested Readings

Diddee R, Shaw IH. Acquired tracheoesophageal fistula in adults. *Contin Educ Anaesth Crit Care Pain.* 2006;6:105–108.
Grebenik CR. Anaesthetic management of malignant tracheoesophageal fistula. *Br J Anaesth.* 1989;63:492–496.
Grillo HC. Acquired tracheoesophageal and bronchoesophageal fistula. In: Grillo HC, ed. *Surgery of the Trachea and Bronchi.* BC Decker; 2004:341–356.
Reed MF, Mathisen DJ. Tracheoesophageal fistula. *Chest Surg Clin N Am.* 2003;13:271–289.

146 Bronchopleural Fistula Repair

Anoushka Afonso • Vojislava Neskovic

Clinical Scenario: A 72-year-old woman presents to the OR *emergently* for a bronchopleural fistula (BPF) repair. Her medical history is significant for adenocarcinoma of the right lung, for which she underwent a right pneumonectomy 2 months ago. She also had two cycles of chemotherapy and radiation to her right chest. She is currently admitted with significant shortness of breath and productive cough.

1 What are the anesthetic and airway management considerations for this case?

A BPF is defined as a communication between the bronchial tree and the pleural cavity with persistent air leak. An air leak for more than 24 hours confirms the diagnosis. BPF may have different etiologies, but lung resection remains the leading cause, where pneumonectomy carries the highest prevalence (4.5% to 20%) and mortality (11% to 18%). BPF associated with empyema after pneumonectomy is a complication which is shown to be an independent predictor of mortality.

Patients may have clinical presentations of different severity levels. Usually, after chest tube placement, bronchoscopy is performed to identify the BPF, to assess the viability of tissues, and the length of the bronchial stump. Appropriately selected patients can be treated using endobronchial procedures (fibrin glue, occlusive materials, and endobronchial valves), thereby avoiding a major reoperation. Yet, the need for operative reexploration is common (more than 90%). The anesthetic and airway management depends on the planned procedure.

Whenever possible, maintaining spontaneous ventilation is preferred. Local infiltration, regional anesthetics, and intravenous techniques with spontaneous ventilation can be used. Bronchoscopy can be accomplished with the patient breathing spontaneously under topical anesthesia (eg, 4% nebulized lidocaine) and light sedation.

If the planned procedure requires general anesthesia and mechanical ventilation, the goals are to:

- maintain adequate ventilation or oxygenation during positive-pressure ventilation (PPV),
- decrease airway pressure on the bronchial stump, and
- protect the unaffected lung from contamination (spillover) of infectious material, which can be devastating complication for a patient with a single lung after pneumectomy.

A large BPF and the presence of empyema, *is an absolute indication* for lung separation in patients who require general anesthesia and PPV.

In mechanically ventilated patients, BPF is commonly complicated by pneumothorax. Because of that, patients have a chest tube inserted prior to the planned procedure to avoid a tension pneumothorax during PPV and to drain pleural collections. Various methods of lung separation are feasible (double-lumen tubes [DLT], bronchial blockers, modified single-lumen tubes); the approach should be individualized, depending on patient anatomy, tolerability of one lung ventilation, position of the fistula, and ventilation techniques. The DLT (endobronchial lumen on the opposite side than the BPF) is the preferred technique of airway management, as it allows an easy conversion to one lung ventilation and lung separation, particularly when an empyema is present. In order to avoid contamination of the unaffected lung, patient positioning is important. Placing the patient in reverse Trendelenburg, with the affected lung in a dependent position, may avoid lung contamination.

2 How would you manage the airway in this case?

Given the patient's history of prior radiation and chemotherapy following a right pneumonectomy, combined with symptoms of respiratory distress and productive cough, a large defect and presence of infectious process in the right chest cavity is suspected. Spillover of infectious material to the only remaining lung could have disastrous consequences. Since the patient presents for emergency surgery, general anesthesia, PPV, and the use of *a left-sided DLT* without a hook is the safest plan. Placement of the DLT under flexible bronchoscopic guidance is preferred. A correct positioning of the DLT under visual control reduces the likelihood of further damaging of the bronchial stump.

Use of single-lumen ETT is not indicated as it does not prevent contamination of the left lung and increases the pressure on the bronchial stump during PPV. A BB cannot be used in this situation, as it prevents any endotracheal intervention on the right side (suspected fistula site) while ventilating the left lung.

Another option is awake intubation using DLT in spontaneously breathing patient, which may be the technique of choice when both mask ventilation and intubation are anticipated to be difficult. However, this technique is usually poorly tolerated. Adequate upper and lower airway topicalization is required. Intravenous sedation with dexmedetomidine maintains spontaneous ventilation while sedating the patient. In addition, titrating remifentanil and/or adding an inhalational agent during spontaneous ventilation before endotracheal intubation can be useful. The patient should be comfortable at all times since excessive coughing and increased airway pressures can cause further dehiscence of the bronchial stump suture. The use of either flexible bronchoscopes or video laryngoscopes may be considered for an awake intubation with placement of the DLT. Use of video laryngoscopes provides high success rate and may shorten the time to successful intubation.

PPV should only be initiated after lung isolation. Ventilator parameter adjustments should attempt to minimize air leak and enable effective ventilation. These include decrease of the peak inspiratory pressure, limiting positive end-expiratory pressure, lowering tidal volume and respiratory rate, and shortening the inspiratory time. There is no evidence of superiority of one mode of ventilation over another, as long as these ventilatory goals are achieved.

3 What are the potential hazards and complications in regard to the airway?

Risks during anesthesia induction and airway management in patients with BPF involve soiling the nonaffected lung before lung isolation. Impairment of ventilation and oxygenation during PPV in the presence of a large fistula leak is also of concern. Before anesthesia induction, the practitioner must ensure that the inserted chest tube is functional, not clamped or kinked. Otherwise, a tension pneumothorax can develop quickly during PPV, which may cause significant hemodynamic compromise. Large amounts of negative pressure applied to the chest tubes should be avoided, since this can impair effective ventilation during PPV. A difficult airway with the need for lung isolation should always be considered. Placement of a single-lumen ETT followed by DLT placement over an airway exchange catheter may be a rescue plan. However, placing a tube exchanger in a patient with a BPF is a high-risk procedure and must be done with extreme care, as this device can further damage the bronchial stump.

4 Are there special considerations for the emergence or the end of the case?

If the patient is meeting criteria, extubation at the end of surgery is preferred. Avoiding PPV decreases the risk of suture dehiscence. An anesthetic technique that provides the patient with adequate analgesia while breathing spontaneously toward the end of the case, is recommended. Limiting the airway pressure during manually assisted spontaneous ventilation prior to extubation is important. Multimodal analgesic therapy should be initiated to keep the patient comfortable during the postoperative period.

- Effective lung separation is important in the management of a BPF repair.
- Introduction of the DLT under direct vision with a FB allows for optimum positioning and avoids injury to the bronchial fistula or stump.
- Patients presenting for repair of BPF should be converted to spontaneous ventilation and extubated as early as possible in order to avoid positive airway pressures and risking air leak.
- *See Figure 146.1 and* ◉ ***Video 146.1*** *for additional details.*

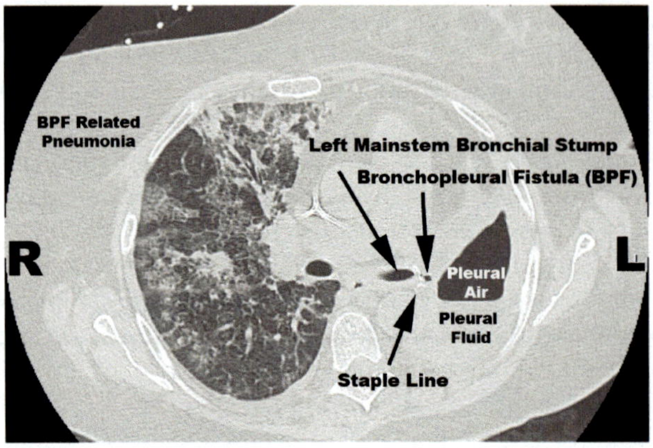

Figure 146.1. An axial CT scan indicating the location of a bronchopleural fistula occurring after a right pneumonectomy.

Suggested Readings

Clark JM, Cooke DT, Brown LM. Management of complications after lung resection: prolonged air leak and bronchopleural fistula. *Thorac Surg Clin*. 2020;30(3):347–358.

Globokar MD, Novak-Jankovic V. Difficult airway and one lung ventilation. *Acta Clin Croat*. 2012;51:477–482.

Goh QY, Kong A. Videolaryngoscope-assisted double-lumen endotracheal tube intubation in an awake patient with known difficult airway and bronchopleural fistula: a case report. *A A Pract*. 2020;14(6):e01186.

Grotberg JC, Hyzy RC, De Cardenas J, Co IN. Bronchopleural fistula in the mechanically ventilated patient: a concise review. *Crit Care Med*. 2021;49(2):292–301.

Left Mainstem Bronchus Resection Via Right Thoracotomy

147

Alessia Pedoto

Clinical Scenario: A 73-year-old man is scheduled to undergo a left bronchial sleeve resection via a right thoracotomy for a left endobronchial carcinoid tumor situated 2 cm below the carina.

1 What are the anesthetic and airway management considerations for this case?

Left mainstem bronchial resection and reconstruction is a challenging procedure that requires careful preoperative planning and close intraoperative communication with the surgical team, especially if done via a contralateral side thoracotomy. In general, the surgical approach is a right thoracotomy because on the left side the heart, the aortic arch, and the descending aorta make access to the left hilum challenging.

The procedure can be divided into three phases: the **dissection**, the **resection**, and the **reconstruction** of the airway. Each step poses specific anesthetic challenges, with the main one being the ability to isolate the right lung and ventilate the left. Due to the left lung disease, a compensatory improved ventilation/perfusion match develops in the right lung. Therefore, right lung collapse, used to facilitate surgical exposure, may not be well tolerated. In addition, left lung ventilation may be difficult due to the ball-valve effect caused by the presence of the endobronchial lesion. The increase in airway pressure and the decrease in lung compliance may limit tidal volume delivery and cause a mismatch between ventilation and perfusion, leading to hypoxemia. In order to improve oxygenation, continuous positive airway pressure, apneic oxygenation, or high-frequency jet ventilation (HFJV) can be attempted on the left side. However, these maneuvers may not be effective due to air trapping beyond the lesion after each inspiration. Resuming two-lung ventilation may be necessary until the airway is opened. At this point, cross-field ventilation or HFJV can be used.

Standard pulmonary function tests and ventilation/perfusion scans should be part of the routine preoperative evaluation to better understand the physiologic implications of lung collapse (right or left). CT scan and MRI with contrast provide additional information regarding the extent of tumor, metastatic spread, as well as vascular involvement. A preoperative bronchoscopic examination of the airway should be done to assess the extent of left bronchial disease, the quality of the mucosa, and to evaluate the contralateral bronchus.

2 How would you manage the airway in this case?

Airway management is customized to each specific phase of the operation and individualized for each patient. Options for lung isolation include bronchial blocker (BB) and double-lumen tube (DLT). Ventilation, depending on the phase of the surgery, can be performed via standard technique, using HFJV or periods of apnea.

If the patient is asymptomatic on the day of surgery, general anesthesia can be induced in a standard fashion. A size 8.0-mm or 8.5-mm endotracheal tube (ETT) is placed via direct laryngoscopy, and a BB is positioned in the right mainstem bronchus under flexible bronchoscope (FB) guidance. In the rare instance of a short take off of the right upper lobe bronchus, two blockers may be necessary to achieve adequate lung collapse. After the patient is placed in left lateral decubitus, the position of the BB is reconfirmed via FB, and the right lung is collapsed. If oxygenation is adequate, OLV can continue until the airway is resected. At this point, a sterile armored ETT tube is placed in the left mainstem bronchus by the surgeon and connected via sterile circuit to the ventilator (see Chapter 148: Carinal Resection). Total intravenous anesthesia is recommended, due to potential leaks around the cuff, or movement or dislodgement of the ETT. Advantages of using BBs include the possibility of selective lobar isolation, in case total lung collapse is not tolerated, and the ease of removal at the end of the case if extubation criteria are not met, thereby avoiding a tube exchange.

Several alternatives to BBs exist to achieve right-sided lung collapse and adequate surgical exposure. If a right-sided DLT is used, it should be placed under direct FB vision to avoid trauma to the left endobronchial lesion. Alternatively, a Hunsaker Mon-Jet catheter or Acutronic LaserJet 40 catheter can be passed through the ETT in the left bronchus distal to the tumor, and HFJV initiated while the right lung is apneic and allowed to collapse.

At the conclusion of the procedure, a flexible bronchoscopy is usually performed to evaluate the viability of the anastomosis, the presence of fistulas, and for pulmonary toileting.

3 What are the surgical issues that impact the anesthetic management?

Left mainstem bronchial resection and reconstruction is reserved for inflammatory, benign, or low-grade malignant lesions (ie, carcinoid tumors) or benign stenosis of the bronchus. The main advantage of this surgical approach is the avoidance of a pneumonectomy, sparing functional lung parenchyma. When feasible, patients may undergo rigid bronchoscopic resection and tumor debulking prior to the definitive surgical treatment, with an immediate improvement of ventilation and symptomatology, and the final result of facilitating surgical resection. Depending on the location of the lesion, a median sternotomy or a left/right thoracotomy can be used. A right thoracotomy is the preferred approach for proximal endobronchial lesions, because it provides better visualization of the carina and avoids the dissection and potential injury of the aortic arch, the intercostal vessels, and the recurrent laryngeal nerve. A right thoracotomy offers access to the first 3 cm of the left main bronchus. On the other hand, the left thoracotomy approach may be better suited for distal bronchial resections, even though it involves significant manipulation of major vascular structures and is associated with increased surgical trauma. A median sternotomy is used for either left or right sleeve resection surgery if the patient does not tolerate OLV.

Contraindications to a sleeve resection include the use of high-dose steroids, an active inflammatory process, and a remote history of high-dose chest radiation, as these could contribute to postoperative airway stenosis or anastomotic dehiscence.

4 Are there any special considerations for the emergence at the end of the case?

Extubation at the end of the surgery is desirable, as prolonged positive-pressure ventilation can lead to an anastomotic leak, barotrauma, or a bronchopleural fistula. Prior to extubation, flexible bronchoscopy is performed for airway toileting and anastomosis evaluation. Possible airway edema and/or the presence of copious amounts of blood or secretions may contraindicate extubation. A detailed extubation plan is essential, including the presence of the surgeon as well as all the airway equipment for emergency reintubation in the OR. During ETT replacement, it is imperative to avoid endobronchial injury (even though rare) or damage to the anastomosis.

- The right thoracotomy approach for left mainstem proximal bronchial resection and reconstruction avoids a pneumonectomy, allowing maximal parenchymal sparing.
- This is a challenging procedure that requires careful preoperative planning and close intraoperative communication with the surgical team.
- During the dissection and resection phases of the surgery, right lung collapse can be accomplished with a BB, right DLT, or passive deflation.
- During the reconstruction phase of the surgery, ventilation of the left lung can be accomplished by cross-field ventilation or HFJV.
- *See Figure 147.1 and* ⊙ ***Video 147.1*** *for additional details.*

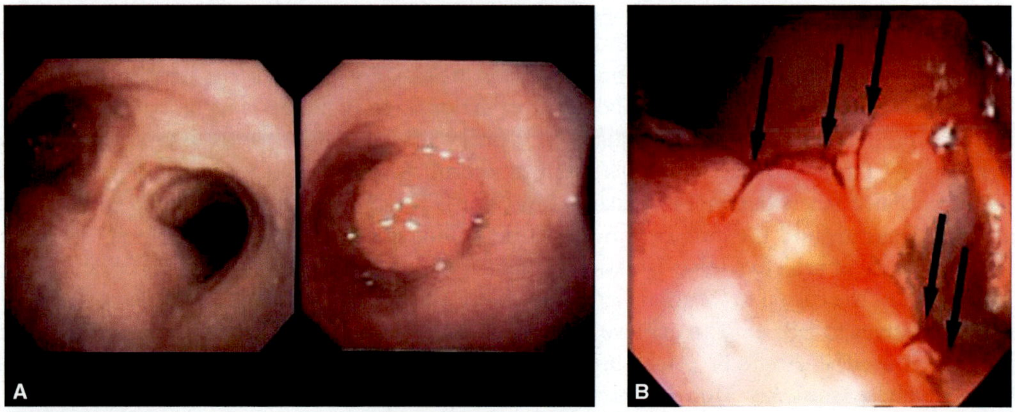

Figure 147.1. A: View of carina with left mainstem mass (**left**). View of mass within left mainstem bronchus (**right**). **B:** Suture line (*arrows*) after left mainstem resection and reanastomosis.

Suggested Readings

Behringer EC, Wilson R. Tracheal resection and reconstruction. In: Cohen E, ed. *Cohen's Comprehensive Thoracic Anesthesia*. Elsevier Inc. 2022:609–622.

Cerfolio RJ, Deschamps C, Allen MS, Trastek VF, Pairolero PC. Mainstem bronchial sleeve resection with pulmonary preservation. *Ann Thorac Surg*. 1996;61:1458–1463.

Detterbeck FC. Management of carcinoid tumors. *Ann Thorac Surg*. 2010;89:998–1005.

Huybrechts I, Tuna T, Szegedi LL. Lung separation in adult thoracic anesthesia. *Saudi J Anaesth*. 2021;15(3):272–279.

Mantovani S, Gust L, D'Journo XB, Thomas PA. Left main bronchial sleeve resection with total lung parenchymal preservation: a tailored surgical approach. *Eur J Cardiothorac Surg*. 2020;57:596–597.

Mathisen DJ. Main and lobar bronchoplasty. In: Grillo H, ed. *Surgery of the Trachea and Bronchi*. 1st ed. BC Decker; 2004: 619–636.

Matsuura N, Igai H, Kamiyoshihara M. Carinal resection and reconstruction. *Transl Lung Cancer Res*. 2021;10(10):4039–4042.

148 Carinal Resection

Eryn Thiele • Randal S. Blank

Clinical Scenario: A 20-year-old, previously healthy female reported to her primary care provider with symptoms of dyspnea and a dry cough. A chest x-ray was completed, which demonstrated right lung collapse with mediastinal shift (Figure 148.1). A subsequent computed tomography revealed a large intraluminal mass, completely occluding the right main bronchus (Figure 148.2).

Rigid bronchoscopy identified a distal tracheal tumor occluding the right mainstem bronchus, adherent to the posterior wall of the carina and the right upper lobe (Figure 148.3). The bronchus intermedius was found to be normal. Using the rigid bronchoscope, the right main bronchus tumor was debulked, reestablishing patency. Tumor samples were collected, which subsequently revealed a diagnosis of carcinoid. Following her diagnosis, the patient was scheduled to undergo a carinal resection, with recreation of a neocarina from the bronchus intermedius and left main bronchus (Figure 148.4).

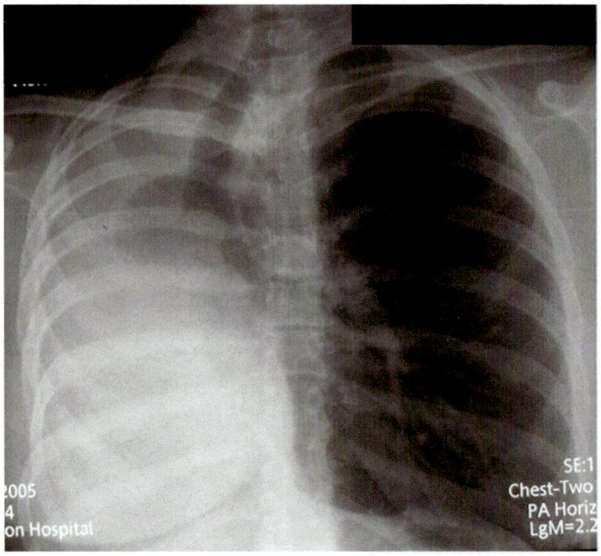

Figure 148.1. Initial chest x-ray demonstrating right lung collapse and mediastinal shift.

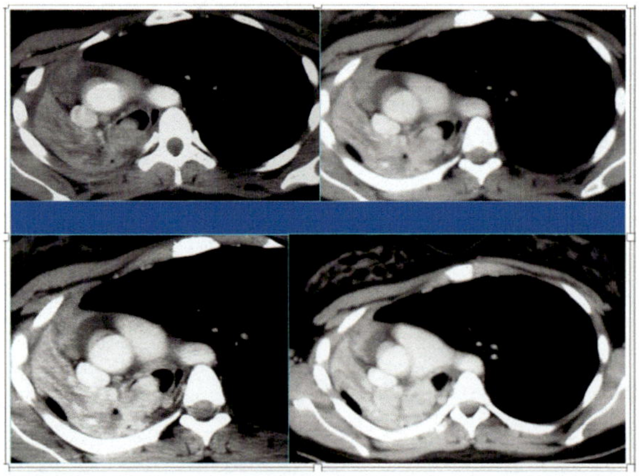

Figure 148.2. CT imaging demonstrating large intraluminal mass completely occluding the right main bronchus.

1 What are the anesthetic/airway management considerations for the case?

A carinal resection is defined as a resection of the tracheobronchial bifurcation, with or without a concomitant lung resection. The evaluation of a patient undergoing major airway surgery, such as a carinal resection, should focus on airway anatomy and functional status of the respiratory system. It is essential for the preoperative evaluation to assess the type and location of the airway tumor, with attention to the residual lumen of the pathologic airway segment. This is generally accomplished via computed tomography (CT) or magnetic resonance imaging (MRI), as well as direct visualization via bronchoscopy. Respiratory function of patients with narrowing of the ventral airway should always be assessed in the supine position to identify dynamic airway changes.

Distal airway surgery involving the carina is complex, requiring careful airway management and multidisciplinary preoperative planning by the perioperative team. Intraoperative monitoring should include electrocardiogram, continuous arterial blood pressure monitoring, pulse oximetry, and waveform capnometry. The arterial line is pertinent for repetitive intra- and postoperative blood gas analysis as well as close hemodynamic

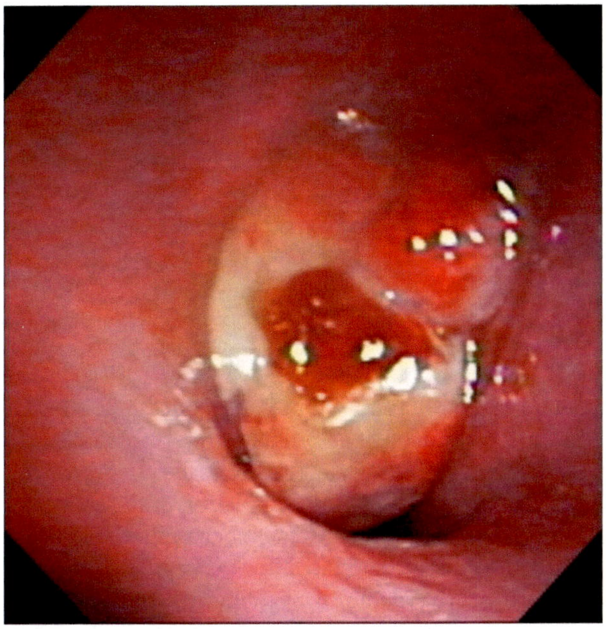

Figure 148.3. Bronchoscopy reveal a distal tracheal tumor occluding the right mainstem bronchus.

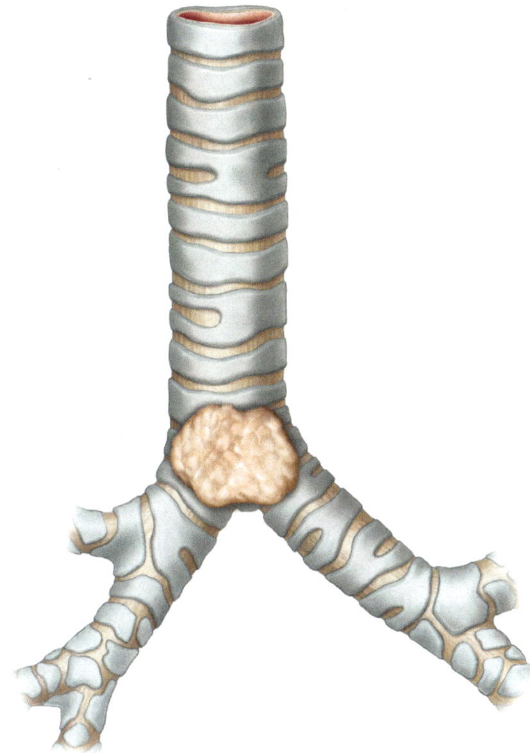

Figure 148.4. Carinal tumor. (Reprinted with permission from Wain JC. Neocarina. In: Mathisen DJ, Morse CR, eds. *Master Techniques in Surgery: Thoracic Surgery: Lung Resections, Bronchoplasty*. Wolters Kluwer; 2015:423–430. Figure 42.1.)

monitoring. Total intravenous anesthesia (TIVA) is desirable to accommodate interruptions in ventilation without risk of awareness. This can be accomplished with short-acting and titratable medications such as propofol and/or remifentanil. However, if ventilation interruptions are rare and brief, adequate anesthesia can be accomplished using volatile agents.

Many carinal resections include an accompanying partial or full lobectomy, or even pneumonectomy. Lung-protective ventilation is of great importance; effort should be made to avoid unnecessarily high inspiratory oxygen concentrations, to utilize appropriate tidal volumes, particularly during one-lung ventilation, to individualize positive end expiratory pressure, and to minimize the number of lung collapse and reexpansion events. In addition, care should be taken to avoid excessive fluid administration.

Carinal resections are generally performed mainly via a right posterolateral thoracotomy. Thoracic epidural or paravertebral analgesia remains the gold standard for pain control for procedures requiring posterolateral thoracotomy. However, multilevel intercostal nerve blockade with liposomal bupivacaine may provide similar efficacy when combined with adjunctive subarachnoid morphine and a regimen of nonopioid analgesic medications.

2 How would you manage the airway in this case?

The patient can initially be intubated with a single-lumen reinforced endotracheal tube (40 cm; Fuji Systems Corporation, Fukushima, Japan) in the proximal trachea. This tube is designed to facilitate endobronchial intubation as it has sufficient length, a short cuff, and a short cuff to tip distance. The tube is then advanced under bronchoscopic guidance into the left main bronchus. The right lung is allowed to passively collapse, while the surgical team gains access and visualization via a right-sided thoracotomy. Following adequate surgical exposure of the airway structures, the endobronchial tube is withdrawn into the distal trachea, and the left mainstem bronchus is incised to facilitate cross-field intubation and ventilation. In anticipation of this period of apnea, the patient is placed on 100% FiO_2 for a brief period. Ventilation is paused, and a sterile, reinforced tube is inserted by the surgical team, attached to a sterile extension, which is then advanced to the anesthesiologist via a small slit in the drapes (Figure 148.5).

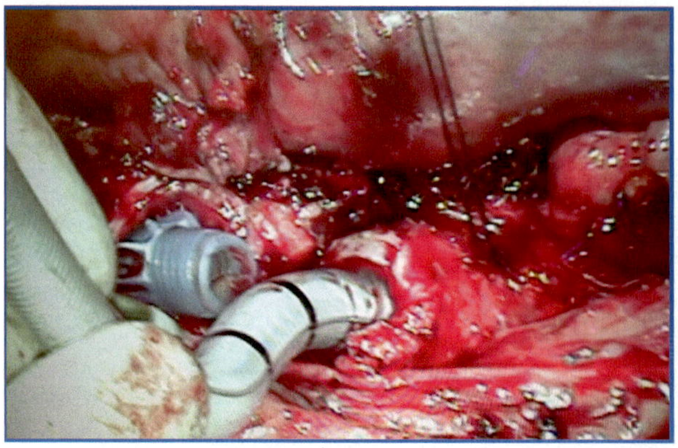

Figure 148.5. After adequate exposure to the airway structures was obtained, the endobronchial tube was withdrawn into the distal trachea, and the surgeon incises the left mainstem bronchus to facilitate on-field intubation.

Cross-field ventilation of the left lung commences. After resection of the right upper lobe, the right main bronchus, and the carina, a neocarina is created between the distal trachea, the bronchus intermedius, and the remaining left main bronchus. Brief periods of apnea and surgical withdrawal of the cross-field left bronchial endotracheal tube are required to facilitate the posterior anastomosis. Following completion of the anastomosis, the surgeon-placed left cross-field tube is removed, and the tracheal tube is readvanced into the left main bronchus guided by flexible bronchoscopy. One-lung ventilation is reinitiated to allow procedure completion. Subsequently, this tube is again withdrawn into a tracheal position, the remaining right lung (middle and lower lobes) reexpands, and two-lung ventilation is reestablished. Following diagnostic and toilet bronchoscopy, the patient emerges from anesthesia and can be extubated in the operating room and transported to the intensive care unit for overnight observation. This patient was discharged 4 days later without complication.

3 What distinct airway device (eg, specialized tracheal tube, rigid bronchoscope, bronchial blocker) might be used in this case, and what are the special considerations?

A distinctive airway device, which is uniquely formed to facilitate lung isolation and one-lung ventilation via endobronchial intubation for such a resection, is the single-lumen endobronchial tube (Figure 148.6). Standard single-lumen endotracheal tubes have a long cuff in addition to a long cuff-to-tip distance, rendering

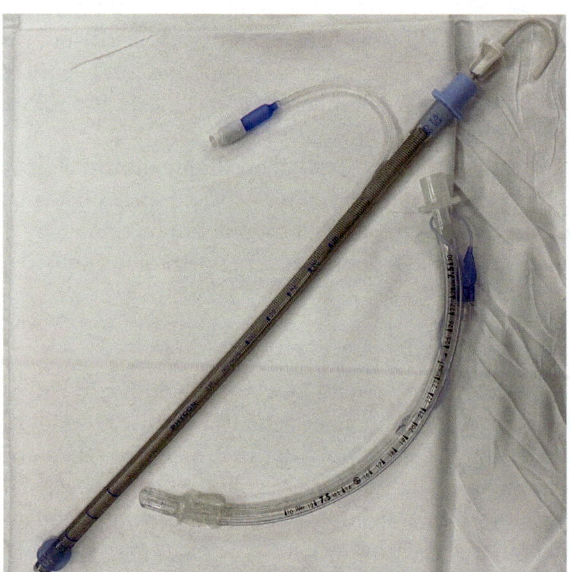

Figure 148.6. The endobronchial tube, compared to the traditional endotracheal tube, has a longer length (40 cm), a pliable and wire-reinforced silicone construction, a smaller cuff, as well as a short cuff-to-tip distance.

them inadequate for endobronchial placement, particularly on the right side where upper lobe blockage is likely inevitable. The development of tubes compatible with endobronchial placement has improved the management of single-lung ventilation in such clinical contexts. For example, the endobronchial tube (used in the above case) has a longer length (40 cm), a pliable and wire-reinforced silicone construction, a smaller cuff, as well as a short cuff-to-tip distance. The tube can be placed within either mainstem bronchus to achieve one-lung isolation and is particularly beneficial in distal tracheal and carinal surgery, as a double-lumen tube would distort tracheobronchial anatomy and impede the carinal dissection.

Other means to facilitate gas exchange during carinal resection include jet ventilation, extracorporeal membrane oxygenation (ECMO), and or cardiopulmonary bypass (CPB). Jet ventilation can be used during the resection and reconstruction phase of surgery via small-bore catheters placed in either the distal trachea or across the surgical field via an existing tracheal tube or supraglottic airway device. Potential disadvantages to this approach include the development of hypercapnia, hypothermia, mucosal desiccation, as well as interference with the surgical field. If surgical manipulation obstructs the passive expiratory outflow of air, there is an increased risk of volutrauma/barotrauma. Both venovenous ECMO and CPB can be used to augment or completely supplant ventilation for gas exchange. However, extracorporeal support is accompanied by an increased risk of vascular injury, coagulopathy, and systemic inflammatory response. The choice of complex lung isolation and ventilation techniques versus extracorporeal support is heavily influenced by surgeon preference. It may be desirable for more complex and extensive resections and in patients with critical airway obstruction or severely impaired pulmonary or cardiac function.

4 Are there special considerations for the emergence or the end of the case?

Postoperatively, patients should be weaned from mechanical ventilation and extubated as soon as safely feasible. If postoperative mechanical ventilation is required, the endotracheal tube cuff should be positioned well away from the anastomosis to minimize injury. Neck extension, coughing, and vomiting should be avoided to minimize tension on the anastomosis. If reintubation is required, smaller tracheal tubes should be used, to mitigate risk of anastomosis dehiscence. The tubes should be placed above the anastomosis and under bronchoscopic guidance.

- Carinal resections are complex procedures which require careful preoperative evaluation, including CT or MRI as well as direct visualization via bronchoscopy, in addition to rigorous operative planning between the surgical and anesthesia team.
- Rigid bronchoscopy equipment and a skilled practitioner should be immediately available for airway rescue.
- Depending on the operative plan, airway management generally includes lung isolation and one-lung ventilation via a bronchoscopically guided endobronchial tube, followed by cross-field ventilation to allow for mobilization and dissection of the carina.
- Endobronchial tubes are uniquely structured to facilitate one-lung ventilation, including their longer length, flexible reinforced structure, smaller cuff, and shorter cuff-to-tip distance.
- Postprocedurally, these patients should be extubated in a timely manner, and subsequent airway management should focus on protecting the fresh anastomosis.
- *See* ⊙ ***Video 148.1*** *for additional details.*

Suggested Readings

Collins SR, Titus BJ, Camps JH, Blank RS. Lung isolation in the patient with a difficult airway. *Anesth Analg*. 2018;126:1968–1978.

Gonfiotti A, Jaus MO, Barale D, Macchiarini P. Carinal resection. *Thorac Surg Clin*. 2014;24:477–484.

Matsuura N, Igai H, Kamiyoshishara M. Carinal resection and reconstruction: now and in the future. *Transl Lung Cancer*. 2021; 10:4039–4042.

Schieren M, Wappler F, Defosse J. Anesthesia for tracheal and carinal resection and reconstruction. *Curr Opin Anaesthesiol*. 2021;35:75–81.

149 Extracorporeal Membrane Oxygenation in Thoracic Surgery

Bhoumesh Patel • Andrew Notarianni

1 Describe in detail the device or technique.

Extracorporeal membrane oxygenation (ECMO) is a temporary artificial extracorporeal therapy that can provide respiratory, cardiac, or combined cardiopulmonary circulatory support. A standard ECMO circuit consists of vascular access (cannulas), a mechanical blood pump, a gas exchange device (an oxygenator), a heat exchanger, all connected together with the conduit tubing (Figure 149.1).

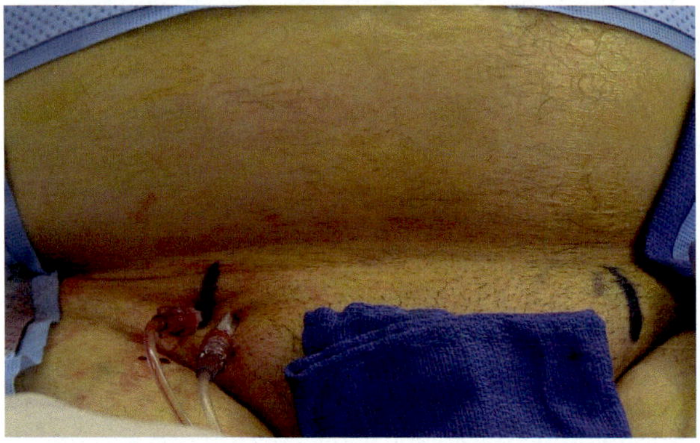

Figure 149.1. Extracorporeal membrane oxygenation (ECMO) cannulas in place. ECMO cannulas placed prior to the induction of anesthesia in the groin vessels of a patient to undergo extensive *tracheal resection*.

There are two main types of ECMO: venovenous (VV)-ECMO and venoarterial (VA)-ECMO. In VV-ECMO, deoxygenated venous blood is drained from a cannula that is usually inserted into the femoral vein. The venous blood goes through the oxygenator for oxygenation and carbon dioxide removal, and then the oxygenated blood is returned into the right atrium via the right internal jugular vein. Dual-stage, single-catheter systems have also been developed that both drain and return blood simultaneously. These integrated catheters are inserted through a single site, most often the right internal jugular vein, and direct the return of oxygenated blood across the tricuspid valve. VV-ECMO only provides respiratory support without any cardiac support. Therefore, it relies on the patient's native cardiac output to pump oxygenated blood into the systemic circulation. In VA-ECMO, deoxygenated blood is drained from the venous system, and oxygenated blood is returned into the arterial circulation, similar to standard cardiopulmonary bypass. VA-ECMO can provide total systemic circulatory support (Figure 149.2). The femoral veins are commonly used for venous cannulation, while arterial cannulation sites include the femoral arteries, axillary arteries, or ascending aorta. The native and artificial membrane lungs are in series in VV-ECMO, whereas they are parallel in VA-ECMO. In both situations, the function of the native lung can be replaced totally or partially.

2 Where or when is the device used in airway management?

ECMO can be utilized during two crucial phases of intraoperative care. It can be electively used prior to induction of general anesthesia, postinduction to facilitate surgery or emergently to manage a crisis. ECMO should be initiated prior to induction of anesthesia in patients with critical airway stenosis, airway distortion, or significant cardiovascular compression who are at risk of acute respiratory or hemodynamic decompensation despite conventional airway management techniques. Intraoperatively, it can play a significant role in facilitating complex high-risk airway or lung resection surgeries that may not be possible utilizing conventional airway techniques due to inadequate gas exchange or significant hemodynamic instability, especially in patients with low cardiopulmonary reserve. In addition, ECMO can be utilized to eliminate the need for cross-field ventilation, thereby creating an unobstructed and motionless view of the surgical field and allowing for unlimited time to complete extended resections and reconstructions. For surgeries where extensive manipulation of

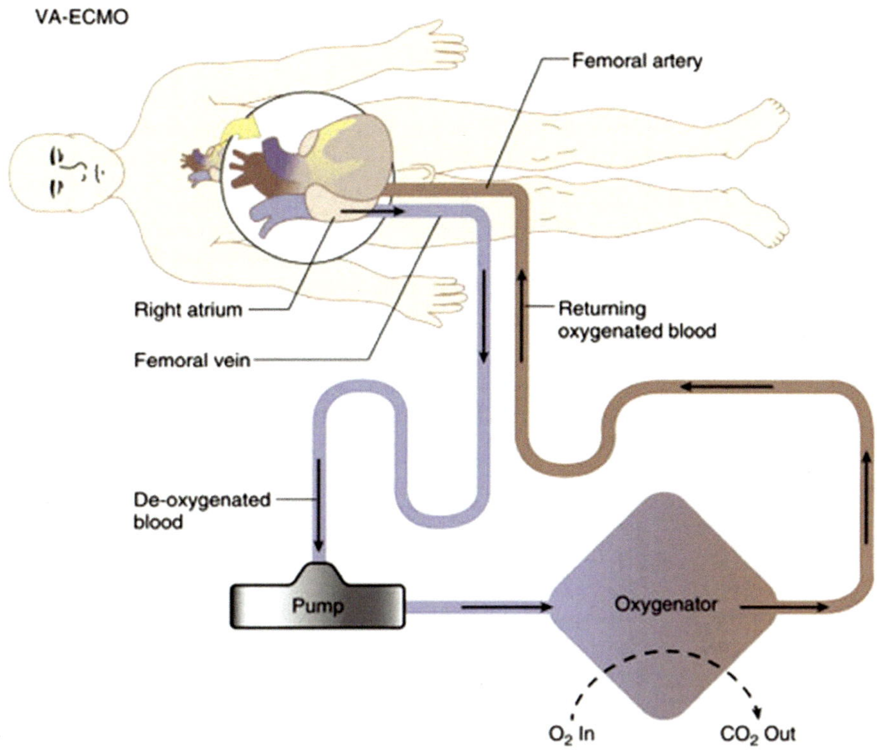

Figure 149.2. Extracorporeal membrane oxygenation (ECMO) circuit components. (Reprinted from Razo-Vazquez AO, Thornton K. Extracorporeal membrane oxygenation–what the nephrologist needs to know. *Adv Chronic Kidney Dis*. 2016;23(3):146–151. Figure 1. Copyright © 2016 The National Kidney Foundation, Inc. With permission.)

the heart and great vessels is anticipated, VA-ECMO should be utilized to maintain adequate global perfusion and prevent hemodynamic stress.

In addition, ECMO can be continued into the postoperative phase to manage complications and to provide the opportunity for ultraprotective mechanical ventilation. Continuation of ECMO support in the postoperative phase can allow an early extubation, which facilitates anastomosis healing and reduces the risk of developing a stenosis due to prolonged intubation or tracheostomy. Dual-lumen catheters placed in the jugular vein can be especially helpful for this purpose.

3 What distinguishes this device or technique from similar airway management methods?

Conventional airways management is challenging, particularly in cases of low cardiopulmonary reserve and in cases of complex tracheobronchial or superior vena cava resections and reconstructions. By providing either partial or complete respiratory and circulatory support during these high-risk surgeries, ECMO eliminates the need for intermittent cross-field ventilation, periods of hypoxemia, hypercarbia, and hemodynamic instability during cardiovascular manipulation.

ECMO differs from conventional cardiopulmonary bypass (CPB) in multiple ways. Modern ECMO circuits are more biocompatible, simpler, and safer. Advantages of ECMO over CPB include the miniaturized circuit that requires lower priming volumes resulting in less hemodilution, closed circulation circuit without the venous reservoir and cardiotomy suction which eliminates air–blood contact and lowers the inflammatory response. The ECMO circuit tubing is coated with a biocompatible lining that decreases the systemic inflammatory response, requires lower anticoagulation levels resulting in less coagulopathy therefore lowering the risk of thrombosis and bleeding. There is no risk of tumor cell dissemination due to the closed system being devoid of cardiotomy suction as during CPB. Moreover, when peripheral ECMO cannulation is used, the surgeon has a clean operative field, without disturbing lines. Finally, in case of an emergent situation, it is possible to convert VA-ECMO into conventional CPB by adding a venous reservoir connected to the ECMO device. However, ECMO, unlike CPB doesn't allow air filtration, so CPB should be utilized if the venous or cardiac chambers will be dissected.

Author Caveats

Transesophageal echocardiography (TEE) or fluoroscopy must be utilized to confirm cannula positioning and prevent any complications. Bispectral index monitor should be utilized to assess anesthetic depth as higher doses of intravenous anesthetics may be needed in ECMO patients, due to a larger volume of drug distribution and drug loss resulting from adsorption in the circuit. ECMO flows should be maintained at greater than 3 L/min to avoid any circuit thrombosis when anticoagulation is held. VV-ECMO circuit blood flow should be targeted to be >60% of cardiac output in most patients to maintain adequate blood oxygenation. Sweep gas flow should be titrated to the desirable pH and $PaCO_2$ goal. Sweep should be lower when ventilation is resumed to avoid hypocarbia and cerebral vasoconstriction. Patients on peripheral VA-ECMO should be monitored via pulse oximetry and/or arterial oxygenation measured from the right upper extremity to assess for differential oxygenation in the setting of intermittent apnea. There are no special respiratory or hemodynamic monitoring considerations in VV-ECMO. TEE should be utilized to assess for intracardiac stasis and ECMO flow should be titrated to achieve a pulse pressure greater than 20 mm Hg in order to avoid any intracardiac stasis.

- ECMO support allows high-risk thoracic surgery in selected patients who would otherwise be considered inoperable.
- VV-ECMO should be considered in all patients with critical upper or lower airway stenosis where a complete airway occlusion can ensue, as well as in patients requiring a complex lower airway resection and reconstruction.
- For procedures involving cardiac manipulations with expected profound hemodynamic instability, VA-ECMO can be utilized for combined respiratory and cardiac support.
- ECMO can provide partial or total cardiopulmonary support without conventional airway management and provide excellent surgical conditions with unobstructed views.
- *See Figures 149.3 and 149.4 as well as* ***Video 149.1*** *for additional details.*

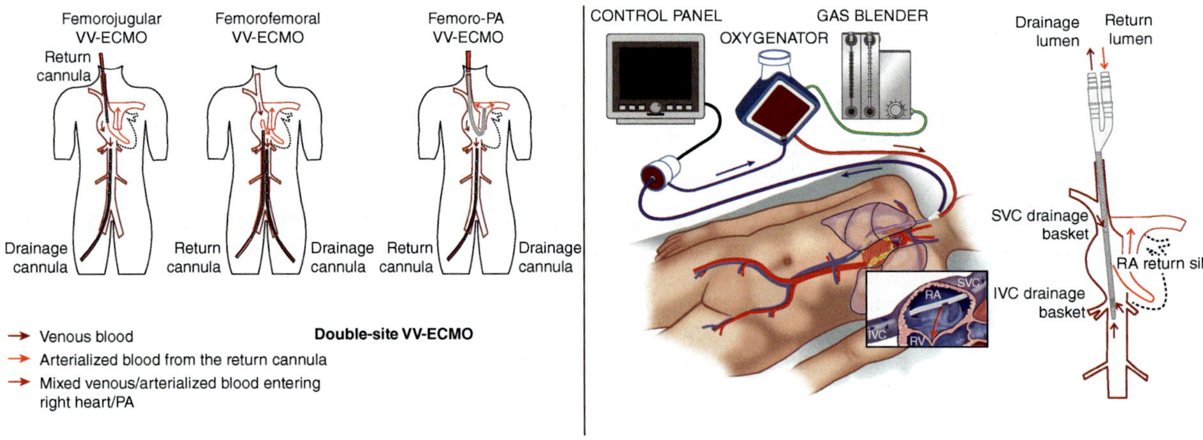

Figure 149.3. Venovenous extracorporeal membrane oxygenation (VV-ECMO) cannulation strategies. (Reprinted with permission from Gajkowski EF, Herrera G, Hatton L, Velia Antonini M, Vercaemst L, Cooley E. ELSO Guidelines for adult and pediatric extracorporeal membrane oxygenation circuits. *ASAIO J*. 2022;68(2):133–152. Copyright © ELSO 2022.)

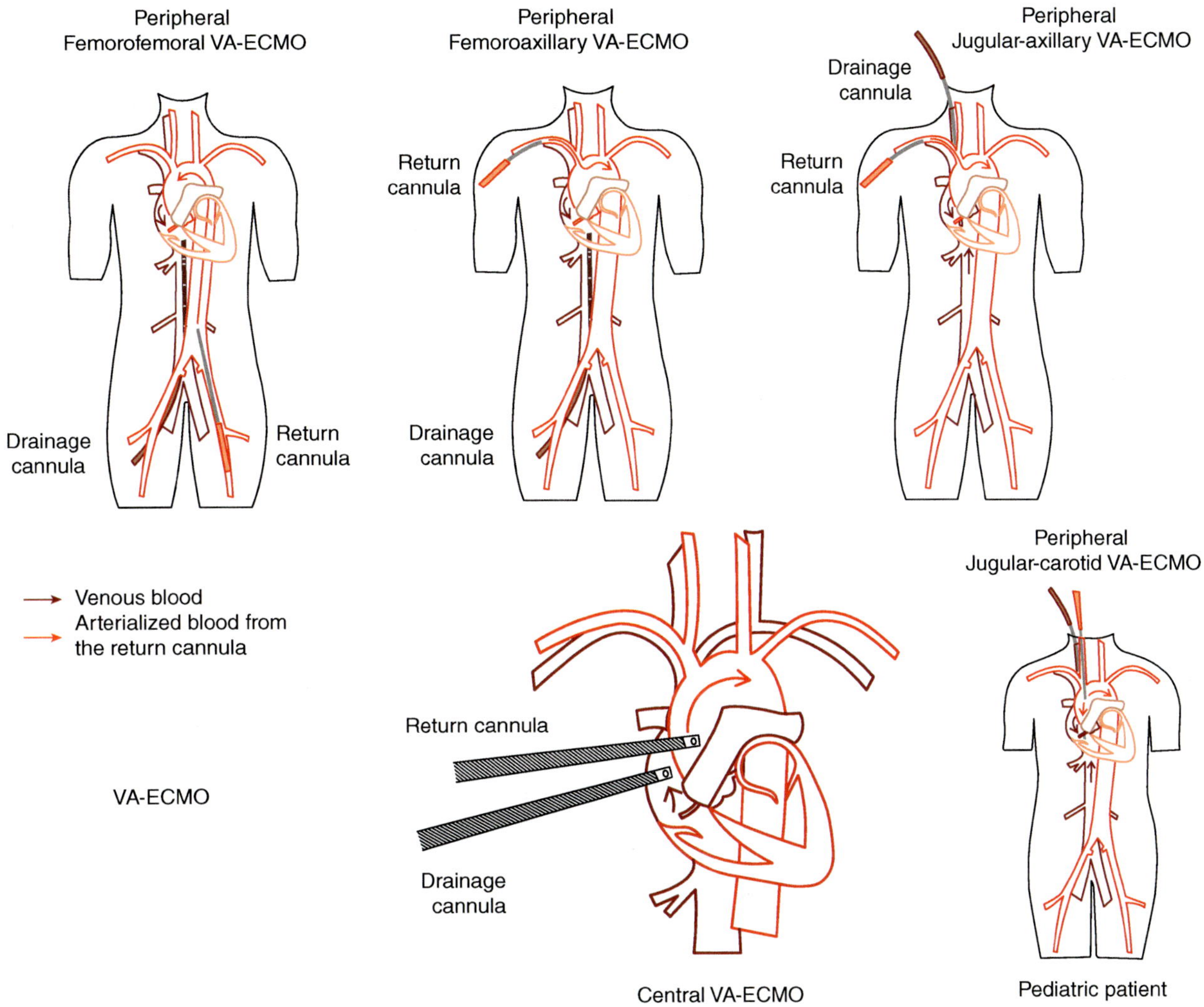

Figure 149.4. Venoarterial extracorporeal membrane oxygenation (VA-ECMO) cannulation strategies. (Reprinted with permission from Gajkowski EF, Herrera G, Hatton L, Velia Antonini M, Vercaemst L, Cooley E. ELSO Guidelines for adult and pediatric extracorporeal membrane oxygenation circuits. *ASAIO J*. 2022;68(2):133–152. Copyright © ELSO 2022.)

Suggested Readings

Chatterjee S, Loor G. Extracorporeal membrane oxygenation during and after pulmonary resection. In: Sugarbaker DJ, Bueno R, Burt BM, Groth SS, eds. *Sugarbaker's Adult Chest Surgery*. 3rd ed. McGraw Hill; 2020:853–862.

Hoetzenecker K, Klepetko W, Keshavjee S, Cypel M. Extracorporeal support in airway surgery. *J Thorac Dis*. 2017;9(7):2108–2117.

Mazzeffi MA, Rao VK, Dodd-O J, et al. Intraoperative management of adult patients on extracorporeal membrane oxygenation: an expert consensus statement from The society of Cardiovascular Anesthesiologists-Part I, technical aspects of extracorporeal membrane oxygenation. *Anesth Analg*. 2021;133(6):1459–1477.

Mazzeffi MA, Rao VK, Dodd-O J, et al. Intraoperative management of adult patients on extracorporeal membrane oxygenation: an expert consensus statement from the Society of Cardiovascular Anesthesiologists-Part II, intraoperative management and troubleshooting. *Anesth Analg*. 2021;133(6):1478–1493.

150 Mediastinoscopy and Video-Assisted Thoracic Surgery

Diana Anca

Clinical Scenario: An 80-year-old woman with a 3-cm left lower lobe nodule presents to the OR for a flexible bronchoscopy and mediastinoscopy, followed by a left lower lobectomy via a video-assisted thoracic surgery (VATS).

1 What are the anesthetic and airway management considerations for this case?

Flexible bronchoscopy and mediastinoscopy are common procedures used in the diagnosis and staging of lung cancer. The flexible bronchoscopy precedes mediastinoscopy and is performed to identify anatomy and possible tumor involvement of the tracheobronchial tree. Occasionally, biopsies or bronchial lavages may be required. The typical mediastinoscopy approach is cervical, via a small incision above the sternal notch. Mediastinal lymph nodes from different locations are collected to identify tumor involvement. If the pathology of the lymph nodes is negative for malignant disease, the mediastinoscopy is followed by lung resection surgery. A previous mediastinoscopy or a history of radiation therapy is a contraindication to the procedure. In such cases, endobronchial ultrasound (EBUS) with transbronchial biopsies can be performed.

Of note, the complication rate is significantly lower with EBUS, and it yields similar results as far as staging, however, the operator experience is important. Paraesophageal lymph nodes can be accessed via endoscopic ultrasound (EUS). Often, the mediastinoscopy and EBUS are combined for an overall sensitivity of 85% to 94% and a negative predictive value of 93%.

This combined surgical procedure requires general anesthesia with endotracheal intubation and positive-pressure ventilation. The anesthetic management of the patient has to take into consideration the fact that the procedure will start with a bronchoscopy, that potentially requires a large endotracheal tube (ETT), and that following the mediastinoscopy, the VATS will require one-lung ventilation (OLV). In extremely rare and unique situations when patients are too sick for a general anesthetic, bronchoscopy and mediastinoscopy can be performed under local anesthesia.

In crafting the anesthetic plan, the overall pulmonary status of the patient and the appearance of the airway (easy vs difficult) will play a role. Nevertheless, a discussion with the surgeon should take place preoperatively to map out the plan and available options.

2 How would you manage the airway in this case?

In managing the airway for this procedure, the clinician should consider that it is a complex, combined surgery and that different parts of this procedure require different airway management devices. When deciding the optimal airway management plan, the patient's airway appearance as well as the surgical requirements must be considered.

The airway can be managed either with an ETT followed by placement of a bronchial blocker (BB) when lung isolation is needed, or with an ETT followed by exchange to a DLT or by using a DLT throughout the entire procedure. However, the flexible bronchoscope required for bronchoscopy is larger and the fit via a DLT is difficult, especially since this patient is a female and smaller-sized DLT would be utilized (35 Fr or 37 Fr). Alternatively, a supraglottic airway device can be initially utilized for the bronchoscopy part of the surgery and then exchanged to a DLT.

If the airway appears normal, the surgeon desires to perform just a surveillance bronchoscopy, and the lung resection is considered routine, then any of the presented options of airway management can be utilized. If, during bronchoscopy, the surgeon plans on performing additional procedures, then a larger-sized bronchoscope is used. Therefore, a minimum 8.0 mm ETT or a supraglottic airway device is required. Following bronchoscopy and mediastinoscopy, the team needs to decide if the lung resection surgery is expected to be straightforward. If chest adhesions are expected or the patient has significant emphysematous disease, it is likely that a BB would not provide adequate and timely lung deflation. In such cases, exchanging the ETT for a DLT would be the best option (see Chapter 140: Single Lumen Tube to Double Lumen Tube Exchange). In all other situations, a BB can be placed via the ETT into the desired bronchus.

If the airway appears to be challenging, then an ETT is placed using either an awake or an asleep intubation technique. Placing a BB should be the lung isolation device of choice for the VATS part. Only significant surgical reasons could compel the anesthesiologist to take into account exchanging a secure airway for a DLT. BBs are viable alternatives to DLTs, as they have a lower incidence and severity of airway injury and comparable quality of lung deflation, though DLT can be placed faster and are less likely to be displaced.

3 What are the surgical considerations that impact anesthetic management?

Several surgical factors need to be considered when deciding the optimal airway management. An important concern is the purpose of the flexible bronchoscopy. If this is performed as a routine surveillance procedure, it is likely that a regular-sized intubating flexible bronchoscope (FB) (3.8 mm) can be used. This scope fits through an ETT as well as a DLT. However, if interventional procedures are required, such as biopsies, bronchoalveolar lavages, or EBUS, a much larger FB (6.0 mm) is used. In such cases, a minimum 8.0 mm ETT will be required. A DLT cannot accommodate the passage of this bronchoscope.

Though mediastinoscopy has a low mortality, it carries risks for serious complications. They are related to the insertion and manipulation of the mediastinoscope. Potential problems that can occur during the procedure are hemorrhage, stroke, air embolism, pneumothorax, recurrent laryngeal or phrenic nerve injury, and tracheal or esophageal laceration. Some directly impact the upper and lower airway. As this patient is undergoing a combined procedure, before manipulating the airway or initiating OLV, the anesthesiologist should evaluate for the presence of such complications and promptly address them if needed.

Another surgical concern is the perceived degree of difficulty of the lung resection surgery. In situations of severe lung emphysema, when it is expected that the patient has significant lung hyperinflation and may have a poor tolerance of OLV, then probably a DLT is a better option. In such cases, use of a BB, with its narrow channel, requires a longer time for complete lung deflation. Moreover, if the patient needs intermittent two-lung ventilation, this problem is augmented. Conversely, if the patient is expected to remain intubated after the procedure, probably the BB is a better lung isolation device as it can be removed at the end of the procedure.

All these considerations should be carefully weighed and discussed with the surgeon preoperatively.

4 Are there special considerations for the emergence at the end of the case?

The considerations at the end of the case are related to the complexity of the procedure, and the presence or absence of complications. Before proceeding to extubation, the anesthesiologist should consider a quick checklist of potential problems: complexity and length of procedure, presence and severity of intraoperative complications, pain control, and overall patient frailty and pre-existent respiratory status.

A large pneumothorax can be easily ruled out by checking for the presence of increased airway pressures, hypoxemia, and decreased blood pressure. However, small pneumothoraxes may take a long time to become clinically evident. Therefore, postoperative radiologic evaluation is indicated. In prolonged dissections, there is an increased risk of recurrent laryngeal nerve injury and airway edema. In such cases, prior to extubation, assessing for vocal cord motion and for the presence of an air leak with cuff deflation is indicated. Although rare, tracheobronchial laceration manifested with subcutaneous emphysema is a serious complication. In such cases, extubation should be postponed until further evaluation. Another rare but serious occurrence is a stroke. It might not be immediately apparent in an elderly patient emerging from general anesthesia, but any delayed emergence or focal deficit should alert the anesthesiologist to this possibility. Some complications take a longer time to fully declare themselves. Therefore, careful monitoring in the postoperative period is considered standard management for these cases.

- Mediastinoscopy can be performed alone or in combination with lung resection surgery.
- EBUS has a lower complication rate than mediastinoscopy, but the choice of staging method depends on the location of lymph nodes, operator experience, and frequently the two techniques are combined for a higher sensitivity.
- Lung isolation is needed if the surgeon proceeds with a VATS; either BB or DLT can be used.
- Complications are rare, but could be severe and must be diagnosed and promptly addressed.
- Complexity and length of procedure, presence of complications, and patient's preoperative pulmonary and functional status should all be taken into consideration when deciding if to extubate the patient.
- *See Figures 150.1 and 150.2 as well as* **Video 150.1** *for additional details.*

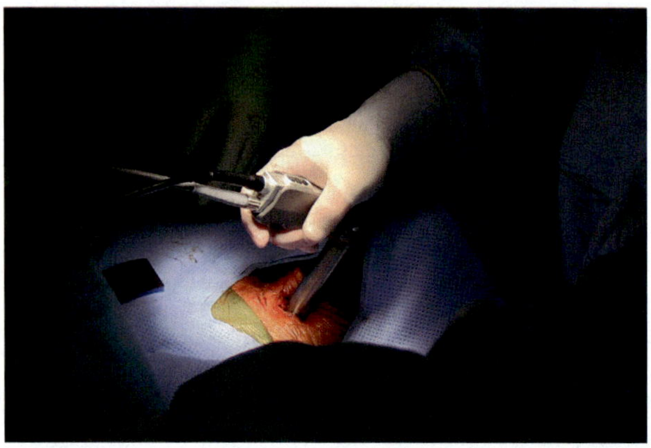

Figure 150.1. The Mediastinoscope is inserted via an incision above the sternal notch.

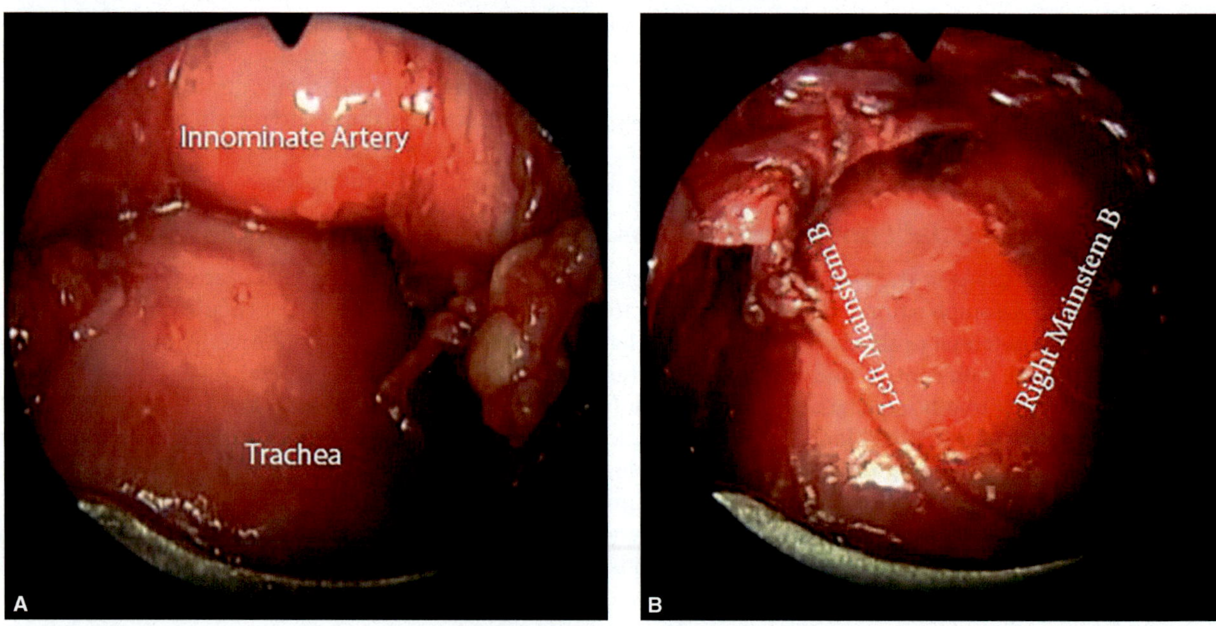

Figure 150.2. **A:** Surgeon's view from the Mediastinoscope. **B:** Surgeon's view of the right and left mainstem bronchi.

Suggested Readings

Anesthesia for Video-Assisted Thoracoscopic Surgery (VATS). https://www.uptodate.com

Campos JH. *Separation of the Lung: Double Lumen Endotracheal Tubes and Endobronchial Blockers in Cohen's Comprehensive Thoracic Anesthesia*. Elsevier; 2021:213–239.

Clayton-Smith A, Bennett K, Alston RP, et al. A comparison of the efficacy and adverse effects of double-lumen endobronchial tubes and bronchial blockers in thoracic surgery: a systematic review and meta-analysis of randomized controlled trials. *J Cardiothorac Vasc Anesth*. 2015;29(4):955–966.

Finlayson GN, Hughes BG. Bronchoscopic procedures. In: Slinger PD, ed. *Principles and Practices of Anesthesia for Thoracic Surgery*. Springer; 2011:197–218.

Lin JL, Fernandez F. Indications for invasive mediastinal staging for non-small cell lung cancer. *J Thorac Cardiovasc Surg*. 2018; 156(6):2319–2324.

Pedoto A, Heerdt PM, Yao FS. Bronchoscopy, mediastinoscopy, and thoracotomy. In: Yao FS, ed. *Yao & Artusio's Anesthesiology: Problem-Oriented Patient Management*. 7th ed. Lippincott Williams & Wilkins; 2011:43–59.

151 Robotic-Assisted Thoracic Surgery

Sarah McDonald • Peter Slinger

Clinical Scenario: A 69-year-old woman with a right upper lobe mass presents to the OR for a robotic-assisted right upper lobectomy. She has moderate chronic obstructive pulmonary disease (COPD). The surgeon requires CO_2 insufflation for improved visualization.

1 What are the anesthetic and airway management considerations for this case?

Robotic-assisted thoracic surgery (RATS) has become relatively common for numerous thoracic procedures, including diaphragmatic repair, esophagectomy, lung resection, and mediastinal tumor resection. This necessitates a level of familiarity for the anesthesiologist involved in robotic procedures and the subsequent issues which may arise. Patient positioning presents a major consideration for airway management. In order to facilitate access of the robotic arms to the thoracic cavity for a lobectomy, the patient is positioned in a flexed, lateral decubitus position. The OR table is rotated away from the anesthesiologist and the robotic system is docked at the head of the patient. Ensuring adequate and stable lung isolation prior to docking the robot is required. During repositioning of the OR table and robot docking, care should be exhibited to avoid circuit disconnection and inadvertent airway device dislodgement. Furthermore, once the robot is docked, neuromuscular monitoring and adequate depth of anesthesia is essential to avoid bucking, which can lead to significant lung/mediastinal injury. A remifentanil infusion, along with adequate muscle relaxation, is beneficial in this regard. At the end of the case, sugammadex should be used if there is any concern of impaired neuromuscular function.

In this patient with moderate COPD, another consideration is the possibility of desaturation at the institution of one-lung ventilation (OLV). In such situations, the initial step in troubleshooting the hypoxemic event is to verify the position of the lung isolation device. A recruitment maneuver may be administered to the ventilated lung. An alternative measure is to transiently insufflate 5 L/min of oxygen via the suction port of a bronchoscope to the bronchopulmonary segments which are not involved in the surgical resection, while being mindful of the risk of barotrauma. Other measures employed to optimize oxygenation, such as passive insufflation of oxygen to the collapsed lung or application of continuous positive airway pressure, would likely interfere with visibility in the surgical field and may be of decreased value in RATS. Furthermore, insufflation of CO_2 may increase airway pressures, making ventilation of the dependent lung more challenging in a patient who is already predisposed to CO_2 retention at baseline (baseline hypercapnia should be assessed with a preinduction blood gas). Finally, should pre-existing pulmonary hypertension exist, it will provide an additional challenge during insufflation and the subsequent decrease in venous return. In this situation, attention must also be made to sudden increases in pulmonary vasculature afterload, which may not be tolerated by an impaired right ventricle.

2 How would you manage the airway in this case?

The aim of airway management is to provide appropriate lung isolation for surgical visualization. Due to limited access to the patient's airway resulting from bed position as well as the robotic chassis, a left-sided double lumen tube (DLT) provides the largest margin of safety. Bronchial blockers (BBs) have a higher tendency to be dislodged during surgical manipulation. The use of a DLT allows more reliable lung collapse, and facilitates flexible bronchoscopy, which may be necessary to confirm the patency of the adjacent airways prior to stapling of the involved bronchus. In patients with moderate and severe COPD, lung collapse may not be optimal due to air trapping. The use of a DLT allows active suctioning of the gas content from the lung to be collapsed.

DLT placement should be checked after the patient has been placed in the final surgical position (for lung resection the most common position being lateral). Prior to instituting OLV, denitrogenation with 100% oxygen expedites lung collapse and provides a margin of reserve before the full onset of hypoxic pulmonary vasoconstriction. The use of alveolar recruitment maneuvers on the ventilated lung prior to docking of the robotic arms is recommended.

3 What are the surgical considerations that impact anesthetic management?

During RATS, insufflation of low-flow CO_2 into the thoracic cavity improves visualization. The effects of CO_2 insufflation can be divided into pressure effects on the mediastinum and on both hemithoraces, and systemic effects related to CO_2 absorption. Insufflation pressures should not exceed 15 mm Hg, as the increase in intrathoracic pressure may result in deleterious effects on the cardiovascular and respiratory systems. These hemodynamic effects are more pronounced on the right hemithorax. Increased pressures on the right atrium and vena cava result in decreased venous return, stroke volume, and cardiac index.

CO_2 insufflation increases peak airway pressure and decreases the compliance of the ventilated lung. A high index of suspicion for tension pneumothorax in the ventilated lung should be maintained if a sudden decrease in lung compliance, desaturation, and increased airway pressure occurs.

Systemic effects resulting from hypercarbia include respiratory acidosis, pulmonary vasoconstriction, and increased sympathetic stimulation. In the setting of RATS, the avoidance of barotrauma while on OLV provides additional challenges to the management of hypercarbia. Inadvertent insufflation of CO_2 into the venous system will result in gas embolism. The pulmonary capillaries filter small volumes of venous gas emboli, producing ventilation–perfusion mismatches, which manifest as worsening hypoxemia. However, a large venous gas embolus may result in circulatory collapse due to the development of a gas lock in the right ventricle. Therefore, CO_2 insufflation should be instituted after the confirmation of the appropriate port position. It should be initiated gradually with close monitoring of vital signs as the insufflation pressures are increased. Intraoperative arterial blood gases are used to assess oxygenation and ventilation. In the event of hemodynamic instability or difficulty with the management of hypercarbia, the surgeon may be required to utilize a lower insufflation pressure.

Of key importance is the fact that the docked robot does not adjust to any patient movement. Thus, adequate muscle relaxation is important to avoid tissue injury and potential bleeding. Furthermore, should significant bleeding occur, hemostasis and visualization is particularly challenging and a plan for urgent undocking of the robot and adequate preparation for opening must be in place. For this reason, patients should have an arterial line and adequate intravenous access (two large IV's) to ensure optimal safety.

4 What are the potential hazards and complications in regard to the airway?

A high level of vigilance is required for dislodgement of circuitry and the airway itself during patient positioning and docking and undocking of the robotic chassis. To avoid disconnections, it is helpful to secure the circuit and the gas sampling line together and elevate them away from the robotic foot. As the OR table is rotated away from the anesthesiologist and surgical drapes and the robot chassis obscure the patient's head, inadvertent dislodgement of the airway isolation device may occur. Loss of lung isolation is best managed by planning in advance for the potential need to perform bronchoscopy during the procedure. This entails having a portable bronchoscope and a mode of accessing the patient's airway under the drapes. An assistant is often beneficial should this need arise.

Intraoperative monitoring of spirometry is helpful in detecting an early air leak, and a decrease in the expired tidal volume should prompt reconfirmation of the lung isolation device placement.

- Usage of a DLT for lung isolation will facilitate optimal lung collapse, especially in a patient with underlying COPD.
- CO_2 insufflation impacts the cardiovascular and respiratory systems and may have particularly deleterious effects in patients with underlying lung or cardiac disease.
- Complications of CO_2 insufflation occur from intraoperative hypercarbia and inadvertent gas embolism into vascular structures.
- The entire surgical team must be familiar with RATS and protocols for urgent undocking of the robot, and potential surgical opening must be in place should an emergency occur.
- *See Figure 151.1 and* ***Video 151.1*** *for additional details.*

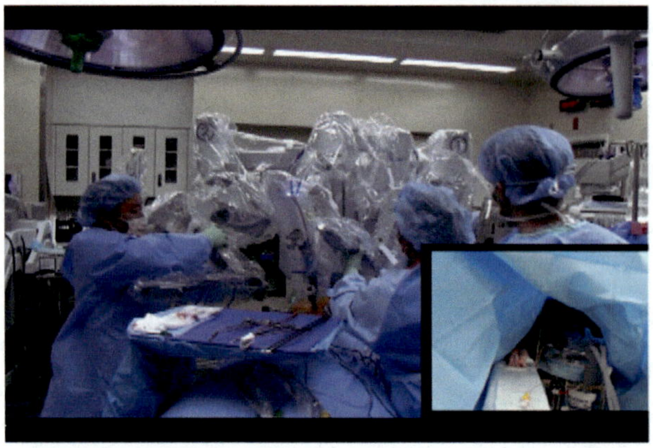

Figure 151.1. The patient is draped and the robot is positioned for thoracic surgery. There is limited access to the patient's airway during the procedure (*inset*).

Acknowledgments

We gratefully acknowledge the contributions of previous edition author, Su Lin Maureen Cheng, as portions of those chapters have been retained in this revision.

Suggested Readings

Campos J. Anesthesia for robotic thoracic surgery. In: Slinger P, ed. *Principles and Practice of Anesthesia for Thoracic Surgery*. 2nd ed. Springer; 2019:651–659.

Pauli H, Eladawy M, Park J. Anesthesia for robotic thoracic surgery. *Ann Cardiothorac Surg*. 2019;8(2):263–268.

Ruan A, Kulkarni V. Anesthesia considerations for robotic thoracic surgery. *Video Assisted Thoracic Surg*. 2020;5.

Robotic-Assisted Thymectomy

152

John B. Pawlowski • Sapna Govindan

Clinical Scenario: A 28-year-old female with myasthenia gravis (MG) controlled on medications presents for robotic-assisted thymectomy.

1 What are the anesthetic/airway management considerations for this case?

Anesthetic concerns for patients with MG include increased sensitivity to nondepolarizing muscle relaxant and resistance to succinylcholine, a depolarizing muscle relaxant, myasthenic/cholinergic crisis resulting in the need for prolonged mechanical ventilation, and rarely airway compromise with induction of anesthesia due to the thymic mass compression.

Minimally invasive robotic thoracoscopic thymectomy has become increasingly popular because of its similar efficacy, safety, and morbidity and decreased hospital stay compared with conventional open surgery. Usually, a left-sided surgical approach is performed, using three or four thoracoscopic ports and CO_2 for insufflation. Either a double-lumen tube (DLT) or a bronchial blocker (BB) placed under flexible bronchoscopy guidance is used for one-lung ventilation, which is required for optimal surgical exposure. The docking of the robot limits free accessibility to the patient's airway and arms.

2 How would you manage the airway in this case?

Special concerns include patient positioning, minimal patient access after docking, capnothorax, and resulting high airway pressures, and compression of the heart and major vessels during surgical dissection. A left-sided DLT is placed and its position is confirmed with an FB. The patient is positioned in the right lateral decubitus or supine position. Both arms may be tucked or the ipsilateral arm may be abducted, extended, and externally rotated. This position can lead to neurovascular compression of the left upper limb. Use of an extra foam pillow to protect the patient's face from the wide-ranging robot arms is advised. The surgeons are positioned between the anesthesiologist and the patient, and the anesthesiologist has to be mindful of the circuit tubing. Access to the patient's airway is limited.

3 What are the surgical considerations that impact anesthetic management?

Intraoperatively, most patients experience transient episodes of arrhythmias (bradyarrhythmias, ventricular or atrial ectopy) and hypotension. This is probably caused by direct compression of the major blood vessels and the heart, stretching of the overlaying structures by the instruments or capnothorax.

During robotic thymectomy, various structures have to be dissected to gain access to the thymus. These include the vagus, recurrent laryngeal, and phrenic nerves and major blood vessels such as the innominate and subclavian arteries, superior vena cava, brachiocephalic, and azygos veins. Neurovascular compression (brachial plexus injury) in the arm of the surgical side approach has been reported. Thus, the pulse oximeter and arterial blood pressure monitoring should be done on the ipsilateral arm. The major complication of this case is pulmonary artery rupture with major hemorrhage.

Undocking the robot and opening the equipment for the surgeons to convert to an open procedure may take up to 15 minutes. During this time, the anesthesiologist should confirm that the airway is secure.

4 Are there special considerations for the emergence or the end of the case?

Most, if not all patients, are extubated at the end of the surgery once they meet extubation criteria.

Recurrent laryngeal nerve injury leads to ipsilateral vocal cord paralysis, resulting in hoarseness. Bilateral recurrent laryngeal nerve injuries result in bilateral vocal cord paralysis, which manifests as laryngospasm at extubation due to the vocal cords being in midline position. The situation represents an airway emergency.

- Lung isolation is essential during thoracic robotic thymectomy. The surgeon may also require CO_2 insufflation, which can significantly restrict venous return and result in hypotension.
- The major complication of robotic thymectomy is the need for emergent conversion to an open procedure due to massive hemorrhage. Fundamental procedures of dedocking the robot should be understood and practiced by all personnel involved.
- Bilateral recurrent laryngeal nerve injuries result in laryngospasm at extubation; this is an airway emergency which needs to be addressed promptly.
- *See Figure 152.1 for additional details.*

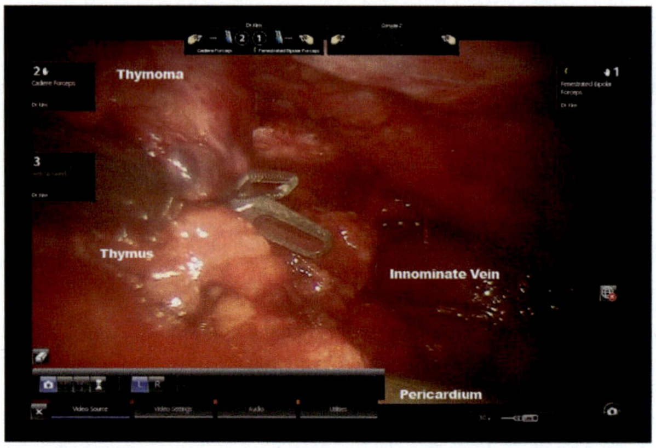

Figure 152.1. Monitor view during robotic-aided thymectomy with superimposed anatomic labels.

Acknowledgments

We gratefully acknowledge the contributions of previous edition author, Galina Korsunsky, as portions of those chapters have been retained in this revision.

Suggested Readings

Kveraga R, Pawlowski J. Anesthesia for the patient with myasthenia gravis. https://www.uptodate.com/contents/anesthesia-for-the-patient-with-myasthenia-gravis

Marulli G, Schiavon M, Perissinotto E, et al. Surgical and neurologic outcomes after robotic thymectomy in 100 consecutive patients with myasthenia gravis. *J Thorac and Cardiovasc Surg*. 2013;145(3):730–736.

Mohamed A, Shehada SE, van Brakel L, et al. Anesthetic management during robotic-assisted minimally invasive thymectomy using the Da Vinci system: a single center experience. *J Clin Med*. 2022;11:4272.

Renaud S, Santelmo N, Renaud M, et al. Robotic-assisted thymectomy with Da Vinci II versus sternotomy in the surgical treatment of non-thymomatous myasthenia gravis: early results. *Rev Neurol (Paris)*. 2013;169(1):30–36.

Lung Resection after Previous Lung Surgery

153

Viji Kurup • Prianka Desai

Clinical Scenario: An 80-year-old woman with a medical history of chronic obstructive pulmonary disease and squamous cell carcinoma of the lung, presents for right upper lobectomy. She has undergone a left upper lobectomy in the past. Preoperative review of the patient's imaging and perfusion tests (V/Q scan) revealed that the right lung receives 71% of the total perfusion.

1 What are the anesthetic and airway management considerations for this case?

This patient's perioperative course presents a variety of challenges, the most important of which is centered on maximizing intraoperative oxygenation. Given her surgical history of a left upper lobectomy, her anatomy presents the unique challenge of trying to maintain adequate perfusion to her dominant lung, which in this case is the same as the surgical side. Under typical circumstances, the use of a double-lumen tube (DLT) or a bronchial blocker (BB) essentially removes an entire lung from ventilation, thereby creating a large shunt with ensuing physiologic sequelae. Upon review of the V/Q scanning results, it seemed abundantly clear that this patient would not tolerate the hypoxemia or hypercarbia resulting from standard implementation of an one-lung ventilation (OLV) technique.

2 How would you manage the airway in this case?

In this particular case, a preoperative conversation between the anesthesiologist and the surgeon is of utmost importance. It should address methods of lung isolation, the optimal surgical approach, and the possible requirement of postoperative ventilatory support.

Due to the patient's previous lung resection and compensatory distribution of perfusion, complete collapse of the right lung would undoubtedly cause significant hypoxia. In this case, the best alternative would be to isolate only the right upper lobe, which is the surgical site, while keeping the remaining right lung and the left lower lobe ventilated. This can be achieved by placing a BB in the right upper lobe bronchus. This technique allows the right upper lobe to be isolated from ventilation and collapsed. It also allows for continued ventilation to the right lower and middle lobes, which are receiving most perfusion, and to the left lower lobe.

Another suitable approach is to purposely position a left-sided DLT in the right mainstem bronchus, so that the bronchial cuff occludes the right upper lobe bronchus takeoff. This essentially excludes the right upper lobe from ventilation, but does not allow the lobe to deflate. Therefore, surgical visualization may be inadequate.

However, in either of the two approaches, if the right middle and lower lobes are being ventilated, visualization via a video-assisted thoracoscopic approach is hindered. Therefore, better surgical approaches are open thoracotomy and sternotomy. In addition to maximizing surgical exposure, the decision to perform the procedure under sternotomy provides physiologic advantages. The typical changes of V/Q mismatch incurred with lateral decubitus will not be present in supine position, therefore contributing to the improved oxygenation and ventilation.

3 What distinct airway device (eg, specialized tracheal tube, rigid bronchoscope, BB) might be used in this case, and what are the special considerations?

Patients presenting for repeat surgery after previous lung resection surgery (lobectomy, pneumonectomy) present unique challenges for isolation of the surgical lobe and ventilation of the remaining lung tissue. Purposeful occlusion of the right upper lobe bronchus has been described in the literature. There are case reports describing a similar technique in patients undergoing emergent surgery for hemorrhage. Blockade of the individual bronchus with a BB through a standard endotracheal tube is a possibility. However, possible dislodgement of the BB should be considered and frequent visualization to guard the position of the blocker may be

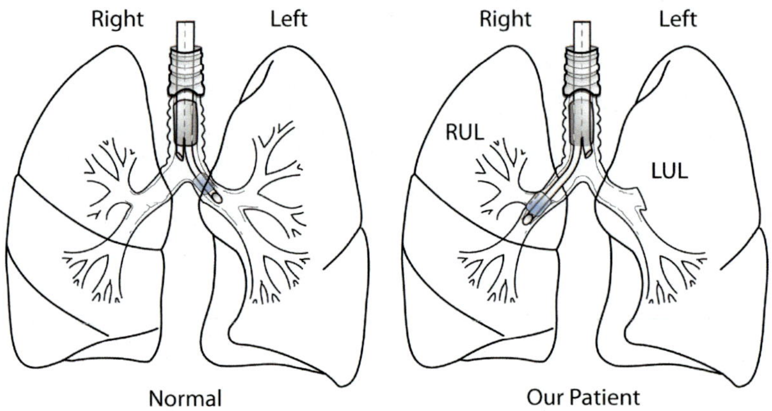

Figure 153.1. Standard placement of a left-sided double-lumen tube versus placement of left-sided double-lumen tube in our patient.

necessary. In this case, placing a left-sided DLT in the right bronchus is another method that could be considered (Figure 153.1).

4 Are there special considerations for the emergence at the end of the case?

Patients with a history of previous lung resection surgery are at particular risk for hypoxia at the end of surgery. Careful consideration of the preoperative lung function tests and, in particular, of predicted postoperative FEV_1 is an important measure to determine whether the patient can withstand further lung resection. For patients with borderline preoperative pulmonary function, keeping them intubated and slowly weaning ventilatory support in the ICU is an alternative.

- Patients with previous lung surgery are vulnerable to hypoxia during subsequent procedures requiring OLV.
- Preoperative lung function tests predict how the patient will behave intraoperatively after lung isolation and postoperatively.
- In patients with previous lung resection surgery, nonstandard methods of lung or lobe isolation must be considered in order to proceed with minimal morbidity.
- In thoracic surgery, in particular in challenging situations, preoperative communication between the surgeon and the anesthesiologist to devise the optimal plan for each patient is critical.
- *See Figure 153.2 and* ◎ ***Video 153.1*** *for additional details.*

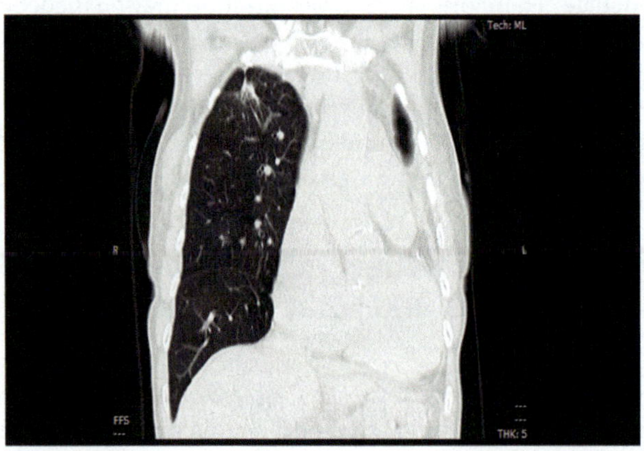

Figure 153.2. The patient's preoperative CT scan demonstrates near total obliteration of the left lung.

Acknowledgments

The authors would like to thank Erica Zador for her artistic assistance with the figures in the chapter.

Suggested Readings

Alfrey DD. Use of a left-sided double-lumen tube to occlude the right upper lobe orifice. *Anesthesiology*. 1995;83:1131.

Campos JH, Massa FC, Kernstine KH. The incidence of right upper-lobe collapse when comparing a right-sided double lumen tube versus a modified left double-lumen tube for left-sided thoracic surgery. *Anesth Analg*. 2000;90:535–540.

Chu LF, Traynor AJ, Kurup V. Thoracic anesthesia. In: Chu LF, Traynor AJ, Kurup V, eds. *Manual of Clinical Anesthesiology*. 2nd ed. Wolters Kluwer; 2021;1129–1142.

Scholten KJ, Kulkarni V, Brodsky JB. Isolation of the right upper-lobe with a left-sided double-lumen tube after left-pneumonectomy. *Anesth Analg*. 2007;105:330–331.

154 Lung Decortication

Diana Anca

Clinical Scenario: A 37-year-old man with a loculated left pleural empyema presents to the OR for lung decortication. He was involved in a motor vehicle accident 1 week ago. He sustained multiple left rib fractures and has a severe pulmonary contusion. He is currently intubated, having failed several extubation trials.

1 What are the anesthetic and airway management considerations for this case?

Lung decortication is the treatment for persistent lung empyema and consists of removal of the fibrous scar layer that covers the lung and diaphragm, restricting lung expansion.

The anesthetic considerations can be divided into patient related, airway management, and procedure related. Given the patient's condition, an extensive discussion with both the critical care and the surgical teams should take place before formulating the anesthetic plan.

The patient-related considerations arise from his critical illness, the fact that he was intubated for 1 week, has multiple rib fractures, and has failed several extubation trials. It is very important to obtain information regarding both the initial intubation and the extubation trials.

One-lung ventilation (OLV) will be required to facilitate surgical exposure. However, any airway manipulation (ie, change from endotracheal tube [ETT] to double-lumen tube (DLT)) should take into consideration the potential airway edema secondary to prolonged intubation, and possible associated cervical spine injuries. The previously failed extubation attempts suggest that postoperative ventilation will be needed. This fact will also impact the decision regarding the choice of the best lung isolation method. Therefore, should a DLT be placed, an exchange to ETT would be necessary at the conclusion of the surgery.

While this patient does not have a COVID-19 infection, the scenario of such patients needing to undergo procedures requiring OLV, can pose a risk for the practitioners. Hence, it is prudent to consider decreasing the aerosol formation. This is obtained by maintaining a "silent airway" with complete neuromuscular blockade and stopping gas flow during airway manipulation and by adding a filter to the "open" airway during suction.

Procedure-related complications include lung injury and bleeding, which might require transfusion of blood and blood products such as fresh frozen plasma and platelets. Also, the availability of point-of-care testing intraoperatively should be considered.

A preprocedure discussion with the surgeon is useful to address the considerations for OLV, options and alternatives, as well as the possibility of open thoracotomy, possible bleeding, and the need for transfusion. Equally important is to set expectations as far as lung deflation extent, since empyema and adhesions usually make lung deflation suboptimal.

2 How would you manage the airway in this case?

The planned procedure, whether performed open or thoracoscopically, is an acknowledged indication for OLV. Before proceeding to lung isolation, detailed information regarding the initial intubation difficulty, size of the existing ETT, current ventilatory parameters (FiO_2, positive end-expiratory pressure [PEEP]), oxygenation level, and degree of secretions should be obtained.

Based on these data, the optimal lung isolation device for this patient can be identified. OLV can be achieved using a DLT, bronchial blocker (BB), or ETT. Placement of a DLT would involve exchanging the existing ETT. This procedure carries several risks, such as airway loss secondary to edema, hypoxemia, airway trauma, and bleeding, potentially compromising other airway maneuvers. Therefore, if this method of lung isolation is chosen, the use of a tube exchanger represents a safer approach. Emergency airway equipment should be immediately available. The tube exchanger should subsequently be used at the end of the case for replacing the DLT with an ETT (see Chapter 139: Double-Lumen Tube to Single-Lumen Tube Exchange).

In a patient with a difficult airway, the BB is a more suitable option for lung isolation. Similarly, if the patient requires high PEEP and FiO_2 settings to maintain adequate oxygenation, or if no air leak is heard with ETT cuff deflation, the use of a BB is a safer technique for OLV. However, if the patient has an in situ ETT smaller than 7.5 mm, only a 7Fr Arndt BB or an EZ-Blocker can be used to assure lung isolation.

Alternatively, the ETT can be advanced into the mainstem bronchus, requiring ventilation. This option is particularly useful in patients where a tube exchange or even placement of BB is deemed unsafe. It must be emphasized that a small-sized ETT is not long enough to be placed endobronchially. In addition, when the ETT is advanced endobronchially and significant airway edema is present, there is not enough space to allow the gas from the nonventilated lung to egress. In such situations, deflating the ETT cuff, disconnecting the patient from the ventilator, and allowing a complete exhalation achieves lung collapse. If this maneuver is not performed, the nonventilated lung cannot deflate adequately. However, if the patient is on high PEEP levels, this maneuver produces lung decruitment and will result in significant hypoxemia.

Patients with marginal respiratory status may not tolerate OLV. In such instances, using high-frequency two-lung jet ventilation may be an attractive alternative. This technique would allow for adequate oxygenation and provide a motionless surgical field, but surgical exposure may be suboptimal.

In patients such as our patient, critically ill, with prolonged mechanical ventilation, empyema, lung isolation options have to carefully be considered, and lung deflation will most likely be suboptimal. It is important to discuss with the surgeon the options of lung isolation and set expectations.

3 What are the surgical considerations that impact anesthetic management?

The procedure is performed via either a thoracoscopic or an open thoracotomy approach. Due to loculations and adhesions, the decortication of an empyema is a more complex procedure than the drainage of a pleural effusion.

The extent and laterality of the surgery (unilateral versus bilateral) dictates not only the patient's positioning but also the required lung isolation device. If a bilateral decortication is considered, then either a DLT or an EZ-Blocker would be the best-suited device for OLV. Regardless of the technique employed, significant adhesions decrease the ability of the lung to collapse, making the procedure technically difficult. This fact not only prolongs surgical dissection, but also increases the risk of blood loss and lung injury, with development of subsequent air leaks and delayed healing.

If surgical exposure using a thoracoscopic approach is suboptimal, conversion to an open thoracotomy is performed. However, in the setting of multiple rib fractures, chest-wall stabilization and rib fixation may be required.

While this patient is intubated, an open thoracotomy will be associated with higher pain levels, and plans to address it should be made preoperatively.

4 What distinct airway device might be used in this case, and what are the special considerations?

In this case, the key decision is choosing the optimal lung isolation device. As previously mentioned, available options include DLTs (right, left), BBs (Arndt, Fuji, Cohen, EZ-Blocker), or ETTs. As described in the reference chapters, all these devices have their advantages and disadvantages. The selection of one over the others needs careful consideration of the clinical details of each patient and of the surgical requirements. In addition, operator experience is a factor that heavily impacts the final decision. Of note, in a study of 100 cases in a surgical center over 4 years, the EZ-Blocker was successfully used for all intubated and tracheostomized patients as a safe way for OLV.

Although tube exchangers are not devices used for lung isolation, they have a critical role either at the beginning or at the end of a case, when the ETT and DLT are exchanged. Aside from representing a guide to the airway, tube exchangers are designed with a central lumen through which apneic oxygenation or jet ventilation can be performed.

- Lung decortication in a ventilated patient requires diligent, multidisciplinary consultation and planning.
- The preoperatively intubated patient will most likely remain so postoperatively.
- Choosing the optimal lung isolation device needs careful consideration of the clinical particulars of each patient and of the surgical requirements, and a preoperative discussion should always take place to address options, possible complications, and set expectations.
- In tedious dissections, lung injury with subsequent air leaks should be expected, as well as the distinct possibility of significant bleeding and necessity of blood transfusion.
- In patients or suspects of COVID-19, careful consideration should be paid to measures to ensure minimizing time and generation of aerosols.
- Plans for postoperative pain control should be in place especially in open thoracotomy cases.
- *See Figure 154.1 and* ***Video 154.1*** *for additional details.*

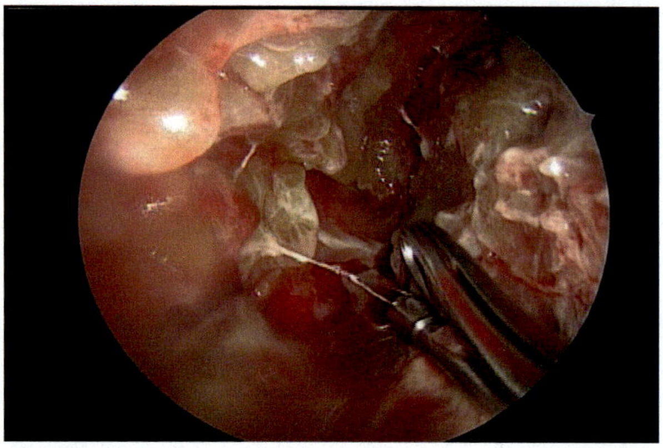

Figure 154.1. Video-assisted image during a decortication procedure.

Suggested Readings

Campos JH. Lung isolation. In: Slinger P, ed. *Principles and Practices of Anesthesia for Thoracic Surgery*. Springer; 2011:227–246.

Campos JH. Separation of the lung: double-lumen endotracheal tubes and endobronchial blockers. In: Cohen E, ed. *Cohen's Comprehensive Thoracic Anesthesia*. Elsevier; 2021:213–239.

Cassina PC, Hauser M, Hillejan L, Greschuchna D, Stamatis G. Video-assisted thoracoscopy in the treatment of pleural empyema: stage-based management and outcome. *J Thorac Cardiovasc Surg*. 1999;117;234–238.

Moritz A, Irouschek A, Birkholtz T, Prottengeier J, Sirbu H, Schmidt J. The EZ-Blocker for one-lung ventilation in patients undergoing thoracic surgery: clinical applications and experience in 100 cases in a routine surgical setting. *J Cardiothorac Surg*. 2018; 13:77.

Ott Q, Popescu WM. Overview of anesthesia for patients with pleural disease. https://www.uptodate.com

Tryphonopoulos, P, McFaul C, Gagne S, Moffett S, Byford L, Thompson C. COVID-19 and one-lung ventilation. *Anesth Analg*. 2020;131(2):e90–e91.

Open Descending Thoracic Aortic Aneurysm Repair

155

Diana Anca

Clinical Scenario: A 60-year-old man with a 6.5-cm descending thoracic aortic aneurysm presents to the OR for open repair via a left thoracotomy.

1 What are the anesthetic and airway management considerations for this case?

Descending thoracic aortic aneurysms involve any portion of the descending aorta distal to the left subclavian artery and can extend throughout the abdominal aorta. The repair can be performed open, via a left thoracotomy, or endovascularly via a thoracic endovascular aortic repair (TEVAR). The anesthetic management of these cases is very challenging, both due to the extent and complexity of the open procedure, as well as the patient's associated comorbidities.

Anesthetic two crucial considerations for the open repair involve the airway management intra and postoperatively, and spinal cord protection. Open surgical repair is associated with increased postoperative mortality but reduced late risk of death and reintervention and should be considered the first line of repair for intact aneurysms. Open surgical repair of the descending aorta is a complex, extensive procedure, with significant fluid shift, large surgical incision, severe postoperative pain, and potential bleeding, and the need of transfusion.

The approach to airway management should consider the fact that an open repair via left thoracotomy requires lung isolation. In addition, the patient will need postoperative ventilation and adequate pain control. Airway management for a patient undergoing open repair, whether emergent or elective, has a dual objective: to secure the airway with minimal hemodynamic changes, avoiding aneurysm rupture, and to provide adequate OLV for surgical exposure. The long procedure duration with significant fluid shifts, blood loss, and hemodynamic fluctuations, makes the requirement for postoperative ventilation almost a certainty.

In this case, lung isolation can be achieved using either a DLT or a BB. Each one of these lung isolation devices has advantages and disadvantages. DLTs are less likely displaced, offer better suction capabilities, but are more rigid. While a left DLT might be considered easier to place, due to compression by the aortic aneurysm, placement might be difficult and even carries a risk of aneurysm rupture, so a right DLT or a BB might be required. At the conclusion of the surgery, the DLT needs to be exchanged for an ETT to allow safe postoperative ventilation. However, significant airway edema is frequently present and should be considered when changing the DLT to an ETT. BBs can be difficult to position in the left mainstem bronchus (due to compression/distortion), can be displaced during surgical manipulation, and can get blocked with secretions. Another pitfall is that due to heparinization during the case, the view might be too bloody, and repositioning the BB might not be easy. Nevertheless, at the end of the case, the BB is removed and the patient is left with an ETT.

2 How would you manage the airway in this case?

When deciding upon the optimal lung isolation device, the fact that large descending aortic aneurysms produce left mainstem bronchus distortion should be considered. Proper preoperative evaluation, review of the CT scan, and bronchoscopy help determine the extent of the compression. In addition, the displacement risk incurred with surgical manipulation, and the need of postoperative ventilation should play a role in the airway management plan.

If the left mainstem bronchus is not compressed or distorted, then a left DLT can be placed. Even if there is no evidence of airway compression, caution should be used during DLT placement. Forceful advancement of this rigid device can lead to aneurysm rupture.

If the left mainstem bronchus is compressed, distorted, or occluded, then a right DLT can be utilized. However, frequent bronchoscopic verification of the right upper lobe ventilation slot is required. Misalignment of the right DLT or obstruction of the right upper lobe bronchus takeoff causes atelectasis and poor tolerance of OLV. Alternatively, considering that this patient will remain intubated at the conclusion of the case, a BB placed through the ETT is a suitable option.

Given the design of the EZ-Blocker straddling the carina, there is less chance of displacement, and might be a preferred option.

3 What are the surgical considerations that impact anesthetic management?

Several additional procedure-specific factors should be considered in the overall airway management plan. Surgical manipulation can lead to lung isolation device dislodgement and loss of OLV. If this occurs at critical times (left atrial appendage cannulation, posterior aortic wall anastomosis), it can have a devastating impact. However, as the procedure is performed via a large thoracotomy, overall left lung collapse is not as critical for surgical exposure as in a VATS, where maneuvering space and visualization are limited. Therefore, in situations when OLV is poorly tolerated, intermittent dual lung ventilation using small tidal volumes and rapid rates can be utilized. In such cases, the left lung can be retracted out of the surgical field.

Due to the use of either full or partial cardiopulmonary bypass (left atrial-femoral bypass), heparinization is required. Therefore, surgical manipulation can provoke airway bleeding. This makes maintenance of OLV or repositioning of the DLT or BB extremely challenging.

4 Are there special considerations for the emergence at the end of the case?

Given the length and extent of surgery, it is expected that the patient requires postoperative mechanical ventilation. If a BB was used as a lung isolation device, then its removal renders the patient with a single-lumen ETT.

If, however, a DLT was used, then the anesthesiologist will need to decide if it is safe to perform the exchange to an ETT. This maneuver should not be taken lightly. Significant airway edema and the removal of the DLT could lead to airway loss. The strategy employed by most practitioners takes into consideration the initial intubation difficulty and the presence or absence of a cuff leak. If the airway was considered challenging at the initial time of intubation, the risks incurred with changing the DLT to an ETT outweigh the benefits. If the initial intubation was considered routine, then the degree of airway edema needs to be assessed. Deflating the DLT's cuff and applying positive pressure to the airway allows for an air leak test. If a leak is heard, then a tube exchanger is used to change from a DLT to an ETT (see Chapter 139: Double-Lumen Tube to Single-Lumen Tube Exchange). When performing the exchange, emergency airway equipment should be readily available. In addition, it is important to have a surgeon in the OR, who can rapidly perform an emergency tracheostomy. Conversely, if no leak is heard, then it is safer to leave the DLT in place, as the risk of airway loss is high. The bronchial cuff should be deflated before transferring the patient to the ICU. The DLT can be changed at a later time when the edema has decreased. If the patient is transferred to the ICU and intubated with a DLT, the nursing personnel require instructions regarding the specifics of this particular tube. An adequate size FB should be readily available at bed side to check correct DLT position in cases of desaturations.

- In this challenging case, detailed airway management planning, both for intraoperative as well as postoperative ventilation, is required for performing a safe anesthetic.
- Both the DLT and BB can be used for OLV; selecting one device over the other depends on the operator's experience and the patient's upper and lower airway anatomy.
- Left DLT might be difficult to place, and it might lead to aneurysm rupture due to left mainstem compression.
- "To change or not to change the DLT to an ETT," this is the question! This issue should not be taken easily.
- *See Figure 155.1 for additional details.*

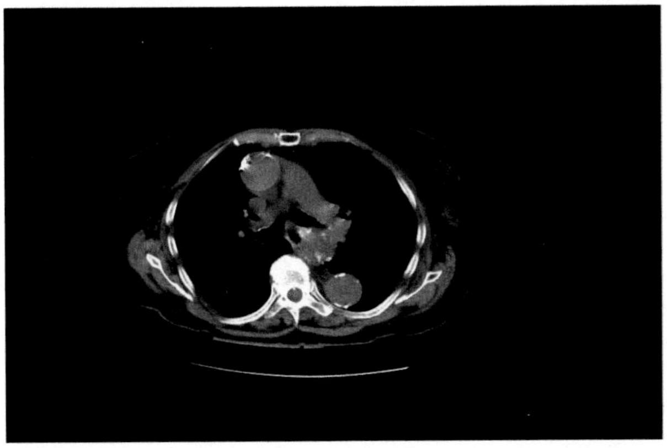

Figure 155.1. Axial CT scan showing a descending thoracic aortic aneurysm.

Suggested Readings

Agarwal S, Kendall J, Quaterman C. Perioperative management of thoracic and thoracoabdominal aneurysms. *BJA Educ.* 2019; 19(4):119–125.

Puskas F, Clendenan N. Anesthesia for open thoracic aortic surgery. https://www.uptodate.com

Silvay G, Lurie JM, Casale M. The anesthetic management of patient with thoracic ascending aortic aneurysm: a review. *J Perioper Pract.* 2021;31(7–8):281–288.

156 Minimally Invasive Esophagectomy

Zyad J. Carr

Clinical Scenario: A 60-year-old man with an esophageal adenocarcinoma at 25-cm distance from the teeth is presenting for a minimally invasive esophagectomy. The surgeon considers performing the chest dissection in the prone position.

1 What are the anesthetic and airway management considerations for this case?

Esophagectomy is still the mainstay of therapy for esophageal cancer, but is hampered by high perioperative morbidity and mortality. The traditional open esophagectomy can be performed using different surgical approaches. Transhiatal esophagectomy is performed through a midline laparotomy with blunt dissection of the thoracic esophagus, a gastric pull-up procedure, and a cervical anastomosis. The Ivor–Lewis procedure consists of an upper midline laparotomy followed by a right thoracotomy and intrathoracic anastomosis. This technique can also be modified with an additional left cervical incision. Finally, a left thoracophrenicolaparotomy in combination with a left neck dissection is also an optional open surgical approach.

Since the end of the 1990s, minimally invasive esophagectomy (MIE) has been introduced and rapidly adopted. Several techniques were developed using a combination of laparoscopy, thoracoscopy, video-assisted minilaparotomy or minithoracotomy, as well as variants of hand-assisted, robot-assisted, or hybrid techniques. The most recent innovation is the use of the prone position for the right thoracoscopic dissection phase instead of lateral decubitus. This procedure is performed using a combination of laparoscopy, right prone thoracoscopy, and neck anastomosis. Prone positioning during the thoracic dissection enhances operative exposure of the esophagus compared to lateral thoracoscopic MIE, which is often suboptimal due to bleeding and lung position.

Anesthetic management of these procedures may require one-lung ventilation (OLV) during the right thoracoscopic phase, although techniques utilizing two-lung ventilation with an artificial pneumothorax have been described. In comparison to lateral positioning, the cardiac index and stroke volume index seem to be lower during a prone procedure. Ventilatory pressures (peak and plateau airway pressures) might be higher with a subsequent reduction in static compliance. However, these hemodynamic and ventilatory changes cumulatively result in improved gas exchange caused by a more uniform distribution of the pulmonary perfusion with superior ventilation/perfusion ratios. Furthermore, thoracoscopy in the prone position has shown to improve oxygenation and reduce mean pulmonary shunt fraction in comparison to a traditional lateral thoracotomic approach. Lower incidences of respiratory complications and improved postoperative oxygenation have been reported after MIE in the prone compared with the lateral decubitus position. Improved clearance of airway secretions during prone positioning might also have an overall beneficial impact on perioperative outcomes.

Other advantages of prone MIE technique, similar to the other minimal invasive approaches, include less blood loss, reduced operative time, decreased hospital stay, and reduced postoperative pain. Many of these observations and theoretical advantages should be further studied in randomized clinical trials.

2 How would you manage the airway in this case?

In order to maximize the surgical exposure, OLV will likely be utilized for the thoracic phase of this procedure. The prone position poses various challenges. To achieve OLV, intubation is performed with either an armored endotracheal tube (ETT) with a bronchial blocker (BB) or double lumen endotracheal tube (DLT) is positioned. Tube position is verified with flexible bronchoscopy. The authors also recommend the EZ-Blocker BB, which has two distal extensions that resemble the bifurcation of the trachea. Each extension has an inflatable cuff for each mainstem bronchus. Displacement of this device is less frequent compared with other BB, assuming a minimal distance of 4 cm is present between the carina and the tip of the ETT. After prone positioning, the device should be rechecked for correct position. Complete collapse of the lung is often not necessary for surgical exposure. Surgical manipulation of the airway during thoracic lymph node dissection increases the risk for BB or DLT displacement. Following the thoracic exposure phase, the patient is turned supine, and the laparoscopic phase and neck anastomosis are completed.

3 What are the surgical considerations that impact anesthetic management?

Unexpected bleeding during the prone thoracoscopic phase can be dangerous and rapid conversion to thoracotomy might be indicated. We recommend ramping the left side of the patient with a negative pressure bag. This bag is further supported with braces attached to the surgical table. In case urgent conversion is needed, the table can be tilted 30 degrees and optimal lateral position is easily achieved for thoracotomy. The prone positioning requires careful support of the head, and continuous ophthalmic pressure monitoring may be recommended. A hard-shell protective helmet with a mirror (ProneView) is recommended. The use of a Mayfield head clamp, which avoids direct facial pressure, has also been reported. To optimize surgical exposure, intrathoracic carbon dioxide may be insufflated at pressures (6 to 14 mm Hg) to create an artificial pneumothorax. The anesthesiologist should be aware of the potential hemodynamic impacts of increased intrathoracic pressure and respiratory acidosis from excessive carbon dioxide absorption.

4 What distinct airway device might be used in this case, and what are the special considerations?

The use of a single-lumen ETT in combination with other commercially available BBs is also feasible. The use of a DLT has also been described. However, displacement of the DLT due to postural changes may be challenging to manage in the prone position. Due to a higher rigidity of these devices, repositioning may be challenging due to the limited space between the mouth and the head-supporting device. Pressure on the DLT might increase the risk for bronchial and tracheal injury. Although thoracoscopic surgery often requires OLV, some have adopted a simplified anesthetic management using a single-lumen ETT and two-lung ventilation with or without an artificial pneumothorax. In their clinical experience, gravity-based exclusion of the lungs in combination with the artificial pneumothorax is sufficient for optimal surgical exposure.

- OLV during prone positioning has different physiologic implications to the supine position.
- Airway management for prone thoracoscopy can be safely performed using an EZ-Blocker or other BB, in combination with a single-lumen ETT, or a DLT.
- Although more challenging for intraoperative management, downstream benefits of prone positioning, like improved operative exposure and reduced operative time, may see its use increase in the management of MIE.
- *See Figure 156.1 and* **Video 156.1** *for additional details.*

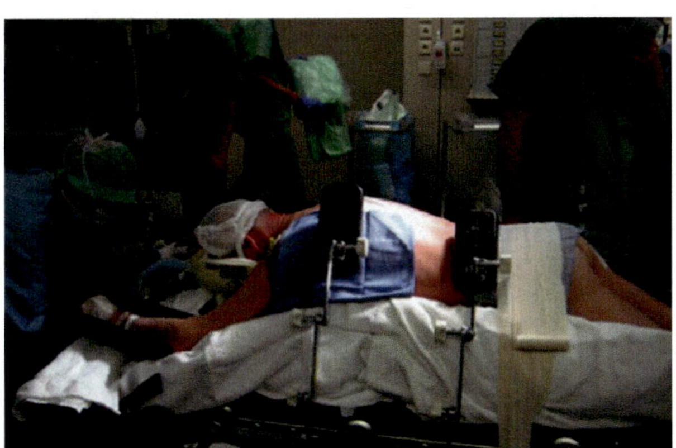

Figure 156.1. Patient in the prone position in preparation for a minimally invasive esophagectomy.

Acknowledgments

We gratefully acknowledge the contributions of previous edition author, Arne Neyrinck, as portions of those chapters have been retained in this revision.

Suggested Readings

Bonavina L, Laface L, Abate E, Punturieri M, Agosteo E, Nencioni M. Comparison of ventilation and cardiovascular parameters between prone thoracoscopic and Ivor Lewis esophagectomy. *Updates Surg*. 2012;64:81–85.

Jarral OA, Purkayastha S, Athanasiou T, Darzi A, Hanna GB, Zacharakis E. Thoracoscopic esophagectomy in the prone position. *Surg Endosc*. 2012;26:2095–2103.

Levy RM, Trivedi D, Luketich JD. Minimally invasive esophagectomy. *Surg Clin North Am*. 2012;92:1265–1285.

Noshiro H, Miyake S. Thoracoscopic esophagectomy using prone positioning. *Ann Thorac Cardiovasc Surg*. 2013;19:399–408.

Saikawa D, Okushiba S, Kawata M, et al. Efficacy and safety of artificial pneumothorax under two-lung ventilation in thoracoscopic esophagectomy for esophageal cancer in the prone position. *Gen Thorac Cardiovasc Surg*. 2014;62:163–170.

Tanigawa Y, Nakamura K, Yamashita T, Nakagawachi A, Sakaguchi Y. Changes in respiratory mechanics of artificial pneumothorax two-lung ventilation in video-assisted thoracoscopic esophagectomy in prone position. *Sci Rep*. 2021;11(1):6978.

Esophagectomy for Achalasia

157

Valentin Calu • Madalina Dutu

Clinical Scenario: A 54-year-old man with a long-standing history of achalasia is presenting to the OR for minimally invasive esophagectomy. Previously, he underwent a failed laparoscopic Heller myotomy. After surgery, he refused a redo-myotomy, and a POEM (PerOral Endoscopic Myotomy) procedure was attempted without relief of symptoms. He has a history of multiple aspiration pneumonias. After proper workup, he was diagnosed with end-stage achalasia and, due to his age and risk of malignancy, esophagectomy was offered as the best option of treatment in this case.

1 What are the anesthetic and airway management considerations for this case?

Achalasia is an esophageal motor disorder characterized by the incapacity of the lower esophageal sphincter to relax and by loss of esophageal peristalsis. Dysphagia is the main symptom. Left untreated, the esophagus dilates significantly, resulting in a "megaesophagus." Due to repeated episodes of aspiration pneumonias, most patients have compromised pulmonary function. There is a higher risk for squamous carcinoma of the esophagus than in uncomplicated achalasia, especially in patients with a longer than 10-year history of symptoms and multiple previous failures of myotomy and/or dilatation. The association of a previous moderate/severe COVID-19 infection can add to the challenge.

The biggest anesthetic challenge during an esophagectomy performed for achalasia derives from the need to safely secure the airway in a patient with a high risk of aspiration. In addition, this procedure requires one-lung ventilation (OLV). Another anesthetic concern is the patient's frail respiratory status, leading to rapid desaturations during intubation and decreased tolerance of OLV. Efficient postoperative analgesia is needed to allow a timely extubation.

A preoperative assessment of the patient's airway determines whether an awake intubation or an rapid sequence induction (RSI) is performed. Lung isolation can be accomplished using a double-lumen tube (DLT) or an endotracheal tube (ETT) with a bronchial blocker (BB).

2 How would you manage the airway in this case?

Despite appropriate fasting, patients with end-stage achalasia presenting for surgery should be assumed to have 300 to 500 mL of esophageal content. Therefore, they are at a particular high risk of massive pulmonary aspiration. In order to safely secure the airway, either an RSI or an awake intubation should be used.

For those patients with airways judged to be easily manageable, the use of a rapid sequence induction with a thorough preoxygenation is prudent. The head of the patient should be elevated at 30 to 45 degrees before induction of anesthesia. If direct laryngoscopy does not offer a good glottic view, a video laryngoscopic technique can be utilized. Lung isolation can be achieved either by placing a DLT or by using an ETT and a BB positioned in the right mainstem bronchus. Both methods of lung isolation produce a similar degree of lung collapse, but the BB incurs a higher incidence of displacement during surgery. Correct device position should be verified using flexible bronchoscopy. Recently, the video DLT has been introduced, with an integrated high-resolution camera.

If there is evidence to suggest a difficult intubation, serious consideration should be given to an awake intubation. In patients with airway abnormalities and difficult intubation BB may be the preferred lung isolation of choice. The best way to obtain lung isolation is to place an awake oral ETT followed by an asleep insertion of the BB. For awake techniques, the airway requires a thorough topicalization. Probably, the best-tolerated technique of awake intubation requires the use of an flexible intubating scope (FIS). However, other awake techniques, such as direct or video laryngoscopy, can be employed. Another alternative is to place an awake FIS-guided DLT. The FIS is passed through the bronchial lumen of the DLT, and advanced into correct position under direct vision. This strategy is difficult to execute because the DLT tends to "hang" at the entrance of the glottis due to its large size.

If the patient has been intubated with an ETT and the right mainstem bronchus is too short to fit a BB, as a last resort, two-lung high-frequency jet ventilation can be employed. However, this strategy may not allow optimal visualization in a thoracoscopic approach, as the right lung will not collapse completely. In such situations, the surgeon decides whether a conversion to an open procedure is required, although the open approach should be looked at as the last resort. Alternatively, the ETT could be exchanged to a left DLT over a tube-exchanging catheter, but the airway would be unprotected, allowing possible aspiration.

3 What are the surgical considerations that impact anesthetic management?

The treatment for achalasia is pneumatic balloon dilation or surgical myotomy, and, recently added, POEM. The most commonly used initial therapeutic approach is laparoscopic Heller myotomy. However, up to 20% of the patients experience therapeutic failure after myotomy with persistent disabling symptoms, such as dysphagia, regurgitation, nutritional failure, and respiratory complications, and 5% will develop end-stage achalasia. The standard treatment for this condition remains esophagectomy, although surgeons are reluctant to perform a major operation for a "benign" disease. Esophagectomy is reserved only for those patients who have failed other less invasive interventions.

Due to an increased risk of aspiration during the surgical manipulation of the esophagus, an upper endoscopy to clear the esophageal content is performed after induction and prior to beginning the surgery. However, if the esophagus cannot be completely emptied, case cancellation should be considered.

Esophagectomy, with the gastric interposition as the best choice for reconstruction, can be performed using different approaches: thoracotomy, transhiatal, or minimally invasive (thoracoscopic or robotic). When a thoracotomy is utilized, the postoperative morbidity and mortality are higher. Thoracoscopic or robotic approaches offer better visualization than the transhiatal approach. Therefore, the minimally invasive approach (thoracoscopic or robotic) is preferred, combining the thoracoscopic esophagectomy with the laparoscopic preparation of the gastric conduit.

The anastomosis between the gastric conduit and the esophageal remnant can be performed in the chest, when the esophagus is removed partially, or in the neck, when the entire thoracic esophagus is removed, and this option is highly influenced by the surgeon's experience. If a prone position for the thoracoscopic approach is considered, its feasibility should be discussed with the anesthesiologist.

4 What are the potential hazards and complications in regard to the airway?

The most feared complication of this procedure is the aspiration of esophageal content into the lungs, during induction of anesthesia, during esophageal surgical manipulation, and at extubation. This can lead to airway obstruction, pneumonia, and acute respiratory distress syndrome, and may be fatal. Therefore, safety measures are employed prior to, during, and at the completion of the procedure.

Even though the optimal NPO period in patients with severe gastroesophageal pathology is unknown, fasting for solid food is recommended for 24 to 48 hours prior to surgery. Clear liquids are stopped 8 hours in advance. Although placement of a nasoesophageal tube prior to induction of anesthesia was thought to be useful in removing the esophageal content, it may stimulate retching, vomiting, and potentially increases the aspiration risk. Frequent oropharyngeal suctioning during the case is strongly recommended. At extubation, the patient should be placed in a sitting position and be wide awake, following commands. An epidural or paravertebral block provides efficient analgesia, avoiding respiratory splinting and the potential need for reintubation.

- Achalasia patients presenting for esophagectomy have an extremely high risk of aspiration.
- Minimally invasive esophagectomy requires OLV. Either a DLT or an ETT with a BB positioned in the right mainstem bronchus can be used for lung isolation.
- An RSI is required, provided that the airway anatomy is normal. In a patient with a known or anticipated difficult airway, the safest way to secure the airway is represented by an awake technique.
- A previous moderate/severe COVID-19 infection can make the procedure more challenging.
- *See Figure 157.1 and* ***Video 157.1*** *for additional details.*

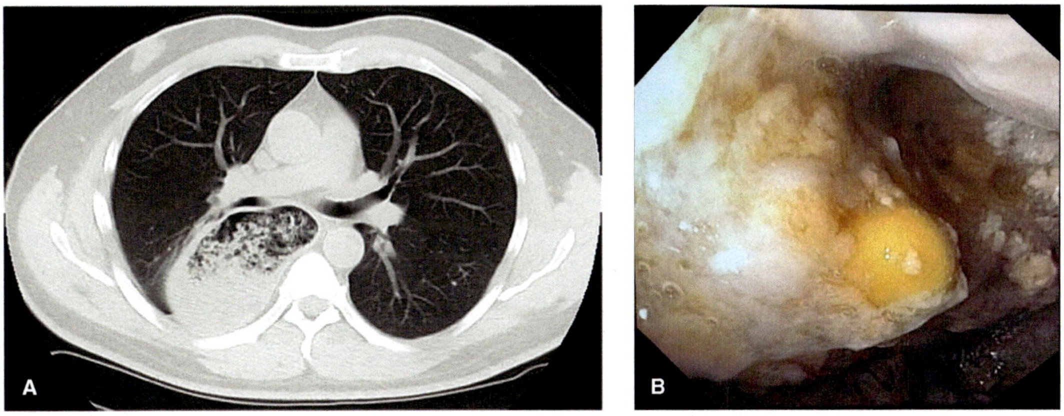

Figure 157.1. **A:** Megaesophagus with entrapped contents. **B:** Endoscopic view of esophageal contents.

Suggested Readings

Campos JH. Lung isolation techniques for patients with difficult airway. *Curr Opin Anaesthesiol.* 2010,23:12–17.

Felix VN, Murayama KM, Bonavina L, Park MI. Achalasia: what to do in the face of failures of Heller myotomy. *Ann N Y Acad Sci.* 2020;1481(1):236–246.

Rucklidge M, Sanders D, Martin A. Anaesthesia for minimally invasive oesophagectomy. *Crit Care Pain.* 2010;10(2):43–47.

Veelo DP, Geerts BF. Anaesthesia during oesophagectomy. *J Thorac Dis.* 2017;9(Suppl 8):S705–S712.

158 One-Lung Ventilation in a Pediatric Patient

Elizabeth S. Reinhart

Clinical Scenario: A 4-year-old, 18-kg girl presents to the operating room for right thoracoscopy for excision of a right lower lobe lung nodule. She has a past medical history significant for Wilm tumor treated with chemotherapy and radiation.

1 What are the anesthetic and airway management considerations in this case?

A thorough preoperative evaluation is essential when caring for a child undergoing thoracic surgery. Important considerations are airway management with potential lung isolation, any need for invasive monitoring, and a comprehensive postoperative plan including pain management. The clinician should discuss with the surgeon any airway concerns and develop a plan to optimize surgical exposure. The type of induction (inhalational vs intravenous) should be carefully considered for thoracic procedures due to potential for difficult intubation and any compression of airway structures. In general, an inhalational induction with maintenance of spontaneous ventilation is often preferred when there is concern for airway compression, and a rigid bronchoscope should be available to bypass potential tracheal compression. For this patient, an inhalational induction or intravenous induction would be appropriate. Placement of invasive monitoring is considered based on the type of surgery (thoracotomy vs thoracoscopy), potential for blood loss, and for monitoring hemodynamics and/or adequate ventilation.

Similar to adults, indications for one-lung ventilation in the pediatric population fall into both absolute and relative categories. Regardless of the indication, thoracoscopic approaches depend on lung isolation to achieve adequate operating conditions. Once lung isolation is achieved, it is essential to optimize ventilation (V) and perfusion (Q). Patient positioning, general anesthesia, mechanical ventilation, and surgical exposure affect the V/Q ratio. Pediatric patients are predisposed to hypoxemia as a result of high oxygen consumption, the relative compressibility of the conducting airways compared to adults, and the increase in chest wall compliance that can make ventilating the dependent healthy lung more challenging.

2 How would you manage the airway in this case?

Because of the smaller size of the pediatric airway, it is critical that clinicians have a range of devices available to provide one-lung ventilation as well as the knowledge of the tracheobronchial anatomy in order to optimize placement and achieve appropriate lung isolation. Options for lung isolation include placing a single-lumen tube into the desired bronchus, bronchial blockers (Uniblocker, Arndt blocker, vascular balloon catheters such as the Fogarty), Univent tube, and double-lumen tube. When choosing the type of lung isolation device, it is essential to know the limitations of each technique.

The simplest method remains endobronchial intubation with a standard endotracheal tube, which can be used in any age and remains the preferred method for infants (up to 6 months). Disadvantages of this technique include poor lung isolation (especially if an uncuffed tube is used), and the challenge of quickly converting to two-lung ventilation.

Bronchial blockers are an acceptable technique from 6 months to 18 years, however, it is the *preferred* method for ages 6 months to 2 years (parallel placement) and 2 to 8 years (coaxial placement). Parallel and coaxial refer to the placement of the blocker relative to the endotracheal tube (ETT), either within the lumen or parallel to it. Both the 5Fr Uniblocker and Ardnt bronchial blockers are suitable for children up to 8 years and should be placed extra-luminal for ETT sizes less than 4.5 internal diameter. Ardnt blockers do come in bigger sizes (7 and 9Fr) which can make their use in older children possible. Fogarty catheters come in a variety of sizes with size 3F suitable for children up to 4 years old (may be placed luminal or coaxial) and size 5Fr for children 5 to 12. Uniblockers and Fogarty catheters do not have a central lumen, which negates the use of continuous positive airway pressure (CPAP), an important consideration for management of hypoxemia during thoracic surgery. Univent tubes are endotracheal tubes that contain a bronchial blocker within a separate lumen and are available in two sizes (3.5- and 4.5-mm ID), which are best utilized in children 6 to 8 years old. The main disadvantage of Univent tubes is that the lumen for ventilation is inevitably smaller (in order to accommodate the blocker lumen channel), which can increase airway resistance.

Double-lumen tubes remain the gold standard for lung isolation due to the ability to quickly convert from single to double-lung ventilation, ease of insertion, application of CPAP, and ability to utilize suction. The smallest size double-lumen tube is a 26Fr, which is equivalent in diameter to a 5.5 to 6.0 cuffed endotracheal tube. Therefore, double-lumen tubes are generally an option only for children over the age of 8. Disadvantages of the double-lumen tube include its use in patients with difficult airways as a result of its bigger size and configuration, and the need to replace the tube with a single-lumen tube if continued postoperative mechanical ventilation is needed.

Successful placement of any device to achieve lung isolation generally requires bronchoscopy to place the tube, confirm placement, and troubleshoot ventilation issues during the surgery. When choosing a bronchoscope, two questions must be asked: "What size bronchoscope will physically fit?" and "What size bronchoscope will allow me to use and still ventilate the patient?" If there is a need to ventilate the patient while performing bronchoscopy, the diameter of the bronchoscope should occupy <50% of the cross-sectional area of the inner diameter of the endotracheal tube. If bronchoscopy is used briefly during apnea to confirm placement, the diameter of the bronchoscope must be <90% of the inner diameter of the endotracheal tube. The smallest pediatric bronchoscope has a 2.2-mm outer diameter and can be used in endotracheal tubes as small as 2.5 mm, however, this size lacks a suction channel and is therefore limited in its utility. A range of bronchoscope sizes accommodates endotracheal tubes of varying sizes for use within the pediatric population.

For this 4-year-old patient with normal tracheobronchial anatomy having right-sided thoracic surgery, a 5Fr bronchial blocker placed in the right mainstem bronchus through a 5.0 cuffed ETT should provide adequate lung isolation.

3 What are the surgical considerations that impact anesthetic management?

Common indications for thoracoscopic procedures in pediatrics include lung biopsy, lobectomy, lung decortication, thymectomy, esophageal atresia repair, mediastinal mass resection, and patent ductus arteriosus ligation. The use of video-assisted thoracoscopic surgery (VATS) in children continues to increase due to its advantages (less postoperative pain, fewer intraoperative complications, and shortened hospital stays) and requires well-executed lung isolation. It is important to note that insufflation of the thoracic cavity with carbon dioxide may not be tolerated by young infants. The physiologic effects of insufflation (especially with higher pressures of 10 to 15 mm Hg) include a decrease in mean blood pressure, decrease in left ventricular stroke index, and increased central venous pressure. Because of this, lower pressures are often used in children (4 to 6 mm Hg). In the young population (<2 years old), surgical exposure can also be achieved with just CO_2 insufflation/pneumothorax and retraction of the operative lung without the need for lung isolation.

4 Are there special considerations for the emergence or the end of the case?

Assuming there is no need for continued controlled ventilation in the postoperative setting, extubation should generally be expected following thoracic surgery. This is a critical part of anesthesia management, particularly if it has been a long and/or complicated procedure, if there was preexisting lung disease, or if the patient has a difficult airway. Considerations for optimizing a successful extubation include recruitment maneuvers delivered to the operative lung, thorough suctioning of the airway, and careful oxygen titration. A comprehensive pain management strategy should be executed in order to maintain adequate analgesia and adequate ventilation postoperatively without excessive sedation.

- There is an increasing use of video-assisted thoracoscopic procedures being performed in the pediatric population.
- Lung isolation in pediatrics can be challenging due to the varying physiologic and anatomical differences compared to adults.
- It is critical to understand the advantages and limitations of each lung isolation technique.
- *See Figure 158.1 and* ***Video 158.1*** *for additional details.*

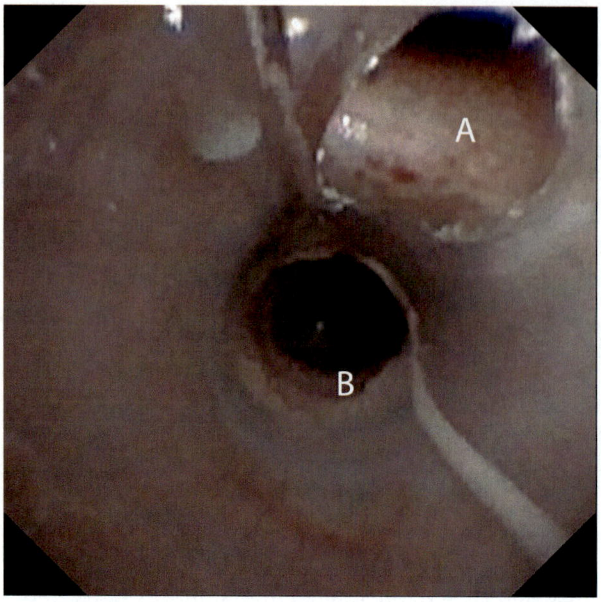

Figure 158.1. Right-sided double-lumen tube in a child. Right upper lobe seen through tracheal tube Murphy eye (*A*). Bronchus intermedius (*B*).

Suggested Readings

Fabila TS, Menghraj SJ. One lung ventilation strategies for infants and children undergoing video assisted thoracoscopic surgery. *Indian J Anaesth*. 2013;57(4):339–344.

Letal M, Theam M. Paediatric lung isolation. *BJA Education*. 2017;17(2):57–62.

Piccioni F, Templeton TW, Morris B, Valenza F. Pediatric thoracic anesthesia: airway management for lung isolation and post-operative analgesia. *Pediatr Med*. 2019;2:23.

Templeton TW, Piccioni F, Chatterjee D. An update on one-lung ventilation in children. *Anesth Analg*. 2021;132(5):1389–1399.

Airway Management for a Large Anterior Mediastinal Mass Resection in Adults

159

Javier H. Campos • Philip M. Hartigan • Sergey Karamnov

Clinical Scenario: A 37-year-old woman with a large thymic mass presents for thymectomy. The patient complains of hoarseness and inability to lay flat. The chest X-ray is depicted in Figure 159.1

Her history is significant for myasthenia gravis treated with pyridostigmine and prednisone. Previously, she has had an episode of breathing difficulty requiring intubation. Currently, her symptoms are controlled. Her CT scan shows a large anterior mediastinal mass, measuring 16 cm in length, compressing, and deviating the trachea to the right (Figure 159.2A).

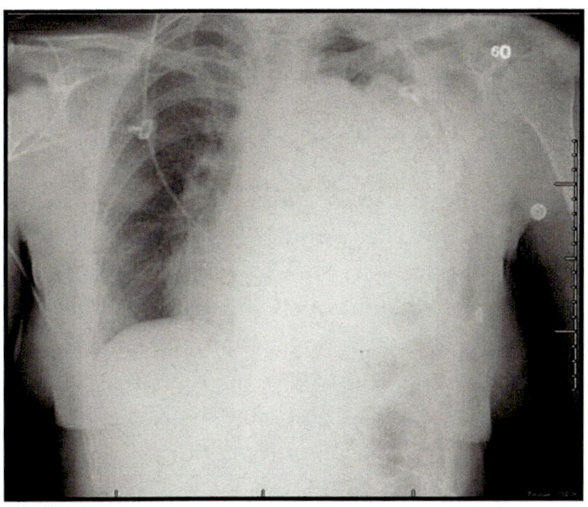

Figure 159.1. Chest x-ray of a 36-year-old woman with a very large mediastinal mass on the left hemithorax.

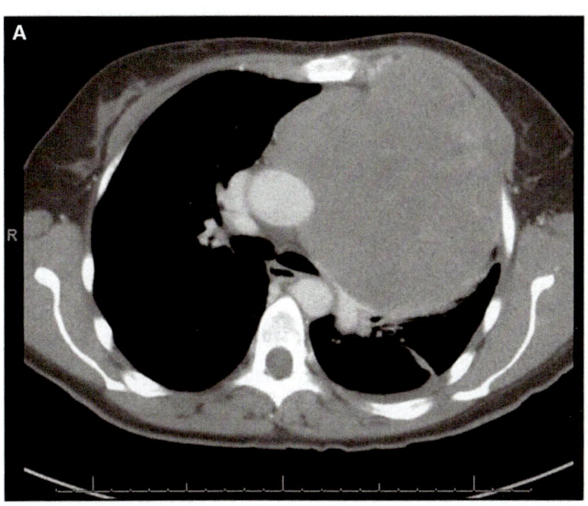

R L

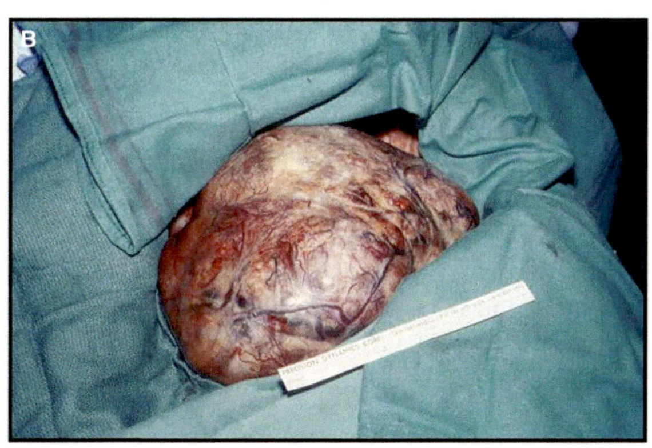

Figure 159.2. A: CT scan of the chest showing a large mediastinal mass on the left hemithorax. **B:** The large mediastinal mass during left-sided thoracotomy.

1 What are the anesthetic and airway management considerations for this case?

Although anterior mediastinal masses are uncommon in adults, they present significant challenges to the anesthesiologist because of their impact on the airway and cardiovascular system. The anatomic location and size of the mediastinal mass has significant implications related to compression of the airway (mainly in the lower third of the trachea and main bronchi), major vessels (including superior vena cava and pulmonary vessels), and adjacent organs.

Airway compression can occur when the patient is placed supine, at induction of anesthesia, intraoperatively, at extubation, or postoperatively. Another concern in this patient population is the length of airway compression with potential bronchial involvement. In patients with extensive airway obstruction, it may be necessary to advance the endotracheal tube (ETT) into the bronchus or to place a stent into the distal airway in order to maintain ventilation of the lung distal to the obstruction. Compression of the large airways can manifest with significant changes in gas exchange and patient morbidity. Some patients with large anterior mediastinal masses develop severe hypoxemia caused by a total obstruction of the main bronchus and pulmonary artery compression. Another potential complication related to airway obstruction is the development of noncardiogenic pulmonary edema, particularly in patients with severe airway obstruction either before or after the surgical intervention.

2 How would you manage the airway in this case?

The airway management approach depends on the perceived degree of risk of airway collapse. Factors associated with mediastinal mass-related severe airway compression have been identified, but they lack high predictive specificity. They include orthopnea, large mass-to-chest size ratio, preoperative tracheal cross-sectional area decreased to <50%, a maximum expiratory flow <50% predicted, and mixed obstructive/restrictive pulmonary function tests.

Patients deemed to be *low risk* may undergo standard IV induction with immediate paralysis, intubation, and conversion to positive pressure ventilation. Following intubation, bronchoscopic examination of the airway should be performed to reassess patency.

Those deemed to be of *intermediate or indeterminant risk* are recommended to undergo a staged induction in the semi-fowlers position, with a spontaneously breathing induction and asleep intubation, followed by stepwise conversion to supine position, positive pressure ventilation, and paralysis. Should ventilatory difficulty occur, advancing the endotracheal tube over a fiberoptic bronchoscope to stent open the airway is the most reliable rescue maneuver. Other rescue maneuvers include reverting to the prior stage, changing patient position to off-load the mass effect, advancing a rigid bronchoscope to stent open the airway, or emergent extracorporeal support (eg, extracorporeal membrane oxygenation [ECMO] or cardiopulmonary bypass). Reverting to the prior stage is only supported by anecdotal case reports, and it may be difficult to reduce inhalational anesthetic levels quickly with an obstructed airway. Position changes may be impractical except in pediatric patients. Rigid bronchoscopy may be very challenging in unparalyzed patients, and emergent extracorporeal support requires more time than is generally available. For these reasons, we advocate advancing a tube over a bronchoscope to stent open the airway, allowing ventilation distal to the compressed airway if necessary.

Although airway compression is only moderate in this patient, she should be considered intermediate/indeterminant risk due to the size of the mass, the presence of orthopnea, the degree of parenchymal compression, and the position of the mass threatening compression of the left pulmonary artery (Figure 159.3). A nuance of this case is that stenting open and selectively ventilating the left lung with a single-lumen tube or endobronchial tube may not provide adequate gas exchange because of left pulmonary artery and parenchymal compression. Thus, a left-sided DLT which stents the left mainstem but also enables bilateral ventilation would be the best choice.

In *high-risk* patients, when general anesthesia cannot be avoided, we recommend awake fiberoptic intubation with topical local anesthesia and judicious sedation, in the semi-Fowler position. This provides an immediate bronchoscopic assessment of the degree of airway compression, as well as a means to monitor changes and advance the tube (single or double-lumen tube [DLT]) across the stenosis if necessary. Depending on how reassuring the airway compression appears, one can proceed with induction, positive pressure ventilation, paralysis, and supination, either before or after stenting the airway with a tube. Intubating patients with a DLT while awake is possible with judicious sedation and "spray-as-you-go" local anesthesia below the vocal cords via the working channel of the bronchoscope. Alternatively, one could preemptively place wires or cannulate for ECMO support under local anesthesia.

It is emphasized that simply maintaining spontaneous ventilation does not guarantee airway patency during anesthesia. The common assumption that spontaneous ventilation and intact muscle tone are superior to positive pressure ventilation and/or paralysis for maintaining patency of extrinsically compressed central airways has been challenged by recent direct observational evidence and remains a matter of controversy as of this writing (**Video 159.1**).

3 What are the potential hazards and complications in regard to the airway?

Intraoperative life-threatening airway compression is the main concern in such cases. In this situation, a rapid diagnosis using a flexible intubating scope (FIS) is required, followed by the rescue maneuvers as discussed above.

4 What distinct airway device (eg, specialized tracheal tube, rigid bronchoscope, BB) might be used in this case, and what are the special considerations?

The type of ETT used to manage the airway depends on the surgical approach. If a sternotomy is planned, a single-lumen ETT may be used. If a patient requires thoracotomy, once the airway is secure with a single-lumen ETT, a bronchial blocker (BB) can be used to facilitate lung isolation. For patients with distal tracheal/bronchial compression, a DLT provides the optimal ability to stent open the compressed bronchus, ventilate both lungs, and isolate ventilation to one lung if a thoracotomy approach is planned. An extrinsically compressed bronchus will generally admit the bronchial lumen of a DLT, but occasionally, one might need to use a right-sided DLT with left mainstem bronchial compression, or vice versa. Endobronchial tubes, like DLTs also have sufficient length to advance across a bronchial stenosis, but cannot allow bilateral ventilation without withdrawing above the carina. The use of the rigid bronchoscope is limited only to cases where the airway is lost due to compression of the lower third of the trachea. Special attention should be given to patients who have a tracheal or bronchial stent due to the potential to dislodge it while placing the ETT (Table 159.1).

TABLE 159.1 Basic Components for Managing the Airway in Patient with a Large Mediastinal Mass
Rigid bronchoscope
FIS
Video laryngoscopes
Armored single-lumen ETTs
DLTs
BBs
Surgical team

5 Are there special considerations for the emergence or the end of the case?

Extubation after removal of a large mediastinal mass can present significant challenges. Some patients will experience tracheomalacia and might need to remain intubated in the early postoperative period. One study demonstrated that if the preoperative CT scan shows more than 50% tracheal compression and a mixed obstructive and restrictive pattern on pulmonary function tests, the likelihood for postoperative reintubation is high. Therefore, all intubating equipment should be available at bedside. This includes video laryngoscope, laryngeal mask airways, and FIS.

Myasthenia gravis (MG) is an autoimmune disorder of the neuromuscular junction. The muscle-type nicotinic receptors are destroyed by autoantibodies, resulting in muscle weakness and fatigue.

Patients with thymomas may develop MG, while 15% of MG patients have thymomas. Patients taking anticholinesterase or steroid therapy should continue them until the day of surgery. If the patient has a mediastinal mass that is not compressing the airway, then succinylcholine can be used for intubation. Nondepolarizing neuromuscular blockers should be used with caution in patients with MG due to their unpredictable effects. A peripheral nerve stimulator must be used in order to administer the appropriate dose of muscle relaxants. Extubation should be performed only when the patient is completely reversed from muscle relaxants.

- A preoperative chest CT scan that assesses the relationship between the mediastinal mass, trachea, bronchi, and major vessels is required.
- Compression of the airway due to large mediastinal mass can occur when the patient is placed supine, at induction of anesthesia, intraoperatively, at extubation, or postoperatively.
- Large anterior mediastinal masses compressing the airway require FB evaluation prior to intubation.
- After resection of a large anterior mediastinal mass, the potential for tracheomalacia exists. This puts the patient at a high risk of failing immediate postoperative extubation.
- *See Figure 159.3 for additional details.*

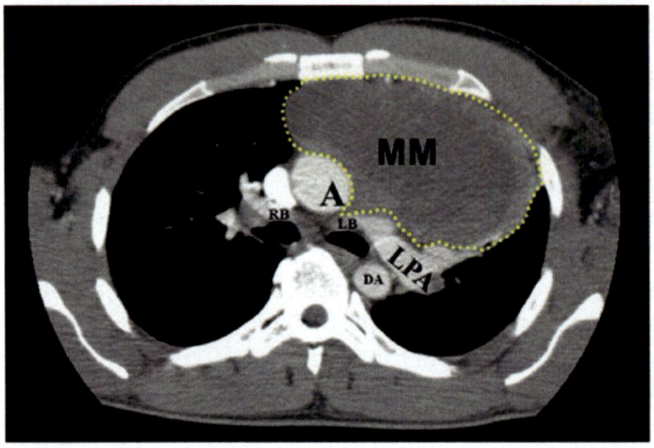

Figure 159.3. Anatomic location of the mediastinal mass in relation to airway and great vessels. MM, mediastinal mass; A, aorta; LPA, left pulmonary artery; DA, descending aorta; LB, left bronchus; RB, right bronchus.

Suggested Readings

Bechard P, Letourneau L, Lacasse Y, Côté D, Bussières JS. Perioperative cardiorespiratory complications in adults with mediastinal mass: incidence and risk factors. *Anesthesiology*. 2004;100:826–834.

Campos JH. Monograph SCA. In: Cohen NH, ed. *Medically Challenging Patients Undergoing Cardiothoracic Surgery*. Lippincott Williams & Wilkins; 2009:285–302.

Chow L. Anesthesia for patients with mediastinal masses. In: Slinger P ed. *Principles and Practice of Anesthesia for Thoracic Surgery*. 2nd ed. Springer; 2019:251–263.

Hartigan PM, Karamnov S, Gill RR, et al. Mediastinal masses, anesthetic interventions and airway compression in adults: a prospective observational study. *Anesthesiology*. 2022;136:104–114.

Ng J, Hartigan PM. Anterior mediastinal mass. In: Hartigan PM, ed. *Practical Handbook of Thoracic Anesthesia*. 2012;335–353.

Shin JH, Song HY, Ko GY, et al. Treatment of tracheobronchial obstruction with a polytetrafluoroethylene-covered retrievable expandable nitinol stent. *J Vasc Interv Radiol*. 2006;17:657–663.

Zhou J, Allen P, Pessah NI, et al. Neuromuscular disorders and malignant hyperthermia. In: Miller RD, ed. *Miller's Anesthesia*. 7th ed. Churchill Livingstone Elsevier; 2009:1171–1196.

Lung Isolation in a Patient with Difficult Airway

160

Diana Anca

Clinical Scenario: An 85-year-old man with a 1.5-cm right middle lobe nodule presents to the OR for a right middle lobectomy via video-assisted thoracoscopic surgery (VATS). The patient has severe kyphosis and cannot extend his neck.

1 What are the anesthetic and airway management considerations for this case?

Patients with severe kyphosis have restrictive lung disease with a limited respiratory reserve. This decreases tolerance to prolonged apnea and one-lung ventilation (OLV) and increases the likelihood of postoperative mechanical ventilation. In addition, airway manipulation in patients with severe kyphosis should be performed cautiously, as degenerative changes of the cervical spine can be present as well.

VATS requires the use of general endotracheal anesthesia with OLV, accomplished by using either double-lumen tube (DLT) or an endotracheal tube (ETT) with a bronchial blocker (BB). In the setting of severe kyphosis and neck immobility, safely securing the airway represents the most important anesthetic consideration. In addition, the need for lung isolation further augments the problem because DLTs may be more difficult to place than ETTs. Careful thought should be given to the method used for lung separation. A discussion with the surgical team is helpful in outlining their requirements in relation to the airway management alternatives. However, in a patient with difficult airway requiring OLV, "less is more"; BBs are perhaps a safer alternative than DLTs. The immediate availability of various airway equipment, such as laryngeal mask airway, video laryngoscope, flexible intubating scope (FIS), tube exchangers, and different-sized ETTs, DLTs, and BBs is important.

Of note, the "difficult airway" potential encompasses few other entities, of special considerations being radiation therapy to neck, hemi-glossectomy/mandibulectomy, limited mouth opening, which might render the possibility of initial or subsequent DLT placement impossible or very risky and traumatic. Ultimately, our primary objective is to "secure the airway."

2 How would you manage the airway in this case?

When devising an airway management plan for this patient, the first step is to decide whether the intubation can be performed with an awake or an asleep technique. The choice of the optimal lung isolation device follows after.

Assuming the patient is appropriately fasted, the decision regarding an awake versus an asleep intubation needs to consider at least two factors: the perceived difficulty of mask ventilation and the presence or absence of significant gastroesophageal reflux disease (GERD).

If mask ventilation is expected to be easily attained and the patient has no significant GERD, then an asleep technique is utilized. The patient's neck immobility may preclude the use of direct laryngoscopy. Either a video laryngoscope or a FIS can be utilized to intubate the trachea. An ETT followed by placement of a BB is easier to employ than a DLT because the latter is bulkier, less flexible, and cannot be used in conjunction with an intubating airway. In addition, a DLT blind intubation cannot be performed. After the trachea is intubated with an ETT, prior to placing the BB, the length of the right mainstem bronchus should be evaluated. A short takeoff of the right upper lobe bronchus may preclude the use of a BB, as the blocker's cuff may herniate above the carina. In such situations, a tube exchanger can be used to replace the ETT with a left DLT (see Chapter 140: Single-Lumen to Double-Lumen Tube Exchange). Alternatively, an EZ blocker could be used which is less likely to displace due to the fact that it straddles the carina.

When using a FIS to place the DLT, the tube needs to be loaded on the scope through the bronchial lumen. This will allow the DLT to follow the passage of the FIS. Direct laryngoscopy, even if it cannot expose the larynx, is very helpful by displacing the tongue and epiglottis and increasing the room to manipulate the FIS and advance the DLT. The techniques utilized to place a DLT using either a Glidescope or a McGrath video laryngoscope are described in Chapter 129: DLT Placement Using the Glidescope and Chapter 130: DLT Placement Using the McGrath Blade.

Conversely, if either the mask ventilation is predicted to be difficult or the patient has significant GERD, then an awake technique should be considered. Either a DLT or an ETT can be utilized. In situations of severe kyphosis, a nasal intubation offers easier access to the airway for an ETT. A DLT is too large to pass nasally. Following placement of an awake oral or nasal ETT, the patient is anesthetized, and lung isolation is achieved by placing a BB. Alternatively, after an awake intubation the ETT can be replaced with a DLT using a tube exchanger (see Chapter 140: Single-Lumen to Double-Lumen Tube Exchange). However, during the tube exchange process, the airway is left unprotected from aspiration and/or may be completely lost. Therefore, only serious reasons should compel the anesthesiologist to perform this maneuver. Regardless of the chosen method, the awake technique requires thorough airway topicalization (see Chapter 11: Preparation for Awake Intubation). Minimal sedation and a slightly elevated head and back position, help the patient maintain adequate ventilation and oxygenation during the awake intubation. Probably the easiest and most comfortable technique for the patient is to place an ETT using the FIS. Awake DLT placement under FIS guidance can be performed, but it is challenging, as the large tube size occasionally impedes the smooth entrance into the trachea. Other awake intubating techniques can be considered.

3 What are the potential hazards and complications in regard to the airway?

The main concern in the care of this patient is the loss of the airway. Due to severe kyphosis and limited neck mobility, the access to the airway via an emergency tracheostomy may be very challenging. Therefore, a secure airway should be always regarded with "respect."

It is important to emphasize that personal experience and comfort with DLT and BB is crucial in deciding which path to take. While both have their advantages and disadvantages, it is best to choose the ones you are more familiar with. The newer models of both DLT and BB are more user friendly. Also, continuous practice improvement, either via thoracic workshops, simulating exercises, or the free online simulator at www.thoracicanesthesia.com could increase the level of proficiency.

4 Are there special considerations for the emergence at the end of the case?

In view of the difficulty in performing an emergency tracheostomy, a premature extubation may lead to complete airway loss. A successful extubation requires thorough intraoperative planning. It entails meeting all the usual ventilatory criteria and proper pain control, which allows deep breathing and maintenance of airway reflexes.

Devising a postoperative pain control plan is an integral part of the extubation process. A solely opioid-based method carries the risk of oversedation and respiratory depression. A thoracic epidural is extremely difficult to place in the setting of severe kyphosis. Therefore, multimodal pain therapy needs to be considered. Continuous intercostal blocks offer an excellent pain management solution, in particular, for patients undergoing VATS. In addition, careful opioid titration and use of adjuvant analgesics, such as intravenous acetaminophen and nonsteroidal anti-inflammatory drugs, are strongly recommended. Enhanced recovery after surgery protocols, well established for thoracic surgery, with opioid sparing techniques, have brought a greater level of safety in these cases.

An elevated head position optimizes ventilation and oxygenation. The intraoperative use of an ETT with a BB has the advantage that, if postoperative ventilation is required, a tube exchange is not required.

- In a patient with a difficult airway, safely securing the airway represents the first priority, while assuring optimal lung isolation is a secondary issue.
- In the case of a difficult airway requiring OLV, "less is more"; BBs are perhaps a safer alternative to DLTs.
- In a patient with severe kyphosis and limited neck mobility, an emergency tracheostomy may be difficult to perform.
- Workshops and simulating labs are a way of improving skills with both DLT and BB.
- An optimal postoperative pain management plan is essential for a successful extubation; multimodal pain therapy is recommended.
- *See Figure 160.1 and* ***Video 160.1*** *for additional details.*

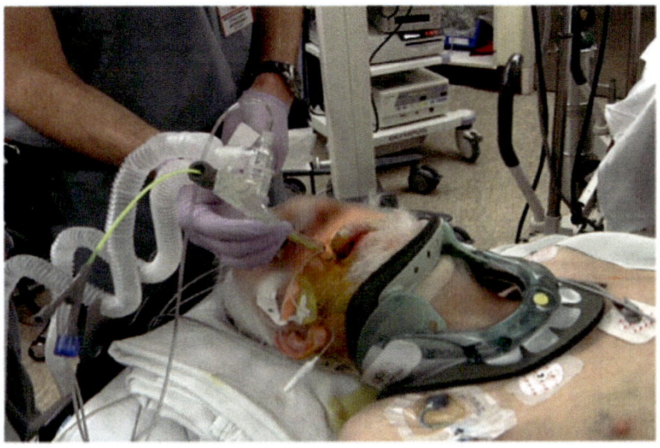

Figure 160.1. A patient with an unstable cervical spine injury is undergoing lung isolation with a single-lumen tube and a bronchial blocker.

Suggested Readings

Batchelor TJP, Rasburn NJ, Abdelnour-Berchtold E, et al. Guidelines for enhanced recovery after lung surgery: recommendations of the Enhanced Recovery After Surgery (ERAS) Society and the European Society of Thoracic Surgeons (ESTS). *Eur J Cardiothorac Surg*. 2019;55(1):91–115.

Brodsky JB. Lung isolation and the difficult airway. *Br J Anesth*. 2009;103:66–75.

Campos JH. Lung isolation in patients with a difficult airway in thoracic anesthesia. In: Cohen E, ed. *Cohen's comprehensive Thoracic Anesthesia*. Elsevier; 2021.

Campos JH. Lung isolation techniques for patients with difficult airway. *Curr Opin Anesthesiol*. 2010;23:12–17.

Campos JH. Which device should be considered the best for lung isolation: double-lumen endotracheal tube versus bronchial blockers. *Curr Opin Anesthesiol*. 2007;20:27–31.

161 Esophageal Dilation

Adriana Herrera

Clinical Scenario: A 58-year-old man who is status post esophagectomy 6 months ago presents for upper endoscopy with esophageal dilation.

1 What are the anesthetic and airway management considerations for this case?

Esophageal stenosis is a very common complication encountered after esophagectomy. In patients with advanced esophageal stenosis, the quality of life is significantly affected. Patients can be malnourished or dehydrated. Esophageal dilation provides an effective therapy to improve oral intake and nutritional status.

In patients with tight esophageal stenosis, oral secretions cannot be properly swallowed, and food may be impacted above the level of the stricture. More importantly, patients who have had an esophagectomy do not have a lower esophageal sphincter. All of the above put such patients at a high risk of pulmonary aspiration. Many patients exhibit dyspnea due to impaired oxygenation, reflecting chronic aspiration. Therefore, standard NPO guidelines should be strictly followed. Pretreatment with H2-receptor blockers, proton-pump inhibitors, or metoclopramide may also be used. Head elevation at 30 to 45 degrees is essential.

Comorbidities related to smoking and alcohol consumption are common in this patient population. Pulmonary, liver, and coronary artery disease may be present. A history suggestive of a possible difficult airway (ie, head and neck cancer, cervical fusion, radiation therapy, etc.) and a known history of difficult airway are important issues to consider in designing the optimal strategy for airway management. Review of previous anesthetic records is useful.

2 How would you manage the airway in this case?

Anesthetic choices include monitored anesthesia care (MAC) with or without topicalization of the oropharynx, and general endotracheal anesthesia. Most procedures last 15 to 60 minutes.

Whenever MAC is the technique of choice, an adequate level of sedation must be provided in order to facilitate a safe and efficient esophageal endoscopic examination and dilation. However, the patient may still have a strong gag reflex. A combination of intravenous sedation and oropharynx topicalization ensures that smaller doses of sedatives are needed to maintain the patient comfortable and more cooperant. A major advantage of this anesthetic technique is represented by a decrease of intraprocedural episodes of oversedation with subsequent desaturation, which can potentially degenerate in losing the airway. On the other hand, in patients who are undersedated, passing the endoscope may be difficult, resulting in mechanical trauma to the teeth and/or the airway or endoscope damage.

Patients are placed in supine position with the head elevated at 30 to 45 degrees to decrease aspiration risk. Topicalization of the oropharynx can be done by gargling and swallowing 2% viscous lidocaine (usually 10 mL) or use of atomized or nebulized 4% lidocaine. Benzocaine spray (cetacaine) has been used for this purpose, but is not currently recommended due to the potential development of methemoglobinemia. Any patient who presents with cyanosis, respiratory distress, mental status changes, headache, dizziness, and a chocolate-brown color of blood after receiving oropharyngeal anesthesia with benzocaine, should be suspected of having methemoglobinemia and treated empirically with methylene blue.

The total dose of local anesthetics is an important consideration as there is a potential for toxicity. Absorption of local anesthetic is fast and reliable, allowing patients to tolerate the placement of an oral airway easily. The bite block should be placed before deepening the level of sedation, as trying to open the mouth afterward may prove challenging. This will also prevent biting of the endoscope and potential dental and endoscope damage. Once sedation is started, jaw extension may be necessary to facilitate surgical insertion of the endoscope. Once the endoscope has been placed, it is important that immediate aspiration of any contents in the esophagus or stomach is performed to decrease risk of aspiration. Risk of micro or macro aspiration is still present even with strict NPO guidelines.

The level of sedation is usually achieved with a combination of an intravenous benzodiazepine and an opioid. Propofol used in incremental boluses or as an infusion is a common alternative. Another choice is a dexmedetomidine or remifentanil infusion. Ketamine is not a good choice as it may result in increased secretions and confusion. It is important to ensure an appropriate level of sedation is achieved before manipulating the oropharynx and airway. Alternatively, if airway management becomes difficult, it will increase the aspiration risk. In order to decrease the episodes of desaturation, supplemental oxygen via nasal cannula is recommended. An alternative may be a continuous positive airway pressure nasal mask such as the SuperNO2VA, which has been utilized and shown to be superior than nasal cannula when performing GI procedures under deep sedation. High flow nasal cannula has been successfully used in selected patients with high risk of hypoxemia under sedation for GI procedures. However, there is no data supporting its use in this population that has a higher risk of aspiration.

If a general anesthetic is chosen, the same precautions regarding fasting status, aspiration risk, and head elevation should be applied. Rapid sequence induction with cricoid pressure is preferred. In a difficult airway patient, an awake intubation should be considered. General anesthesia protects the airway and facilitates endoscope passage.

3 What are the potential hazards and complications in regard to the airway?

The risk of aspiration is high. Measures to decrease this risk should be employed. A poorly anesthetized and uncooperative patient undergoing MAC can result in aspiration, a challenging endoscopy, or even an airway emergency. When MAC is performed inappropriately, other possible complications include laryngospasm, bronchospasm, episodes of desaturation, and hypoxia.

Bite blocks are necessary to avoid dental trauma or endoscope damage. Jaw extension allows for an easier insertion of the scope.

Patients identified as having difficult airways may still be candidates for MAC. However, a rescue plan for an airway emergency should be thought ahead. This plan could include immediate availability of various devices such as a Glidescope and/or a flexible bronchoscope. Appropriate communication and planning with the surgeon and other OR staff is strongly recommended.

4 What distinct airway device (eg, specialized tracheal tube, rigid bronchoscope, bronchial blocker) might be used in this case, and what are the special considerations?

The Three-In-One (TIO) is a combination product that incorporates the benefits of an oropharyngeal airway, a bite block, and an oxygen administration port into one disposable device.

This device comes in different color-coded sizes: 90 mm (yellow), 100 mm (blue), and 110 mm (purple). It encompasses a 60Fr bite block that allows the use of a wide range of endoscopes and a standard-size oxygen administration port. The TIO can also be used for other procedures such as transesophageal echocardiography and bronchoscopy. It may also be of great help in patients with obesity or obstructive sleep apnea.

- Risk of pulmonary aspiration is high and common.
- To decrease the aspiration risk, patients should be supine with the head of the bed elevated at 30 degrees.
- MAC with oropharyngeal topicalization is an excellent anesthetic choice for this population; however immediate aspiration through endoscope is required in order to decrease the risk of aspiration.
- Blunting the gag reflex is a priority in order to avoid oversedation resulting in oxygen desaturation.
- *See Figure 161.1 and* ***Video 161.1*** *for additional details.*

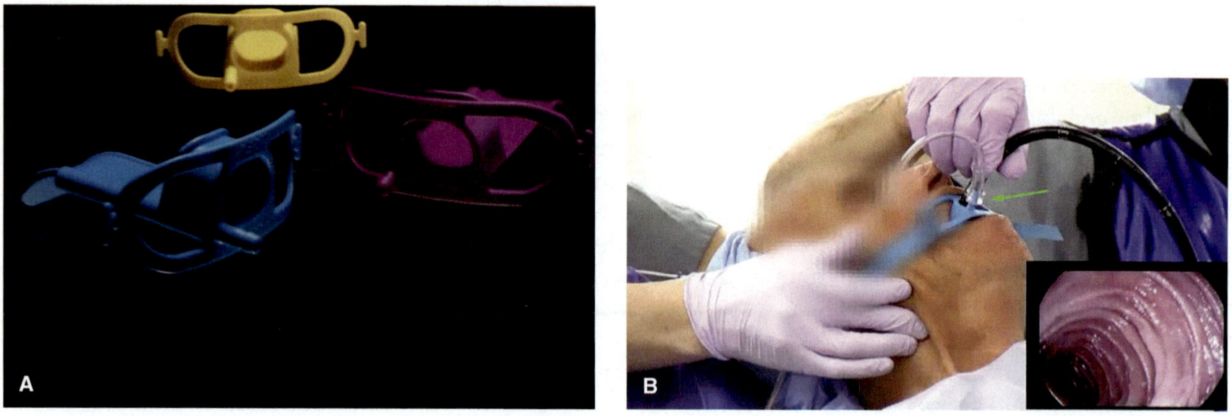

Figure 161.1. **A:** The Three-in-One bite block acts as an oral airway, a bite block and allows oxygen insufflation. **B:** A gastroscope is passed through the bite block while oxygen is being insufflated (*arrow*).

Suggested Readings

Bhavani SS, Abdelmalak B. Nonoperating room anesthesia: anesthesia in the gastrointestinal suite. *Anesthesiol Clin*. 2019;37:301–316.

Evans LT, Saberi S, Kim HM, Elta GH, Schoenfeld P. Pharyngeal anesthesia during sedated EGDs: is "the spray" beneficial? A meta-analysis and systematic review. *Gastrointest Endosc*. 2006;63:761–766.

Heuss LT, Hanhart A, Dell-Kuster S, et al. Propofol sedation or in combination with pharyngeal lidocaine anesthesia for routine upper GI endoscopy: a randomized, double-blind, placebo-controlled, non-inferiority trial. *Gastrointest Endosc*. 2011;74:1207–1214.

Ng A, Smith G. Gastroesophageal reflux and aspiration of gastric contents in anesthetic practice. *Anesth Analg*. 2001;93:494–513.

Rice TW. Anastomotic stricture complicating esophagectomy. *Thorac Surg Clin*. 2006;16:63–73.

One-Lung Ventilation in a Patient with Dextrocardia

162

Loreta Grecu

Clinical Scenario: A 23-year-old woman presents for the revision of a colonic interposition used for the repair of esophageal atresia when she was an infant. Her medical history is significant for dextrocardia and left-lung hypoplasia.

1 What are the anesthetic and airway management considerations for this case?

A relatively common finding, dextrocardia has an incidence of 0.1 per 1000 live births, and is an important diagnosis that should be carefully evaluated preoperatively. Dextrocardia must be differentiated from dextroposition, which means that the heart is in the right chest but is displaced due to causes such as right-lung agenesis or hypoplasia, right pneumonectomy, absence of the pericardium, or diaphragmatic hernia, and is not due to embryologic abnormalities.

The second aspect that needs to be assessed is the position of the abdominal organs and how they correspond to the position of the heart, that is, if the liver is on the right (situs solitus) or on the left (situs inversus) side of the abdomen. There are four possible combinations: normal heart position with situs solitus (heart on the left and liver on the right), dextrocardia with situs inversus (heart on the right and liver on the left), dextrocardia with situs solitus (heart and liver on the right), normal heart position and situs inversus (heart and liver on the left).

The tracheobronchial tree may have several types of abnormalities as well, and identifying them is important due to possible associated pathology. Normally (situs solitus), the right bronchus is wide and short, while the left bronchus is long and narrow and descends more horizontally, with the opposite being true for cases of situs inversus (Figure 162.1). Bilateral morphologic right-type bronchi are associated with asplenia syndrome, while bilateral left-type bronchi are associated with polysplenia syndrome.

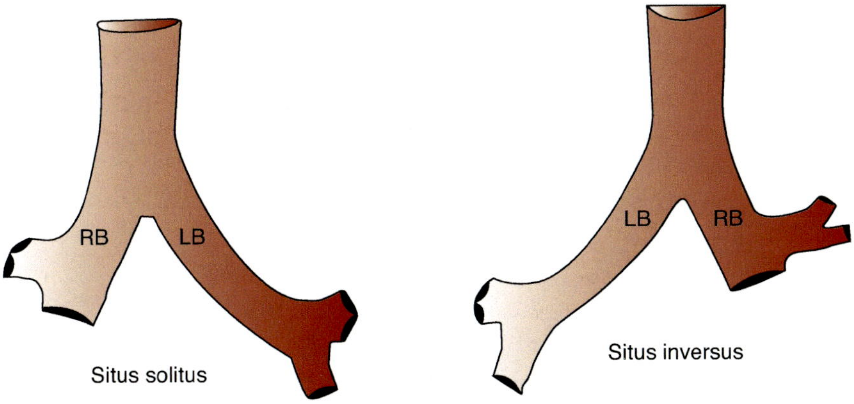

Figure 162.1. In situs solitus (**left**), the morphologic right bronchus (RB) is short, wide, and straight, and the morphologic left bronchus (LB) is long, thin, and curved. In situs inversus (**right**), the morphologic right bronchus is left sided, and the morphologic left bronchus is right sided. (Reprinted from Perloff JK. The cardiac malpositions. *Am J Cardiol.* 2011;108(9):1352–1361. Copyright © 2011 Elsevier. With permission.)

2 How would you manage the airway in this case?

Esophageal atresia with colonic interposition is, by definition, an esophagus without sphincters. In such cases, the patient's airway should be managed similarly to any patient with a "full stomach." For the revision of her colonic interposition, it is most likely that a right-sided thoracic surgical approach will be used, therefore necessitating lung isolation and one lung ventilation.

Prior to the beginning of the case, a discussion with the surgeon is important. Depending on the location of the repair, lung isolation may be necessary for this case. Commonly, this is done with a left double-lumen tube (DLT). For this particular patient with left-lung hypoplasia this may not be the ideal lung isolation device, since the left bronchus may be narrower than usual and may be unable to sustain the tension of the DLT balloon.

Although the bronchial tree anatomy may be well known from previous imaging studies (chest radiography, chest CT), a bronchoscopy is essential to evaluate the anatomy and to rule out the presence of bronchiectasis, which are associated with increased secretion production and respiratory infections.

Taking into consideration the history of a hypoplastic left lung, there are two alternatives to obtain lung isolation in this patient: using a bronchial blocker in the right mainstem bronchus or a DLT. However, because of dextrocardia, it is highly probable that the bronchial tree is reversed as well, and what we expect to find on the right, will be on the left and vice versa. In this case, a left DLT may be able to fit perfectly into this patient's right bronchial tree (which anatomically may be identical to the normal left bronchial tree). While both lung isolation devices could be used in this patient, considering the high aspiration risk and the initially unknown tracheobronchial anatomy, it may be prudent to intubate the airway with a single-lumen ETT in a rapid sequence fashion, bronchoscopically evaluate the lower airway, and then place a bronchial blocker on the right side.

3 What are the potential hazards and complications in regard to the airway?

Possible aspiration of gastric content during airway manipulations is an important concern. Placement of the OR table in reverse Trendelenburg and rapid sequence induction may mitigate this risk.

In a patient with dextrocardia, the tracheobronchial anatomy may be reversed, or may be totally anomalous. For this reason, intraoperative bronchoscopy is useful in identifying the airway device of choice and verifying its correct placement in the bronchus. The presence of bronchiectasis with increased respiratory secretions poses an increased risk for development of atelectasis, lobar collapse, desaturation, and respiratory infection.

The diagnosis of left-lung hypoplasia suggests that there are other associated anatomic abnormalities. Structurally, this lung may be imperfect, with a narrower bronchus unable to sustain the same airway cuff pressure as a normal one. These facts would preclude the use of a DLT due to possible tracheobronchial disruption. In addition, for a patient with hypoplastic lung, in order to prevent the development of a pneumothorax, maintenance of low tidal volumes without extreme increases in airway pressures is recommended. It should be emphasized that with right-lung deflation, the occurrence of a left pneumothorax may be followed by severe desaturation. In such cases, until the cause of desaturation is identified and treated, the right lung should be ventilated.

4 Are there special considerations for the emergence or the end of the case?

It is essential that a patient be awake, able to follow commands and achieve expected respiratory parameters, prior to extubation. Prevention of atelectasis and suctioning of secretions, with careful reinflation of the lungs, while maintaining low airway pressures, are the most important aspects of a successful extubation. Of course, the usual parameters (normothermia, reversal of muscle relaxation, elimination of inhaled anesthetics, normal hemodynamics, adequate pain control) are the mainstay of this important anesthetic step. More than ever, all extubation criteria should be fulfilled prior to proceeding with ventilatory support weaning.

- Dextrocardia may be associated with tracheobronchial anomalies.
- Bronchoscopy is important to evaluate the bronchial anatomy, and to rule out bronchiectasis.
- Lung hypoplasia may be associated with a narrower bronchus, which may preclude the use of a DLT.
- In a patient with hypoplastic lung, in order to prevent the development of a pneumothorax, maintenance of low tidal volumes without extreme increases in airway pressures is recommended.
- *See Figure 162.2 for* ⓒ ***Video 162.1*** *for additional details.*

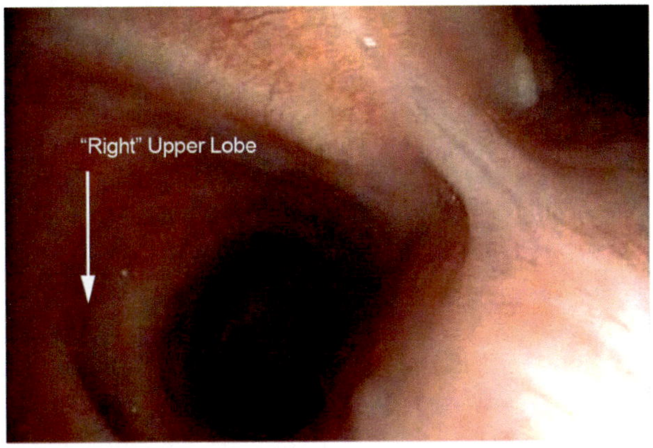

Figure 162.2. The physiologic right upper lobe is seen within the left side bronchus.

Suggested Readings

Duong SQ, Godown J, Soslow JH, et al. Increased mortality, morbidities, and costs after heart transplantation in heterotaxy syndrome and other complex situs arrangements. *J Thorac Cardiovasc Surg*. 2019;157(2):730–740.e11.

Perloff JK. The cardiac malpositions. *Am J Cardiol*. 2011;108(9):1352–1361.

Rao PS. Dextrocardia: systematic approach to differential diagnosis. *Am Heart J*. 1981;102(3 Pt 1):389–403.

Teeter EG, Barrick BP, Kumar PA, Haithcock BE, Karenz AR, Martinelli SM. Anesthetic management of a patient with situs inversus for bilateral orthotopic lung transplantation. *J Cardiothorac Vasc Anesth*. 2016;30(6):1641–1644.

163 One-Lung Ventilation in a Patient with Tracheal Bronchus

Loreta Grecu

Clinical Scenario: A 54-year-old woman presents for a right video-assisted thoracoscopic middle lobectomy for a right middle lobe mass. The preoperative CT scan is suggestive for possible tracheal bronchus (bronchus suis).

1 What are the anesthetic and airway management considerations for this case?

Tracheal bronchus (TB), bronchus suis, or "pig bronchus" is a rare congenital anomaly seen in general population with an incidence of 0.001% to 2%. It is characterized by the fact that the right upper lobe (RUL) bronchus originates from the trachea, at or above the carinal level. This is different from the typical right bronchial mainstem trifurcation which occurs below the carina.

Identification of the TB anatomy can be done with imaging studies (CT scan, MRI), as well as with flexible bronchoscopy. There are three types of possible TB anomalies: an additional (supernumerary) RUL bronchus, a high RUL bronchus takeoff (most common type) that can be associated with a stenosis of the remainder right bronchus, and a diverticular type (underdeveloped RUL bronchus). The TB is usually located in the middle to distal third of the trachea on the right lateral wall. If the opening of the RUL bronchus is found on the posterior wall, the presence of a tracheobronchial fistula should be evaluated.

TB may be asymptomatic and discovered as an incidental finding. It may also cause atelectasis and recurrent pneumonias due to retained secretions, manifesting as cough and stridor. In such cases, resection of the anomalous lobe may be required.

The main anesthetic concern for a patient with TB undergoing surgery that requires one-lung ventilation is providing adequate lung isolation. Placement of any type of endotracheal tube (ETT) can lead to the occlusion of the RUL bronchus takeoff, with potential desaturation. In the rare event when the ETT migrates into the TB, there is an increased risk of pneumothorax, secondary to volutrauma and barotrauma. Hence, it is important to place the ETT higher than the distal third of the trachea to avoid this possible complication. Additionally, providing RUL collapse required for surgical exposure will represent a significant anesthetic challenge. In order to develop an appropriate airway management plan, a bronchoscopic evaluation of the TB anatomy is required.

2 How would you manage the airway in this case?

In order to decide on the best airway device to be utilized in this case, communication with the surgeon prior to the beginning of the procedure is recommended. Depending on the exact anatomy of the anomaly, the location of the lesion, and the surgical approach, various options of lung isolation are available. They include the use of a double-lumen tube (DLT), a bronchial blocker (BB), or an ETT.

If the TB is represented by a carinal takeoff of the RUL bronchus, a left DLT is a good option for lung isolation. If the RUL bronchus takeoff is situated in the distal third of the trachea, then a left DLT appears a less desirable option. In this situation, the tracheal lumen may obstruct the RUL, resulting in not only a nonventilated lobe, but also a not fully collapsed lobe. If the surgeon considers that this would not impede visualization, then the left DLT can be used for the planned procedure. If lung collapse is inadequate, then the tracheal cuff is deflated, the tube disconnected from the circuit, while a suction catheter de-airs the right lung. The tracheal cuff is reinflated, and ventilation of only the left lung is resumed.

Employing a BB in the right mainstem bronchus is another alternative. As the RUL origin is tracheal, it would still be ventilated. Using intermittent ventilation may allow the surgeon to proceed. However, if surgical visualization is deemed suboptimal, then two BBs are needed; one is placed in the anomalous RUL bronchus, and the other one is advanced into the right mainstem bronchus.

Alternatively, an ETT or a single-lumen endobronchial tube is placed into the left mainstem bronchus using a flexible bronchoscope. Since the left mainstem is smaller in caliber than the trachea, the adequate ETT size should be carefully chosen. However, a regular ETT may be too short to be advanced into the left mainstem. When using this technique, if right lung collapse is suboptimal, the cuff is deflated, the tube is disconnected from the circuit, and the lungs are allowed to passively collapse. Subsequently, the cuff is reinflated and left lung ventilation is initiated.

3 What are the potential hazards and complications in regard to the airway?

Due to anomalous anatomy with potentially stenosed or underdeveloped bronchi, the placement of BBs may injure the mucosa. BB dislodgement may occur more frequently, given the different angles at which anomalous bronchi arise. This may manifest as loss of lung isolation, increased airway pressures, and desaturation. Therefore, the differential diagnosis of a sudden, unexpected decrease in oxygen saturation is complex. The first step in the management of desaturation should be a bronchoscopic examination to confirm the DLT, BB, or ETT position.

If the ETT or endobronchial tube migrates into the anomalous RUL bronchus, a pneumothorax may occur, because the entire tidal volume is delivered to one lobe. Auscultation of bilateral lung fields, and radiographic evaluation, is necessary. Caution to the set ventilatory parameters (airway pressures and tidal volume) is indicated. Due to the possible increases in airway pressures associated with changes in overall lung compliance (caused by blood, mucus, or secretions), pressure-controlled ventilation may be a better strategy for this case.

4 Are there special considerations for the emergence or the end of the case?

In a patient with a TB anomaly, prior to extubation, it is necessary to assess that all pulmonary lobes are adequately ventilated. In order to decrease atelectasis and prevent further RUL collapse, depending on the exact anatomy, the ETT or DLT may be required to be withdrawn. A bronchoscopic inspection establishes RUL patency and facilitates clearing of residual secretions or blood.

- The TB is usually located in the middle to distal third of the trachea on the right lateral wall.
- Choosing the optimal airway management device is done in concordance with the assessed anatomy and in close communication with the surgeon.
- Flexible bronchoscopy at the beginning and at the end of the procedure is recommended to assess anatomy, and patency of the RUL.
- *See Figure 163.1 and* **Video 163.1** *for additional details.*

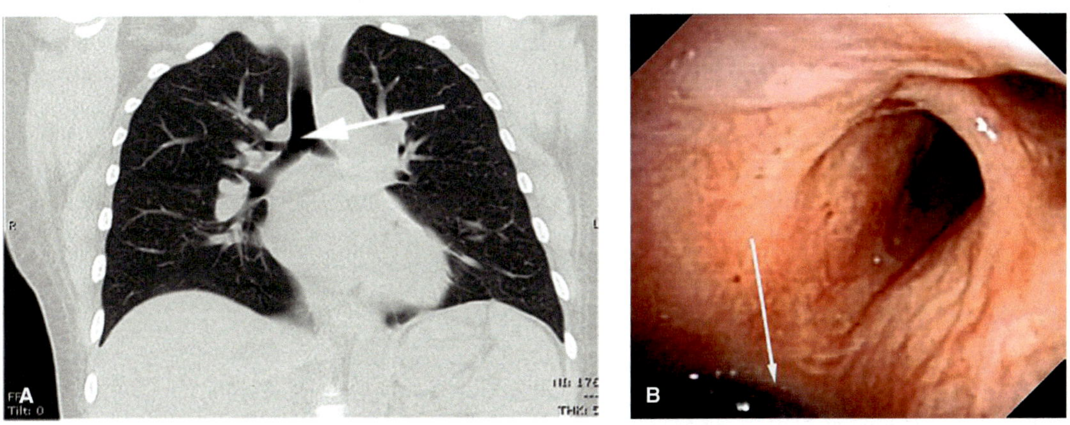

Figure 163.1. **A:** The right upper lobe bronchus is seen originating from the trachea (*arrow*). **B:** Pig trachea balloon in left with *arrow*. Lung isolation is achieved, in a patient with bronchus suis with the double-lumen tube cuff noted (*arrow*).

Suggested Readings

Doolittle AM, Mair EA. Tracheal bronchus: classification, endoscopic analysis, and airway management. *Otolaryngol Head Neck Surg*. 2002;126:240–243.

Friedlander DA, Panigrahi R, Palaniappan D. Tracheal bronchus with difficult lung isolation: a case report. *Semin Cardiothorac Vasc Anesth*. 2022;26:237–240.

Hwang BY, Kwon JY, Kim E, et al. The E-Z blocker for one lung ventilation in a patient with Kartagener syndrome and tracheal bronchus—a case report. *Korean J Anesthesiol*. 2023;76:67–71.

Panzironi G, Noce V, Ammendola RM, Fiorelli A, Carbone I. Tracheal bronchus: high resolution computed tomography diagnosis in a symptomatic patient. *Eur J Radiol Open*. 2014;2:1–2.

164 Bilateral Sequential Lung Transplant

Archer Kilbourne Martin

Clinical Scenario: A 42-year-old female with primary pulmonary hypertension is presenting for bilateral sequential lung transplant. Her baseline echocardiogram shows severe right ventricular enlargement with severely decreased function, and she presents to the operating room with inability to lie flat and on 50 L of oxygen per minute.

1 What are the anesthetic and airway management considerations for this case?

Lung failure can arise from multiple etiologies of end-stage lung disease (ESLD), and the ultimate treatment in medically refractory failure is lung transplantation. The four general categories of ESLD are primary pulmonary hypertension (PPH), restrictive, obstructive, or suppurative disease. PPH is one of the most challenging due to concomitant end-stage cardiac disease that may often present in these patients, arising from the pathophysiology of elevated right ventricular afterload leading to anatomical changes in the right ventricle. This combination of physiologic and anatomical aberrations leads to tenuous cardiopulmonary status throughout the entire perioperative period. A multidisciplinary approach is required, with careful perioperative planning involving the anesthesiologist, surgeon, perfusion, and transplant pulmonary team.

Induction of anesthesia can be particularly challenging, given the sensitivity of the failed right ventricle to abrupt changes in preload, afterload, rate, rhythm, and contractility. The concept of a cardiopulmonary unit should be considered a foundational principle when planning induction, where changes in intrathoracic pressure directly impact right ventricular cardiac output. Positive pressure ventilation, with resultant changes in intrathoracic pressures, decreases cardiac preload and impedes optimal ventricular filling.

Primary graft dysfunction (PGD), a form of acute lung injury characterized by pulmonary edema, diffuse alveolar damage, and insufficient gas exchange, can arise within the first 72 hours following lung transplantation. It is a leading cause of early morbidity and mortality. Risk factors include high pulmonary artery pressures, ischemic-reperfusion injury, and autologous blood transfusions.

2 How would you manage the airway in this case?

PPH has very specific considerations for airway management in bilateral lung transplantation. Even brief episodes of hypoxia or hypercapnia are poorly tolerated and can result in rapid hemodynamic collapse. Adequate oxygenation and ventilation always should be of utmost importance.

Prior to induction, an assessment needs to be considered regarding whether the patient will tolerate induction of general anesthesia. Often, these patients require femoral venous and arterial sheath placement prior to induction, in order to facilitate rapid placement of extracorporeal membrane oxygenation (ECMO) cannulae to provide cardiopulmonary support. In rare cases, awake ECMO cannulation is performed prior to induction of anesthesia, requiring a balance of maintaining spontaneous ventilation with very light sedation.

If the patient is deemed a candidate for induction without ECMO cannulation, the principles of rapid airway acquisition, avoidance of hypoxemia/hypercarbia, and balance of intrathoracic pressure changes secondary to positive pressure ventilation with right ventricular cardiac output are paramount. A particular challenge in PPH patients is positioning, due to their frequent inability to lay flat. Therefore, the positioning of the anesthesiologist, patient, and airway equipment should take these factors into consideration.

Following extensive preoxygenation and induction of anesthesia, adequate mask ventilation should be established before the airway is instrumented. A rapid sequence intubation is recommended in order to obtain the airway as soon as possible, and if there is any concern for achieving rapid airway placement, a single-lumen endotracheal tube (ETT) should be the device of choice for airway management. Subsequently, this single-lumen tube should be exchanged to a double-lumen endotracheal tube (DLT) after invasive monitors are placed, to allow for a real-time assessment of pulmonary arterial pressures. Rarely, this exchange may need to occur after placement of mechanical cardiopulmonary support in order to facilitate a stable cardiopulmonary environment.

Bilateral lung transplantation is performed by sequential single-lung transplantation with an airway anastomosis at the level of both the left and right mainstem bronchi. This procedure requires lung isolation and one-lung ventilation, requiring a DLT be in place prior to explantation of the lungs. The correct position is confirmed using a FB. However, visualization and identification of anatomical structures can be extremely difficult due to secretions and surgical field manipulation.

For ease of placement and maintenance, a left-sided double-lumen tube (LDLT) is recommended and can be used for both the left and right lung implantation. The bronchial reimplantation is performed distally to allow adequate vascularization at the level of the sutures. Therefore, the bronchial lumen of the LDLT allows sufficient distal space for the anastomosis. In case the position is too distal, the LDLT should be slightly retracted as guided by the surgeon. The reimplantation of the right bronchus results in contraction of the bronchus intermedius and the right–upper-lobe bronchus. This changed anatomical position makes it difficult to correctly position the right–upper-lobe bronchial orifice of a right DLT.

Extensive surgical manipulation during the procedure often necessitates frequent repositioning of the DLT. Before resuming ventilation of the implanted donor lung, careful aspiration of secretions and blood should be performed to avoid airway obstruction. Initial reinflation of the implanted lung should occur with the lowest inspired fraction of oxygen that the patient may tolerate, and a lung-protective ventilatory strategy utilizing limited inspiratory pressures should be employed.

Reperfusion of the transplanted graft can induce PGD with possible severe pulmonary edema. Therefore, strict lung isolation is indicated to avoid contamination of the contralateral side. The bronchial cuff should remain inflated during the entire procedure.

The anesthesiologist should be able to access the left and right bronchus at any time to aspirate blood and edema fluid and to inspect the sutures. The use of a bronchial blocker is less optimal for this purpose and should be reserved for patients with a difficult airway when a DLT cannot be introduced.

3 What are the surgical considerations that impact anesthetic management?

The utilization of ECMO has recently emerged as the preferred method for intraoperative cardiopulmonary support in lung transplantation. The utilization of some form of intraoperative cardiopulmonary support is nearly always required in PPH, and this may be provided by a stand-alone ECMO circuit, a hybrid ECMO-cardiopulmonary bypass (CPB) circuit, or a CPB circuit. When full CPB is instituted during the procedure, ventilation becomes theoretically unnecessary. However, in case partial support by ECMO is used, additional lung ventilation is still mandatory to guide ongoing cardiopulmonary resuscitation.

During implantation, clamping of the left or right pulmonary artery might further increase the right ventricular afterload. Performing the venous anastomosis by partial clamping of the left atrium can dramatically decrease left ventricular preload and is associated with low cardiac output and significant hypotension. Maintenance of adequate organ perfusion during this phase is of critical importance.

4 Are there special considerations for the emergence or the end of the case?

At the end of the procedure, the patient is transported to the intensive care unit, intubated, and ventilated. When the pulmonary function is acceptable and if there is no risk for contamination of either side by pulmonary edema or blood, the DLT is typically switched to a single-lumen ETT to decrease the risk of airway injury and to facilitate ventilatory support weaning. In order to avoid airway contamination, a thorough aspiration of the pharynx should be performed. The use of a tube exchanger is not advised routinely, due to the risk of bronchial anastomotic dehiscence with manipulation. However, if there are concerns regarding distortion of the normal anatomy of the upper airways due to edema and mucosal injury, then a tube exchanger is advised. The diameter of the ETT should be sufficient to allow passage of an adult bronchoscope.

In a patient with unilateral ischemia–reperfusion injury where the risk of contralateral contamination is high, the DLT is left in place until the edema is resolved. The DLT will also permit differential lung ventilation using two ventilators, which results in optimal lung protection.

When PGD is present in association with increased pulmonary artery pressures, inhaled nitric oxide (NO) is often started as supportive therapy. The anesthesiologist should be careful not to interrupt the inhaled NO therapy during transport to the ICU since rebound PPH can ensue.

In critical reperfusion injury, ECMO can be considered in order to maintain gas exchange, allow "lung rest," and provide a stable cardiopulmonary environment as the biventricular anatomy remodels secondary to normalization of pulmonary arterial pathophysiology.

- Lung transplantation requires strict cardiovascular and respiratory management by a multidisciplinary team.
- Management of lung transplantation should be tailored to the recipient's etiology of ESLD.
- PGD is a major cause of morbidity and mortality early after implantation.
- Airway management requires strict lung isolation and is optimally performed using a left-sided DLT.
- *See Figure 164.1 and* ***Video 164.1*** *for additional details.*

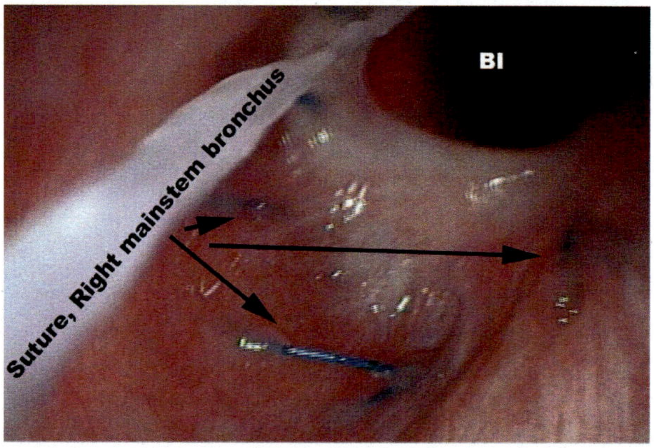

Figure 164.1. Suture line is seen in the right mainstem bronchus in a patient undergoing bilateral, sequential lung transplant.

Suggested Readings

Diamond JM, Lee JC, Kawut SM, et al. Clinical risk factors for primary graft dysfunction after lung transplantation. *Am J Respir Crit Care Med.* 2013;187:527–534.

Hoetzenecker K, Schwarz S, Muckenhuber M, et al. Intraoperative extracorporeal membrane oxygenation and the possibility of postoperative prolongation improved survival in bilateral lung transplantation. *J Thorac Cardiovasc Surg.* 2018;155(5):2193–2206.

Martin AK, Fritz AV, Wilkey BJ. Anesthetic management of lung transplantation: impact of presenting disease. *Curr Opin Anaesthesiol.* 2020;33(1):43–49.

Martin AK, Harrison BA, Fritz AV, et al. Intraoperative management of a hybrid extracorporeal membrane oxygenation circuit for lung transplantation. *J Card Surg.* 2020;35(12):3560–3563.

Martin AK, Yalamuri SM, Wilkey BJ, et al. The impact of anesthetic management on perioperative outcomes in lung transplantation. *J Cardiovasc Anesth.* 2020;34(6):1669–1680.

Moser B, Jaksch P, Taghavi S, et al. Lung transplantation for idiopathic pulmonary arterial hypertension on intraoperative and postoperatively prolonged extracorporeal membrane oxygenation provides optimally controlled reperfusion and excellent outcome. *Eur J Cardiothorac Surg.* 2018;53(1):178–185.

Rigid Bronchoscopy with Stent Placement after Bilateral Lung Transplant

165

Sarah McDonald • Peter Slinger

Clinical Scenario: A 65-year-old woman status post double-lung transplant 5 years ago, presents with worsening shortness of breath secondary to bronchus intermedius stenosis in the allograft. Her postoperative course was complicated by bronchiolitis obliterans syndrome (BOS) for which she has been managed on prednisolone and azathioprine. Her pulmonary function tests show a decreased FEV_1 of 55%. She presents for rigid bronchoscopy and laser therapy with stent placement.

1 What are the anesthetic and airway management considerations for this case?

Overall survival rates in lung transplant recipients have improved over the years, based on a decline in the incidence of airway complications. However, bronchial stenosis remains the most frequent complication encountered. Other airway complications that may arise include granulation tissue formation, tracheobronchomalacia, and infectious complications, which may result in necrosis, dehiscence, or fistula formation. Complications arising post lung transplant will directly affect airway management, and overall lung function must be taken into account when devising an anesthetic plan. Other complications, not related to airway, may arise from long-term immunosuppression and include renal dysfunction, diabetes mellitus, as well as hypertension.

The native blood supply of the tracheobronchial tree consists of collaterals from the bronchial and pulmonary circulation that anastomose in the submucosal plexus. However, the bronchial circulation is not routinely reestablished in the donor lung after transplantation. Collateral revascularization by the recipient's bronchial arteries may take up to 4 weeks. In the interim, the bronchial anastomosis is solely dependent on perfusion from the poorly oxygenated pulmonary arterial circulation, resulting in an increased ischemic risk at the anastomotic site. Other perioperative factors, such as positive-pressure mechanical ventilation with the use of positive end-expiratory pressure, low cardiac output, primary graft dysfunction, infections, and use of immunosuppressive agents, may also have adverse effects on anastomotic healing. Common symptoms from bronchial stenosis include dyspnea, wheezing, recurrent chest infections, and abnormal pulmonary function tests.

Considerations for anesthetic and airway management must take into account that this is a shared airway case, and the proceduralists performing rigid bronchoscopy need full access to the airway and stable operative conditions. Adequate muscle relaxation is a necessity in order to ensure an immobile patient and minimize the risk of trauma associated with manipulation of the bronchoscope. Train-of-four monitoring and adequate reversal of neuromuscular blockade at the end of the case is essential for this highly vulnerable population. Airway topicalization while under anesthesia will assist with coughing once the patient is no longer anesthetized. A total intravenous anesthetic (TIVA) should be utilized for the maintenance phase of anesthesia as inhalational agents cannot be reliably delivered during rigid bronchoscopy.

In this particular patient, the presence of BOS must be taken into account as well. BOS is a manifestation of chronic rejection that results in lymphocytic infiltration of the airway submucosa, followed by epithelial cell necrosis and proliferation of granulation and stenotic scar tissue. The end result is airway lumen obliteration with a reduction in air passages. The International Society for Heart and Lung Transplantation proposed a clinical classification based on the severity of airflow obstruction as measured by the decrease in FEV_1 (that is not caused by other known and potentially reversible causes of posttransplant loss of lung function). The clinical presentation can be nonspecific and includes worsening exertional dyspnea and recurrent chest infections. In advanced disease, high-resolution CT scans may demonstrate air trapping due to obstructive bronchiolar inflammatory and fibrotic changes. Patients with severe disease will not tolerate long periods of apnea and optimal management during a shared airway procedure such as rigid bronchoscopy requires meticulous communication, planning, and execution.

2 How would you manage the airway in this case?

Prior to anesthesia induction, the proceduralist and anesthesiologist should have a comprehensive discussion regarding the surgical plan. Several ventilatory management strategies are possible and the plan may need to be adapted to patient tolerance. Intermittent apneic oxygenation may be utilized with the caveat being that these patients will not tolerate long apneic periods, likely resulting in frequent procedural interruptions. Another option is positive-pressure ventilation via the rigid bronchoscope. A standard anesthetic circuit can be connected to the side port of the rigid scope and high-flow oxygen is then used for ventilation. Ventilation is not particularly effective, especially if smaller-diameter bronchoscopes are used, due to large leaks and the inability to generate adequate ventilatory pressures. To decrease the leak, throat packs may be placed. A third option, which requires adequate time for expiration and careful monitoring, is jet ventilation.

Following induction, neuromuscular blockade should be administered after establishing adequate bag mask ventilation. To decrease the reactivity of the airway during insertion of the rigid bronchoscope, the airway should be topicalized with aerosolized lidocaine via direct laryngoscopy. If the proceduralist desires to assess the airway with flexible bronchoscopy, a supraglottic airway device (SGA) is used for ventilation. The anesthesiologist should remain vigilant to the possibility of SGA dislodgement or malposition caused by maneuvering of the fiberoptic scope. Circuit leaks will necessitate higher gas flows and an FiO_2 of 100% is used to minimize the incidence of desaturation (prior to initiation of laser treatment). If stent deployment is required during rigid bronchoscopy, jet ventilation will be most beneficial to minimize disruption of the procedure.

3 What are the potential hazards and complications in regard to the airway?

This patient has multiple risk factors for airway complications related to their underlying disease as well as the surgical procedure. The use of jet ventilation poses a risk for tension pneumothorax, specifically in a patient with potential for gas trapping and requiring a prolonged expiratory time. This complication should be suspected in the presence of subcutaneous emphysema or signs of hemodynamic instability. In cases where laser therapy is employed, there is a risk of endobronchial burns, hemorrhage, airway perforation, and hypoxemia. The risk of airway fire must be taken into account and the FiO_2 adjusted accordingly. An oxygen blender can be used to decrease the FiO_2 to 30% to 40%. However, due to this patient's intrinsic lung disease, a balance between the lowest FiO_2 the patient can tolerate and the risk of airway fire is required.

5 Are there special considerations for the emergence or the end of the case?

After positioning of the stent, an SGA device should be inserted while transitioning to spontaneous ventilation. Caution should be taken after the relief of chronic airway obstruction, as patients who have underlying recurrent chest infections or bronchiectasis have a risk of tracheobronchial tree contamination. Bleeding or sloughing of tissue after laser therapy further contributes to potential contamination. If jet ventilation was used, radiologic examination to rule out an occult pneumothorax is recommended. The anesthetist should be prepared for a potential period of postoperative ventilation should complications arise.

Corticosteroids should be administered, particularly in this patient who has chronic steroid exposure. Once the patient is awake and following commands, while generating adequate tidal volumes with a satisfactory respiratory rate, the SGA may be removed. A low threshold for the use of sugammadex should be employed in order to ensure adequate return of neuromuscular function. Once the SGA is removed, the patient can then be transitioned to a facemask with oxygen and observed in the operating room until the anesthetist is satisfied that they are fully awake and stable.

- Bronchial stenosis is the most common airway complication in patients post lung transplant and often requires procedural intervention.
- Familiarity with the use of jet ventilation and the associated risks allows for effective oxygenation with minimal interruptions to bronchoscopic procedures.
- Rigid bronchoscopy and stent placement in a patient with poor lung function is a demanding procedure, requiring flexible airway management skills, excellent preparation, as well as clear communication among all team members.
- *See Figure 165.1 and* **Video 165.1** *for additional details.*

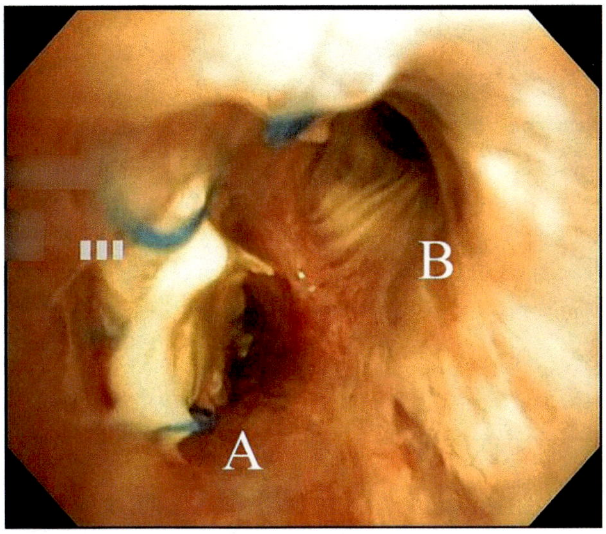

Figure 165.1. *A*, Suture lines are seen at the partially obstructed bronchus intermedias; *B*, entrance to the right upper lobe appears unobstructed.

Acknowledgment

We gratefully acknowledge the contributions of previous edition author, Su Lin Maureen Cheng, as portions of those chapters have been retained in this revision.

Suggested Readings

Consta J, Benvenuto LJ, Sonett JR. Long-term outcomes and management of lung transplant recipients. *Best Pract Res Clin Anaesthesiol.* 2017;31:285–297.

Finlayson GN, Shaipanich T, Durkin C. Bronchoscopic surgery. In: *Slinger P, ed. Principles and Practice of Anesthesia for Thoracic Surgery.* 2nd ed. Springer, 2019:197–217.

Meyer KC, Raghu G, Verleden GM, et al. An international ISHLT/ATS/ERS clinical practice guideline: diagnosis and management of bronchiolitis obliterans syndrome. *Eur Respir J.* 2014;44:1479–1503.

166 Airway Management Post–lung Transplant

Adriana Herrera

Clinical Scenario: A 45-year-old man presents to the OR for open abdominal surgery. He has scleroderma with CREST syndrome. He underwent bilateral lung transplant 2 years ago. His postoperative course was complicated by respiratory failure requiring tracheostomy and placement of a left bronchial stent. At the same time, he had a vocal cord paralysis, which was treated with vocal cord injection and speech therapy. He has since recovered well and the tracheostomy is currently healed.

1 What are the anesthetic and airway management considerations for this case?

Scleroderma is a collagen vascular autoimmune disease characterized by inflammation, vascular sclerosis, and fibrosis of the skin and internal organs (ie, lung fibrosis, etc.). Scleroderma patients have skin thickening with nonpitting edema, presenting with limited oral aperture, decreased jaw extension, limited mobility of the neck, and flexion contractures. Other important considerations include the presence of oral or nasal telangiectasias that increase the bleeding risk during intubation. Gastrointestinal problems include esophageal fibrosis and abnormal motility, dysphagia, and reflux, all of which increase the aspiration risk. The chronic steroid treatment and subsequent diabetes is associated with a higher incidence of an unanticipated difficult intubation due to the diabetes-related stiff joint syndrome at the atlanto-occipital level.

Due to pulmonary fibrosis, this patient had a bilateral lung transplant. Usually, an improvement of respiratory function, gas exchange, and exercise tolerance is seen, but the compromise of other organs remains. It is important to understand the surgical technique used for the double-lung transplant. This can be done as an "en bloc" technique that includes a tracheal anastomosis, or as bilateral sequential single lung transplants. The technique is important because the level of denervation is different. In the bilateral sequential lung transplant technique, the denervation occurs distal to the bronchial anastomosis, so the distal bronchi will not respond to stimulation, but the cough reflex at the carinal level will remain intact. The "en bloc" technique causes denervation at the level of the carina, resulting in loss of the cough reflex and increased risk of aspiration and infection. Airway tone, primarily mediated via parasympathetic efferent nerves on bronchial smooth muscle, is not affected by the denervation. The hypoxic pulmonary vasoconstriction reflex is usually not affected by the airway denervation. An exception occurs during a rejection episode where this response may be attenuated, leading to shunting of blood flow from healthy to pathologic areas of the transplanted lung.

Transplanted lungs are susceptible to fluid overload, since tracheal or main bronchi resection during harvesting interrupts the lymphatic drainage, increasing the risk of developing pulmonary edema with minimal fluid overload.

2 How would you manage the airway in this case?

Airway evaluation in this patient population is of critical importance. The history of a previous tracheostomy and of a difficult airway should be considered in the overall airway management plan.

Ventilation and tracheal intubation may be difficult. Orotracheal intubation is preferred, as there is an increased risk of severe nasal bleed due to telangiectasias. Antisialogogues are useful for drying secretions, especially if a flexible intubating scope (FIS) technique is chosen. These patients are at increased risk of pulmonary aspiration, which is a devastating complication after lung transplant. Semiupright position, preoperative use of antacids, H2 blockers, and metoclopramide are recommended measures to diminish this risk. If on physical examination, no concerns related to the airway examination arise, rapid sequence induction is an option. An awake FIS technique may be required if the patient has a tenuous airway with a very small oral aperture, limited jaw, and neck extension.

Airway stenting (with metallic mesh or silicone stents) is done frequently in patients post–lung transplant due to airway stenosis at either the tracheal or the bronchial level. Therefore, in lung transplant patients, tracheal intubation should be done under FIS guidance to avoid trauma to previous anastomosis (especially in an en bloc transplant technique) or stent migration. After intubation, a flexible bronchoscopic examination identifies endotracheal tube (ETT) and stent position, and evaluates the anastomosis. Bigger size ETTs facilitate suctioning of secretions and lower airway resistance.

3 What are the potential hazards and complications in regard to the airway?

Double-lung transplantation patients who do not have pulmonary complications do not require particular ventilatory precautions. Barotrauma and volutrauma are of concern in patients with reduced compliance, such as those with pulmonary infections, rejection, or obliterative bronchiolitis. These situations cause increased airway resistance with high peak and plateau pressures and pose a risk of respiratory failure and anastomosis dehiscence. Protective lung ventilation, consisting of small tidal volumes (4 to 6 cc/kg IBW), peak inspiratory pressures of 30 to 35 cm of H_2O, plateau pressures of 20 to 25 cm of H_2O, and positive end-expiratory pressure of 5 to 10 cm of H_2O, may be associated with a lower incidence of postoperative lung complications and less stress on suture lines. Pressure-controlled ventilation is preferred over volume control.

Different considerations apply for recipients of single-lung transplant, as they have different degrees of V/Q mismatch and different lung compliances.

The history of a previous tracheostomy is relevant as tracheal stenosis may be present. Placement of smaller ETTs may be necessary, thus impacting the ventilatory management with increased airway resistance and difficulty suctioning secretions.

4 Are there special considerations for the emergence or the end of the case?

These patients have a higher risk for respiratory infections. Early postoperative extubation is encouraged. Reversal of muscle relaxants is necessary, as minimal residual blockade may impair adequate respiratory function. In addition, as these patients have compromised airway reflexes, they should be awake and able to cough before extubation.

Adequate pain control allows better coughing, expectoration, and early mobilization, avoiding atelectasis and respiratory infections. The use of epidural analgesia (low-dose narcotic with local anesthetic) decreases the side effects of systemic opioids (somnolence, respiratory depression, decreased cough reflex). Acetaminophen, nonsteroidal anti-inflammatory drugs, and peripheral blocks can be considered.

Intensive care admission is necessary only if the respiratory function is inadequate.

- Patients with lung transplants with well-functioning grafts usually tolerate anesthesia uneventfully. If patients have infections, rejections, or obliterative bronchiolitis, the risk of postoperative respiratory failure increases significantly.
- In patients with post–lung transplant, the use of a FIS allows correct placement of the ETT, evaluation of suture lines, and stent position.
- In patients with single or complicated double-lung transplants, protective lung ventilation is recommended.
- *See Figure 166.1 and* ***Video 166.1*** *for additional details.*

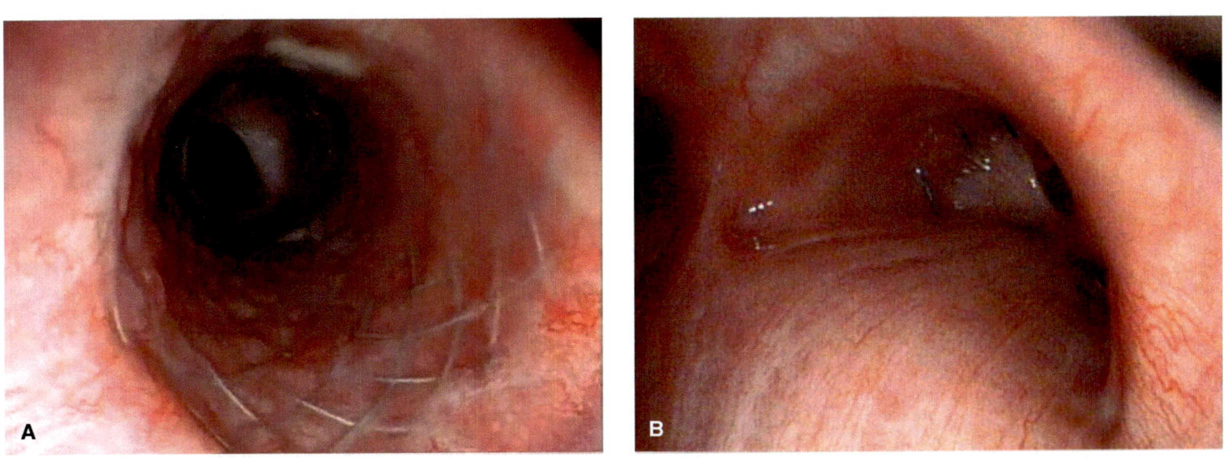

Figure 166.1. A: Left-sided mainstem bronchus is stented with a wire mesh device. **B:** The right-sided anastomosis of a transplanted lung is seen.

Suggested Readings

Dempsey ZS, Rowell S, McRobert R. The role of regional and neuroaxial anesthesia in patients with systemic sclerosis. *Local Reg Anesth*. 2011;4:47–56.

Feltracco P, Falasco G, Barbieri S, Milevoj M, Serra E, Ori C. Anesthetic considerations for nontransplant procedures in lung transplant patients. *J Clin Anesth*. 2011;23:508–516.

Machuzak M, Santacruz JF, Gildea T, Murthy SC. Airway complications after lung transplantation. *Thorac Surg Clin*. 2015; 25:55–75.

Roberts JG, Sabar R, Gianoli JA, Kaye AD. Progressive systemic sclerosis: clinical manifestations and anesthetic considerations. *J Clin Anesth*. 2002;14:474–477.

Massive Airway Bleeding During Transbronchial Biopsy

167

Gaetane C. Michaud

Clinical Scenario: A 75-year-old male with a left lower lobe mass presents for a flexible bronchoscopy with a transbronchial biopsy performed under moderate sedation. During the biopsy procedure a massive airway bleed occurs.

1 What are the anesthetic/airway management considerations for this case?

Transbronchial biopsy (TBBx) is one of the most common bronchoscopic procedures performed. Indications for TBBx include evaluation of endobronchial masses, solitary pulmonary nodules, bacterial or fungal infections, granulomatous disease, vasculitis, inflammatory lung conditions (rheumatoid, hypersensitivity pneumonitis), or surveillance of transplanted lung. Complications of TBBx are rare and include pneumothorax, hemoptysis, and infection. The procedure is typically performed in the outpatient setting using a flexible bronchoscope, with/without fluoroscopy, endobronchial ultrasound, electromagnetic navigation, or robotic bronchoscopy. The patient is typically given both local anesthesia and moderate sedation. In more complex navigational cases patients may require general anesthesia to minimize movement while patients are in the electromagnetic field. During the procedure, the patient is intubated with the bronchoscope and the scope is advanced to the site of the lesion using one of the aforementioned imaging modalities. A biopsy forceps is passed through a working channel within the bronchoscope to the lesion and a sample is taken for histologic analysis.

The risk of serious bleeding occurs in 1% to 2% of patients undergoing TBBx, although death is extremely rare. As removal of tissue is performed in a partially blinded manner, it is possible to inadvertently biopsy structures such as vessels or the chest wall. Patients with highly vascular tumors, including some lung cancers or metastases from renal cell carcinoma or melanoma, are at an increased risk of bleeding. Immunocompromised patients and patients with renal insufficiency are also at higher risk for bleeding complications during TBBx. In addition, patients with severe pulmonary hypertension are at high risk of bleeding during a TBBx. Considering the overlap between lung cancer, venothromboembolic disease, and coronary artery disease, many patients take anticoagulants and antiplatelet agents. These agents have varying half-lives and it is essential for the bronchoscopist and anesthesiologist to be aware of the necessary time to be off each drug in advance of the procedure to minimize bleeding risk. Careful preoperative evaluation by the bronchoscopist is essential to avoid such risk in the setting of suspected malignancy. In the case of a major airway bleed, the major concerns include maintenance of adequate oxygenation, ventilation, and hemodynamic stability. Many of these patients have limited cardiopulmonary reserve due to comorbid illness and thus hemodynamic compromise could be devastating. Previously undiagnosed coagulopathies can further impair the ability to achieve hemostasis. If the patient bleeds into the pleural space, there is potential for developing a hemopneumothorax. This may require immediate evacuation by tube thoracostomy, particularly in the setting of severe hemodynamic compromise.

2 How would you manage the airway in this case?

The initial control of the airway during an iatrogenic bleed is important as the bronchoscopist evaluates the location of the bleed, the options for management, or the necessity to pursue more invasive means to achieve hemostasis. Once the site of the bleed has been identified, the patient can be positioned in a lateral decubitus position with the shoulders and hips perpendicular to the floor and with the bleeding lung in the dependent position. This is accomplished to protect the noncompromised lung from becoming soiled and potential worsening gas exchange. Some very easy and rapid means to achieve hemostasis include wedging the bronchoscope within the bleeding airway, lavage with small aliquots of iced saline, topical use of vasoconstricting agents (1:20,000 epinephrine or vasopressin). If these methods fail, one should consider placing a hemostasis balloon catheter, such as a Fogerty catheter or a bronchial blocker. In the unlikely event that this maneuver also fails, the next step is to consider intubation. In a briskly bleeding airway, it is essential to have the most experienced person intubate the patient and adjuncts such as a glide scope or flexible bronchoscope (FB) may be used if immediately available. A single-lumen large bore endotracheal tube directed into the unaffected mainstem bronchus is the preferred modality to secure the airway. A double-lumen tube also allows for lung isolation, however it has the major disadvantage of having two small lumens. This small caliber of each lumen can render aspiration of blood and clot from the unaffected side quite difficult. Ventilation has to be optimized to avoid further hypoxia and hypercapnia. Once the airway is stabilized even temporarily, the cardiovascular compromise needs to be addressed. All potentially correctable coagulopathies need to be addressed. Volume resuscitation or blood products may be required in the setting of hypotension. Bronchoscopic evaluation of the airway, whether rigid or flexible, may be performed once it is thought that hemostasis has been achieved. If a flexible bronchoscopy is to be performed, a large-bore (therapeutic) bronchoscope should be used to allow for aspiration of clot. The endotracheal tube is slowly withdrawn into the trachea under direct visualization. The bronchial blocker is slowly deflated while monitoring for ongoing bleeding. If bleeding persists, the blocker is reinflated. Should a rigid bronchoscopy be performed, the rigid is advanced down beside the endotracheal tube and once at the level of the vocal cords, the cuff is deflated and the rigid scope passed through the vocal cords as the endotracheal tube is removed.

3 What distinct airway device (eg, specialized tracheal tube, rigid bronchoscope, bronchial blocker) might be used in this case, and what are the special considerations?

A bronchial blocker may be helpful in the setting of a significant airway bleed. Some of the concerns with its use include the need to insert it using a bronchoscope. The Arndt bronchial blocker can be employed in this setting. A loop on the end of the catheter is used to guide the catheter into place. The loop is placed over the tip of the flexible bronchoscope in a sort of "piggy-back" fashion. Alternatively, a pair of forceps advanced through the working channel and guided with the bronchoscope may hold it.

4 Are there special considerations for the emergence or the end of the case?

Suppression of cough is a significant postoperative consideration in patients with massive hemoptysis. Cough can increase the likelihood of a rebleed and dislodge a tamponade balloon or endotracheal tube. In these cases, monitoring patients for adequate sedation is important during transfer and in the postoperative period. It is very important to note that bronchial blockers may only remain in place for 24 to 48 hours and should be placed as distally as possible to maintain hemostasis while minimizing the occlusion of functional airways proximal to the site of bleeding. In addition, it is very important to keep patients with bronchial blockers in situ intubated, sedated, and calm to avoid accidental displacement.

- TBBx is one of the most common bronchoscopic procedures performed and the risk of massive hemoptysis is 1% to 2%.
- The initial management of patients with massive hemoptysis includes optimizing positioning, attempting to use local therapies to achieve hemostasis, and then considering selective intubation or a bronchial blocker.
- Massive hemoptysis can often be managed bronchoscopically through the use of tamponade balloons and vasoconstricting agents.
- Postoperative sedation and cough suppression are essential to achieve and maintain hemostasis.
- *See Figure 167.1 and* ***Video 167.1*** *for additional details.*

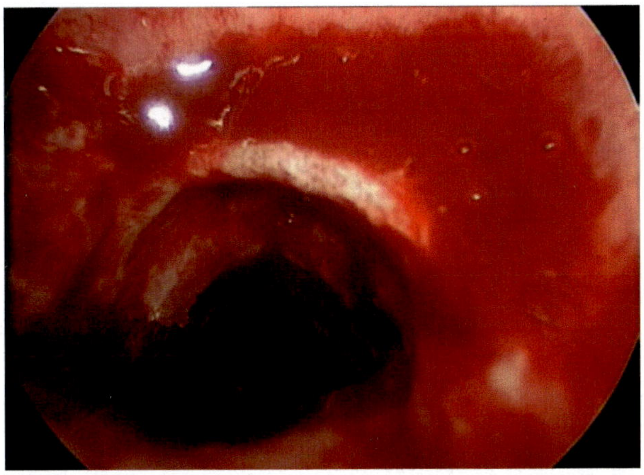

Figure 167.1. Blood contamination of the airway is seen during flexible scope inspection of the airway. In this patient, bleeding from the contralateral lung has been isolated with a bronchial blocker.

Suggested Readings

Davidson K, Shojaee S. Managing massive hemoptysis. *Chest.* 2020;157:77–88.
Semmelman A, Loop T. Anesthesia for interventional pulmonology. *Curr Opin Anesthesiol.* 2022;35:82–882.

168 Chest Trauma

Shamsuddin Akhtar

Clinical Scenario: An 18-year-old man with a gunshot to the right chest presents emergently to the OR for a right thoracotomy for exploration and possible lung resection. The patient is agitated and combative. He is coughing blood. The surgeon informs you that OLV is required during the case.

1 What are the anesthetic and airway management considerations for this case?

This is a noncooperative patient with a tenuous airway and potential injury to lung parenchyma, proximal airways (trachea and bronchi), esophagus, major blood vessels, and the heart. Clear communication with the surgical team is very important to determine the exact location and type of injury they are expecting. Coughing blood should not be assumed to be originating solely from the tracheobronchial tree. Upper airway, oral, or laryngeal trauma may present as hemoptysis. Subcutaneous emphysema in the neck may represent injury to the cervical trachea. Patients with distal tracheal or bronchial lesions may present with a very large pneumothorax rather than subcutaneous emphysema. In the presence of tracheal or bronchial injuries, the lung may not expand completely, even after successful placement of thoracostomy tube. Hemoptysis can also occur due to significant parenchymal lung contusion. Hemoptysis and hemothorax are frequently present if major vessels are injured. Hemoptysis warrants a bronchoscopy to rule out tracheal or bronchial injury. This can be performed in the OR, once the airway is secured. In this case, a right thoracotomy is planned, which suggests unilateral thoracic or mediastinal injury.

Typically, the first question anesthesiologists will address is whether to keep the patient spontaneously breathing or not. In a cooperative patient who is not coughing blood, inhalational induction with spontaneous ventilation maintained until the airway is secured and evaluated is a fine option. However, this plan is unlikely to be successful in this patient as he is agitated and combative. Although lung isolation may be desirable, in an acute trauma situation, securing the airway and ventilation are of prime importance. The surgeon should be prepared to do an emergency tracheostomy. After placement of an endotracheal tube (ETT), bronchoscopy is conducted to rule out other injuries. If tracheal injury is expected, ETT should ideally be placed under bronchoscopic guidance. Further surgical and anesthetic management will be based on the cardiorespiratory status of the patient and the site and extent of the injuries identified.

2 How would you manage the airway in this case?

A clear, coordinated plan and ongoing communication with the surgical team is essential. All airway management equipment should be ready and confirmed to be functional. In this patient, who is combative, has chest trauma, and coughing blood, airway management can be particularly challenging. The patient can be induced with ketamine or sedated with dexmedetomidine if spontaneous ventilation is desired. Placement of an ETT can be achieved via direct laryngoscopy, flexible bronchoscope (FB), video laryngoscopy, or tracheostomy. Significant blood in the airway and tracheobronchial tree may make the FB techniques more challenging. If the airway can be visualized with a FB, then this technique is ideal, as it allows positioning of the ETT under vision.

After the airway is secured, a thorough bronchoscopy is performed. Blood is cleared from the airway and tracheal and bronchial injuries are assessed. To inspect the cervical and mediastinal trachea during bronchoscopy, the ETT may have to be pulled into the larynx.

Once the integrity of the airway has been confirmed, a BB can be placed to achieve lung isolation. Other options include placing a long endobronchial tube or advancing the ETT in the mainstem bronchus.

Though some institutions place double-lumen tubes (DLT) in emergency situations, most experts recommend placing an ETT. DLTs are large, can be difficult to position, and are potentially harmful when airway integrity is questionable. In this patient, who requires bronchoscopy, placement of a DLT will require removal of the single-lumen ETT after bronchoscopy and reintubation. Such intervention should be performed after thorough assessment and thoughtful communication.

If tracheal and/or proximal bronchial injuries require repair, the anesthesiologist should be prepared for intermittent periods of apnea, as surgeons withdraw the distal ETT for better exposure. Increased oxygen concentration (>70%) is used to prevent or delay desaturation. Periods of moderate hypercapnia are inevitable but are usually well tolerated. The anesthesia team should also be ready for cross-field intubation and ventilation. Sterile ETT or endobronchial tubes should be available to be placed by the surgeon. Alternatively, the ETT balloon can be temporarily deflated, decreasing the chances of puncturing it during suturing. The use of stents in a traumatic airway is considered on case-by-case basis.

Ideally, ventilation should provide adequate oxygenation with low mean airway pressures. Small tidal volumes and pressure-control ventilation are possible options. In rare cases, high-frequency jet ventilation or other specialized modes of ventilation may be required. In severe parenchymal injury, patients develop decreased lung compliance and are difficult to ventilate. Veno-venous extracorporeal membrane oxygenation to oxygenate the patient may be required.

3 What are the surgical considerations that impact anesthetic management?

Surgical incision and positioning are dictated by the type and location of injury. There are four basic types of surgical incisions that can be used to explore the chest: anterolateral, posterolateral, bilateral anterior thoracotomies, and median sternotomy. The anterolateral approach is rapid and can be quickly extended to expose the contralateral lung and anterior mediastinum. The distal half of the trachea, right mainstem bronchus, and left mainstem bronchus are best approached through a right posterolateral thoracotomy.

Significant injury to the lung parenchyma or the hilum may necessitate a lobectomy or even a pneumonectomy. Emergency pneumonectomy can lead to an acute and significant increase in pulmonary pressures with subsequent right heart failure.

Less than 20% of patients who present with chest trauma will require video-assisted thoracoscopic surgery (VATS). Significant thoracic hemorrhage, pulmonary trauma, and major injuries to the mediastinal structures will most likely be managed by open thoracotomies. VATS is used to manage peripheral lung injuries, ligation of intercostal arteries, rib fracture reduction, or evacuation of hemothorax or empyema.

As airway and lung injuries lead to significant leakage of oxygen in the operative field, the anesthesiologist should consider the risk of fire. Cooperation with the surgeon cannot be overemphasized.

4 Are there special considerations for the emergence or the end of the case?

With the exception of complex repairs, early extubation is desirable. If the lower airway was injured and required repair, the ETT cuff and positive-pressure ventilation produce trauma to the freshly placed sutures, predisposing to dehiscence. However, the decision to extubate is based on the type and location of the injury and the performed surgery. Isolated tracheal injuries can be easily extubated at the end of the procedure. If the patient cannot be extubated after the tracheal repair, then the ETT should be placed distal to the repair and potentially sutured, to prevent accidental movement.

- The patient presenting with chest trauma and hemoptysis requires bronchoscopy for full evaluation of lower airway integrity.
- The airway is usually secured with an ETT or a tracheostomy.
- DLTs are large, difficult to position, and are potentially harmful when airway integrity is questionable.
- Except in complex repairs, early extubation is desirable.
- *See Figures 168.1 and 168.2 for additional details.*

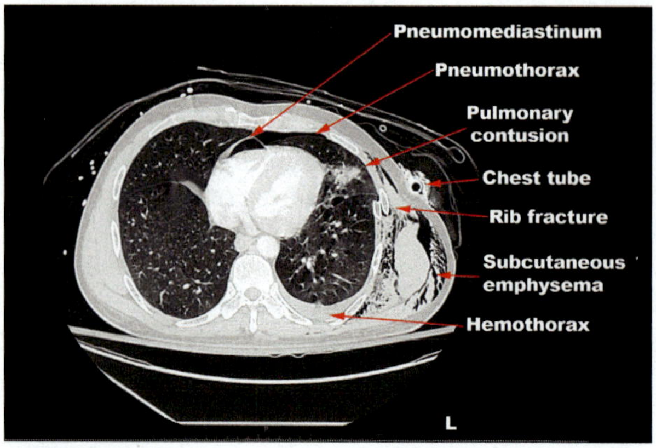

Figure 168.1. CT scan following chest trauma. Labels the multiple indicated injuries seen in this patient. See **Video 168.1** and **Video 168.2**.

Suggested Readings

Dubose JA, O'Connor JV, Scalea TM. Lung, trachea and esophagus. In: Mattox TL, Moore EE, Feliciano DV, eds. *Trauma*. 8th ed. McGraw Hill Medical; 2017:479–492.

Fagenholz P, Velmahos G. Surgical treatment of thoracic trauma: lung. In: Di Saverio S, Tugnoli G, Catena F, et al., eds. *Trauma Surgery, Thoracic and Abdominal Trauma*. Vol 2. Springer; 2014:77–90.

McRae K. Tracheal resection and reconstruction. In: Slinger P, ed. *Principles and Practice of Anesthesia for Thoracic Surgery*. Springer; 2011:181–195.

Rosengart M, Karmy-Jones R. Urgent thoracotomy. In: Karmy-Jones R, Nathens A, Stern EJ, eds. *Thoracic Trauma and Critical Care*. Springer; 2002:63–68.

Airway Management for Potential Tracheal Rupture

169

Jagtar Singh Heir

Clinical Scenario: A 54-year-old man is transferred from an outside hospital to your emergency department with worsening respiratory distress. His medical history includes a large right tonsillar cancer that resulted in right vocal cord paralysis. He received chemotherapy and recently had pneumonia and an asthma exacerbation treated with antibiotics and bronchodilators. Subsequent to his pneumonia, he had intense bouts of productive cough. The family informs you that there is a possible suspicion of a tracheal tear. You are asked to emergently intubate this gentleman for respiratory failure.

1 What are the anesthetic and airway management considerations for this case?

Tracheal disruptions are fortunately rare but can be potentially life threatening. They can occur spontaneously via forceful coughing or vomiting, be secondary to blunt or penetrating trauma, or be iatrogenically induced due to traumatic intubation or associated with certain types of surgery. Patient-related risk factors for tracheal injury can include female sex, short stature, tracheomalacia, tracheal stenosis, and chronic steroid use. Non–patient-related risk factors can include emergent intubation, multiple attempts at intubation, inappropriately large-sized endotracheal tubes (ETTs), positioning of the ETT, use of rigid ETT introducers, cuff overinflation, movement of the head or neck while the patient is intubated, and head/neck/thoracic surgery itself. The American Society of Anesthesiologists' airway disruption algorithm is an excellent resource that can help guide the management of these patients. A key point emphasized within the algorithm is to maintain spontaneous ventilation, particularly until the level and extent of the tear has been determined by chest radiography, CT, and/or fiberoptic bronchoscopy (FOB). During positive-pressure ventilation (PPV), peak airway pressures should be maintained below 25 cm H_2O to avoid further worsening of the injury. After the extent of injury has been determined, the algorithm suggests placing the ETT beyond the tear to avoid increasing the risk for worsening pneumomediastinum and/or subcutaneous emphysema.

2 How would you manage the airway in this case?

Albeit there are multiple approaches that can be utilized to manage this type of airway, transferring this patient to the OR prior to instrumenting the airway increases safety. For example, if all airway interventions are unsuccessful or inadequate, then a surgical airway would be needed, which would be more readily accomplished in the OR environment.

Similarly, in patients with large disruptions in whom the airway cannot be secured, oxygenation and ventilation may require initiation of extracorporeal membrane oxygenation (ECMO). Therefore, examination of the airway should ideally begin in the OR.

If the patient is cooperative and stable, an awake flexible bronchoscope (FB) approach at evaluating and securing the airway, while maintaining spontaneous ventilation, can be utilized. Alternatively, a mask induction technique, with or without a laryngeal mask airway (LMA), while maintaining spontaneous respiration, can also be used. If the patient is uncooperative, a rapid sequence intubation using a combined video laryngoscopy/FB approach can be used to thoroughly evaluate and secure the airway. To prevent desaturation during intubation, the patient should be adequately preoxygenated and apneic oxygenation using high-flow nasal cannula can be used. In either approach, the ETT should be advanced distal to the injury making sure the cuff is inflated past the distal portion of the tear. If the tear involves either bronchus and lung isolation is necessary, a double-lumen tube or a bronchial blocker should be employed. Consideration should be given to the possibility of worsening the tear due to inadequate topicalization/sedation during an awake approach or excessive use of force with laryngoscopy. Therefore, in a patient with tracheal injury, attempts to blindly advance the ETT are contraindicated. In this particular patient, FB examination revealed a large circumferential defect in both the membranous and cartilaginous trachea, extending from about 2 cm below the vocal cords to approximately 4 cm into the left mainstem bronchus. Given the magnitude of the defect and bronchial involvement requiring lung isolation, consideration was given to advancing a small-sized single-lumen ETT to the right mainstem bronchus or using a small-sized right-sided double-lumen tube. A 6.0-mm single lumen was ultimately chosen because it would minimize the chances of further worsening airway injury. However, it should be kept in mind that insertion of either type of tube could lead to the creation of a false passage, potentially leading to acute worsening of oxygenation and ventilation.

3 What are the surgical considerations that impact anesthetic management?

The fact that the surgeon and anesthesiologist share the airway requires dynamic communication and coordination. The importance of meticulous planning of airway management preoperatively cannot be overemphasized, as it would ensure maximal patient safety.

Diagnostic evaluation can include a chest x-ray and CT. However, the preferred modality is FB, as it will define the tear in terms of length, depth, and location, thus helping to determine surgical versus conservative management. Despite lack of universally accepted guidelines, lesions measuring less than 2 cm can potentially be managed conservatively with administration of empiric antibiotics and steroids to prevent infection and decrease inflammation, respectively. Conversely, larger lesions will require a surgical approach, in which case, an intraoperative FB examination is indispensable in facilitating surgery. Furthermore, lesions that need to be excised and require primary reanastomosis, particularly those involving carinal reconstruction, may warrant cross-field ventilation. Cross-field ventilation involves the surgeon inserting a sterile ETT directly into the intact bronchus, which is used to temporarily ventilate the patient while the tracheobronchial defect is being repaired. Additionally, if appropriate, airway stents may sometimes be deployed by the surgeon or interventional pulmonologist. Occasionally, disruptions may be so large that both the central trachea and the mainstem bronchi have disruptions, necessitating ECMO support during repair.

4 What are the potential hazards and complications in regard to the airway?

Care must be taken to avoid excessive PPV until the location of the lesion is determined. PPV via mask ventilation, LMA, ETT, or jet ventilation above the lesion can worsen pneumomediastinum and subcutaneous emphysema, potentially leading to a tension pneumothorax. As volatile anesthetics leak via the defect, a total intravenous anesthetic is preferred.

5 What distinct airway device (eg, specialized tracheal tube, rigid bronchoscope, bronchial blocker) might be used in this case, and what are the special considerations?

The FB is the preferred airway tool to characterize the extent and location of the defect. This evaluation subsequently helps determine the most appropriate type of airway device to be used. In this particular case, due to the nature of the defect, lung isolation was necessary. Therefore, a small-sized single-lumen tube was advanced into the right mainstem bronchus to secure the airway under FB guidance, thus avoiding inadvertent worsening of the airway defect. This also allowed surgical access to the left mainstem and central trachea for repair. Furthermore, care was taken to position the tube in a manner that allowed ventilation of the right upper lobe. Regardless of which airway device is ultimately chosen, it is imperative that the provider have comfort and experience in using it.

6 Are there special considerations for the emergence or the end of the case?

Depending on the location and repair of the tracheal defect, consideration must be given to extubating the patient as soon as possible after surgical repair. Prolonged intubation can cause mucosal ischemia due to endotracheal cuff pressure. Moreover, prolonged PPV promotes dehiscence of the repair. A deep extubation may be a viable strategy, as it would avoid coughing and bucking on the ETT. However, consideration must be given to the patient's respiratory status and degree of difficulty in initially securing the airway. Another FB examination can help assess the presence of edema, secretions, airway stenosis, as well as vocal cord function. This FB examination can be more readily facilitated with the placement of an LMA either before or after extubation. Since postoperative pain, as well as opioid overuse, can impact recovery, a multimodal analgesic approach is recommended to help optimize postoperative respiratory function.

- Maintaining spontaneous ventilation is crucial, as PPV above the tear can worsen the injury, exacerbating pneumomediastinum or subcutaneous emphysema.
- Performing a diagnostic FB examination determines the extent and location of the tear.
- If an ETT is used, placing it beyond the level of the tracheal tear under FB guidance is recommended.
- Surgical airway capability should be available; consider ECMO support for major tears.
- *See Figure 169.1 and* ⓥ ***Video 169.1*** *for additional details.*

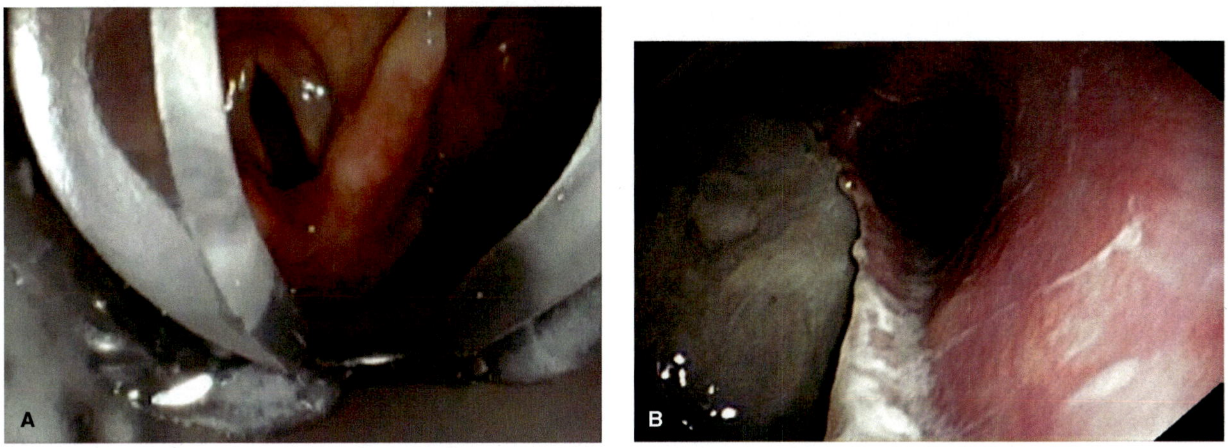

Figure 169.1. **A:** The patient was initially managed with an LMA and spontaneous ventilation so that a flexible bronchoscope could be used to examine the ruptured trachea. **B:** The segment of ruptured trachea is reexamined and includes both membranous and cartilaginous portions.

Suggested Readings

Hagberg CA, Kaslow O. Difficult Airway Management Algorithm in Trauma Updated by COTEP. *ASA Newsletter.* 2014;78:56–60.

Jain U, McCunn M, Smith CE, Pittet JF. Management of the traumatized airway. *Anesthesiology.* 2016;124(1):199–206.

Khan SA, Ekeoduru RA, Tariq S. Traumatic tracheobronchial laceration causing complete tracheal resection: challenges of anesthetic management. *A A Pract.* 2018;11(4):109–111.

Menard C, Pierce S, deTar TR. Difficult airway management in trauma: a review of current guidelines. *Emerg Med Pract.* 2025;27:1–40.

Wei P, Yan D, Huang J, et al. Anesthetic management of tracheal laceration from traumatic dislocation of the first rib: a case report and literature of the review. *BMC Anesthesiol.* 2019;19:149.

PART C COVID-19

SECTION I AIRWAY CONSIDERATIONS IN COVID-19

170 Airway Management in the COVID-19 Patient

Felipe Urdaneta

Clinical Scenario: A 65-year-old female with multiple chronic comorbidities presents in respiratory distress secondary to an active COVID-19 infection. She has failed a trial of bi-level positive airway pressure (BiPAP) ventilation. You have been called to the ICU to intubate this patient.

1 What are the anesthetic and airway management considerations for this case?

A pulmonary infection from Coronavirus SARS-CoV-2 often results in severe hypoxemia requiring airway management intervention. These interventions are usually carried out on an emergent basis on critically ill patients that may have coexisting medical issues such as airway edema, acute respiratory distress syndrome (ARDS), acute kidney injury, myocardial dysfunction, and coagulation abnormalities. These patients may have failed non-invasive positive pressure ventilation or oxygenation (NIPPO/HFNO). They are vulnerable to potential hemodynamic and ventilatory instability, putting them at higher risk of suffering cardiac arrest during or after airway instrumentation.

The SARS-CoV-2 virus is spread via aerosolization, so any airway instrumentation procedures place health care workers (HCWs) at risk for viral exposure. Appropriate personal protective equipment (PPE) use and standardized PPE protocols reduce the incidence of exposure and contamination during airway instrumentation. However, the use of PPE leads to decreased physical mobility of HCWs and diminished communication between team members, which may lengthen the time needed to secure the airway. Other barriers such as airway boxes and plastic cover shields are not recommended. These barriers may increase the difficulty of intubation and are associated with higher failure rates and prolonged intubation times.

2 How would you manage the airway in this case?

The intubation and extubation of patients with COVID-19 pulmonary infections will be discussed in this chapter. Other techniques such as the use of supraglottic airways (SGAs) as primary or conduit for intubation, the use of flexible intubating scope (FIS), and front of neck access (FONA) are described elsewhere in this book.

The general recommendations for intubation in these scenarios are:

1. Optimize patient positioning for airway management.
2. Use disposable airway equipment whenever possible.
3. The most experienced airway provider should perform the procedure.
4. Limit additional personnel to decrease potential viral spread.
5. When possible, preoxygenate with a 100% FiO_2 using a sealed facemask with a high efficiency particulate air (HEPA) filter. Preoxygenate to a target end tidal O_2 of 90% if possible (when a gas analyzer is available). HFNO/NIPPV may be considered as alternative techniques for preoxygenation. If hypoxemic, perform bag-mask ventilation with a well-sealed facemask. If bag-mask ventilation is ineffective or there is a leak, a SGA is an alternative to facilitate ventilation and preoxygenation.
6. Perform rapid sequence induction and intubation using a video laryngoscope as the first-choice tool. A conventional laryngoscope should be immediately available as a backup tool.

7. Once the endotracheal tube is through the cords to the appropriate depth, the cuff should be inflated before connecting the breathing circuit. Capnography is the recommended method for confirmation of endotracheal tube placement.
8. Dirty airway equipment should be placed into a double zip-locked plastic bag for subsequent disposal or decontamination.

3 What are the potential hazards and complications in regard to airway management?

Airway management techniques (including tracheal intubation or extubation, bag-mask ventilation, noninvasive ventilation, administration of high-flow oxygen or nebulized medications, tracheotomy, open suctioning of airways, bronchoscopy, and interventional pulmonology procedures) are aerosol-generating procedures. A key aspect of successful airway management in these patients is planning and preparation. Airway Management bundles have been developed for patients with active COVID-19 infections. These bundles consist of both technical and nontechnical aspects of patient care.

Only necessary equipment and personnel should be present in the airway procedure area to prevent unnecessary viral contamination. Backup and emergency equipment should be kept immediately outside the procedure area and brought in as required by an assistant wearing appropriate PPE. Airway management teams should include a limited number of highly skilled and experienced providers. There should be a predetermined airway management plan, and there should be an immediately available standard supply of medications and airway equipment, including endotracheal tubes (ETT), intubating SGAs, laryngoscopy equipment (VL and DL), FIS, and a kit for invasive FONA. When feasible, these devices should be single-use to limit the amount of cross-contamination after the procedure.

4 Are there special considerations for emergence?

Extubation of patients with an active COVID-19 infection carries a comparable risk of viral aerosolization as intubation. Similar precautions to prevent contamination and exposure should be followed. Only essential personnel should be in the procedure room for reasons described above. Consider the need for nausea and vomiting prophylaxis as retching can produce significant aerosolization. Similarly, coughing will produce significant aerosol particles, so a cough suppressant should be considered if appropriate. Immediately following extubation, it is recommended to cover the patient's face with a surgical mask.

- Airway management of patients with COVID-19 involves conflicting concerns of minimizing HCWs' risk, maximizing first-attempt success, and maintaining patient safety.
- Some airway procedures and practices typically recommended for patients with a difficult airway are not ideal for patients with COVID-19 infections due to the potential increase in the aerosolization of viral particles.
- A tailored, stepwise approach is recommended by experienced and skilled teams that can safely manage airway procedures before, during, and post-crisis.

Suggested Readings

Cook TM. Personal protective equipment during the coronavirus disease (COVID) 2019 pandemic—a narrative review. *Anaesthesia*. 2020;75(7):920–927.

Foley LJ, Urdaneta F, Berkow L, et al. Difficult airway management in adult coronavirus disease 2019 patients: statement by the Society of Airway Management. *Anesth Analg*. 2021;133(4):876–890.

Nauka PC, Chen JT, Shiloh AL, Eisen LA, Fein DG. Practice, outcomes, and complications of emergent endotracheal intubation by critical care practitioners during the COVID-19 pandemic. *Chest*. 2021;160(6):2112–2122.

Schumacher J, Arlidge J, Dudley D, Sicinski M, Ahmad I. The impact of respiratory protective equipment on difficult airway management: a randomised, crossover, simulation study. *Anaesthesia*. 2020;75(10):1301–1306.

Wong DJN, El-Boghdadly K, Owen R, et al. Emergency airway management in patients with COVID-19: a prospective international multicenter cohort study. *Anesthesiology*. 2021;135(2):292–303.

171 Difficult Airway Management in the Patient with COVID-19

Christian R. Tilley • Robert White

Clinical Scenario: A patient hospitalized for a COVID-19 infection requires urgent intubation for worsening respiratory failure. He has a history of prior difficult intubation.

1 What are the anesthetic/airway management considerations for this case?

The airway management of this patient poses several major concerns. This patient with a known difficult airway is experiencing worsening respiratory failure due to COVID-19 pneumonia. Management of a difficult airway often takes advanced planning and time, which may not be possible in this scenario. Prior anesthetic records and a thorough clinical airway exam should be reviewed in patients with a documented difficult airway. However, given the urgent/emergent need for tracheal intubation in a rapidly decompensating patient, this may not be feasible. In this case, the most skilled and practiced clinician should manage the airway in this rapidly decompensating patient with COVID-19.

An additional concern is the significant risk of COVID-19 viral exposure to involved medical personnel due to increased aerosolization of the virus during airway management procedures. While the practice of personal protective equipment (PPE) varies globally, the clinician should wear at minimum a fit-tested N95 respirator, eye protection, fluid-resistant full body gown, and gloves. Donning and doffing procedures should be followed per institution protocol, with a second individual verifying the correct procedures.

2 How would you manage the airway in this case?

In this patient with COVID-19–induced respiratory failure, the decision to secure the airway via tracheal intubation should be made rapidly, and the intubation should be performed by the most experienced airway clinician. After obtaining a second assistant and properly donning PPE (assuming that all airway equipment and medications are available), the application of 100% FiO_2 should be implemented for at least 5 minutes if timing allows. Preoxygenation can be performed via non-rebreather face mask (NRBF), high-flow nasal cannula (HFNC), or bag mask. Patient positioning should be optimized prior to induction. During induction, avoid the use of depolarizing neuromuscular blocking agents (succinylcholine), which cause fasciculations, which can promote further viral aerosolization. Finally, the technique of intubation is important to consider, given the rapid desaturation times and existing hypoxemia in most patients with respiratory failure due to COVID-19. Retrospective studies have shown that modified rapid sequence intubation (RSI) with mask ventilation prior, in combination with video laryngoscopy, achieved the highest first-pass and overall intubation success rates. Video laryngoscopy should be utilized on the initial attempt when available, and a supraglottic airway device should be available in the event of a failed attempt. Especially in a patient with a known difficult airway, an emergency tracheostomy kit and an appropriate specialist should be available as backup. Following intubation, the intubating provider(s) should appropriately doff PPE to avoid self-contamination and perform hand-hygiene per institutional protocol.

3 What are the potential hazards/complications in regard to the airway?

For reasons described above, critically ill patients with COVID-19 have a significant risk of experiencing peri-intubation complications. They have likely already failed noninvasive positive pressure oxygenation. They are also more likely to become hemodynamically unstable during induction of anesthesia and risk experiencing cardiovascular collapse with postintubation positive-pressure ventilation.

The airway in a patient with COVID-19 may be edematous and more prone to bleeding with manipulation. Distorted airway anatomy in a patient experiencing worsening hypoxemia usually makes video laryngoscopy the most appropriate choice for initial intubation attempt. However, video laryngoscopy may be difficult in the case of bleeding in the airway or copious dried oral secretions.

Preoxygenation of a patient with COVID-19–induced respiratory failure is essential prior to intubation attempts. While preoxygenation increases apneic time, it leads to viral aerosolization and increases exposure risk to the health care team. If possible, utilizing an appropriately sized, tightly fitting face mask attached to a high-efficiency particulate absorbing (HEPA) filter can provide optimal preoxygenation while also minimizing viral exposure to staff. Noninvasive positive pressure ventilation or HFNC can also be used. Despite preoxygenation, apneic time will likely be reduced in a patient with COVID-19 pneumonia.

4 Are there special considerations for the emergence or the end of the case?

Patients with COVID-19 should meet all standard extubation criteria. Studies have shown that viral aerosolization occurs more during extubation than during intubation. The reversal of paralytic agent and the initiation of spontaneous ventilation can yield coughing and forceful expiration, which are both highly aerosolizing. These patients notably may have reactive airways secondary to their infection and are at higher risk for laryngospasm and bronchospasm. Creating a tailored extubation plan will be critical to safely extubate while also minimizing viral exposure to staff. It is also important to note that significant changes in airway anatomy may have occurred in patients who have been intubated for prolonged periods.

- Patients with respiratory failure due to COVID-19 have challenging airways and will have significantly shorter apneic times, so conditions should be optimized to increase the chance of first-pass intubation success.
- Airway management procedures are highly aerosolizing, posing a high risk of viral exposure to health care personnel. Adequate PPE should be worn at all times during the airway management of the patient with COVID-19.
- Extubation is highly aerosolizing, so appropriate planning should occur to ensure a smooth and safe extubation.

Suggested Readings

Foley LJ, Urdaneta F, Berkow L, et al. Difficult airway management in adult coronavirus disease 2019 patients: statement by the Society of Airway Management. *Anesth Analg*. 2021;133(3):876–890.

Wenlong Y, Tingting W, Bailin J, et al. Emergency tracheal intubation in 202 patients with COVID-19 in Wuhan, China: lessons learnt and international expert recommendations. *Br J Anaesth*. 2020;125(1):e28–e37.

Wong DT, Dallaire A, Singh KP, et al. High-flow nasal oxygen improves safe apnea time in morbidly obese patients undergoing general anesthesia: a randomized controlled trial. *Anesth Analg*. 2019;129:1130–1136.

172 Thoracic Surgery in Patients with COVID-19

Radu Stoica • Mert Senturk

Clinical Scenario: A 43-year-old man with an active COVID-19 infection presents to the OR for a video-assisted thoracoscopic surgery (VATS) bullectomy. He has a history of chronic obstructive pulmonary disease (COPD) and is currently in the intensive care unit, spontaneously breathing with high-flow nasal oxygen (HFNO) support. Bullectomy is now indicated due to worsening hypoxemia and persistent pneumothorax.

1 What are the anesthetic and airway management considerations for this case?

This case presents multiple challenges to the anesthesiologist. A VATS bullectomy requires one-lung ventilation (OLV) to provide optimal surgical conditions. Adequate oxygenation can be problematic during OLV in certain patients. During OLV, hypoxemia can ensue due to an increased intrapulmonary shunt and/or ventilation-perfusion mismatch, especially in this patient with preexisting COPD.

The other major challenge in this patient presenting for lung surgery, will be his active COVID-19 respiratory infection. The most common and most fatal clinical presentation of a COVID-19 infection is hypoxemia. "High-flow nasal oxygen" (HFNO) therapy has helped to decrease the need for mechanical ventilatory support in some patients with COVID-19 infections, but many patients still require an invasive approach to assure adequate oxygenation. Multiple phenotypes of COVID-19 infections that vary in clinical severity have been described to date, so it is difficult to predict which patients will require mechanical ventilatory support. In addition, the COVID-19 infection should be regarded as a multiorgan infection. The anesthesiologist should be on high alert of the possibility of multiorgan complications ensuing in COVID-19 patients presenting for surgery during the active infection phase.

Another notable challenge in this case will be minimizing the risk of COVID-19 exposure to all staff involved in the care of this patient during his surgery. Lung surgery presents a higher risk of aerosolization and potential transmission of respiratory infections during bronchoscopy and due to an open airway during OLV. Appropriate personal protective equipment (PPE), including respiratory protection with properly fitted respirators, will be crucial in this case to minimize provider exposure to the virus. This procedure should be performed in a negative-pressure OR, if available, to further minimize risk of virus transmission in other ORs.

An active COVID-19 infection and preexisting COPD compound the risk of hypoxemia during OLV in this patient. Ventilator settings and oxygen delivery should be tailored with regard to oxygenation requirements and airway pressures. Lobar isolation using a bronchial blocker (BB) (rather than a complete lung collapse) may be necessary to help alleviate hypoxemia in these patients. If refractory hypoxemia is anticipated during OLV in these patients, preemptive initiation of extracorporeal support can also be considered.

2 How would you manage the airway in this case?

The patient should be maintained on the current HFNO for preoxygenation if feasible. After ensuring all staff in the OR have appropriate PPE, the patient's airway should be secured as quickly as possible to minimize aerosolization. Rapid sequence induction is appropriate to avoid mask ventilation. Video laryngoscopy (VL) is the preferred method to secure the airway in patients with COVID-19 infections because its use is associated with a higher first attempt success rate. In addition, a VL device with a remote screen is preferred to help increase the physical distance between the anesthesiologist and the patient's airway.

The choice of airway device to achieve OLV should be driven by provider proficiency, device availability, and patient characteristics. In this case, a double lumen tube (DLT) or an single lumen tube (SLT) with a BB are equally appropriate choices as they both provide "functional sealing" of the operative lung. A more cumbersome and less preferred method would be initial placement of an SLT followed by exchange to a DLT using an airway exchange catheter (AEC). If a lobar blockade is planned, a BB is the sole option for isolation. If the plan is to continue mechanical ventilation during the postoperative period, then the use of a single endotracheal tube with a BB is preferred.

After the airway is secured, there are additional precautions that can be taken to minimize viral exposure, such as the use of a connector with a valve for placing the flexible bronchoscope (FB). If a DLT is used, separate viral filters can be placed on each lumen. In addition, in order to minimize viral contamination of the environment, the ventilator should be placed in standby mode during any disconnections of the anesthesia circuit.

3 What are the potential hazards and complications in regard to the airway?

Generally, it is well known that DLTs are associated with a higher risk of laryngeal and airway injury compared to SLTs. The risk can be even higher when the airway needs to be secured quickly, as in this case. The use of VL is recommended, as mentioned above, to increase the chance of first attempt success.

For proper and safe placement of both DLTs and BBs, the use of flexible bronchoscopy is inevitably necessary even in a patient with an active COVID-19 infection. Bronchoscopy is undoubtedly a highly aerosolizing procedure, so appropriate PPE should be worn at all times during this procedure.

4 Are there special considerations for the emergence or the end of the case?

This patient will likely require postoperative mechanical ventilation support with a need for ICU care. If a DLT was used for OLV, it should be exchanged to an SLT at the end of the operation. This procedure is more challenging than exchanging an SLT and should be performed with a specialized AEC designed for use with DLTs if available (see Chapter 139: Double-Lumen Tube to Single-Lumen Tube Exchange). If extubation is planned at the end of the procedure, coughing should be prevented as much as possible to minimize viral transmission.

- Patients with an active or recent COVID-19 infection presenting for thoracic surgery are at an increased risk for intraoperative hypoxemia and need for postoperative ventilation.
- COVID-19 viral exposure with possible transmission is a known risk during intubation, bronchoscopy, and lung collapse; therefore, proper PPE should be worn at all times by all OR personnel.
- Optimal airway management includes securing the airway as quickly as possible to minimize aerosolization and placing viral filters at the connection between the endotracheal tube and the ventilator.
- These patients are at high risk for requiring continued postoperative mechanical ventilation and ICU care.

Suggested Readings

COVID Surg Collaborative. Elective surgery cancellations due to the COVID-19 pandemic: global predictive modelling to inform surgical recovery plans. *Br J Surg*. 2020;107(11):1440–1449.

Fraser R, Steven M, McCall P, Shelley B. Anesthetic management for thoracic surgery during the COVID-19 pandemic. *Curr Anesthesiol Rep*. 2021;11(4):405–413.

Şentürk M, El Tahan MR, Shelley B, et al. Thoracic anesthesia during the COVID-19 pandemic: 2021 Updated recommendations by the European Association of Cardiothoracic Anaesthesiology and Intensive Care (EACTAIC) Thoracic Subspecialty Committee. *J Cardiothorac Vasc Anesth*. 2021;35(12):3528–3546.

Thornton M, Reid D, Shelley B, Steven M. Management of the airway and lung isolation for thoracic surgery during the COVID-19 pandemic: a reply. *Anaesthesia*. 2020;75(11):1548–1549.

173 Awake Intubation in Patients with COVID-19

Rita Asuquo

Clinical Scenario: A 62-year-old male presents to the emergency room in acute respiratory failure. He recently presented to an urgent care center for a cough and was prescribed antibiotics. Chest radiograph is significant for bilateral infiltrates, and PCR is positive for COVID-19. His oxygen saturation is declining despite oxygen supplementation using a nonrebreather mask, and intubation is becoming urgent. During your airway evaluation, you learn that the patient has a history of laryngeal cancer treated with a chemoradiation protocol. There are cutaneous radiation changes over the larynx, and the patient has a limited neck range of motion and modest trismus.

1 What are the anesthetic and airway management considerations for this case?

COVID-19, a virus initially discovered and characterized in 2019, caused a pandemic killing millions of people worldwide. Patients infected with COVID-19 present with a broad spectrum of symptoms ranging from asymptomatic to respiratory failure. Physiologic changes may occur to the airway and lungs due to COVID-19. Some presentations include pharyngeal or tracheal edema, decreased functional residual capacity, atelectasis, and pneumonia or pneumonitis. These patients also commonly present with other comorbidities that may impact airway management—cardiovascular disease, diabetes, increased BMI, limited neck range of motion, etc.

Awake intubation is indicated if evaluation of the patient reveals risk of a challenging intubation and at least one of the following risks: (1) difficult mask ventilation, (2) gastric contents aspiration, and/or (3) rapid oxyhemoglobin desaturation. Patients with active COVID-19 infections who require awake intubations pose unique challenges to the anesthesiologist. Cautious and thoughtful management of a difficult airway may take more time, potentially increasing the risk of viral exposure and transmission to health care staff. These considerations must be taken into account when developing an airway management plan for these patients.

2 How would you manage the airway in this case?

An awake tracheal intubation (AI) requires patient cooperation. An AI may be stressful to the patient, especially in the setting of respiratory distress due to a COVID-19 infection. Explaining the rationale and process of AI to the patient is the best approach as this usually establishes trust. The patient should be walked through each step of the AI. He or she should be warned about what they might hear during the process such as monitors, suctioning, conversation, etc. In addition, the patient should be told what to expect physically during the intubation—fullness in mouth or airway, lightheadedness, coughing, etc. Last, emphasis should be placed on needing the patient's cooperation while assuring them that the main priority is their safety.

To "prepare" the airway, we most commonly consider two things: managing secretions and anesthetizing the mucosa. These preparatory steps are paramount in COVID-19 patients. To decrease airway secretions, an antisialagogue will often be administered preoperatively. In most facilities, atropine and glycopyrrolate are readily available. Most commonly, glycopyrrolate is chosen due its mild risk of causing tachycardia or CNS effects. To render the mucosa anesthetized and suppress gagging, multiple routes of local anesthetics are available. Lidocaine can be given as a nebulized aerosol in the preoperative setting, applied as a viscous jelly, or applied into the airway during the procedure. Patients suffering from COVID-19 can present with edematous mucosal tissue that is sensitive secondary to excessive coughing, irritation, etc. Thus, anesthetizing the airway to suppress an already irritable and inflamed airway is important.

Most providers will opt for a flexible intubation scope technique when performing AI. Prior to proceeding, the functionality of all equipment should be checked, and the flexible intubation scope should be preloaded with a lubricated endotracheal tube. Depending on the provider's preferences, (1) suction or (2) oxygen to physically displace secretions and aid in extending safe apnea time, may be applied through the working channels of the scope.

Other intubation modalities are available, such as direct laryngoscopy or indirect laryngoscopy using videoscopes or optical stylets. When choosing a flexible intubation scope, the scope size should match the patient population—adult, adult small, or pediatric scope. A guiding principle when choosing equipment is which size of tracheal tube will be used. The tube size is based on the size of the patient and the clinical situation. For example, a patient who is expected to remain intubated for a prolonged period in the ICU setting and requires vigorous pulmonary toileting will require a larger endotracheal tube internal diameter. If a flexible intubation scope is to be used for the AI, a scope that best matches the internal diameter of the chosen tracheal tube should be sought. Assess the respiratory status of the patient and associated comorbidities—if they are being intubated secondary to impending respiratory failure, then it is reasonable to use a larger tube if you anticipate mechanical ventilation for a longer period.

3 What are the potential hazards and complications in regard to the airway?

Oxygenation during the AI procedure is aimed at prolonging the safe apneic period in the event of airway failure. Patients with respiratory failure due to COVID-19 can desaturate rapidly during apneic periods despite preoxygenation. Studies have shown that High Flow Nasal Cannula can successfully oxygenate a patient without increasing aerosolization and contamination of surrounding areas. However, all personnel should still be wearing protective masks and eyewear to minimize this risk.

For sedation, most providers will use either infusions or intermittent boluses of sedatives to help with patient cooperation and anxiety. For induction, some have opted for intermittent boluses of low-dose remifentanil, a dexmedetomidine bolus followed by infusion, or intermittent propofol boluses. Dexmedetomidine is the only modality of these options that does not cause apnea. The goal of sedation is to suppress the cough reflex and increase patient cooperation and comfort (swallowing on command, suppressing cough, radical movements, etc.).

Personal protective equipment (PPE) should be worn to protect the providers involved with the intubation. At minimum, protective eyewear, a face shield, and an N95 mask or powered air-purifying respirator should be worn. Patient coughing during awake intubations may cause more viral aerosolization. All providers performing and/or assisting in the intubation and any nearby personnel should wear appropriate PPE. Most importantly, donning and doffing the PPE should be done properly to minimize contamination. Personnel in proximity to the patient should be minimized as much as possible.

It goes without saying that performing an awake intubation requires skill and concentration. The plan to perform an awake intubation should be discussed with all present personnel to ensure a calm environment. This includes alerting other staff of the potential risks and complications related to the procedure, as well. It is always beneficial to have more than one anesthesia provider that is familiar with the airway equipment being used. As always, extra personnel should be readily available in case of an airway emergency.

- The presence of an active COVID-19 respiratory infection should not prevent an awake intubation if indicated based on patient comorbidities.
- Appropriate PPE should be worn by all staff involved in the intubation of patients with COVID-19.
- Proper airway preparation and thoughtful sedation can help to minimize viral aerosolization through minimizing patient coughing, etc.

Suggested Readings

Fuchs A, Lanzi D, Beilstein CM, et al. Clinical recommendations for in-hospital airway management during aerosol-transmitting procedures in the setting of a viral pandemic. *Best Pract Res Clin Anaesthesiol.* 2021;35(3):333–349.

Kiss E, Garcia-Marcinkiewicz A, Zhong J, et al. Management of the normal and difficult pediatric airway: unique challenges in the time of COVID-19. *Curr Surg Rep.* 2023;11(6):144–153.

Yadav P, Garg R. The barrier techniques for airway management in COVID-19 patients—review of literature. *J Anaesthesiol Clin Pharmacol.* 2021;37(2):171–178.

174 Intraoperative Management of Subglottic Stenosis in Post COVID-19 Patients

Lauren C. Williams • Jaime B. Hyman

Clinical Scenario: A 60-year-old previously healthy woman has recovered from COVID-19 but has increasing shortness of breath with minimal exercise. She is evaluated with a CT scan, which shows subglottic narrowing thought to be secondary to her tracheal intubation when hospitalized for COVID-19. She is currently scheduled for a direct laryngoscopy with CO_2 laser incision and balloon dilation of subglottic stenosis.

1 How would you manage the airway in this case?

There are several options for airway management in this patient, ranging from endotracheal intubation to more advanced techniques. When subglottic dilation is planned, the endotracheal tube typically must be removed from the operative field. Intermittent apnea is commonly employed in these situations where the endotracheal tube is intermittently removed and the patient remains apneic for a short period of time while dilation or other airway instrumentation is performed. Once the patient's SpO_2 begins to decrease, the procedure is paused, the endotracheal tube is reinserted, and ventilation is maintained until the SpO_2 increases.

Alternatives to intermittent apnea include advanced airway management techniques such as high-frequency jet ventilation and apneic oxygenation with high-flow nasal cannula, also called transnasal humidified rapid-insufflation ventilatory exchange (THRIVE). Jet ventilation can be subglottic, supraglottic, or transtracheal. Subglottic jet ventilation involves placement of a small-caliber tube to deliver a narrow, high-pressure jet of gas into the trachea, which is then passively exhaled. Supraglottic jet ventilation utilizes a side port on the operative laryngoscope. Transtracheal jet ventilation involves transcutaneous insertion of a small catheter through the cricothyroid membrane into the airway. THRIVE is an apneic oxygenation technique using high-flow nasal cannula to deliver up to 100% oxygen at a rate of up to 70 L/min. The use of THRIVE during microlaryngeal surgery is a relatively novel technique which was first reported in 2015. The use of high-flow nasal cannula in this manner can prolong apneic time, and some patients may even maintain SpO_2 throughout the duration of the case. However, if the SpO_2 decreases, a transition to alternative methods of airway management, including intubation or jet ventilation, is always a possibility.

2 What are the anesthetic/airway management considerations for this case?

The patient's airway anatomy, degree of stenosis, and underlying comorbidities should factor into the decision for which airway management technique to use. The normal inner diameter of the trachea ranges from 10 to 21 mm in females and 15 to 25 mm in males. Assuming this patient has an average airway diameter of 15 mm, if she were to have 70% stenosis, for example, her subglottis would have a diameter of 5 to 6 mm. In this scenario, even a size 4 microlaryngeal endotracheal tube, with an outer diameter of 5.6 mm, may not be small enough to pass into the airway.

In addition to the patient's airway pathology, there are other comorbidities that play a role in determining the optimal strategy for intraoperative airway management. Attention should be given to cardiopulmonary comorbidities, as patients with poor cardiac or pulmonary reserve may not tolerate respiratory acidosis during periods of apnea. Patients with lung disease or obesity may have shorter apneic periods and may not receive adequate gas exchange with high-frequency jet ventilation. Communication between the anesthesiologist and surgeon is essential in these instances. In patients with a history of COVID-19–related respiratory failure, there should be a higher level of suspicion for underlying restrictive lung disease as well as poor pulmonary reserve.

3 What are the surgical considerations that impact anesthetic management?

The level of airway stenosis often dictates surgical and airway management planning. Patients with subglottic stenosis, as in this patient, typically undergo balloon dilation procedures, which are often combined with laser incision of subglottic scarring. Open oxygen sources cannot be in use while lasers are being used due to risk of airway fire, so THRIVE would not be an appropriate strategy to use during periods when the laser is in use. In addition, with jet ventilation, it is important to note that exhalation is passive, necessitating a path for gas egress at all times. This means that for balloon dilations, jet ventilation must be paused when the balloon is inflated, as the inflated balloon would prevent gas egress, and severe barotrauma could result. If the airway is managed with intermittent apnea and the endotracheal tube is left in place during the laser portions of the procedure, a laser-resistant endotracheal tube must be used. Last, a team-based approach with discussion between the anesthesiologist and surgeon should always be used when determining an airway management plan for patients with airway stenoses. Differences in institutional practices and anesthesiologist/surgeon experience are important factors in designing a successful plan for management of the difficult airway.

4 I decided to use subglottic jet ventilation, but my patient's SpO_2 is beginning to drop after several minutes. What should I do?

There are several reasons why a patient may not tolerate jet ventilation. In this patient's case, as mentioned earlier, previous severe COVID-19 infection may have led to long-term pulmonary sequelae such as fibrosis, bronchiectasis, or air trapping. These factors may impair gas exchange with jet ventilation. If this occurs, tracheal intubation with intermittent apnea can be used as a rescue method. One problem that the anesthesiologist may encounter when attempting intermittent apnea is that, as mentioned earlier, the subglottis may be too narrow to pass an endotracheal tube through. If the jet catheter is removed and a microlaryngeal endotracheal tube cannot fit past the region of stenosis, balloon dilation can be attempted, which may then allow tracheal intubation. Alternatively, the patient may require mask ventilation for a period of time to achieve adequate oxygenation. Of note, intermittent facemask ventilation requires removal and reinsertion of the laryngoscope each time, which can become cumbersome, particularly in suspension laryngoscopy procedures.

If the patient does not tolerate jet ventilation and cannot be intubated with an endotracheal tube, another option to consider is a supraglottic airway (SGA). This will require adaptation of the surgical plan, however, as direct laryngoscopy cannot be performed with an SGA in place. Instead, a flexible bronchoscope can be inserted through the SGA adapter to visualize the airway. A laser fiber and/or balloon catheter can then be passed through the working channel on the flexible bronchoscope to perform incisions and/or balloon dilations of the region of stenosis. A final option to consider is using high-flow nasal cannula as an adjunctive measure during direct laryngoscopy if the patient's SpO_2 drops quickly after removing the endotracheal tube. This can help prolong apneic times and allow the surgeon more time to work before the patient requires reintubation.

5 What are the potential hazards/complications in regard to the airway?

In this scenario, there are several complications that can arise related to this patient's airway. Although unlikely, the most feared complication is complete loss of the airway. The patient's airway is already significantly narrowed, and further trauma to the subglottis could lead to edema or bleeding, which could cause the airway to become completely obstructed, warranting an emergency surgical airway. It is important to be very gentle with intubation, especially if using a subglottic jet catheter which has a somewhat pointed distal end, to minimize trauma to the airway. Barotrauma-related complications are also important to be aware of, particularly when using jet ventilation. These include pneumothorax, pneumomediastinum, and subcutaneous emphysema. Tracheobronchitis can occur if jet ventilation is employed for prolonged periods without heating and humidifying gases. Finally, there is risk of airway fire whenever lasers are used during surgery. Constant communication between the surgeon and anesthesiologist is essential to ensure that oxygen concentration is below 30% prior to laser use.

6 Are there special considerations for the emergence or the end of the case?

After successful dilation of the subglottis, there are several options for airway management during emergence. The original tracheal tube or one with a slight larger diameter can be placed. Alternatively, an SGA can be placed or mask ventilation can be used until the patient resumes spontaneous ventilation. Regardless of the method chosen, vigilance should be maintained to evaluate for blood or secretions in the airway, bronchospasm, and laryngospasm, and these should be promptly managed if they occur. Analgesia and postoperative nausea and vomiting prevention are also essential for a smooth postoperative course.

- In a patient with subglottic stenosis, options for airway management include intermittent apnea, high-frequency jet ventilation, and THRIVE.
- Patients with long-term pulmonary sequelae from severe COVID-19 infection may be less likely to tolerate jet ventilation, as residual lung pathology may impair gas exchange.
- It is essential to have backup airway management plans in place in the event that the initial airway management strategy fails.
- Complications of airway management in patients with subglottic stenosis include loss of airway, pneumothorax, pneumomediastinum, tracheal injury, or airway fire.
- *See Figure 174.1 and* ***Video 174.1*** *for additional details.*

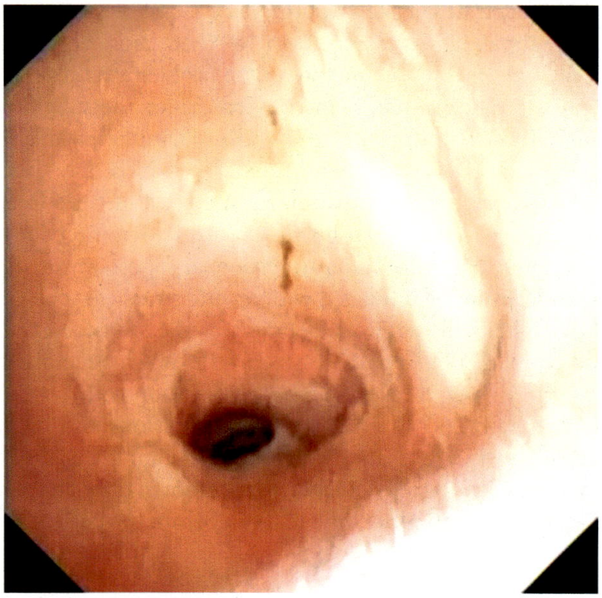

Figure 174.1. Severe subglottic stenosis in a patient intubated during a COVID-19 infection.

Suggested Readings

Chan KC, Yang TX, Khu KF, So CV. High-flow nasal cannula versus conventional ventilation in laryngeal surgery: a systematic review and meta-analysis. *Cureus*. 2023;15(5):e38611.

Kanne JP, Little BP, Schulte JJ, Haramati A, Haramati LB. Long-term lung abnormalities associated with COVID-19 pneumonia. *Radiology*. 2023;306(2):e221806.

Mangahas AM, Talugula S, Husain IA. Anesthesia considerations during management of airway stenosis: a systematic review. *Am J Otolaryngol*. 2022;44(2):103767.

Reed AP, Woo P. Phonomicrosurgery and office-based laryngology. In: Levine AI, DeMaria S Jr, Schwartz A, eds. *Anesthesiology and Otolaryngology*. Springer Science + Business Media; 2013:147–171.

To K, Harding F, Scott M, et al. The use of transnasal humidified rapid-insufflation ventilatory exchange in 17 cases of subglottic stenosis. *Clin Otolaryngol*. 2017;42(6):1407–1410.

Airway Management Consideration in Patients with Lower Airway Sequelae from COVID-19

175

Grace F. Donzelli • Hisashi Tsukada • Gyorgy Frendl

Clinical Scenario: A 60-year-old woman with a history of recent severe COVID-19 pneumonia requiring 13-day intubation, presents with respiratory distress and stridor. In the 3 months following her COVID-19 infection, the patient had experienced increasing dyspnea on exertion, worse for 3 days prior to admission. CT scan revealed narrowing of the proximal trachea measuring 6 mm × 9 mm in diameter (Figure 175.1). She is currently scheduled for a rigid bronchoscopy with dilation and possible stenting.

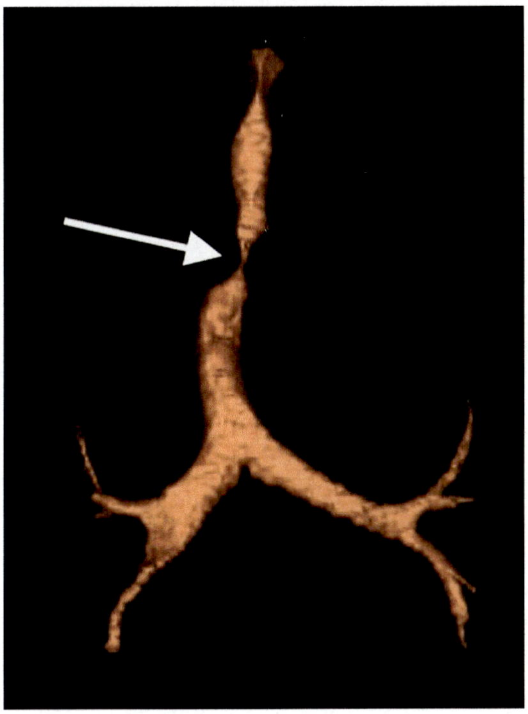

Figure 175.1. 3D CT reconstruction of post-COVID tracheal stenosis.

1 What are the anesthetic/airway management considerations for this case?

The COVID-19 pandemic created an unprecedented worldwide need for prolonged mechanical ventilation for the treatment of ARDS, often combined with prone positioning. As a result, patients not uncommonly present with late airway sequelae of COVID-19, especially tracheal stenosis, an epidemic reminiscent of the post-polio tracheal stenosis of the 20th century. Patients with post-COVID-19 tracheal stenosis typically present 1 to 3 months after the initial COVID-19 infection. Presentation ranges from subtle, with mild respiratory symptoms easily mistaken for the recovery phase of the illness, to acute respiratory distress that requires emergent intervention. Even with mild symptoms, patients can have significant narrowing (70% to 90%) of the tracheal lumen, and some patients may be asymptomatic. This poses a challenge for their airway management due to an inability to pass a normal-sized endotracheal tube, a scenario which requires specialized management. In the worst-case scenario, this challenge may be unanticipated.

When available, preoperative CT scan can help determine the size of the largest endotracheal tube that can safely pass a tracheal lesion, as well as the location of the stenosis. Total intravenous anesthesia with short-acting agents is also customary for these cases with surgical airway manipulation.

2 How would you manage the airway in this case?

To effectively treat the patient's tracheal stenosis, the surgical team will need to be able to visualize and maneuver instruments in the subglottic trachea. Anesthesia may be induced intravenously and the patient mask ventilated. A rigid bronchoscope is then inserted into the airway, and patient is jet ventilated via the side port of the rigid bronchoscope. The tracheal stenosis is visualized under bronchoscopic guidance (Figure 175.2). The stenosis is mechanically dilated with the barrel of the rigid bronchoscope, with the help of balloon dilators, and, occasionally, with the use of cryogenic or laser-based treatment of the scar. Then an hourglass-shaped silicone stent is often placed across the lesion to maintain airway patency (Figure 175.3). At the conclusion of the procedure, the rigid bronchoscope is removed. The airway must now be resecured until emergence, which can be done with the insertion of a supraglottic airway device.

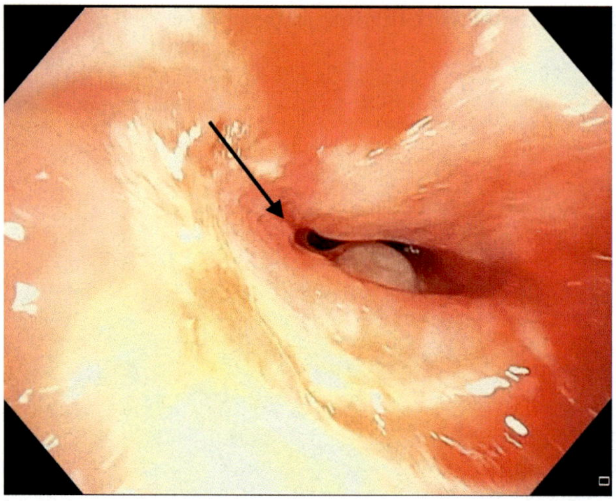

Figure 175.2. High-grade tracheal stenosis visualized with rigid bronchoscopy prior to treatment.

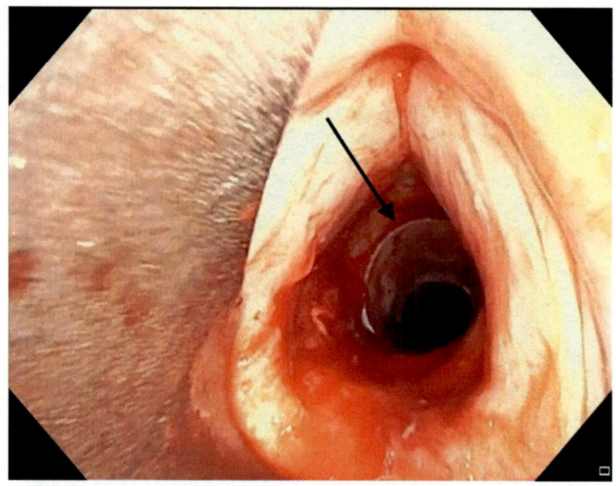

Figure 175.3. Tracheal stenosis after dilation and placement of a silicone stent.

If the patient requires evaluation of the lower airway after treatment of the stenosis, an endotracheal is used to secure the airway. If needed, for one-lung ventilation (OLV) for these patients, a bronchial blocker is the preferred method. This avoids the risk of traumatizing the narrowed airway with a large-diameter double-lumen endotracheal tube. However, patients with a history of severe COVID-19 pneumonia may not tolerate OLV due to subsequent pulmonary fibrosis. These patients have poor lung compliance and impaired gas exchange.

3 What are the potential hazards/complications in regard to the airway?

When using a manual jet ventilator, it is possible to inadvertently administer dangerously high airway pressures and create a tension pneumothorax. For jet ventilation, an egress to the jet must be available, hence, jet ventilation is safer once the airway stenosis is dilated. The pressure gauge should be adjusted to the minimum pressure necessary to achieve bilateral chest expansion. Furthermore, the operator should allow adequate time for chest recoil between breaths. Use of an automated jet ventilator can somewhat mitigate this risk.

There is a risk for airway fire when using jet ventilation combined with laser therapy, as 100% inspired oxygen is typically delivered. Closed-loop communication regarding the start and end of periods of apnea is of paramount importance in facilitating treatment of surgical stenosis while mitigating risks and maintaining sufficient oxygenation.

Despite its name, jet ventilation does not allow for significant exchange of carbon dioxide (ventilation). It may not be suitable for patients who cannot tolerate hypercarbia, such as those with pulmonary hypertension and impaired right ventricular function.

4 What are the surgical considerations that impact anesthetic management?

The various modalities of bronchoscopic treatment of tracheal stenosis have direct implications for anesthetic management. Mechanical dilation with the barrel of the rigid bronchoscope, or balloon dilatation via flexible bronchoscopy, requires different airway management and ventilation strategies. Cryoablation, laser ablation, and local steroid injection may be used. For any modality, periods of apnea may be necessary to facilitate intervention. When using jet ventilation and laser in the airway, periods of apnea are important to prevent airway fire.

Stenting can be performed to bypass long lesions in the trachea. However, if the stent migrates, it can cause complete obstruction of the airway. If this occurs intraoperatively, emergency airway management should include urgent rigid bronchoscopy for the removal of the malpositioned stent or bypassing tracheostomy if the stenosis is proximal. For distal lesions, emergency extracorporeal membrane oxygenation may be necessary.

- The COVID-19 pandemic will likely lead to an increase in patients with tracheal stenosis.
- Anesthesiologists should maintain a high index of suspicion for tracheal stenosis in patients with a history of severe COVID-19 infection requiring prolonged intubation or tracheostomy.
- Emergency airway management should include consideration of mask ventilation, small-bore endotracheal tubes, jet ventilation, and tracheostomy.
- *See* ◎ ***Video 175.1*** *for additional details.*

Suggested Readings

Adeloye D, Elneima O, Daines L, et al; International COVID-19 Airways Diseases Group. The long-term sequelae of COVID-19: an international consensus on research priorities for patients with pre-existing and new-onset airways disease. *Lancet Respir Med.* 2021;9:1467–1478.

Brichet A, Verkindre C, Dupont J, et al. Multidisciplinary approach to management of postintubation tracheal stenoses. *Eur Respir J.* 1999;13:888–893.

Grillo HC, Donahue DM, Mathisen DJ, Wain JC, Wright CD. Postintubation tracheal stenosis. Treatment and results. *J Thorac Cardiovasc Surg.* 1995;109:486–493; discussion 492–493.

Piazza C, Filauro M, Dikkers FG, et al. Long-term intubation and high rate of tracheostomy in COVID-19 patients might determine an unprecedented increase of airway stenoses: a call to action from the European Laryngological Society. *Eur Arch Otorhinolaryngol.* 2021;278:1–7.

Zias N, Chroneou A, Tabba MK, et al. Post tracheostomy and post intubation tracheal stenosis: report of 31 cases and review of the literature. *BMC Pulm Med.* 2008;8:18.

176 Transcutaneous CO_2 Monitoring

William H. Rosenblatt

1 Describe in detail the device or technique.

Transcutaneous CO_2 monitoring ($TcCO_2m$) is a noninvasive method of measuring the partial pressure of CO_2 at the skin surface, providing an approximation of the arterial partial pressure of CO_2. This method can monitor ventilation status in situations where traditional end-tidal CO_2 measurements are not feasible.

Transcutaneous CO_2 monitors were first introduced in 1958 with the Severinghaus electrode. This electrode consisted of a thin membrane of Teflon (commonly silicon polymer today) through which carbon dioxide diffuses into an aqueous, bicarbonate solution. Changes in the pH of the aqueous solution allow for calculation of the pCO_2 (cutaneous CO_2). $TcCO_2m$ devices have been widely used in neonatal ICU care since the 1970s. With the expansion of apneic anesthetic techniques, these monitors have become more popular in the operating room and perioperative care.

Variations in temperature can cause discrepancies in $TcCO_2$ monitoring, so modern versions of this monitor warm the skin around the measurement area. This warming mechanism helps minimize temperature as a variable in the calculations. The real-time measurement provided is corrected to a temperature of 37 °C. It also functionally "arterializes" the capillaries, resulting in a more stable local metabolism, improved gas diffusion, and reproducible readings.

The $TcCO_2m$ is a free-standing monitor that is similar in size to a standard, portable pulse oximeter. The $TcCO_2m$ electrode is fastened to the patient's skin (preferably on the cheek, deltoid, or the skin above the clavicle). After a calibration period lasting around 5 to 10 minutes, $TcCO_2$, SpO_2, and pulse rate are displayed on the monitor. Due to the calibration period, it is important to place and initiate the transcutaneous monitor before airway management is attempted. In the operating room, this requires the clinician to place the probe as soon as the patient is placed on the procedure table.

2 Where or when is this device or technique used in airway management?

The detection and measurement of end-tidal CO_2 is a standard monitor utilized during nearly all forms of airway management, including both natural and instrumented airway techniques. The American Society of Anesthesiologists recommends continuous end-tidal CO_2 monitoring availability in all encounters for airway management.

More recently, apneic techniques of airway management have been introduced into clinical practice. In apneic techniques, end-tidal CO_2 cannot be accurately measured using the traditional method. An example of an apneic technique is Transnasal Humidified Rapid-Insufflation Exchange (THRIVE), which was introduced in 2015 as a means of maintaining both oxyhemoglobin saturation and providing CO_2 ventilation in the muscle-relaxed, apneic patient via high-flow nasal cannula. This technique relies on monitoring of patient blood gases, as hypercapnia from inefficient THRIVE ventilation or intermittently "held" ventilation can result in patient compromise. In this scenario, $TcCO_2$ monitoring provides a minimally invasive option. In studies of patients who were apneic for up to 15 minutes and subsequently intubated, $TcCO_2$ m was found to correlate well with end-tidal CO_2 measurements. $TcCO_2m$ provides a trend of arterial CO_2 measurements, but precise estimates of P_aCO_2 may not be possible.

THRIVE is commonly applied for airway management during procedures involving the larynx. Its application improves operating conditions for the surgeon by eliminating the obstruction of a tracheal tube and minimizing movement of the airway with respiration. By making prolonged periods of apnea possible, THRIVE can also reduce motion artifact for certain fluoroscopically guided procedures. In these scenarios, the advantages of apnea must be weighed against the inability to measure end-tidal CO_2.

$TcCO_2m$ could also be applied in the critical care setting. In cases of hypercarbic respiratory failure in which the patient is not intubated, trends from transcutaneous monitoring could be used along with clinical data to adjust bi-level positive airway pressure settings or as a predictor for the need for intubation. For patients receiving extended extracorporeal membrane oxygenation support, transcutaneous monitoring could help reduce the need for arterial blood gas sampling from the system, potentially reducing infection risk. It is important to note, however, that $TcCO_2m$ measurements may be inaccurate in patients with higher BMI's.

3 What distinguishes this device or technique from similar airway management methods?

The current gold standard of carbon dioxide measurement is arterial blood gas sampling. Although arterial blood gas sampling offers the most precise measurement of P_aCO_2, it is an invasive technique that requires frequent, costly sampling to produce actionable data. Transcutaneous monitoring, however, allows for continuous monitoring of pCO_2 with a decreased risk of operator error or harm to the patient.

Another commonly used mechanism of carbon dioxide measurement is the end-tidal CO_2. Although end-tidal CO_2 and transcutaneous monitoring both offer continuous monitoring, end-tidal CO_2 requires a closed ventilatory system to provide measurements. For airway management techniques that do not involve a closed circuit, such as the application of nonrebreather masks or nasal cannula, $TcCO_2m$ provides a quantitative measure of ventilatory status. Furthermore, as apneic airway techniques continue to grow in popularity, $TcCO_2m$ may become more widely utilized.

End-tidal CO_2 has traditionally been used to monitor airway patency and ventilation. During natural or apneic airway management techniques, continuous breath-to-breath end-tidal CO_2 waveform measurements may not be reliable or accurate, favoring the use of an alternative method such as transcutaneous CO_2 measurement. Although transcutaneous measurements do not directly assess airway patency, trending these values can alert the clinician to interruptions in airway patency and changes to carbon dioxide removal.

Author Caveats

There is a need for future product development as current systems do not reliably reflect arterial gas readings at higher values. In addition, current electrochemical probes require user servicing of the calibration gas and transducer membrane. Training for this servicing is specific to the brand of $TcCO_2m$ being used. The use of optical sensors, which are used in pulse oximeters, is being considered.

- Transcutaneous CO_2 monitoring provides a noninvasive method of measuring trends in arterial CO_2, acting as a surrogate for end-tidal CO_2 monitoring.
- $TcCO_2m$ is useful in natural or apneic airway management cases in which traditional end-tidal CO_2 measurements are not possible.
- Hypoperfusion limits the accuracy of $TcCO_2$ monitoring—a low cardiac index, hypothermia, hypoxemia, edema at the placement site, and the use of vasoactive agents can affect $TcCO_2m$ accuracy.
- $TcCO_2$ is best utilized for monitoring trends in CO_2, not quantitative accuracy.
- *See Figure 176.1 and* ***Video 176.1*** *for additional details.*

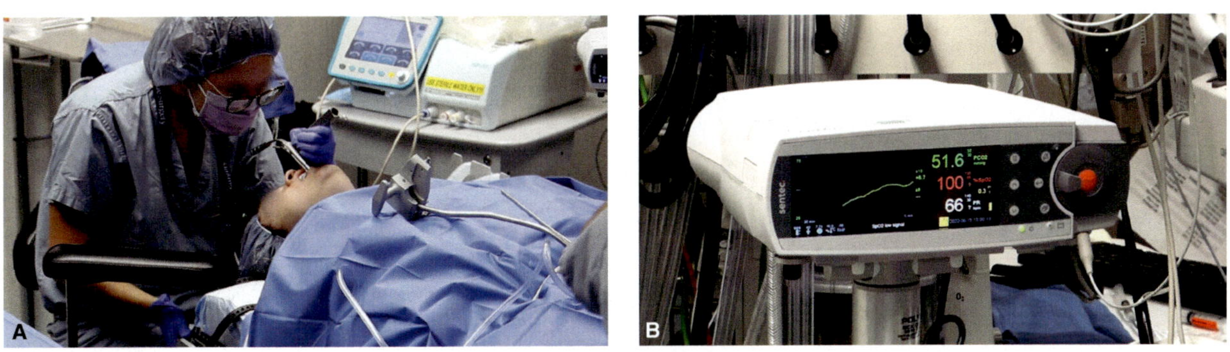

Figure 176.1. A: Suspension laryngoscopy during jet ventilation in a patient with subglottic stenosis. **B:** Sentec transcutaneous CO_2 monitor reads a modest rise in CO_2 during jet ventilation.

Suggested Readings

Apfelbaum JL, Hagberg CA, Connis RT, et al. 2022 American Society of Anesthesiologists Practice guidelines for management of the difficult airway. *Anesthesiology*. 2022;136(1):31–81.

Bernasconi S, Angelucci A, De Cesari A, et al. Recent technologies for transcutaneous oxygen and carbon dioxide monitoring. *Diagnostics (Basel)*. 2024;14(8):785.

Bolliger D, Steiner LA, Kasper J, Aziz OA, Filipovic M, Seeberger MD. The accuracy of non-invasive carbon dioxide monitoring: a clinical evaluation of two transcutaneous systems. *Anaesthesia*. 2007;62(4):394–399.

Ebeling CG, Riccio CA. Apneic oxygenation with high-flow nasal cannula and transcutaneous carbon dioxide monitoring during airway surgery: a case series. *A A Pract*. 2019;12(10):366–368.

Eley VA, Guy L, Woods C, Llewellyn S, Van Zundert AAJ. Transcutaneous carbon dioxide measurements in anesthetized apneic patients with BMI >35 kg/m^2. *J Anesth*. 2023;37(6):971–975.

Barrier Devices to Reduce Aerosol Exposure in the COVID-19 Patient

177

Justine Denomme • Tim Ting Han Jen

Describe in detail the device or technique.

In the beginning of the COVID-19 pandemic, global shortages of personal protective equipment (PPE) put health care providers at risk of airborne viral transmission during airway procedures. This inspired the development of novel, self-made barrier enclosure devices to provide an additional layer of safety and bridge the gap in PPE shortage. The first barrier enclosure device was the "aerosol box" developed by Dr Hsien Yung Lai from Taiwan in March 2020. This was a semi-open, transparent plastic box that covers the supine patient, with two arm holes that allowed for airway manipulation. The "aerosol box" soon achieved worldwide popularity through information sharing on social media and a published correspondence in the New England Journal of Medicine discussing its efficacy in droplet prevention from a simulated patient to the airway provider. Locally, variations of such barrier enclosures (Figure 177.1) were developed with modifications such as arm hole seals, drapes to cover the open end, and suction attachments to remove aerosols. Given its potential protective effects, the U.S. Food and Drug Administration (FDA) issued emergency use authorization (EUA) in May 2020 for barrier enclosures when used in conjunction with conventional PPE.

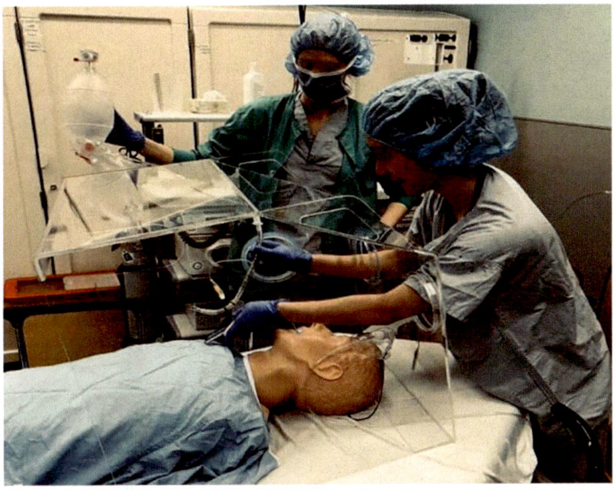

Figure 177.1. An example of a locally developed barrier enclosure used on a manikin. [Reprinted by permission from Springer: Jen TTH, Gusti V, Badh C, et al. The impact of a barrier enclosure on time to tracheal intubation: a randomized controlled trial. *Can J Anaesth*. 2021;68(9):1358–1367. Copyright © 2021 Canadian Anesthesiologists' Society.]

However, further simulation studies evaluating the barrier enclosures' efficacy in reducing aerosol spread to airway providers yielded disappointing results. Only meticulously placed closed barriers, such as the glove box with long gloves sealing the arm holes, consistently reduced aerosol spread to the operator. Incompletely closed devices may paradoxically direct aerosolized particles toward the operator through arm holes. Furthermore, as barrier enclosures are lifted and removed following intubation, concentrated viral particles may aerosolize. To minimize this, either 5 minutes of suction with a smoke evacuator or 15 minutes of hospital suction must be applied prior to device removal, which limits the devices' clinical applicability. Similarly, simple plastic drape barriers over the patient did not reduce aerosol spread to the operator when accounting for drape removal after airway management.

Airway experts also questioned the safety and practicality of barrier enclosures. First, barrier enclosures resulted in prolonged time to intubation and lower first-pass success rates in simulation studies. These results were not replicated in a subsequent randomized controlled trial involving healthy surgical patients with reassuring airway features. Nonetheless, there was an increase in anesthesiologists' perceived difficulty in intubation, as airway maneuvers such as head repositioning and chin-lift are ergonomically challenging within barrier enclosures. Second, in an unexpected difficult airway, it may be challenging to quickly remove a barrier enclosure due to its bulky nature. Third, utilizing barrier enclosures expends the limited mental capacity that airway providers have when intubating critically ill patients at risk of rapid desaturation. Finally, appropriate transport, storage, and disinfection of barrier enclosures can be challenging due to their large size and heavy weight.

In response to the emerging evidence of potential harm, the FDA removed the umbrella EUA for barrier enclosures in August 2020. As a result, any new devices could no longer be distributed or used without a new FDA application and approval. It was recommended that the previously approved barrier devices, if used, incorporate negative pressure to evacuate aerosolized particles and that devices should be immediately removed if there is any difficulty with airway management. It was emphasized that these devices do not replace mandated PPE during aerosol-generating procedures.

Barrier enclosures intended to minimize health care workers' exposure to COVID-19 briefly gained worldwide interest as a stopgap solution to address PPE shortages early in the pandemic. However, with efficacy and safety concerns, barrier enclosures are now primarily of historical interest. In future pandemics or other emergencies, we should aim to systematically evaluate any proposed medical devices and rapidly synthesize evolving efficacy and safety data, while exercising caution when utilizing any untested equipment.

Suggested Readings

Canelli R, Connor CW, Gonzalez M, Nozari A, Ortega R. Barrier enclosure during endotracheal intubation. *N Engl J Med*. 2020; 382(20):1957–1958.

Fidler RL, Niedek CR, Teng JJ, et al. Aerosol retention characteristics of barrier devices. *Anesthesiology*. 2021;134(1):61–71.

Jen TTH, Gusti V, Badh C, et al. The impact of a barrier enclosure on time to tracheal intubation: a randomized controlled trial. *Can J Anaesth*. 2021;68(9):1358–1367.

Mariano ER, Kou A, Stiegler MA, Matava C. The rise and fall of the COVID-19 aerosol box through the lens of Twitter. *J Clin Anesth*. 2021;69:110145.

Sorbello M, Rosenblatt W, Hofmeyr R, Greif R, Urdaneta F. Aerosol boxes and barrier enclosures for airway management in COVID-19 patients: a scoping review and narrative synthesis. *Br J Anaesth*. 2020;125(6):880–894.

Note: Page numbers followed by f denote figures; those followed by t denote tables.

B

G

H

U

V